CONTENTS

KU-061-994

ACKNOWLEDGEMENTS

City & Guilds would like to sincerely thank the following.

For invaluable hairdressing and beauty expertise
Lou Hockings, Sarah Farrell, Anita Crosland and Diane Mitchell

For taking college photos
Andrew Buckle

For supplying pictures for the front cover
Front cover main image: hair by Jennifer Cheyne, styling by Lorraine Adamczuk and photography by Paul Adamczuk; smaller images: Central Sussex College; Hertford Regional College; Istockphoto: Quavondo, Dashek, Valua Vitaly, Paul Adamczuk (photographer), Ashley Kerr (hairdresser) and Lorraine Adamczuk (stylist).

For their help with photoshoots
Kendal Butler, Emma Middleton, Lesley Mercala, Cheryl Moloney and Louise Hemmings at Stephenson College , Denise Johnson, Stephen Beckley, Susan Billington, Diane Flanagan, Jane Clappison, Siobhan Parr, Karen Critchley, Joanne Walsh, Eilidh Sanders, Tim Bolton, Sarah Gannon, Becky Thow, Toni Cansfield, Hayley Cater, Cara Wall, Stephanie Connolly, Chloe Lynch, Lizzy Woodward, Michael D. A. Johnson, Amy Sheridan, Stevie O'Toole, Ray Wright and Lewis Mahei from Hugh Baird College, Melissa Birch and Sue Jane Hartley from Cheynes Training, and Lucy Kaye, Dean Tatum, Lina Davey, Laura Desimone, Sophie Balaam and Rebecca Greenaway from Cambridge Regional College.

Picture credits
Every effort has been made to acknowledge all copyright holders as below and the publishers will, if notified, correct any errors in future editions.

Alamy: © Andrew Twort p237, © blickwinkel p260, © Chloe Parker p58, © Dick Makin p288, © Fabrizio Troiani p287, © itanistock pp202, 203, © jayfish p284, © Lenscap p24, © Oleksiy Maksymenko p325, © Ray Watkins p323, © Tetra Images p14, © Tony Lilley p47; **Camera Press:** © Chris Ashford p302, © Mark Stewart p302; **Charles H. Fox:** pp287, 292, 314, 427, 430; **Corbis:** © Erika Svensson p257, © Imagemore Co p316, © Image Source p258, © Ocean p67; **Hive of Beauty:** p191; **HSE:** p24; **iStockphoto:** © Abel Mitja Varela p253, © acilo p261, © Alina Solovyova-Vincent p35, © Amanda Rohde pp26, 255, © Andrey Popov p436, © Andrzej Burak p320, © Angela Gyorfy p66, © aldra p311, © Brian McEntire p126,© catalina mas sebastián pp225, 228, © cc-stock p287, © Сергей Дашкевич p202, © Chris Gramly p217, © craftvision pp35, 198,© Dmitriy Norov pp347, 355, © DNY59 p225, © eli_asenova p353, © EXTREME-PHOTOGRAPHER p37, © Factoria Singular p250, © Famke Backx pp37, 150, 257, © George Cairns p9, © gilaxia p153, © gruizza p278, © Gubcio p203, © Iconogenic pp37, 216, 218, 293, 153, © Inga Ivanov p153, © isidor stankov p197, © ium kivoart p4, © Jacob Wackerhaus pp4, 144, © Jamie Evans p143, © Jasmina p33, © John Steele p211, © Joshua Hodge Photography pp54, 163, © Juan Monino p240, © Julia Savchenko pp150, 434, 306, 153, © Kamil Krajewski p10, © Kelly Cline p23, © Kris Hanke p335, © kristian sekulic pp23, 347, © lambada p38, © Larysa Dodz p39, © Lebazele p97, © Linda Alstead p199, © Luis Albuquerque p373, © mbbirdy p151, © MorePixels p197, © nelic p298, © Nicholas Monu p14, © Osuleo p183, © Plougmann p199, © Ralf Hettler p6, © ratchanida thippayos p203, © Rhienna Cutler p253, © Robert Pears p148, © Sergey Anatolievich Pristyazhnyuk p126, © Sherwin McGehee p226, © susandaniels p199, © Svetlana Alyuk p211, © Tom Marvin pp173 298, © tuncaycetin p199, © Uwe Merkel p65, © Valua Vitaly pp219, 388, © webphotographeer p13, © WEKWEK p286, © Zlatko Kostic p180; **Mediscan:** pp110, 173, 198, 200, 202, 211, 227, 228, 259, 298; **Professionails:** p438; **Rex Features:** © James McCauley p457, © Startraks p347; **Science Photo Library:** Cordelia Molloy p197, Dr Jeremy Burgess p201, Dr P. Marazzi pp173, 197, 199, 211, Dr Harout Tanielian p200, Lee Samsami/Custom Medical Stock Photo p346, Subbotina Anna p41; **Shutterstock:** © Amy Planz p198, © Cindy Hughes p196; © CURAphotography p253, © Diana Jo Currier p326, © @erics p148, © FXQuadro p390, © Galina Deinega p148, © Iablonskyi Mykola p226, © ifong p24, © Jaimie Duplass p443, © Leonid and Anna Dedukh p22, © Luba V Nel p391, © Malyugin p24, © Melianiaka Kanstantsin p169, © Miramiska p334, © Olga Ekaterincheva p1, © Photoroller p169, © PhotoStock10 p436, © ruzanna p21, © Shyrokova p225, © Slobodan Miskovic p257, © Tania Zbrodko p198, © Valua Vitaly pp161, 301, 391, © Victor Potasyev p67, © Warren Goldswain p168, © wtamas p253; **Snazaroo:** pp40, 312, 319, 320, 323, 324, 325, 326.

This book is dedicated to my dear Mum.

To my Dad: you are my inspiration to keep going even when things are tough. Thank you.

To my beautiful children, Rose and Ashton: thank you for your patience and understanding while I was writing this book. I love you both very much.

To my sisters, Helen, Claire and Sue: thank you for your constant love and support.

To Lynn: sincere thanks for being such a wonderful friend.

Louise

To the many hundreds of students that I have worked with during my long career and whose success has made me so proud. To my family for their support and encouragement. To the future generations of hairdressers that they may achieve rewarding and successful careers. May they always be professional, customer focused, innovative and creative.

John

ABOUT THE AUTHORS

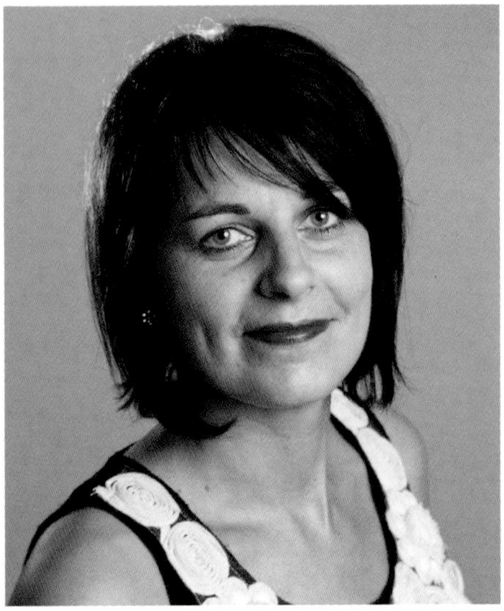

Louise Hemmings has been teaching in further education at Stephenson College, Leicester for the last 20 years. Her career has included working in a hairdressing salon in Leicester and then as a beauty therapist at Ragdale Hall health hydro. She currently manages the beauty and complementary therapies department and also teaches across hair, beauty and complementary therapy courses (from Levels 1, 2 and 3).

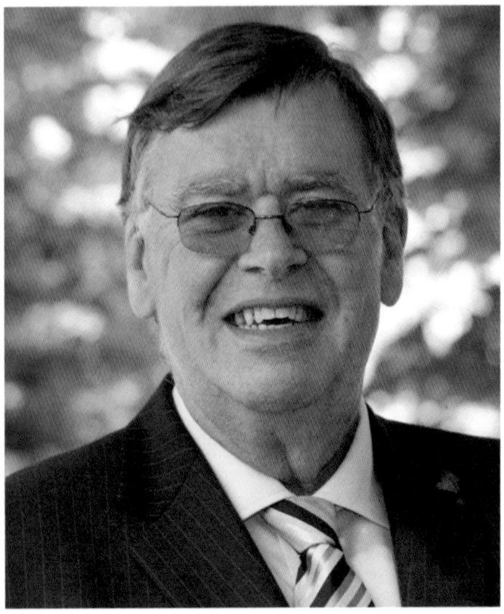

John Armstrong retired in 2011 after a successful career in teaching. He was Head of Hairdressing and Beauty at Great Yarmouth College for 20 years. John qualified as a trichologist in 1982. He is a National Executive Member of the National Hairdressers' Federation and is Chair of their Education Committee. John represents the NHF on the City & Guilds National Advisory Committee for Hairdressing.

FOREWORD

The Hair and Beauty industry is a fantastic place to work! There are lots of different jobs you can choose from, such as working as a Hairdresser, Barber, Beauty Therapist, Nail Technician or Make-up Artist.

This Level 1 qualification is the perfect beginning on the road to your chosen career. It will give you the opportunity to have a taster of many different areas from styling women's hair, to nail art, to themed face painting. This qualification will not only give you some of the creative skills but more importantly will develop your communication and employability skills.

This book captures how exciting and fun our industry can be. It's a great resource to help you through your qualification, giving you handy hints, tips and visual step-by-steps. The revision exercises at the end of each chapter help to prepare you for your assignment work.

John and Louise have put their passion and expertise into developing this book. As tutors who have taught this qualification they are the ideal writers for it.

Between us we have worked in this industry for 60 years! Throughout our careers we have worked with some incredibly talented people and have had the chance to work in colleges, salons, spas, on photoshoots and have judged competitions. We can honestly say every day has been exciting, fun and different.

We would like to take this opportunity to wish you good luck with your qualification and your future career within the Hair and Beauty industry.

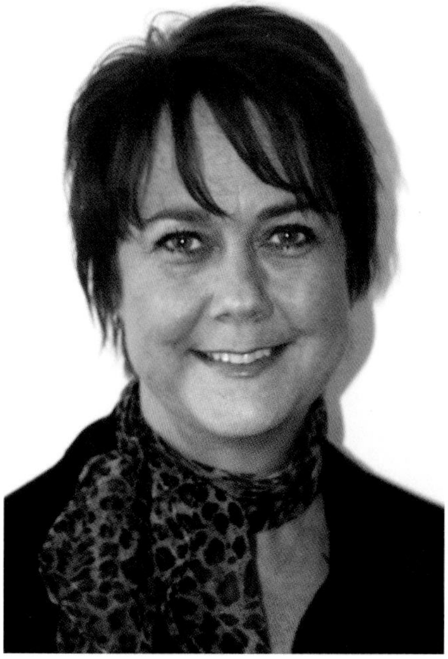

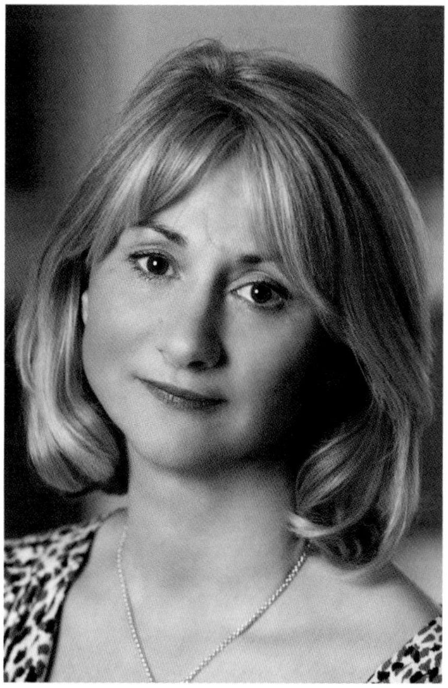

Anita Crosland and Diane Mitchell
Hairdressing and Beauty Therapy Portfolio Managers, City & Guilds

INTRODUCTION – HOW TO USE THIS TEXTBOOK

Each chapter in your textbook covers everything you will need to understand in order to complete your written or online tests and practical assessments.

Throughout this textbook you will see the following features:

HANDY HINTS

Lowlights are colour effects darker than the client's natural depth colour; highlights are colour effects lighter than the natural depth colour.

Handy hints are particularly useful tips that can assist you in your revision or help you remember something important.

Oxidation

A chemical process that combines a substance with oxygen

Words in bold in the text are explained in the margin to aid your understanding.

ACTIVITY

Activities – The activities help to test your understanding and learn from your colleagues' experiences.

SmartScreen GH9 worksheet 5

SmartScreen – These icons refer to the City & Guilds SmartScreen resources and activities. Ask your tutor for your log-in details.

At the end of each chapter are some wordsearches, crosswords and quizzes to test your knowledge.

You need to be aware that throughout this book the word 'client' might also refer to a friend, family member or model.

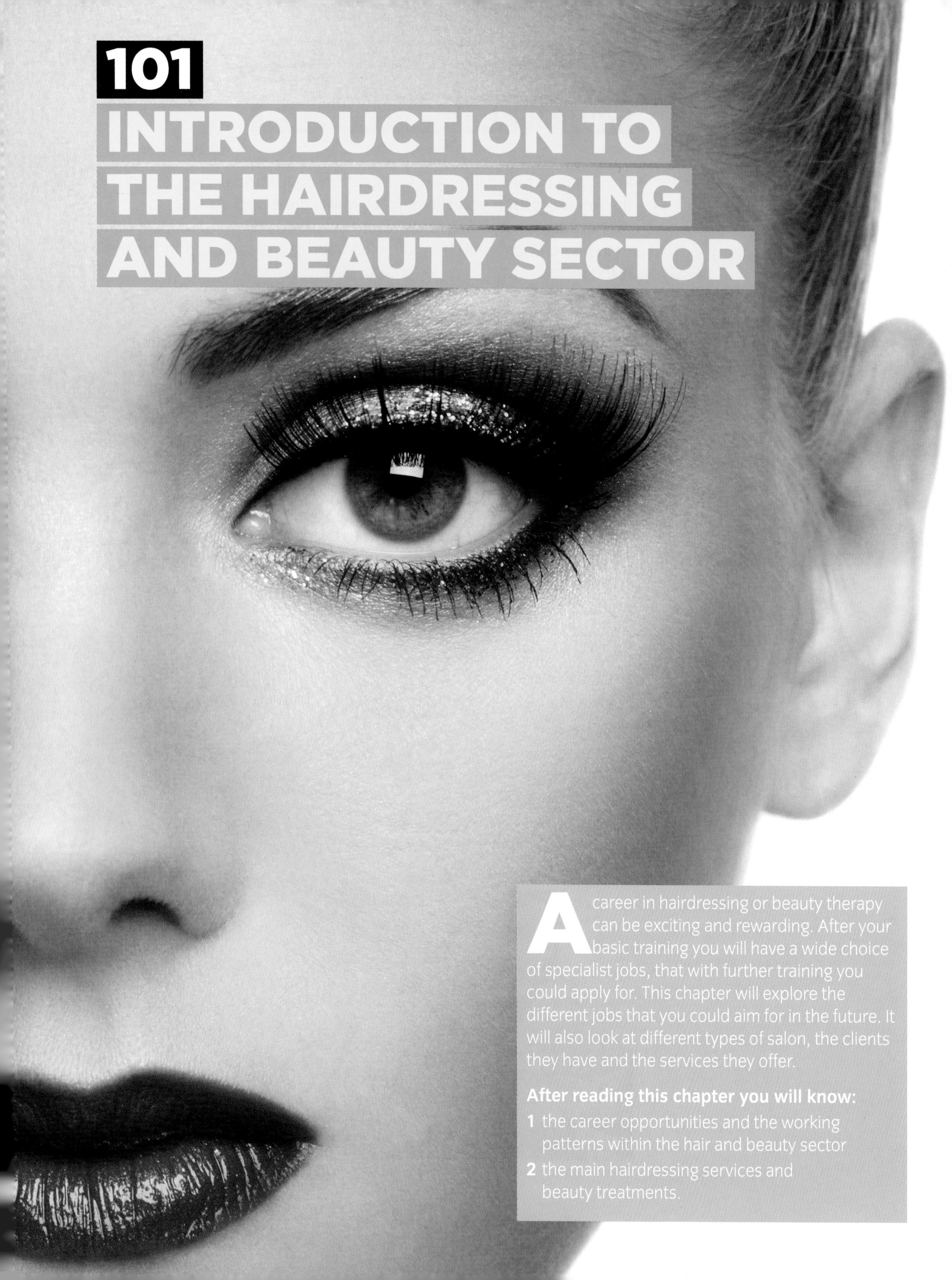

101 INTRODUCTION TO THE HAIRDRESSING AND BEAUTY SECTOR

A career in hairdressing or beauty therapy can be exciting and rewarding. After your basic training you will have a wide choice of specialist jobs, that with further training you could apply for. This chapter will explore the different jobs that you could aim for in the future. It will also look at different types of salon, the clients they have and the services they offer.

After reading this chapter you will know:

1 the career opportunities and the working patterns within the hair and beauty sector
2 the main hairdressing services and beauty treatments.

THE CAREER OPPORTUNITIES AND THE WORKING PATTERNS WITHIN THE HAIR AND BEAUTY SECTOR

In this part of the chapter you will identify **occupational** roles, outline the working patterns and identify the main career opportunities in the hair and beauty sector and related industries. You will also learn examples of sources of information on training and career opportunities in the sector.

Occupational
Relating to the type of job people do

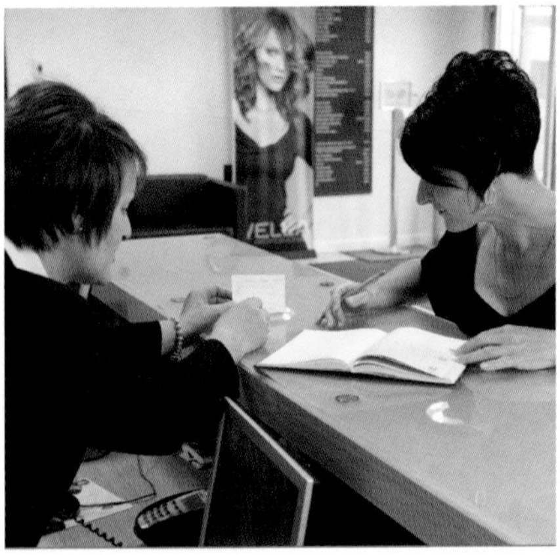

A salon receptionist

OCCUPATIONAL ROLES

There are many jobs that you could do as you progress in your career:

- Salon junior – helping the stylist, barber or beauty therapist while learning your skills and getting your qualifications.
- Hair stylist – working on clients, giving all the services that the salon offers or specialising in cutting, colouring, perming or long hair.
- Barber – working in a gent's salon, providing cutting and styling services on mainly male clients.
- Beauty therapist – after training, working on clients, giving all the massage or beauty treatments offered by the salon/spa.
- Make-up artist – working in areas like the theatre, television and films, in the fashion industry or photography and also in the health service, providing make-up services for people needing make-up to cover skin injuries.
- Nail technician – providing nail services, including nail art and nail enhancements, to clients.
- Salon manager – as you gain more experience and skills you could become the manager and be responsible for running the salon.
- Receptionist – in this role you would make all the appointments for clients, deal with their queries and be responsible for the reception area of the salon.
- Salon owner – owning your own salon is the ambition of many hairdressers and beauty therapists.

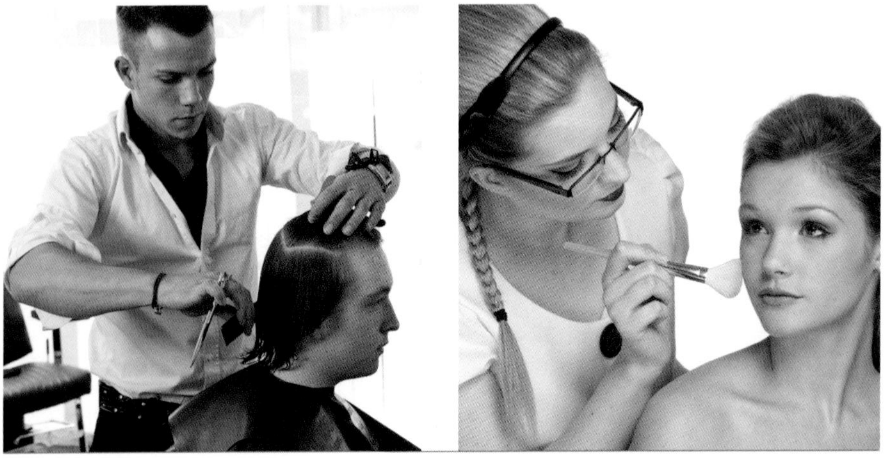

There are so many wonderful career opportunities in the hair and beauty industry!

- Colour technician – if you enjoy colouring, then working for a manufacturer such as L'Oreal or Wella, training other hairdressers in colour skills, could be an ideal career for you.
- Session stylist – this is a high-fashion job, working for photographers, television, fashion houses, magazines, etc.
- Product technician – like the colour technician but demonstrating new products, and training hairdressers and beauty therapists to use them.
- Manufacturer's sales rep. – visiting salons and selling products and equipment.
- Spa therapist – providing specialist beauty services in a health spa, hotel, etc.
- Beauty consultant – selling and giving advice to customers about make-up and beauty products in a retail outlet such as a shop or department store.
- Trainer – training other staff and juniors in both hairdressing and beauty therapy.
- Assessor – working with trainees to help them gain their qualification.
- Tutor – working in a college, teaching students and trainees.

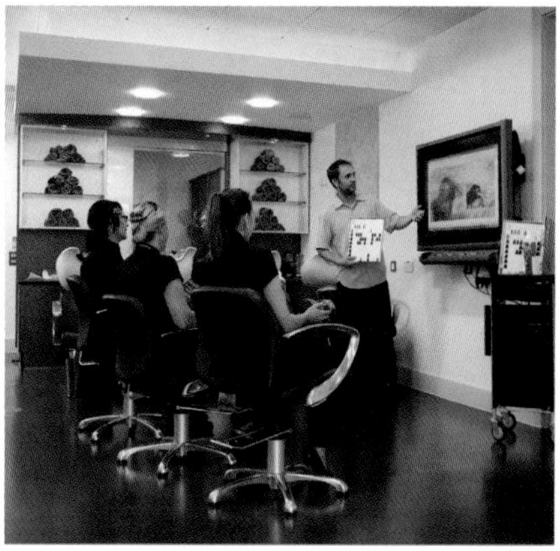

A trainer visiting a salon

HANDY HINTS

Find out more about the jobs that you could work towards as you progress through your training.

HANDY HINTS

Planning your training is very important. Making sure you get the right qualifications you need is also important.

ACTIVITY

Choose one of the above jobs that interests you. Find out what qualifications you might need for that job.

SmartScreen 101 worksheets 1 and 2

WORKING PATTERNS

In our modern marketplace, hairdressers and beauty therapists must be **flexible** in how and when they work.

Many salons will be open 7 days a week and often from early in the morning to late into the evening. Clients may want to book appointments before they go to work or after they finish work in the afternoon.

Working shifts

As a hairdresser or beauty therapist you might be expected to vary the times you go to work.

- You might work early mornings to early afternoon. On other days you may have to work early afternoons to late evenings.
- The owner of the salon will plan the hours the salon will be open. They organise the staff on a **rota** system to make sure they can do the clients' hair during opening hours.

Flexible

Ready and able to change when necessary

Rota

A list showing when each person has to do a particular job

HANDY HINTS

There is a set of regulations called the Working Time Regulations. Your boss has to make sure that he/she abides by this set of guidelines. It will cover such things as when you should have a break in your working day and the numbers of hours that you should work.

ACTIVITY

Find out more about the Working Time Regulations. Make a list of the things that they cover, eg hours, holidays, etc. (Try www.direct.gov.uk for more information.)

Being flexible is necessary for a make-up artist, hairdresser, barber, beauty therapist or nail technician.

- When you are working on a client, you cannot finish work until you have finished the treatment or service.
- Sometimes you may need to do extra work if one of your fellow workers is ill.
- Sometimes you may need to delay your lunch break in order to fit in another client.

HANDY HINTS

Your clients are important. The money they pay for their hair or beauty treatment pays your salary. Keeping them satisfied and ensuring they make another appointment is key to your success.

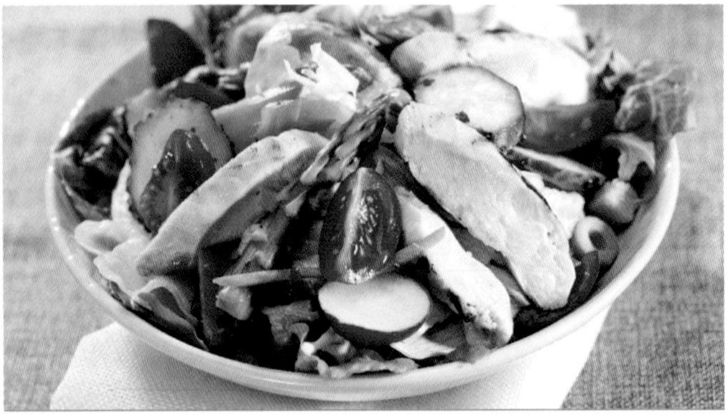

A healthy meal

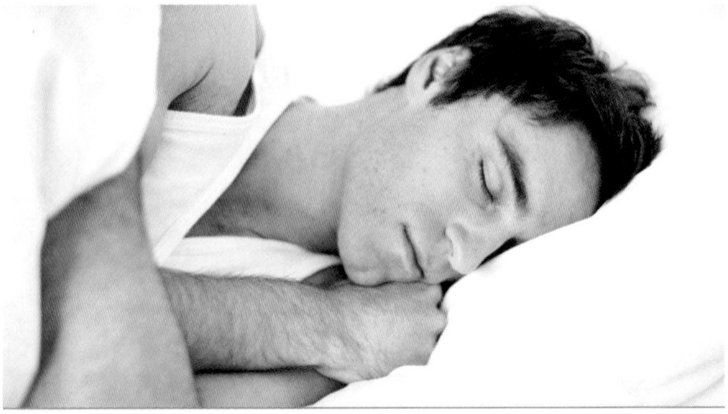

It's important to get lots of sleep

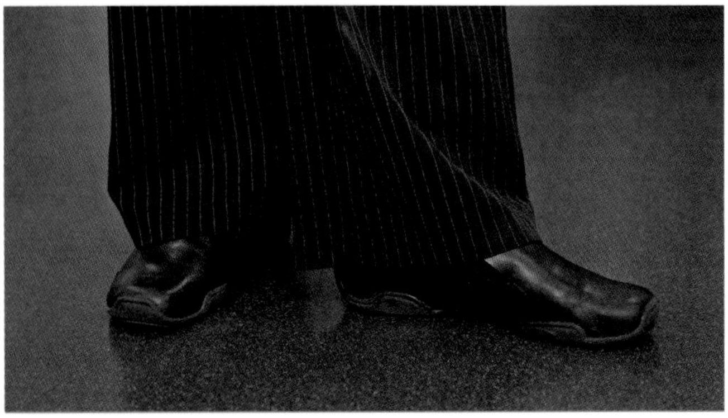

Comfortable footwear

HANDY HINTS

Your client might be offended by body odour or bad breath. Make sure you bathe or shower every day and clean your teeth regularly.

BEING HEALTHY AND FIT

Remember, you need to be fit to work in the hair or beauty sector; you will be on your feet most of the time you are at work.

You should make sure that you:

- eat properly – drink plenty of water, eat fresh fruit and vegetables
- get enough rest – try to get six to eight hours' sleep a night
- keep healthy – exercise regularly
- wear the right shoes – low heeled, so they do not put a strain on your back
- pay attention to your personal hygiene – wash regularly, use deodorant.

By doing all this you will hopefully avoid problems like backache, sore feet and feeling tired. You will be able to go out and enjoy yourself after work instead of just wanting to go to sleep.

ACTIVITY

With a partner, find out about the types of food that you should include in your diet to keep healthy and fit, and those foods you should avoid. Make up a diet sheet of things you that are good for you.

WORKING FULL TIME OR PART TIME

Some hairdressers, barbers, beauty therapists and nail technicians decide not to work full time. There are opportunities to work part time, doing hours and days that suit you and your boss.

CAREER OPPORTUNITIES

When you have finished your training, what opportunities are there for your future? Below are many examples of the places you could work and the jobs you could consider. For some you will need more qualifications, specialist skills, experience and ambition. With hard work you can get there.

- Hairdressing salon – working as a stylist or colour technician. Progressing to a trainer, manager or salon owner.
- Barbers – working as a barber, progressing to manager or owner.
- Beauty salon – opportunities to work as a therapist, progressing to trainer, manager or owner.
- Nail bars – offer careers in manicure, nail art and nail enhancements.
- Specialist salons/spas – these will include jobs for those with skills in areas such as **aromatherapy**, **reflexology** and **reiki**.
- Clinics – opportunities for therapists in remedial massage and other specialist treatments to treat minor injuries and conditions.
- Health hydros/farms – offer a wide range of services for guests, including hairdressing, beauty, specialist treatments, massage, diet and exercise.
- Health and fitness clubs – opportunities for therapists providing specialist massage techniques linked to fitness programmes.
- Leisure centres and hotels – many offer hairdressing and beauty services alongside spa-type facilities.
- Cruise liners – all cruise liners will offer a full range of hair and beauty services to passengers and an opportunity to see the world for staff.
- Theatre, film and television studios – opportunities for highly skilled make-up artists and hairdressers, providing hair and make-up for plays and films in a wide variety of settings.
- Fashion and photography – fashion shows and photoshoots give opportunities for hairdressers and make-up artists to provide hair and make-up services for the models.

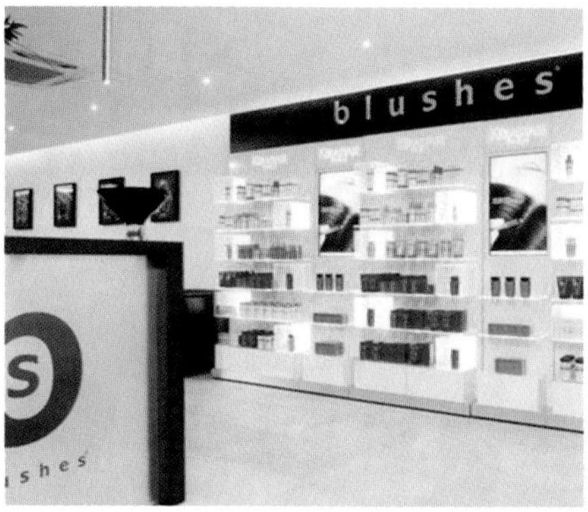

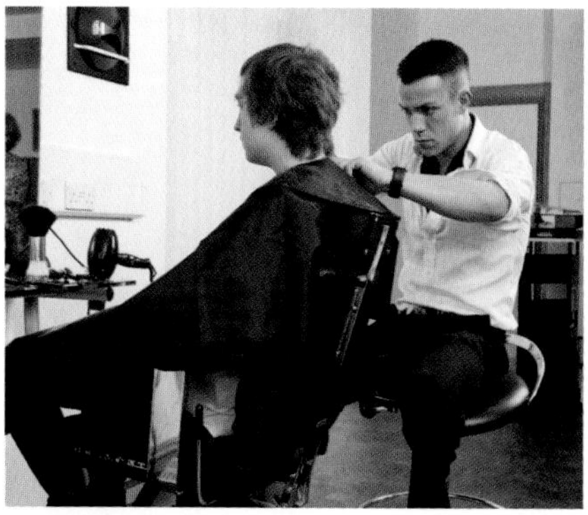

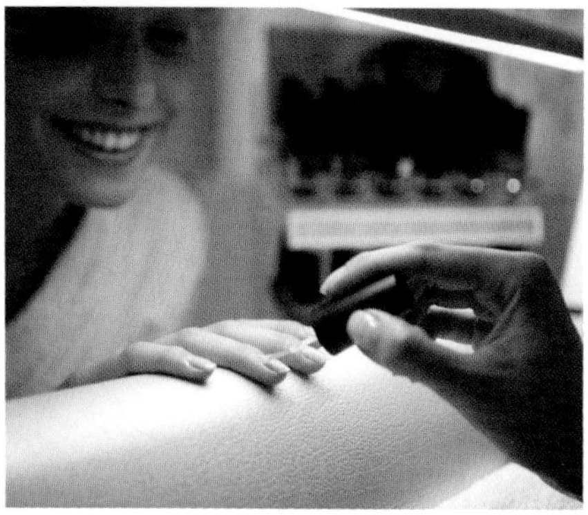

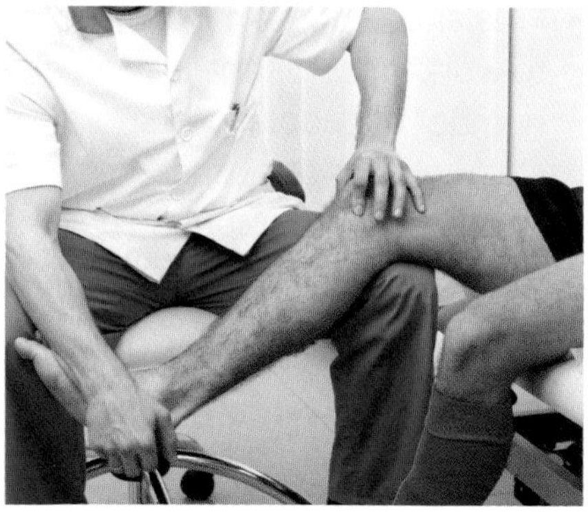

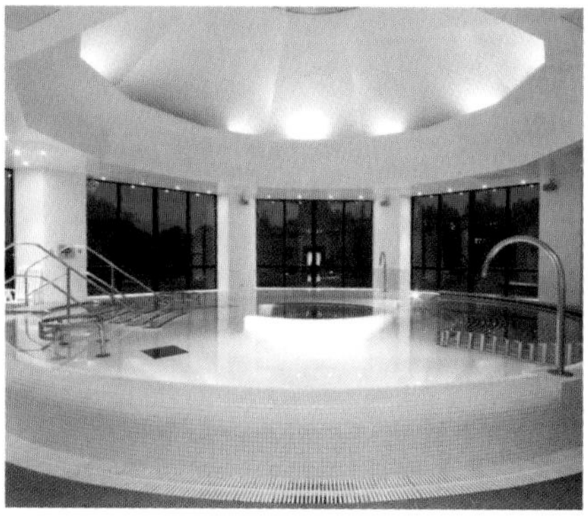

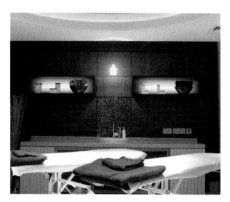

Aromatherapy
Massage with essential oils

Reflexology
Massage of the feet to improve health

Reiki
A healing therapy

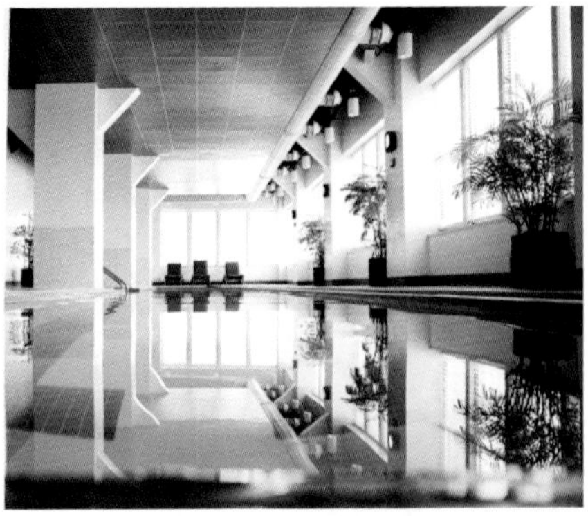
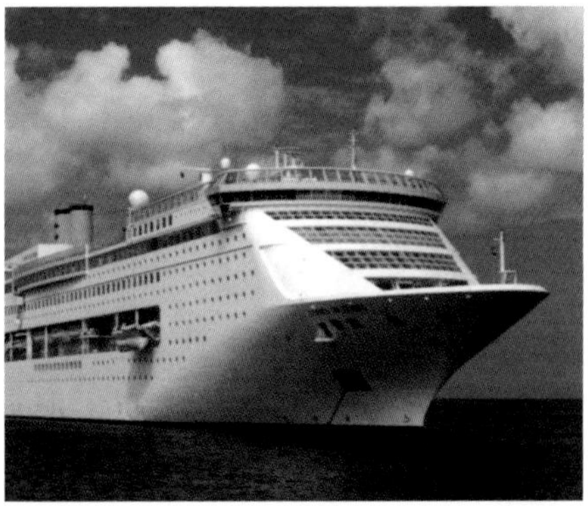
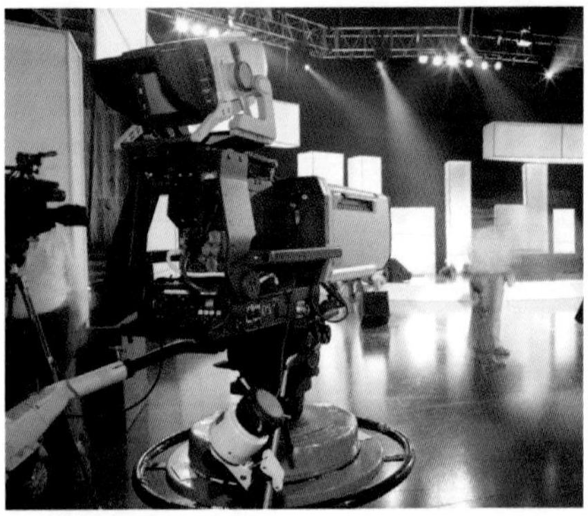
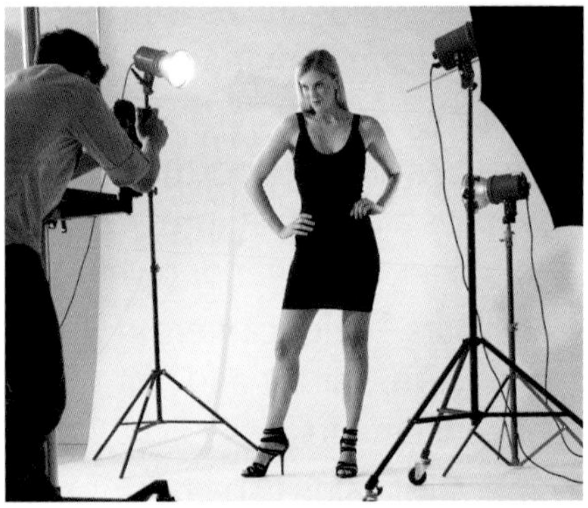

- Hospitals – many hospitals provide hair and in some cases beauty services to staff and patients.
- Mobile salons – some hairdressers and beauty therapists offer their services to clients in the clients' own homes or workplaces. Some companies will contract with therapists to offer services as part of a staff wellbeing service.
- Freelance – some hairdressers and beauty therapists don't want to work for someone else on a permanent basis; they work for a number of people for a short period and then move on, covering staff holidays or sickness for example, or for a project for a fashion house or photographer. They may also have their own clients like those running a mobile salon.

SmartScreen 001 handout 1

SmartScreen 001 handout 2

HANDY HINTS

For some of the opportunities that are in the list there will be lots of applicants. It is important to make sure you have all the qualifications and the personal skills the employer is looking for.

ACTIVITY

Find out more about the places that you could work and the jobs that you would be able to do there. Try using the internet to see what vacancies are available and the skills and qualifications that the owner is asking for.

WHERE TO FIND INFORMATION ON TRAINING AND CAREER OPPORTUNITIES

Now you have looked at the variety of jobs that are available, it would be useful to know where to find out information about how to get the training and qualifications. You will then be able to plan your own development so you can achieve your ambition.

Below you can find out who to go to to find information and where to go to find them.

Who to go to for:

- qualifications – awarding organisations
- education and training – colleges, awarding bodies, Habia, training providers, manufacturers
- apprenticeships – training providers, colleges, employers.

Where to find them:

- Habia – Habia is the Hairdressing and Beauty Industry Authority. It is the industry lead body and has information about the standards for hairdressing, barbering, beauty, nails and spa (www.habia.org.uk).
- Awarding organisations – City & Guilds (www.cityandguilds.com) has lots of information about qualifications and where you can take them.
- Colleges – your local college will have details of courses you can take and qualifications may include apprenticeships.
- Training providers – will have details of apprenticeships available locally.
- Manufacturers – some of the large companies that make hair and beauty products provide courses or training for using products and the latest techniques.
- Employers – your local salon will have opportunities for apprenticeships and for more qualified staff, which is useful when you have finished the various stages of your training.

City & Guilds

dermalogica®
a skin care system researched and developed by The International Dermal Institute

GUINOT
INSTITUT • PARIS

WELLA
PROFESSIONALS

ACTIVITY

Make a list of all the places you can get information from in your area. Include their names, addresses, telephone numbers and email addresses.

SmartScreen 001 handout 3

THE MAIN HAIRDRESSING SERVICES AND BEAUTY TREATMENTS

There are many thousands of hairdressing and beauty salons across the country. They will all be different in the services they offer and the type of client that they have. Here are some examples.

TYPES OF SALON

Salons vary in size from large ones that employ lots of people, to small ones employing no more than five people.

Small salons are not likely to have different specialists. Their hairdressers or beauty therapists will carry out all the different services that the salon offers.

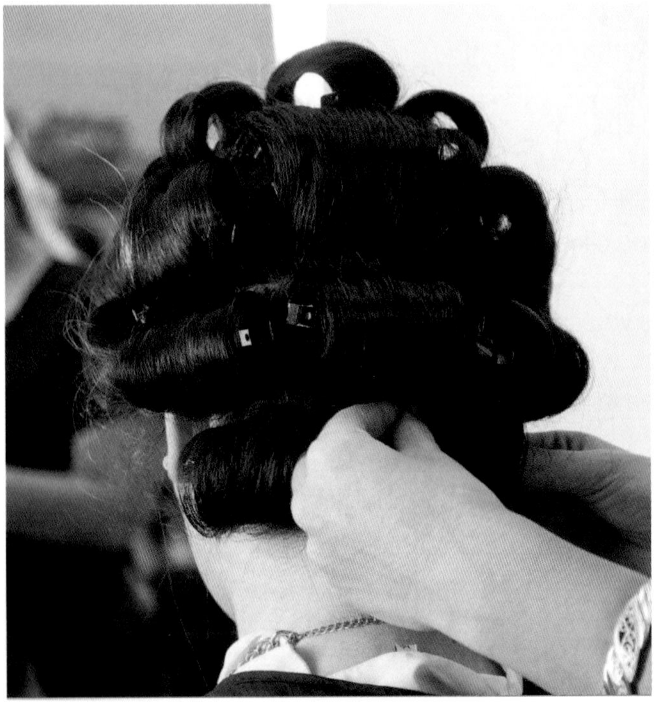

Large hairdressing salons will have a team of staff doing different jobs like this

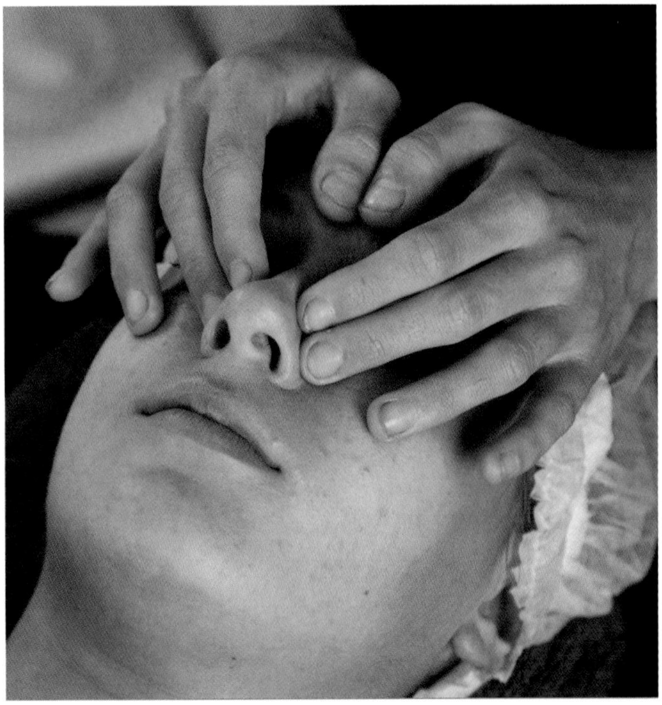

A facial is one of the most popular beauty treatments

SALONS AND THEIR CLIENTS

Decor
Decoration

All salons are competing with each other to attract as many clients as possible. The services they offer, the furniture, the **decor**, even the music they play will be designed to attract particular clients.

HAIRDRESSING SALONS

- The trendy fashionable salon: if the salon wants to attract younger, fashion-conscious clients then it will be bright with modern furniture. The staff will wear the latest fashions and have the latest styles.

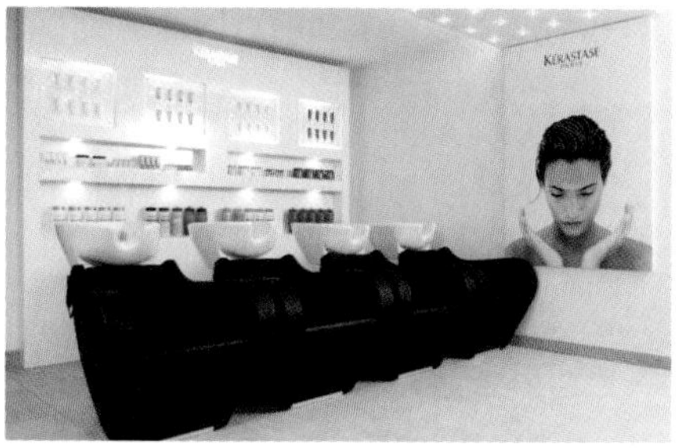

- The traditional salon: if the salon wants to attract clients that are more **conservative**, then the furniture will be comfortable rather than trendy. The colours on the wall will be more **subdued**.

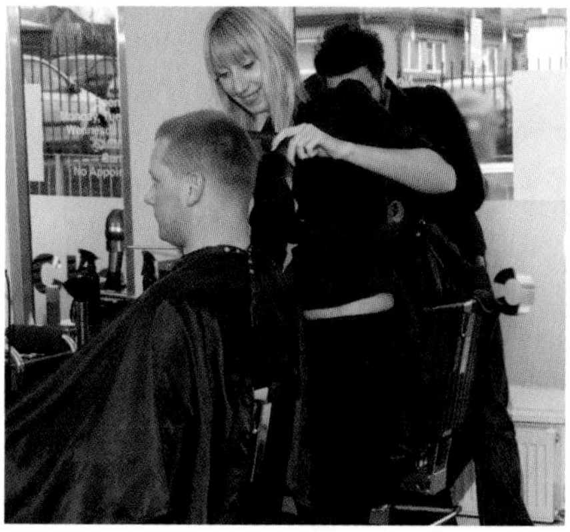

Conservative
Cautious about change

Subdued
Subtle, not bright

- The **'up-market'** salon: if the salon wants to attract the more wealthy client then it will be fitted out with **luxurious** furniture. It will offer lots of additional treatments with the services available. The professional image of the salon will be of a very high standard.
- The franchise salon: salons that have become very successful will let other salon owners buy and run a salon under their name, eg Toni & Guy or Essentials. The main salon will provide everything for the new owner – furniture, training, marketing and more. This will attract clients because of the link to the famous salon.

Up-market
The more expensive or luxury sector

Luxurious
Expensive and high quality

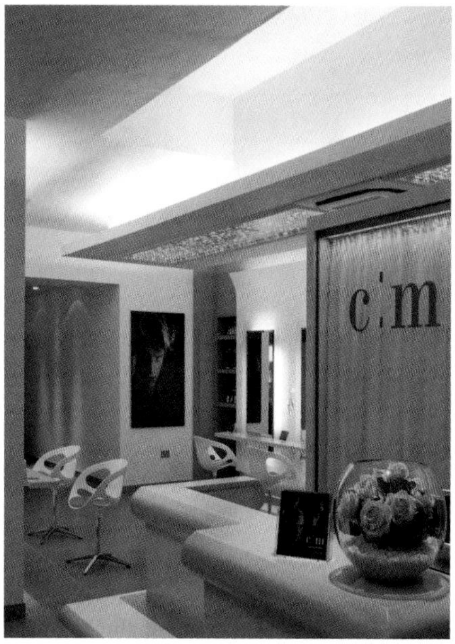

You can tell an 'up-market' salon as soon as you walk in

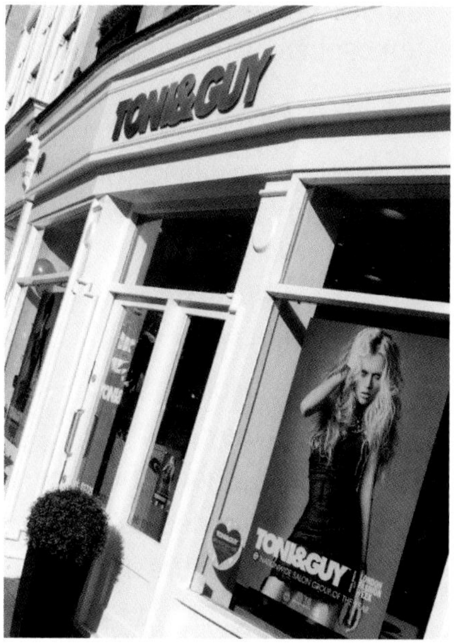

Toni & Guy is one of the most successful salons

BEAUTY SALONS

These will be similar to hairdressing salons:

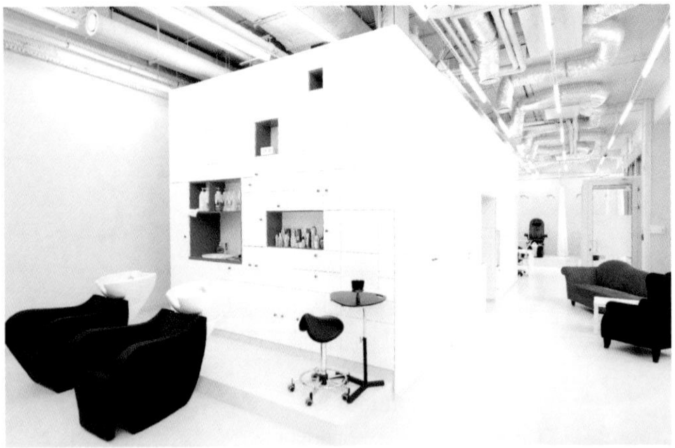

- The combined hair and beauty salon: often there will be a beauty therapy salon within a hairdressing salon. Here, the beauty salon will be similar to the hairdressing part. There may be some differences such as the decor. Some beauty treatments require a relaxing atmosphere as part of the treatment; bright colours and loud music may not be suitable. The therapists should wear appropriate uniforms; trendy, fashionable clothes may not be acceptable to the client and do not look very professional.

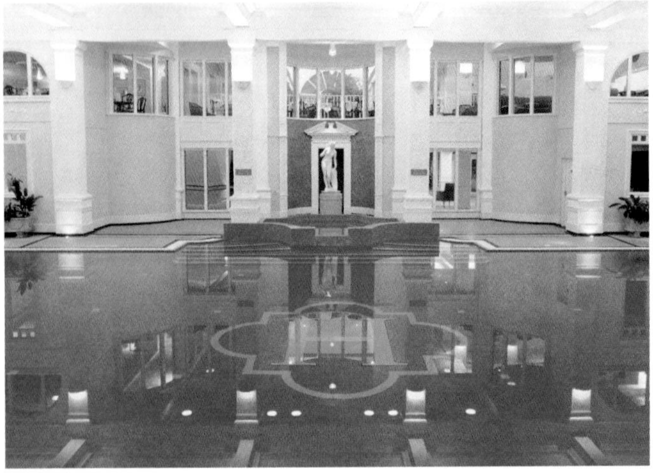

- The 'up-market' salon: this will be luxuriously fitted out and offer many services in addition to the usual beauty treatments. Many of these salons will be part of spas, health farms or hotels.

Complementary therapies
Treatments such as aromatherapy (massage with essential oils), reflexology (massage of the feet to improve health), Indian head massage and reiki (a type of healing)

SmartScreen 101 handout 6

- The specialist salon: these include nail bars, complementary therapy clinics, and clinics offering remedial massage, sports massage and **complementary therapies**. Nail bars are likely to be more colourful, bright and trendy. Sports massage and remedial massage clinics are likely to be more like a doctor's surgery because that is what clients expect. Complementary therapy clinics will tend to have a warm atmosphere with quiet colours.

ACTIVITY

Pick some salons where you live and ask if you can visit them to see how the salon works. You can choose either hairdressing or beauty or both. Things to look for are:

- what the staff are wearing
- the music they play
- how big the salon is
- the services they offer
- the clients they have (their age, the styles and services they are having)
- how the salon is decorated
- what sort of furniture they have.

Make some notes about what you have seen. These will be useful for your fact sheets and reports that you will complete for your assessment.

HAIRDRESSING SERVICES

A hairdressing salon will offer many services. They include:

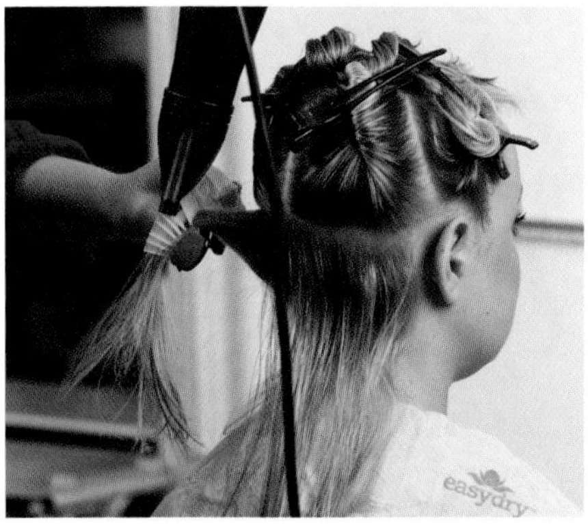

- **Shampoo and blow drying** – clients have their hair shampooed and then styled by blow drying.

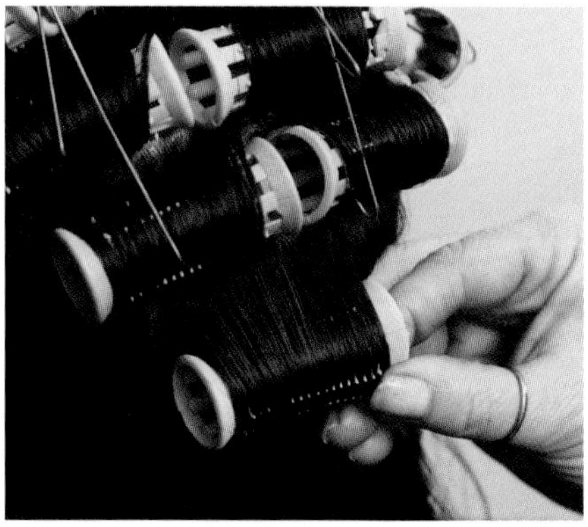

- **Shampoo and setting** – clients have their hair shampooed and set. Their hair is then dressed out.

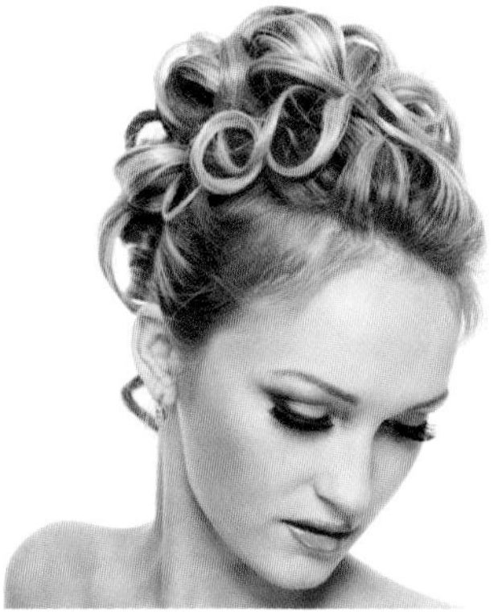

- **Dressing hair for a special occasion** – for a wedding or party or evening out.

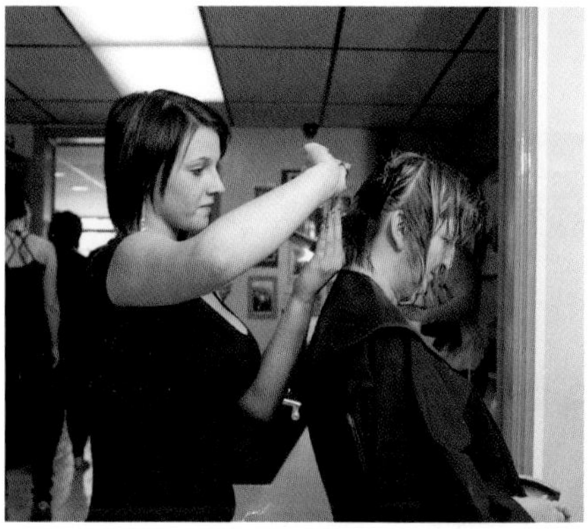

- **Cutting** – cutting the hair into a new style or maintaining the client's current style.

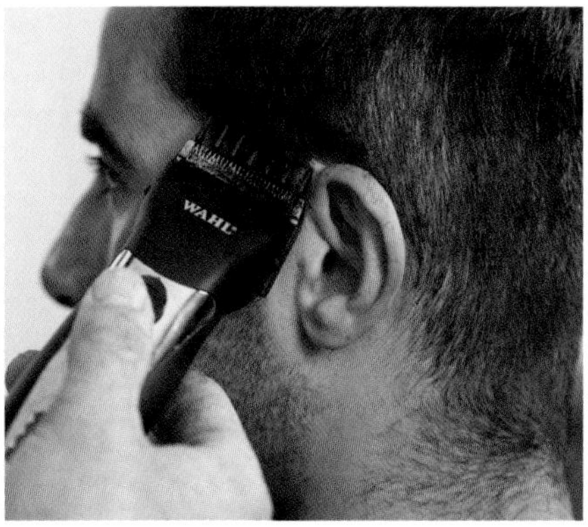

- **Gents' cutting** – cutting shorter styles, sometimes called short back and sides.

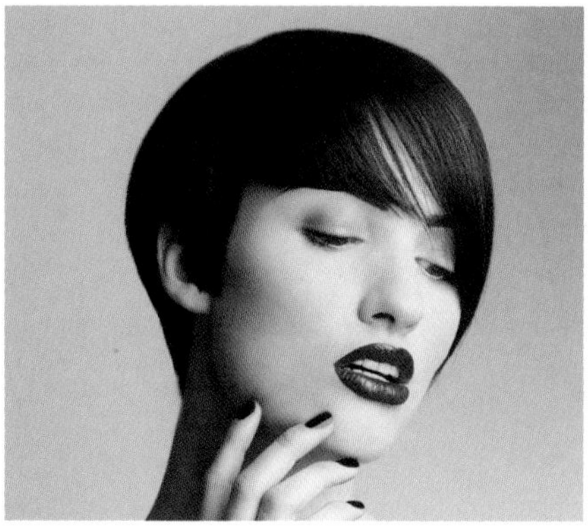

- **Full head colouring** – changing the colour of the client's hair permanently.

SmartScreen 001 handout 4

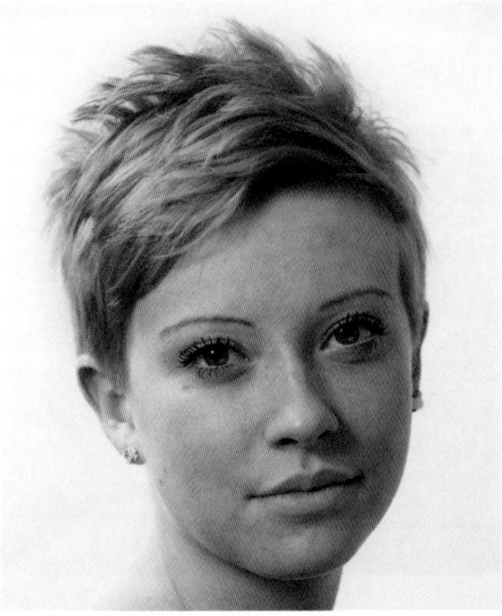

- **Temporary colouring** – changing the colour of the client's hair temporarily. The colour will only last for a few washes.

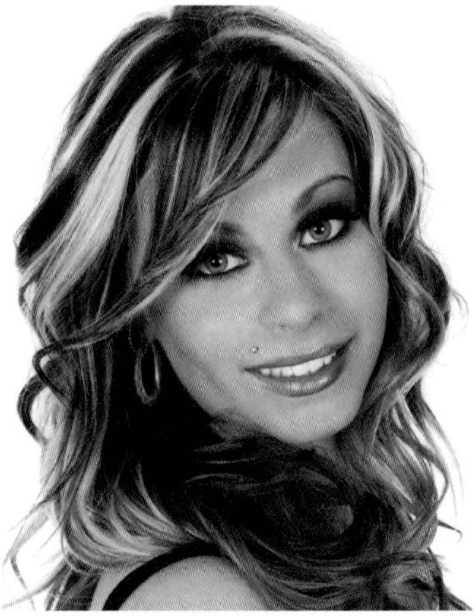

- **Highlighting or lowlighting** – colouring pieces of hair either lighter or darker than the client's natural colour.

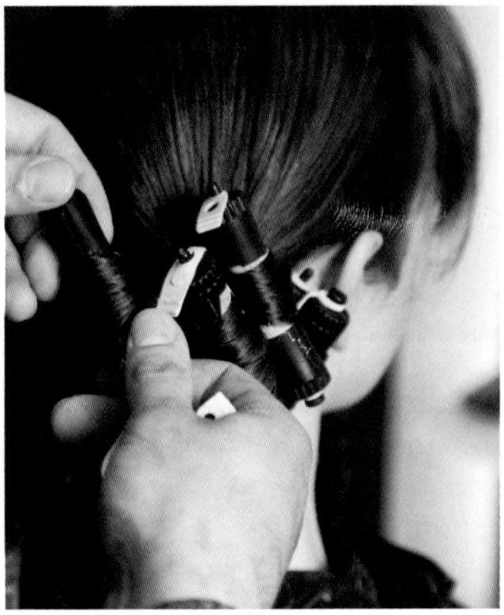

- **Perming** – changing the hair from straight to curly using chemicals.

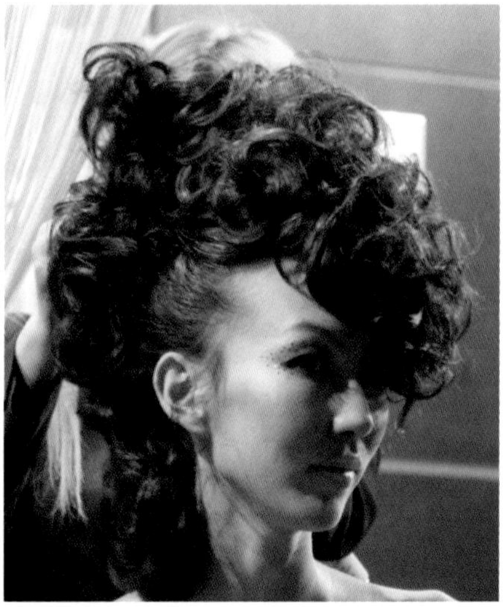

- **Hair extensions** – adding hair to make it look longer or thicker.

BEAUTY TREATMENTS OFFERED

A beauty salon will offer many services. They include:

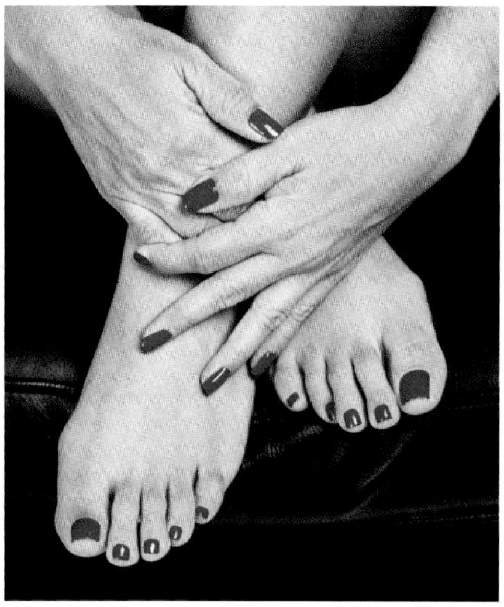

- Manicure and pedicure – improving the nails of the hands and feet.

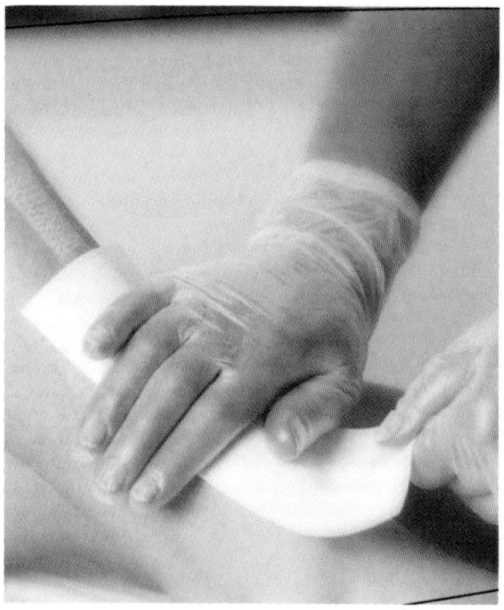

- Waxing – removal of hair using wax.

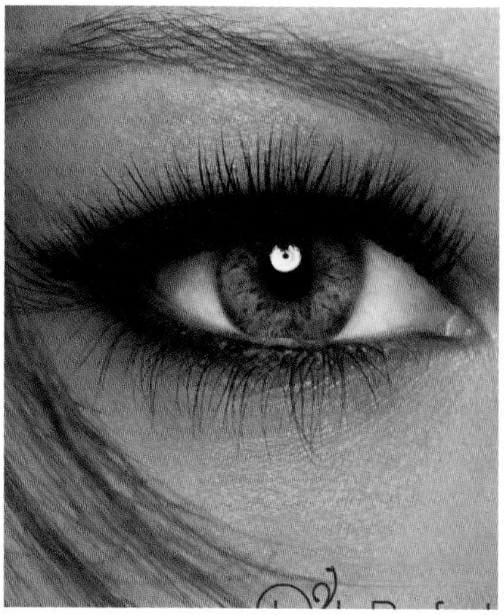

- Eye treatments – improving the look of the eyes and brows.

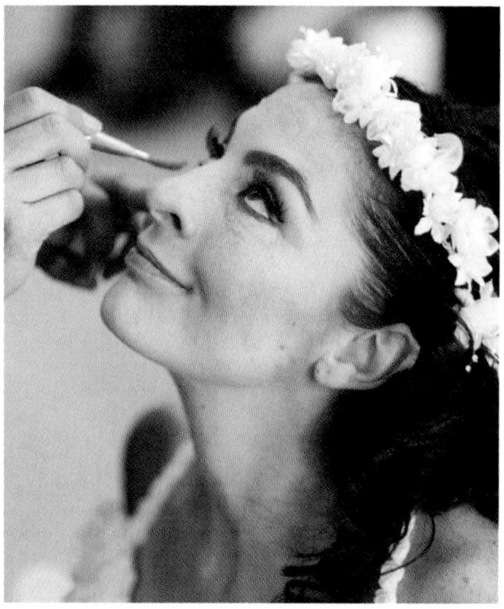

- Make-up for all occasions – such as parties and weddings.

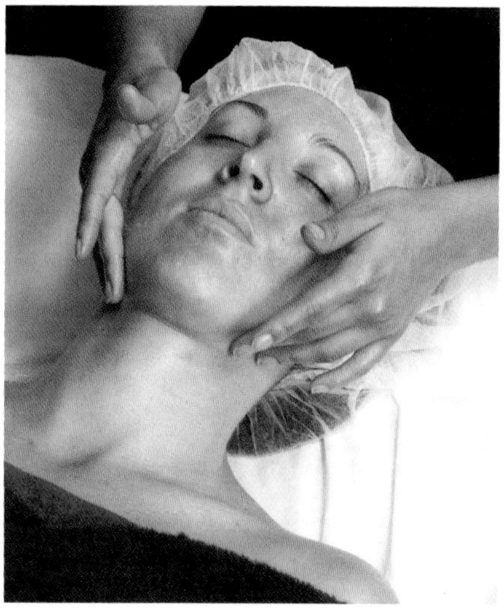

- Facial – treatments to improve the skin of the face.

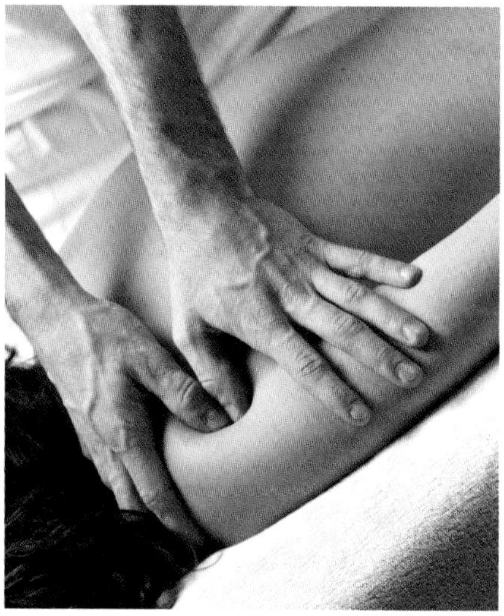

- Body massage – massage to improve the muscle and skin tone.

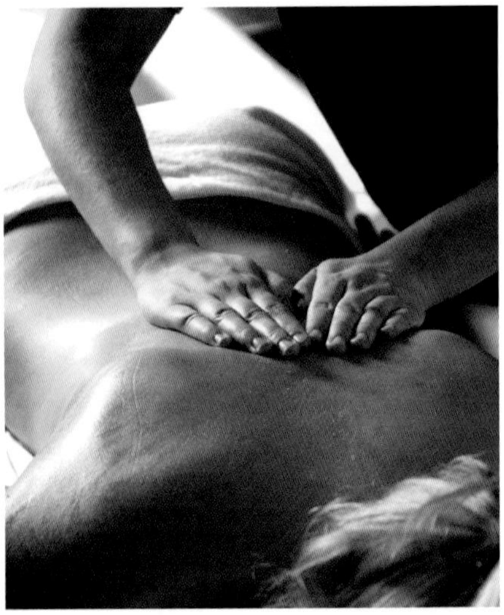

- Aromatherapy – massage using **essential oils**.

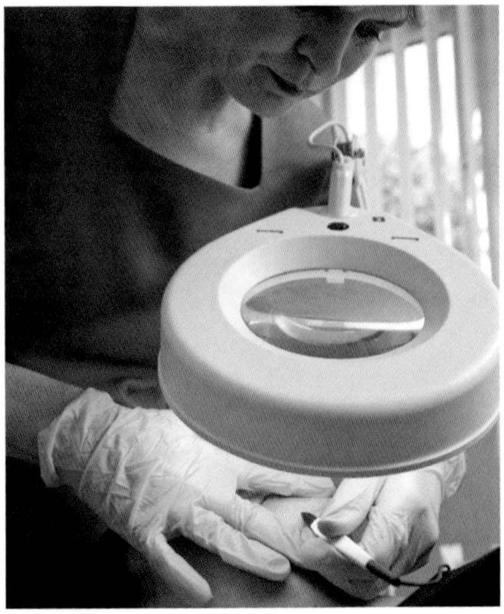

- Electrical epilation – permanent removal of unwanted hair.

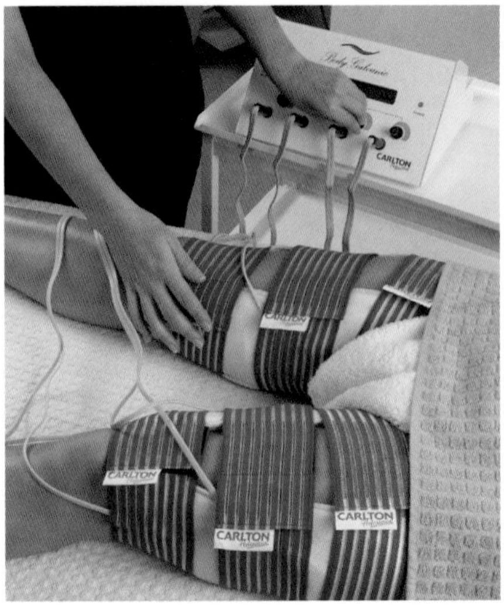

- Body therapy treatments – eg **anti-cellulite** and muscle toning.

Essential oils
Pure plant oils

Anti-cellulite
Reducing fluid retention

SmartScreen 101 handout 5

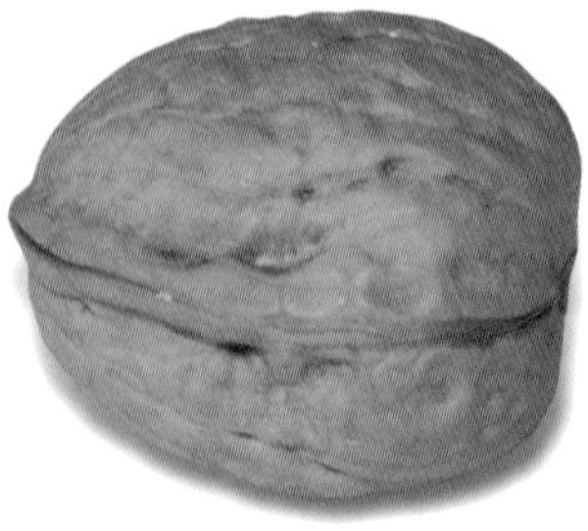

SmartScreen 001 activity assignment

IN A NUTSHELL

You are now at the end of the chapter. Before you test your knowledge with the revision activities, check the following list to see if you feel confident in all the areas covered. If there are still any areas you're unsure of, go back over them in the book and ask your tutor for extra support:

- occupational roles – the range of jobs you can do
- work patterns
- the importance of being fit and healthy
- career opportunities – the places you can work after you have finished training
- types of hairdressing salon
- types of beauty salon
- the services offered by hairdressing and beauty salons.

REVISION ACTIVITIES

Using the questions below, test your knowledge of Chapter 101 to see just how much information you've gained. This can help you to prepare for your assessments.

Turn to pages 480–481 for the answers.

WORDSEARCH

Have a go at finding some of the key words for this unit in the grid below.

By doing this, you will become more familiar with some of the words used in this unit.

barber	facial	colour	perming
waxing	manicure	salon	nail
stylist	therapist	reception	

									Q	W									
									D	E									
								K	X	J	A								
								N	L	P	Z								
							Q	W	I	E	X	X							
							K	K	R	R	U	B							
W	B	A	R	B	E	R	L	B	T	M	J	W	A	X	I	N	G	D	R
I	E	E	T	W	O	S	T	Y	L	I	S	T	B	C	O	L	O	U	R
	N	Z	T	B	A	A	T	S	N	N	U	I	Y	W	T	U	L	E	
		M	V	A	H	E	H	V	B	G	Y	D	W	J	F	T	J		
			S	R	E	C	E	P	T	I	O	N	I	S	T	K			
				D	P	Q	R	Y	C	X	W	I	O	U	H				
			W	J	J	Q	A	M	A	N	I	C	U	R	E	F			
			E	P	A	P	P	N	K	H	S	A	L	O	N	A			
		W	R	Q	H	W	I	A	Q	F	V	N	A	I	L	C	P		
		B	U	T	Q	Y	S	Q			E	A	J	R	R	I	M		
	I	X	F	S	K	F	T					R	H	Q	O	A	V	Z	
	U	Y	M	C	U									I	G	L	B	B	
B	S	U	G													C	Q	G	Y
U	U																	P	T

TEST YOUR KNOWLEDGE FURTHER

1 List **eight** job opportunities in the hairdressing and beauty sector.

2 What is the name of the regulations that cover working hours and breaks?

3 List **three** things that you should do to keep fit and healthy.

4 Give **two** reasons why being flexible is necessary for a hairdresser, barber, beauty therapist or nail technician.

5 Name **eight** places you could work when you have finished your training.

6 Name **two** organisations that could give you information about qualifications.

7 List **six** services provided by a hairdressing salon.

8 List **four** services provided by a beauty salon.

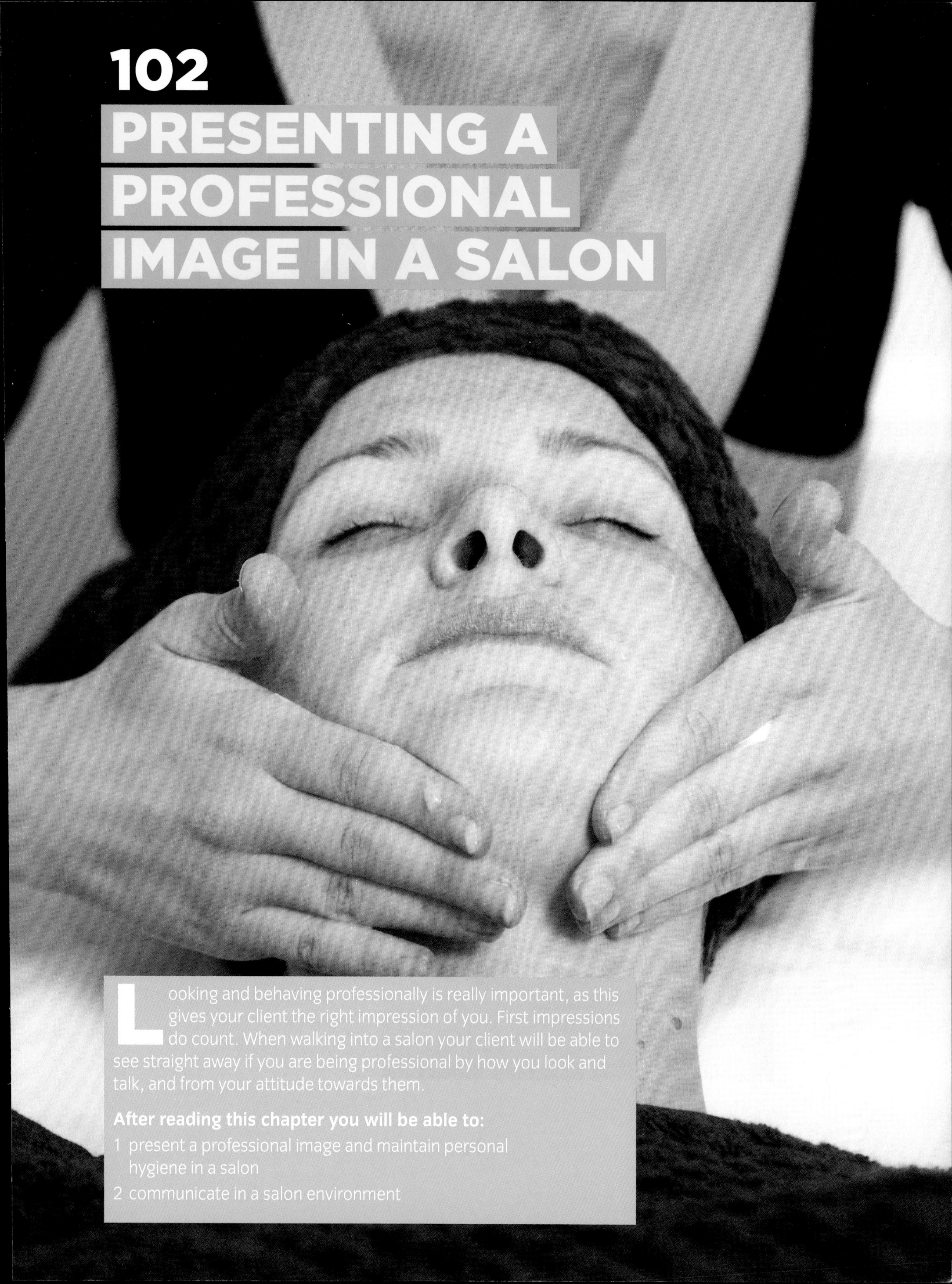

102 PRESENTING A PROFESSIONAL IMAGE IN A SALON

Looking and behaving professionally is really important, as this gives your client the right impression of you. First impressions do count. When walking into a salon your client will be able to see straight away if you are being professional by how you look and talk, and from your attitude towards them.

After reading this chapter you will be able to:

1 present a professional image and maintain personal hygiene in a salon

2 communicate in a salon environment

PRESENT A PROFESSIONAL IMAGE AND MAINTAIN PERSONAL HYGIENE IN A SALON

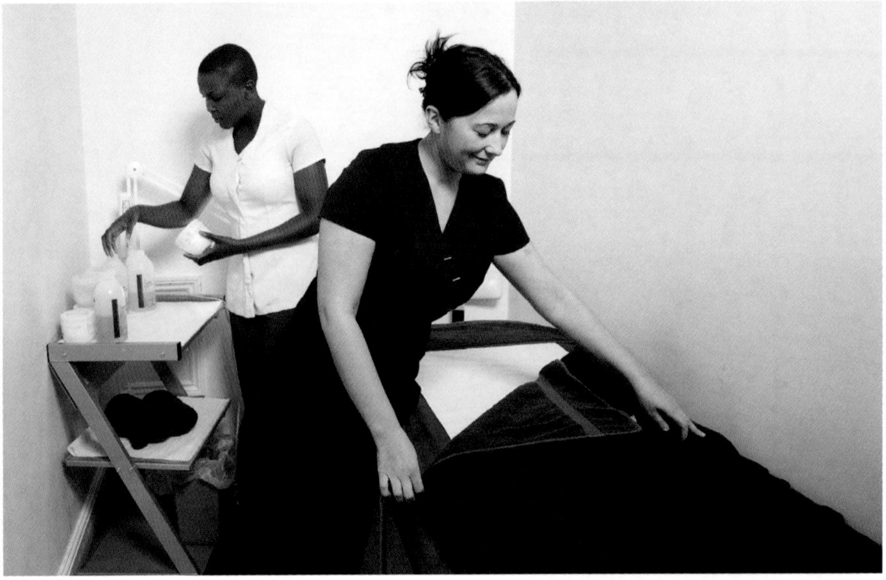

Professional image
Looking clean, tidy and wearing the correct uniform

What is 'a **professional image**'? It is the impression you give to your clients that shows your ability to do your job. Your boss will expect you to present the image that they want for the salon. You might be expected to wear a uniform or clothes that are co-ordinated, to have your hair styled to show the work the salon specialises in and to follow a code of behaviour. Let's look at the things you need to learn about presenting a professional image in the salon.

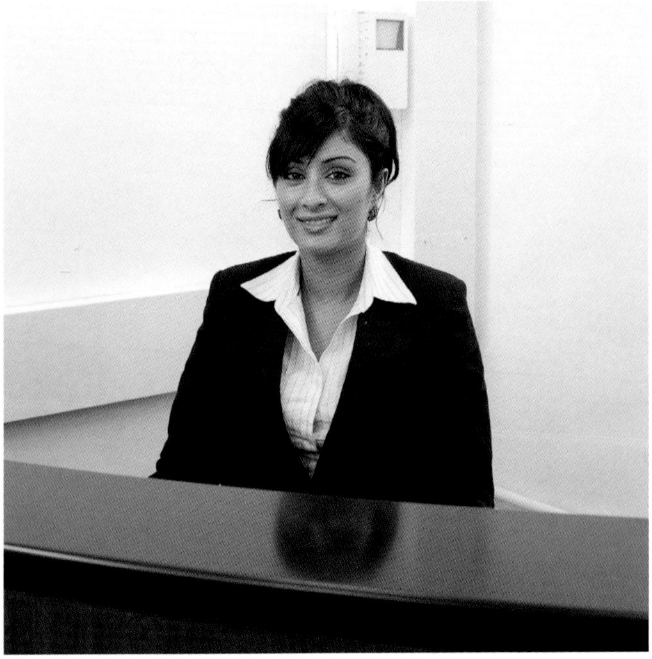

PERSONAL APPEARANCE

How you look in the salon says a lot about 'you'. How you are dressed, your hair and make-up, your hands, etc, will influence what your client thinks about you. If you show them that you care about yourself, then you are also showing that you will care about them when you are working on them.

CLOTHES

What you wear in the salon may be chosen your boss. Whatever you wear, make sure it is always clean, ironed and looks good.

Make sure that your clothes are not too tight. If they are they are likely to make you sweat more and this could cause body odour (BO). This is not very nice for your clients or your **colleagues**. Tight clothes will also be uncomfortable to wear.

Colleagues
People that you work with

In a beauty salon the beauty therapists you work with will wear a professional 'uniform'. A clean, hygienic uniform such as a dress or tunic top with co-ordinated trousers would meet the standard expected in the industry.

SmartScreen 102 worksheet 1

ACTIVITY

In your group, look at the four photos. Discuss which stylist and which therapist you would prefer to do your hair or give you a beauty treatment and why.

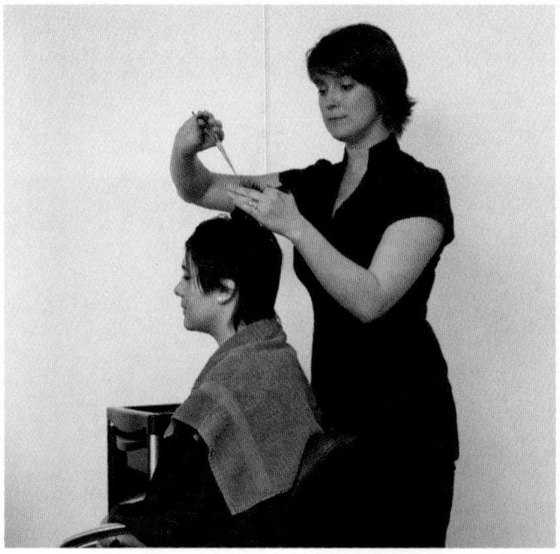

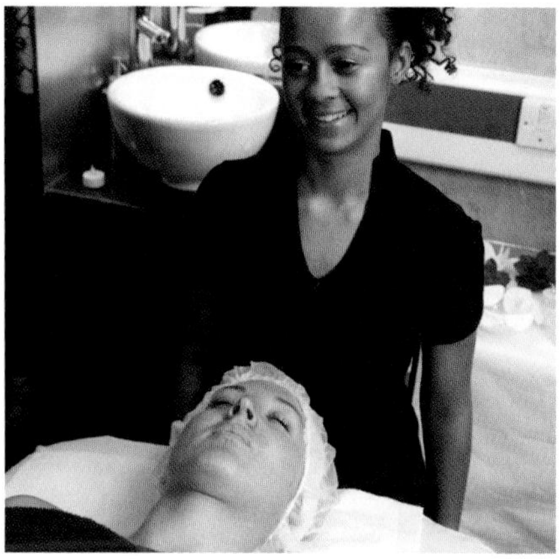

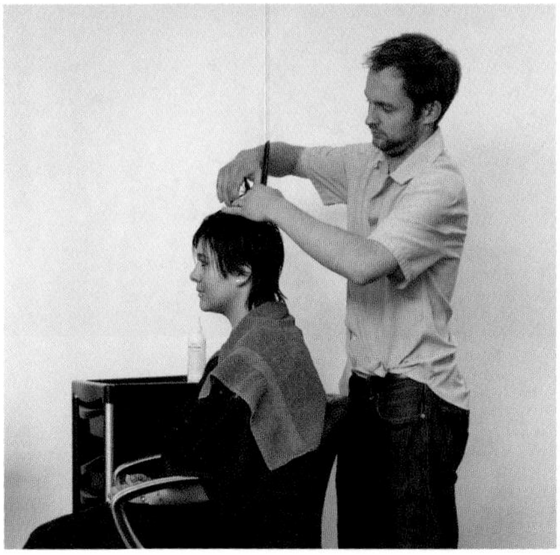

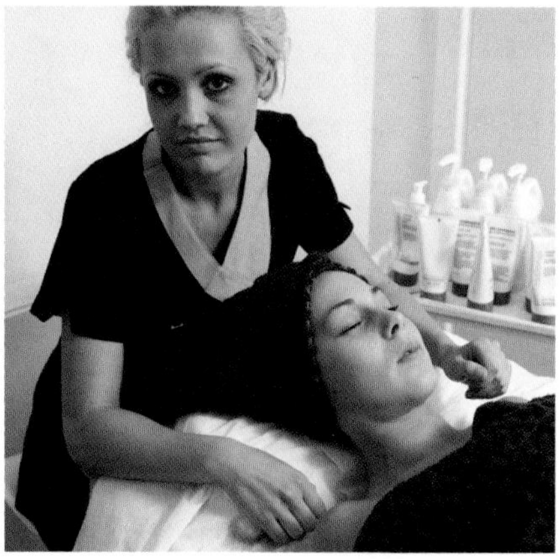

SmartScreen 102 handout 1

HAIR

Whether you are going to be a stylist or a therapist, your hair and how it looks are important to your image. As a stylist your hair is an advert for the work the salon does. Your boss will probably expect you to have a style and colour that complements what the salon is offering its clients.

Always make sure your hair is done before you start work. Use whatever products will help keep it in good condition and styled. This will help you to sell additional products to your clients. They will think that they must be OK if you use them on your hair.

As a therapist, when carrying out beauty treatments it is important that your hair is neat and tidy. It shouldn't get in your way while you are giving a treatment to a client. If your hair is long it should be tied up and off your face and collar.

Always make sure your hair is looking good before you start work. Give yourself enough time to do it properly.

ACTIVITY

Look at the four pictures. Choose which stylist or therapist you would prefer to have work on you.

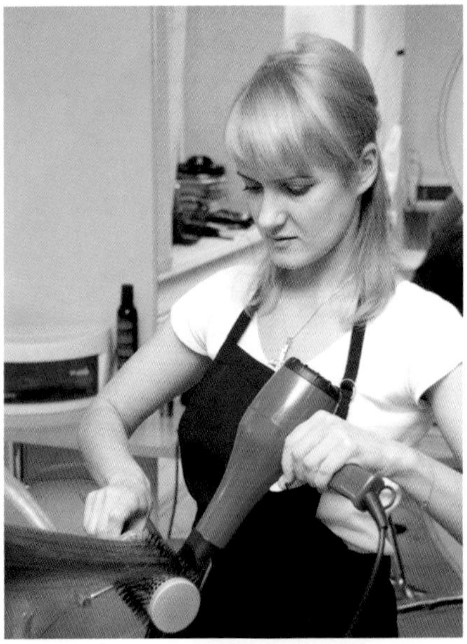

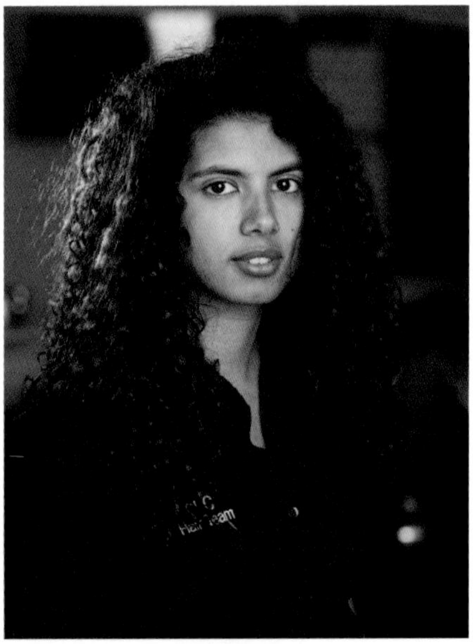

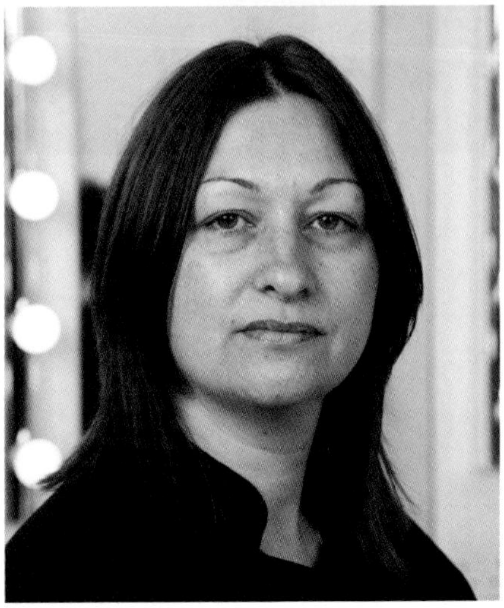

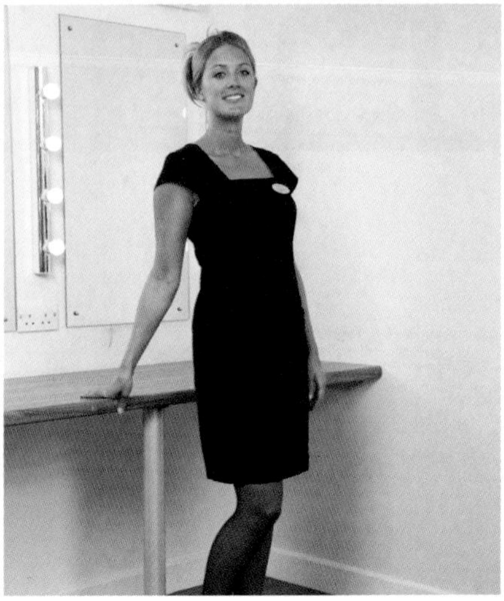

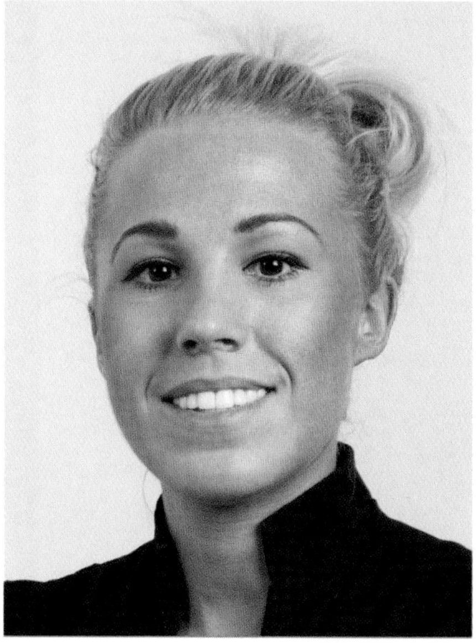

Don't wear too much make-up at work

MAKE-UP AND FACIAL CARE

If you are going to wear make-up then it should look good and go with your hairstyle. It should also fit the salon image. Give yourself time to apply it properly.

Go for an attractive make-up. If you are not going to wear make-up then use the right skin care products to make the skin look as good as possible. As a therapist, your make-up is an advert for your work and that of the salon. As with the stylist's hair it can assist in the selling of products and services.

As with your hair, give yourself enough time to do your make-up ready to start work and refresh it during your work day when necessary so it always looks at its best.

SmartScreen 102 handout 4

HANDS AND NAILS

Your hands are the main tools of the job you do. They will always be close to your client, so making sure they look good is very important to give the client the right impression. They must show that you have pride in your work.

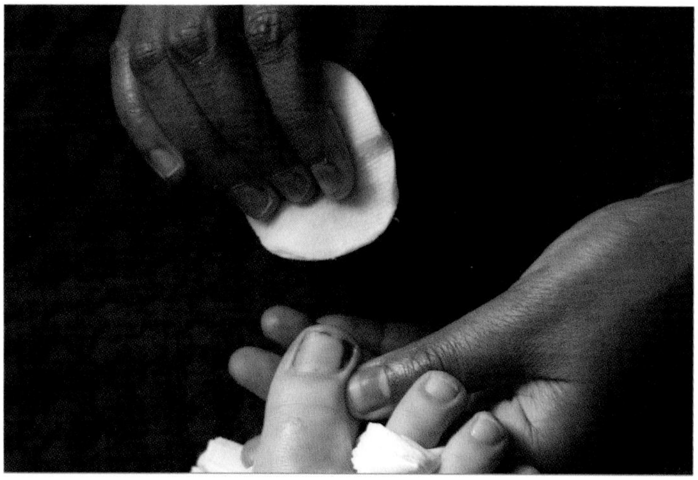

Keep nails short and clean

SmartScreen 102 worksheet 3

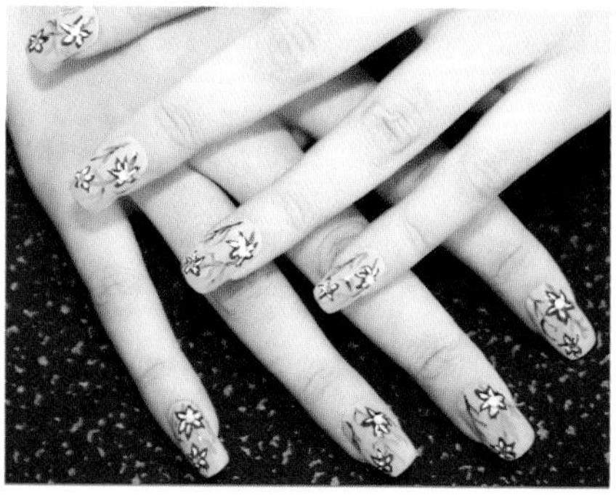

If you're a nail technician you can use your nails to show the services you offer

Your hands should always be very clean. If you have to do dirty jobs, either at work or at home, then wear gloves to protect your hands. Use moisturiser regularly to keep your skin smooth.

The nails are also an important part of your image. A therapist should always have short, neatly manicured nails that are not varnished.

For a nail technician, the nails should be used as an advert for your skills, so nail varnish and nail art are essential. For a stylist, the nails should be short and neatly manicured. If varnish is worn it must not be chipped or smudged.

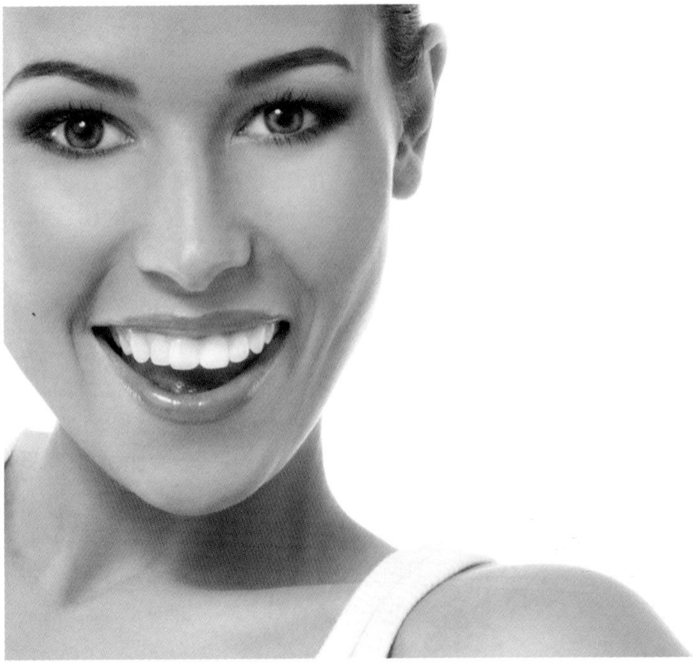

MOUTH

Looking after your teeth and making sure your breath is fresh by brushing your teeth is most important, both for personal health and hygiene and for cosmetic appearance. Regular visits to the dentist will keep your teeth looking good, especially when you smile. Don't chew gum while you're seeing clients.

FEET

All of your effort to look good can be spoiled by wearing the wrong shoes. Don't forget, your client can see your shoes as well as the rest of you. Their style and colour should go with your clothes.

SmartScreen 102 worksheet 4

Don't forget you will be on your feet all day so comfort is a must. The golden rule for shoes is that they should be flat, and if you are a stylist they should be closed toe. Low heels will help prevent backache and closed toes will stop hair cuttings from getting between the toes and on to the soles of your feet. Hair clippings can work their way into the skin and cause infections.

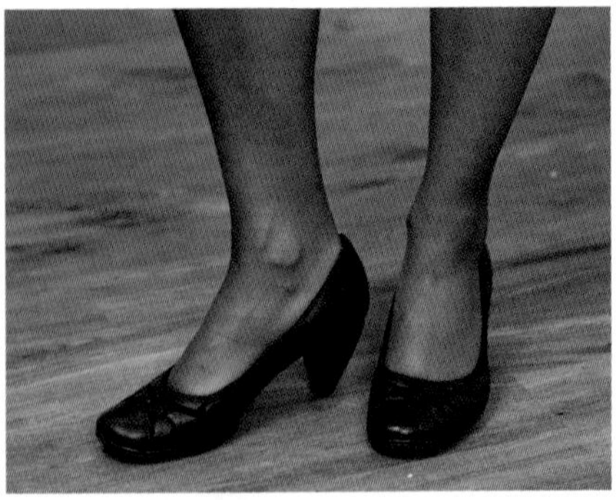

JEWELLERY

Beauty therapists should only wear small stud earrings and possibly a wedding band where appropriate. Hair stylists should wear as little jewellery as possible. The salon is likely to have a policy that you must follow. Remember, jewellery can be a safety hazard. Wearing too many rings can increase the risk of developing dermatitis, which could prevent you from doing your job. Necklaces and bracelets could get tangled in a client's hair. For a therapist, jewellery should not be worn for hygiene and safety reasons.

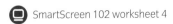

PERSONAL HEALTH AND HYGIENE

Looking after your own health and your personal hygiene is important to the image you give your clients. Having a good health routine will give you the energy to do your work.

SmartScreen 102 handout 2

PERSONAL WELLBEING

Your health routine should include:

- a well-balanced diet – it should include fresh fruit and vegetables and not too much 'junk' food
- enough sleep – between six and eight hours is recommended per night
- regular exercise – although you are on your feet all day this is not enough. Try a sport, or a regular 'workout' or gym session
- good posture – because you are on your feet all day, make sure you stand correctly. Keep your back straight and stand with your feet apart, in line with your shoulders. Your weight should be evenly spread on both legs. Putting your weight on one leg increases the pressure in the veins of that leg and can cause varicose veins to develop.

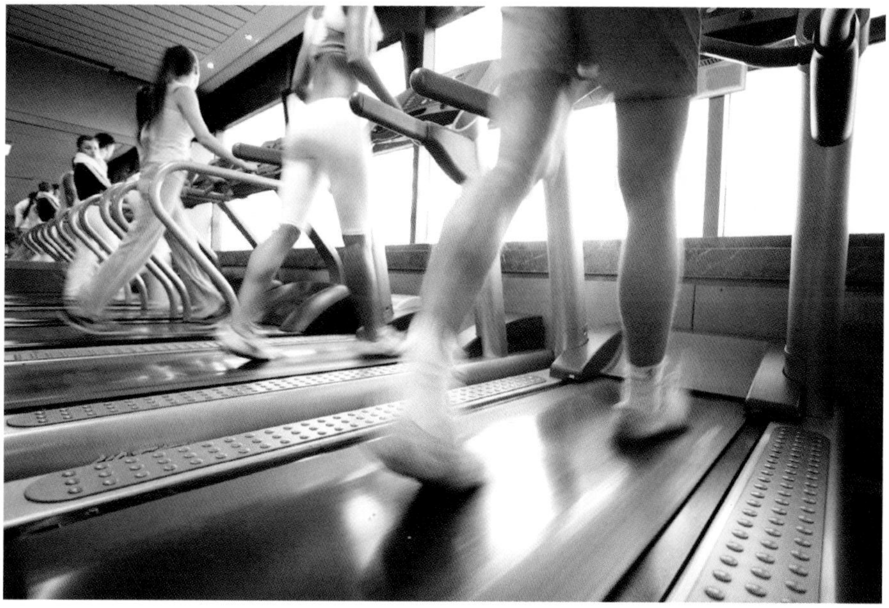

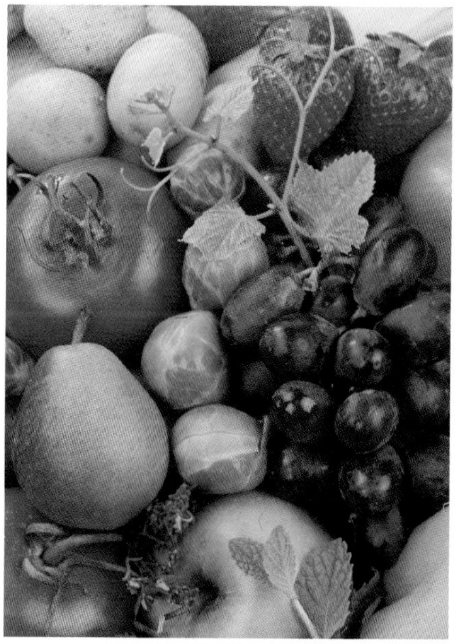

ACTIVITY

Keep a diary for a week. Write down what you had to eat and drink, how much sleep you had, and what exercise you did.

With a partner, discuss whether you could change anything to improve your health and wellbeing.

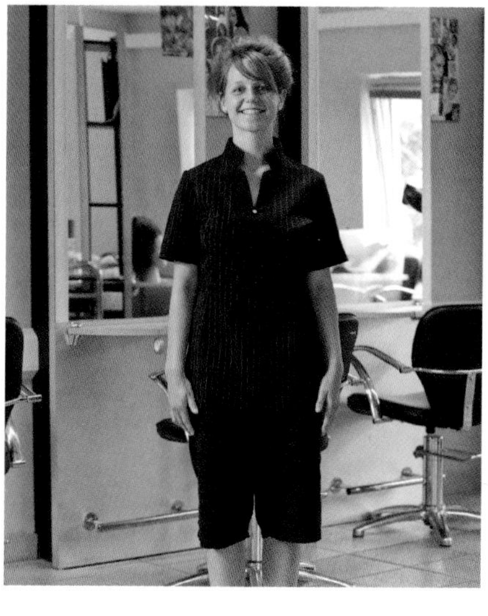

PERSONAL HYGIENE

Body

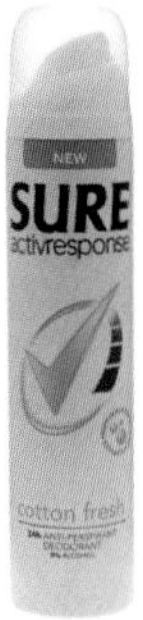

- You should bathe or shower every day.
- Use moisturiser/body lotion to replace lost moisture; this will stop the skin from becoming dry.
- Use deodorant or anti-perspirant regularly; this will help prevent unpleasant body odour (BO) which will be offensive to clients and your colleagues

SmartScreen 102 handout 2

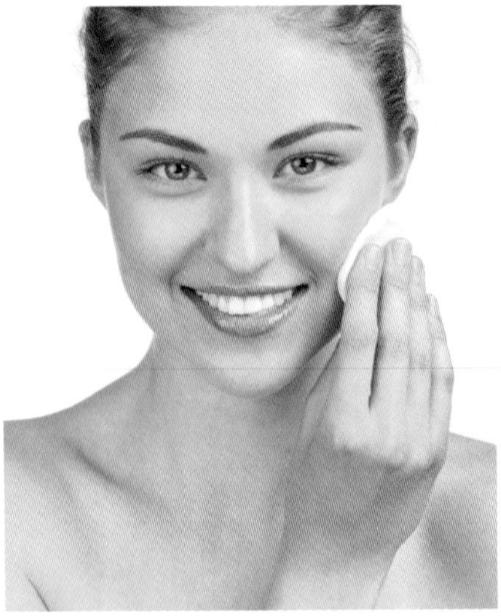

Face

- Use a good cleanser to remove the daily grime that your skin picks up.
- Use a toner or astringent to tone the skin so that it looks its best; you should do this even if you do not wear make-up.
- Moisturise every day to keep your skin supple.
- Treat spots and blackheads as soon as they appear; regular cleansing will reduce this problem.

Hands and nails

- Keep your hands and nails clean and your nails well manicured.
- Use hand cream or moisturiser regularly.
- Always use non-latex gloves when you are using chemicals.
- If your hands get wet, dry them thoroughly; make sure you dry between the fingers.

Using chemicals without gloves and not drying your hands will increase the risk of developing dermatitis. Many budding stylists and therapists have been forced to give up because they did not pay enough attention to looking after their hands.

ACTIVITY

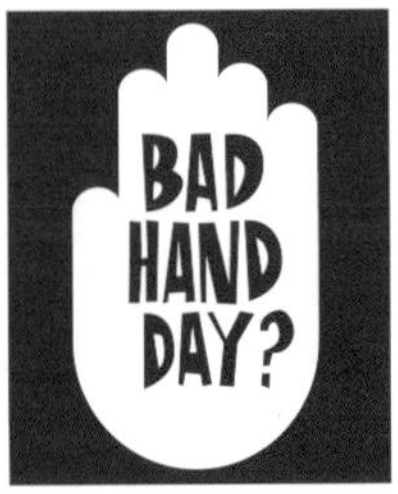

Go to www.badhandday.hse.gov.uk and learn more about reducing the risk of developing dermatitis. When you have visited the site, discuss the importance of looking after your hands with your group.

Mouth

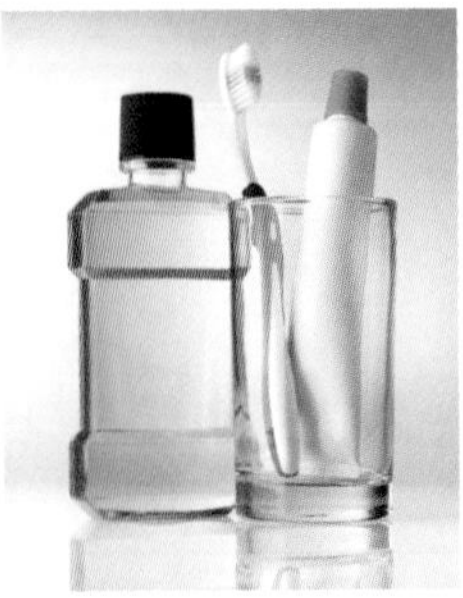

- As well as making regular visits to the dentist, make sure your teeth are clean and your breath is fresh.
- Clean your teeth at least twice a day.
- Use a mouthwash if you need to; bad breath (halitosis) can be offensive to your clients and colleagues.
- Do not chew gum in the salon as it looks unprofessional.

Feet

- Smelly feet can be a problem for some people because their feet sweat. Wash them regularly and use a foot spray if necessary.
- Check your feet for things like veruccas and corns. Get them treated as soon as possible. They can make standing painful.
- Make sure your shoes are a good comfortable fit.
- Do not wear high heels as they damage your back.

ACTIVITY

Make a checklist of things you need to do every day, and at what time, to maintain good personal hygiene.

COMMUNICATE IN A SALON ENVIRONMENT

Your professional image is not just about looking good and having good personal hygiene. **Communication** is important in this industry as you are working with clients. You need to be able to talk to people. These may be people that you have not met before.

In order for clients to feel happy about coming to you for treatments, you will need to feel comfortable with them. This starts with being confident about what you are doing.

Communication

The exchange of thoughts, messages or information, by speech, signals, writing or behaviour

SmartScreen 102 handout 4

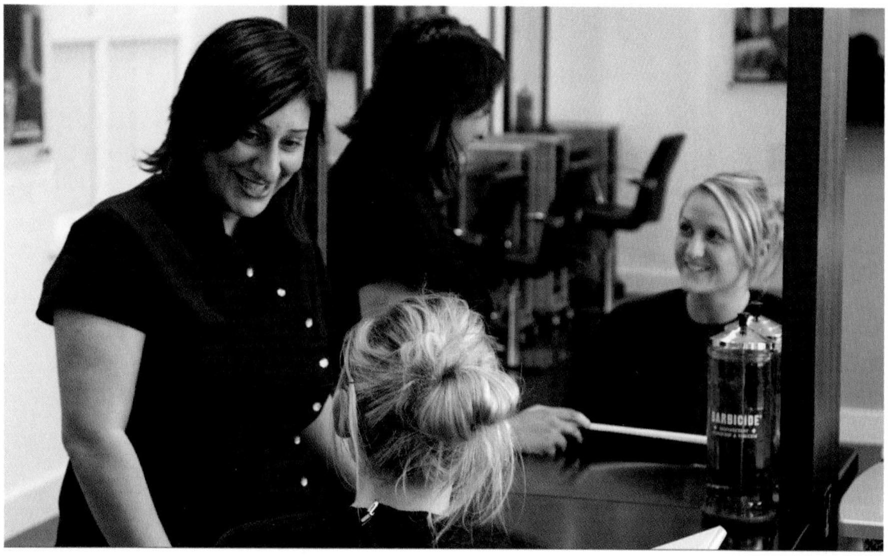

A smile can speak a million words

We communicate in different ways – by speaking and using our voices, which is called verbal communication; by using body language and gestures, which is called non-verbal communication. We can also communicate by writing and by listening.

When dealing with clients it is important that you communicate in a positive and professional way.

- An example of positive verbal communication is speaking *slowly and clearly*.
- Examples of positive non-verbal communication are making *good eye contact, smiling* and *giving the client your full attention*. Your body language should reflect a positive and relaxed manner. Good posture and a smart appearance are also examples of this.

ACTIVITY

Find some examples of pictures showing positive and negative body language. Print them off and then work with a partner to see if they can work out which ones are which. Ask them how they would react to a person showing the types of body language in your pictures.

When we communicate:

- 50 per cent is through our body language
- 40 per cent is through our tone of voice
- 10 per cent is through the words that we say.

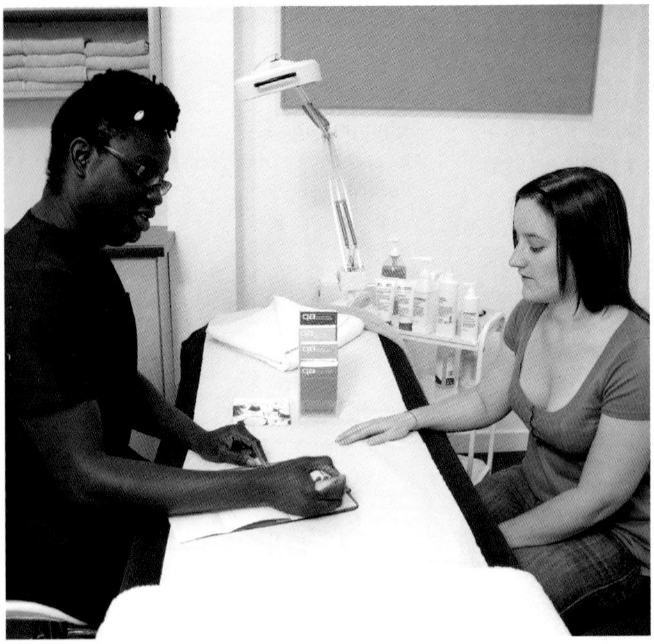

SPEAKING

Talking to people in conversation is a form of verbal communication. Examples of how we can do this in a professional way are:

- Speak clearly (so that the client can understand what we are trying to say).
- Use the right 'tone'. Positive tones will be softer than negative, harsh tones.
- Use the right volume. Don't speak so softly so the client can't hear you. Don't shout.
- Listen to the client talking (so you can understand what they are saying).
- When giving information, try to keep it simple (to help the client understand).
- Never speak to the client when chewing gum or eating (as this is unprofessional).

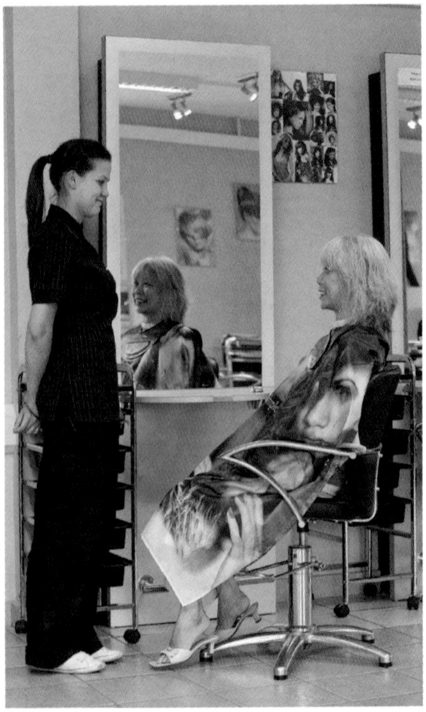

ACTIVITY

Talk to a partner about something you are interested in. Then discuss how well you communicated. Did they understand what you were saying? Did you speak clearly, with the right tone of voice and volume?

BODY LANGUAGE

This is a form of non-verbal communication. It is not what we are saying out loud, but what we are saying through our movements and gestures.

Some examples of positive body language are:

- smiling – will make the client feel welcome
- good eye contact – lets the client know you are interested in what they are saying
- listening – will help you understand what the client is trying tell you
- standing or sitting upright – will give the impression that you are keen and giving the client your full attention.

Some examples of negative body language are:

- frowning – will give the client the feeling that you do not agree with something
- shrugging your shoulders – will give the client the feeling that you are not interested in them or what you are doing.

ACTIVITY

Think of some examples of both good and poor body language. Role play these with a partner, with one of you using poor body language first, and then using good body language. Try to use facial expressions and gestures. Discuss how it made you both feel for each example.

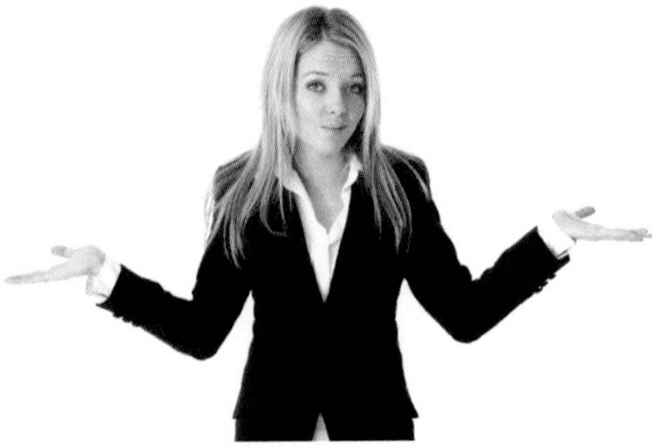

CONSULTING WITH THE CLIENT

In all the practical tasks you do, you will need to have a consultation with your client. The consultation is where you find out what the client wants from the hair service or beauty treatment. This will help you decide how you will do the service or treatment to satisfy the client. You need to communicate with them to find out information. This will involve asking the client questions.

GOOD QUESTIONING TECHNIQUES

Asking the right questions will help you get the correct information to carry out the service or treatment.

Closed questions

Closed questions can be described as:

A question that can be answered with either a single word or a short phrase.

Examples are 'How are you today?' and 'Where do you live?'

Or:

A question that can be answered with either 'yes' or 'no'.

Examples are 'Are you comfortable?' and 'Would you like me to show you how I apply this product, so that you can use it at home?'

Using closed questions

Closed questions are useful for the following reasons:

- They give you *facts* (such as the client's name and date of birth).
- They are good for getting basic information.
- They are easy to answer.

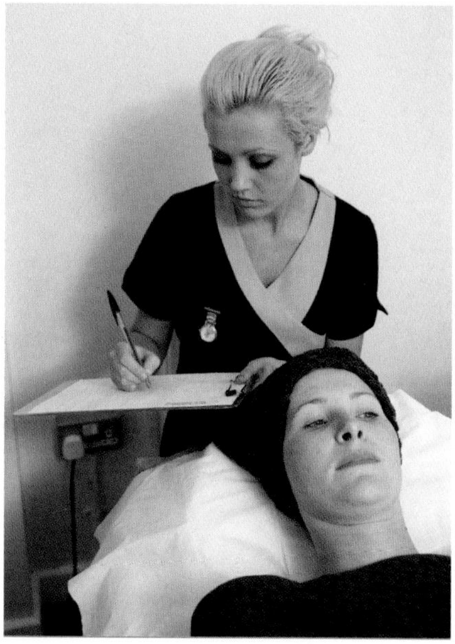

Make sure you ask your client the right questions

Open questions

These types of questions can be described as:

A question that will encourage a long answer.

Open questions can start with the following words: 'who', 'what', 'when', 'which', 'how' and 'would'.

Examples would be 'Why have you booked in for this make-up treatment today?', 'Which eye-shadow colours do you normally wear?' or 'What shampoo do you use at home?'

Using open questions

Open questions are useful for the following reasons:

- You will get a more detailed answer.
- They will give you information about the other person's opinions and feelings.
- They switch control of the conversation to the other person.

ACTIVITY

Start a list of open and closed questions that you could use to find out what the client wants from the service or treatment. Remember to add to the list as you learn your different skills.

ACTIVITY

With a partner carry out a consultation role play. One of you will be the client, the other the stylist or therapist. Carry out two consultations, one using only closed questions, and the second using both open and closed questions. Discuss with each other which one was better at getting the information you needed.

WHAT TO SAY AND HOW TO SAY IT

Communicating with your client is not just about finding out what they want done. It also involves chatting to them. For some clients it is the main reason they come to the salon. Some may be lonely; others may want to get away from the house and the children – to have a little 'me' time.

The way we talk to people in conversation is the same as when we talk to them in the consultation.

- Speak clearly so that the client can understand what you are trying to say.
- Listen to the client talking so you can understand what they are saying.
- When giving information, try to keep it simple, to help them understand.
- Never speak to them when chewing gum or eating, as this is unprofessional.
- Never discuss religion or politics.
- Remember, the client is not paying to listen to your troubles.

Some people are more outgoing whereas others are more quiet and shy. Whatever your personality, you will need to be able to talk to a client. The following tips will help:

- Be confident in what you are doing. Practise the skin care routines and learn about the products. This will help you when you are talking to your client.
- Try to maintain a positive body language. This will help you feel more confident. The client will also feel more confident with you.
- Try to talk slowly and clearly so that they understand what you are trying to say. Remember to listen to them too!
- Use questions that help you to get what information you need from the client.
- Smile so that the client knows that you are happy to be treating them. This will help them to relax.
- Last of all, be yourself! Don't try to be someone you are not. Unless you are a good actor it will come over as false and insincere.

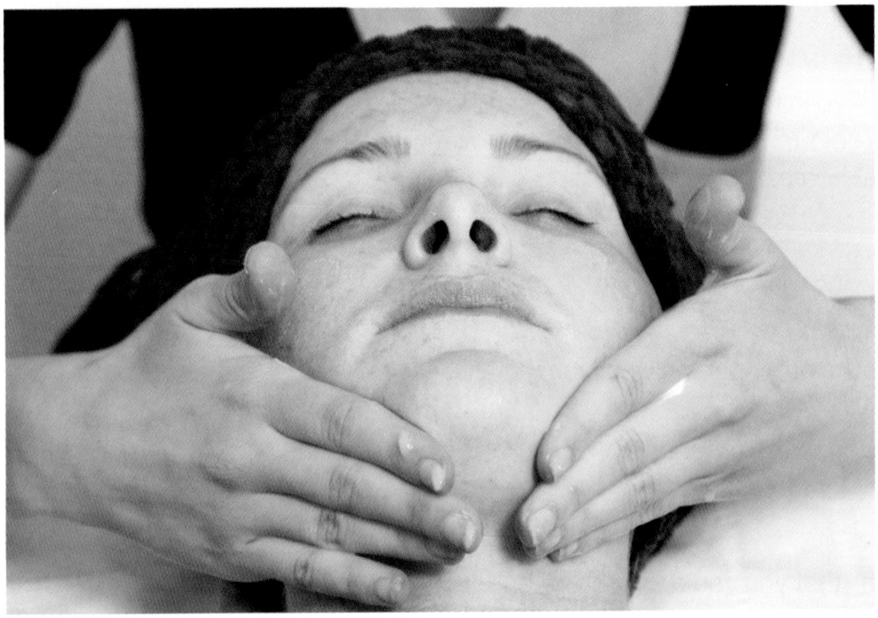

BEHAVIOUR AND ATTITUDE

Good behaviour in the salon is important. How you behave will affect everyone around you. The salon is not the place to mess around, play jokes or sit around doing nothing. Chewing gum, texting and filing your nails are also things to avoid.

It is not just when you are working on a client that you need to think about your professional image. Remember, you can still be seen by other clients and they can be influenced by what you are doing.

To help promote a good atmosphere and image in the salon you need to make sure you do the following.

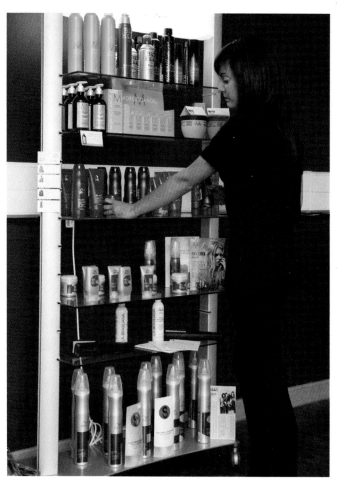

FOLLOW INSTRUCTIONS WILLINGLY

Always follow the instructions from the stylist/therapist when they ask you to do something. Always do it willingly; if you don't the client will notice.

There may be times when your salon manager asks you to do a job that you do not like (such as tidying the towels or emptying the bins). Sometimes being professional means doing things that you do not want to do!

WORK CO-OPERATIVELY WITH OTHERS

It is important to work as a team with your colleagues.

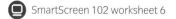

SmartScreen 102 worksheet 6

Always treat each other with respect. Working well together and being respectful will not only make it a happier place to work, but will also mean that the clients feel more comfortable too. Being kind and considerate to each other will improve your relationships with your colleagues.

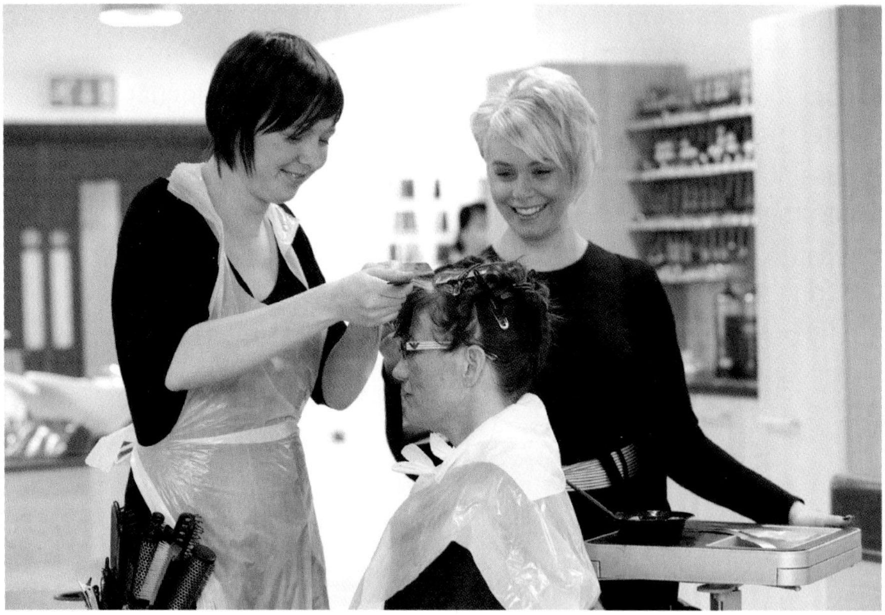

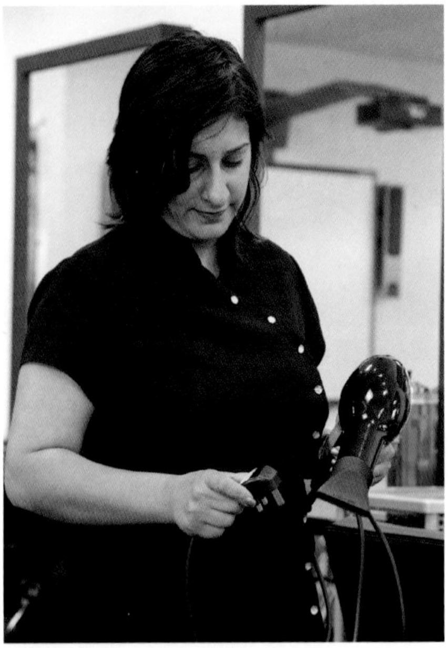

Procedure
Step-by-step

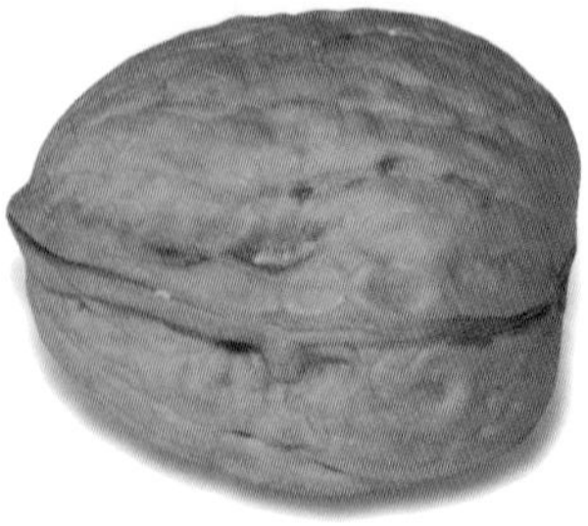

FOLLOW SALON PROCEDURES

A good stylist/therapist will follow salon rules from their salon manager, such as cleaning up after treatments and using the equipment correctly. They also need to follow salon **procedures** such as health and safety standards, eg using hygienic products and equipment. This will make the salon a safer and cleaner place for both staff and clients.

ACTIVITY

Make a list of positive ways in which you can behave in the salon. What effect will they have on you, the clients and your colleagues?

ACTIVITY

Think of some examples of poor behaviour. How would you deal with them if you were the salon manager?

THE IMPORTANCE OF A GOOD PROFESSIONAL IMAGE

Good impressions bring clients back and lead to good business. Communication skills are important for developing good relationships with both clients and colleagues.

If the atmosphere in a salon is good, clients will want to come back.

IN A NUTSHELL

You are now at the end of the chapter. Before you test your knowledge with the revision activities, check the following list to see if you feel confident in all the areas covered. If there are still any areas you're unsure of, go back over them in the book and ask your tutor for extra support:

- what makes a professional image
- wow to maintain your personal appearance – the clothes you wear, your hair, make-up, hands and nails, etc
- how to maintain your personal hygiene – the importance of washing and using deodorants, etc; looking after your skin; keeping your hands and nails clean and moisturised; finding out about the risk of dermatitis from the HSE website; why fresh breath is important
- how you communicate with others – speaking, body language, listening and writing
- consulting the client – using closed and open questions to get information from the client
- what to say and when to say it – the importance of conversation during the client's visit
- why behaviour and attitude are important to the image and atmosphere of the salon.

REVISION ACTIVITIES

Using the questions below, test your knowledge of Chapter 102 to see just how much information you've gained. This can help you to prepare for your assessments.

Turn to pages 482–483 for the answers.

WORDS TO FIND

Copy and complete the sentences below. Use these words to help you fill in the gaps.

attitude	deodorant	closed
professional image	body language	listening
flat shoes	follow instructions	behaviour
salon procedures	speaking	personal wellbeing
open		

1 Presenting a ____________________ to your client is very important.

2 Using ____________________ will help you communicate effectively with your client.

3 Wearing ____________________ will prevent backache and fatigue.

4 To be effective in your work you must know the ____________________ used in your place of work.

5 A well balanced diet, regular exercise and enough sleep are essential parts of your ____________________ .

6 ____________________ and ____________________ will help you communicate effectively with the client.

7 Using ____________________ will help prevent body odour when you are working.

8 ____________________ and ____________________ are types of question you can use when consulting with the client.

9 A good stylist/therapist will always ____________________ from their salon manager.

10 Good ____________________ and ____________________ will help to give your clients the right impression of you.

TEST YOUR KNOWLEDGE FURTHER

1 Name the four things that are important to your professional Image.

2 Why is it important for your hair or your make-up to look good in the salon?

3 Why should you keep your nails short and well-manicured when working in the salon?

4 Why is it important to keep your hands dry and moisturised?

5 What is using facial expression and gestures called?

6 Why is it important to listen when you are communicating?

7 Why is it important to keep good eye contact with your client when you are talking to them?

8 What are questions that require a short answer called?

9 What type of question would you use if you needed to find out about products and equipment the client has used at home?

10 Name **two** things that will promote a good atmosphere and give a good impression in the salon.

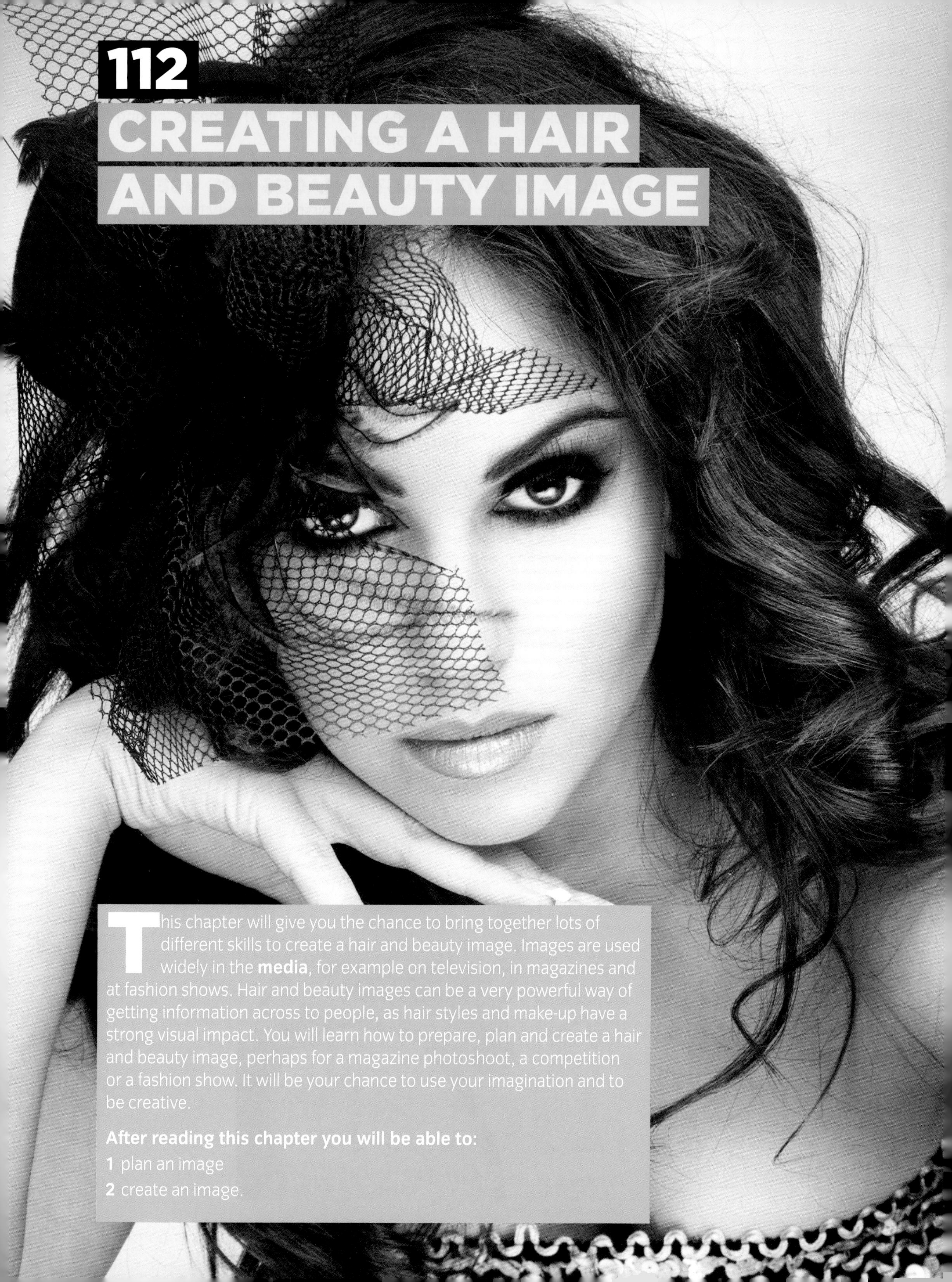

112 CREATING A HAIR AND BEAUTY IMAGE

This chapter will give you the chance to bring together lots of different skills to create a hair and beauty image. Images are used widely in the **media**, for example on television, in magazines and at fashion shows. Hair and beauty images can be a very powerful way of getting information across to people, as hair styles and make-up have a strong visual impact. You will learn how to prepare, plan and create a hair and beauty image, perhaps for a magazine photoshoot, a competition or a fashion show. It will be your chance to use your imagination and to be creative.

After reading this chapter you will be able to:

1 plan an image

2 create an image.

Media
Ways of communicating with people, for example newspapers, radio, television

Inspiration
Using other ideas to come up with your own, unique idea

Image
A total look that may include hair, make-up, clothes and jewellery

Promotion
An event where you can sell products or treatments to your clients

Existing clients
Clients that have had one or more treatments at the salon

PLAN AN IMAGE

You must plan your image before you can create it. This means looking at lots of different images for **inspiration**.

HOW HAIR AND BEAUTY IMAGES ARE USED

There are many different reasons why a hairstylist, beauty therapist, make-up artist or nail technician might need to create an **image**. The following are examples of when images can be used.

AS PART OF A PRESENTATION

An example of a presentation is holding an open evening at a salon, inviting people to come in to see a **promotion** that the salon is offering. This may be for a new service, treatment or products. This is a good way of letting new or **existing clients** know about these products and services. The hair or beauty image would be used on any adverts for the presentation such as a poster on the salon door or in a leaflet that is posted out to local homes.

FOR A PHOTOGRAPHIC SHOOT

This could be for a picture in a magazine. Hair and beauty images are used a lot in magazines to advertise products such as perfume, hair, make-up and skin care products and clothes.

HANDY HINTS

You may decide to present your ideas to the rest of the group by pretending that they are your clients at a salon open evening. You can make a leaflet or poster using the hair and beauty image to advertise the promotion.

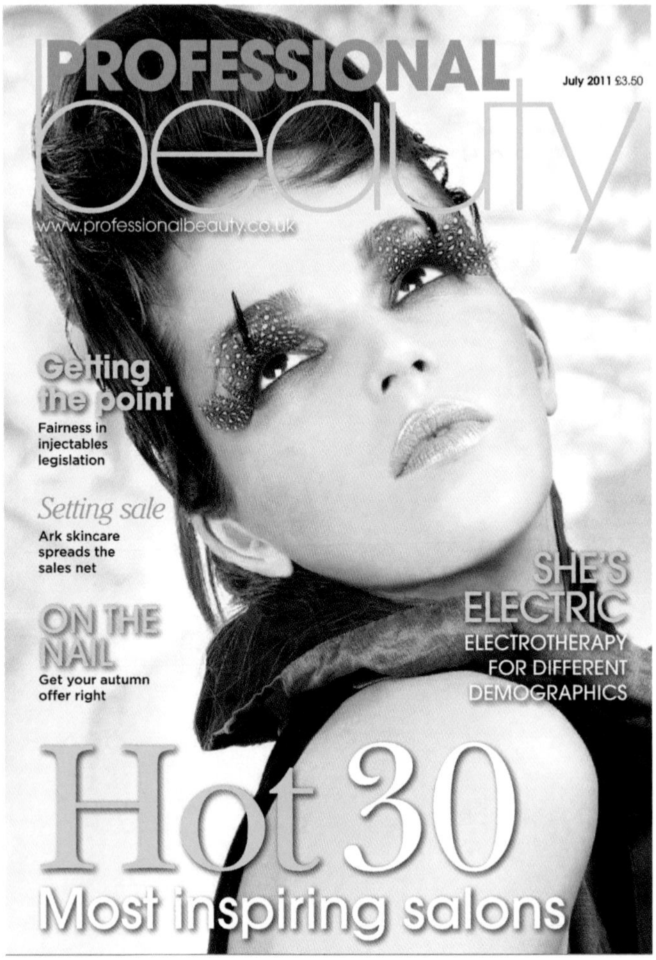

Magazine image

ACTIVITY

Take a look through some magazines and see how hair and beauty images are used to advertise different products. Collect examples of ones that you like, as these may come in useful later when you are planning your image.

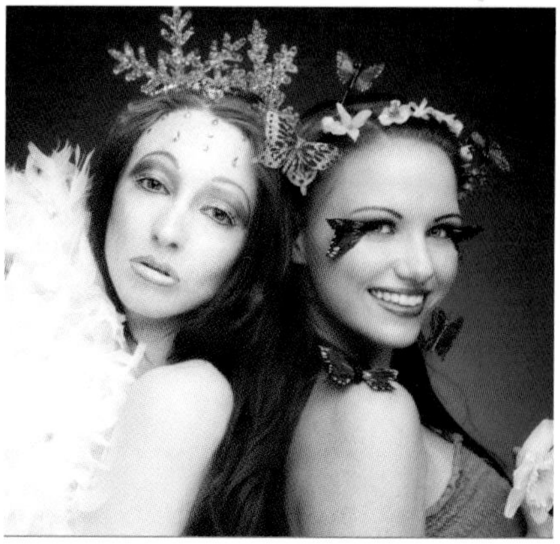

A photographic image

FOR FASHION OR CATWALK SHOWS

The show **organiser** will have an idea of what image they want the models to have in order to create the overall look of the show. This will usually include the total look – the hairstyle, make-up and clothes that are to be worn.

AS PART OF A COMPETITION

In order to make sure it is fair for all who take part, there are usually competition rules that clearly state exactly what the **competitors** have to do. Examples of such rules include:

- what the **theme** of the competition will be
- what you are expected to complete for the competition, for example a hair and beauty image based on the punk era
- whether the hair and beauty image is to be carried out on a head block, model or **peer**
- what tools, equipment and products are needed and allowed
- how long you have to complete the competition.

Organiser
The person in charge

Competitors
The people entering a competition

Theme
The subject or topic, for example Christmas, the seasons, nature, history

Peer
Someone of the same age, for example another student on your course

ACTIVITY

Decide as a group what your hair and beauty image is going to be used for. You can use the information above to help you decide. Your tutor can also help you. Once you have made this decision, you can start to plan what it is that you need to do next. The following information will help you to develop your ideas further.

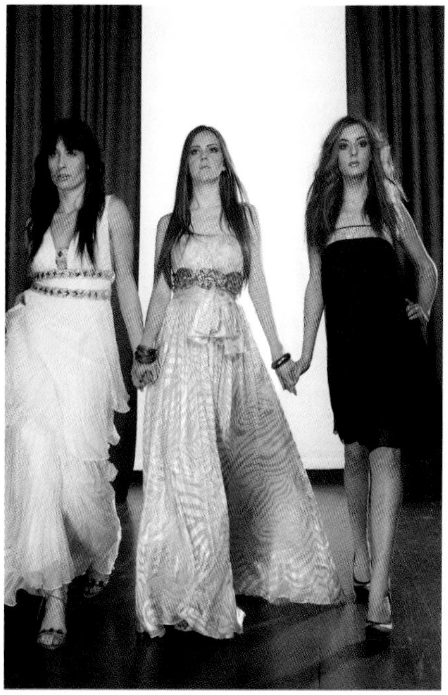

An image from a catwalk

HANDY HINTS

You must always say where you got your information from.

SOURCES OF INFORMATION

The following is a list of different places that you can go to for information. These **sources** will help to give you ideas and inspiration for your hair and beauty image. It is important to take the time to carry out research for your image, as this will help you decide:

- what you want the completed image to look like
- what planning is needed to help you create the finished image
- whether the information that you are using is up to date and correct.

Sources

Somewhere you go for information, eg a book or the internet

Sources of information for creating an image

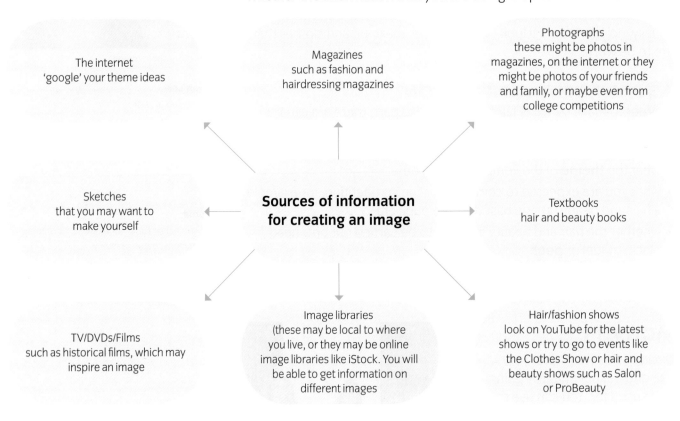

- The internet – 'google' your theme ideas
- Magazines – such as fashion and hairdressing magazines
- Photographs – these might be photos in magazines, on the internet or they might be photos of your friends and family, or maybe even from college competitions
- Textbooks – hair and beauty books
- Hair/fashion shows – look on YouTube for the latest shows or try to go to events like the Clothes Show or hair and beauty shows such as Salon or ProBeauty
- Image libraries (these may be local to where you live, or they may be online image libraries like iStock. You will be able to get information on different images
- TV/DVDs/Films – such as historical films, which may inspire an image
- Sketches – that you may want to make yourself

HANDY HINTS

To help create your overall image, you also need to think about the clothing, accessories, hairstyle, nails and make-up (colours and styles).

Accessories

Extra items that make up an outfit, such as jewellery and hair decorations

ACTIVITY

Include in your research all of the following (this will help you get all the information you need to plan for your total look):

- hair colour and style
- make-up colours and how they are applied, for example either a more natural-looking make-up or a more dramatic look using darker colours
- nail colours or nail art designs
- style of clothes and colours
- **accessories** needed, for example bags, jewellery, hair clips and ornaments, etc
- face or body painting needed to create the final look.

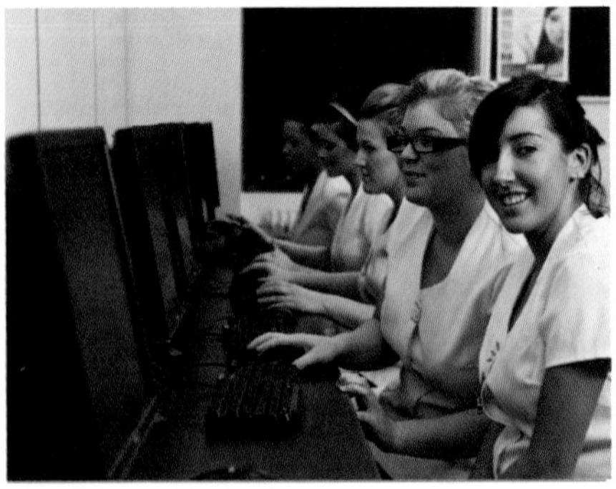

Students carrying out internet research

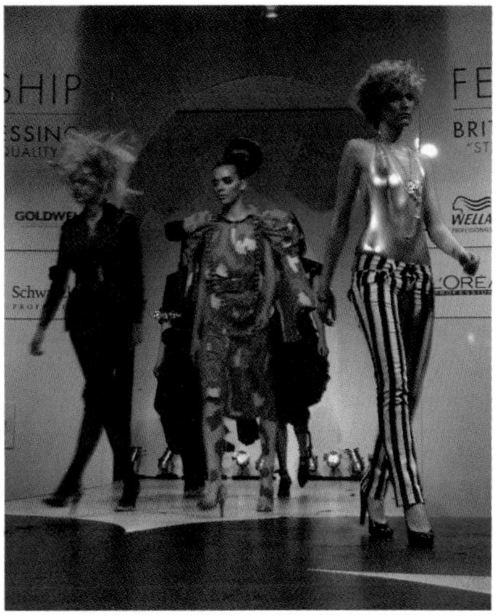

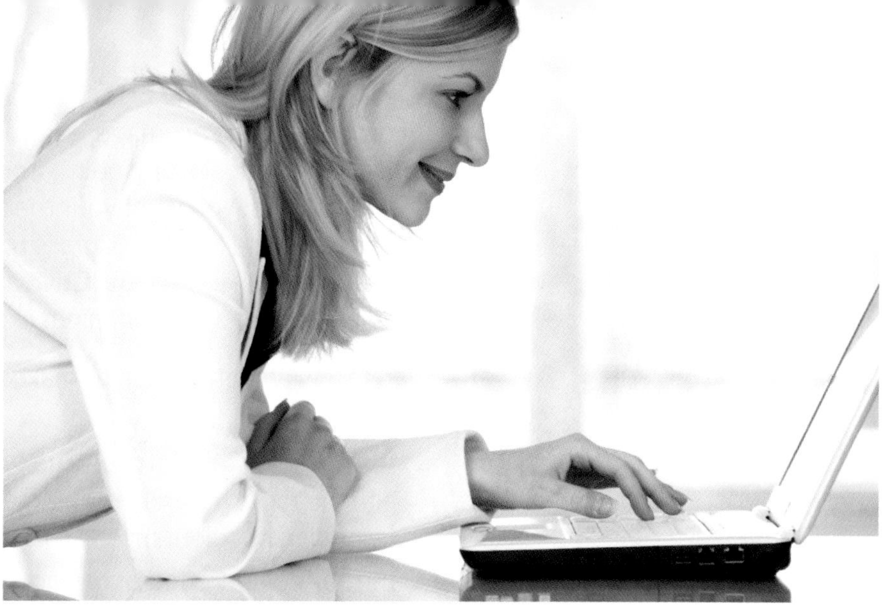

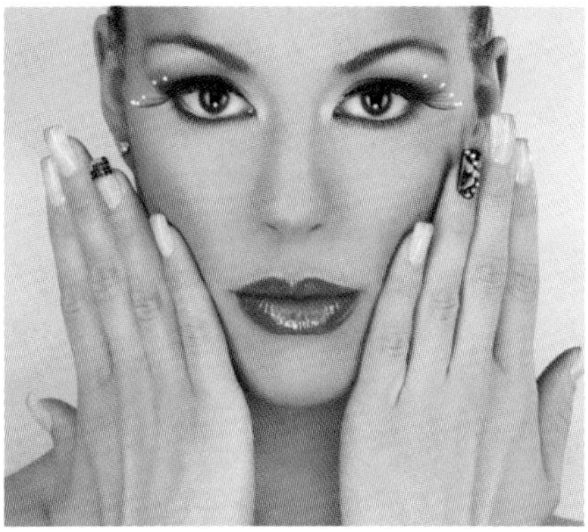

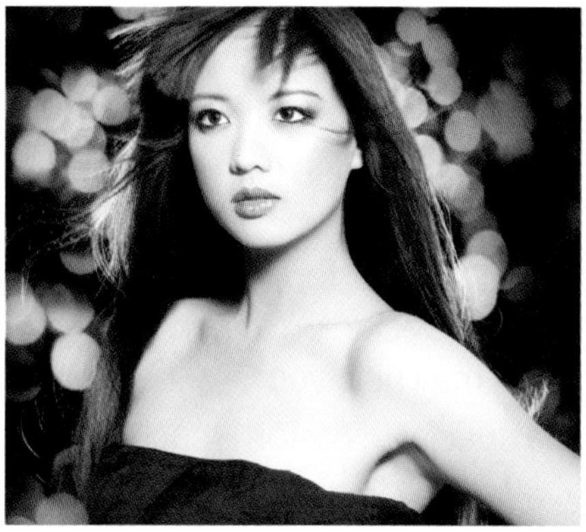

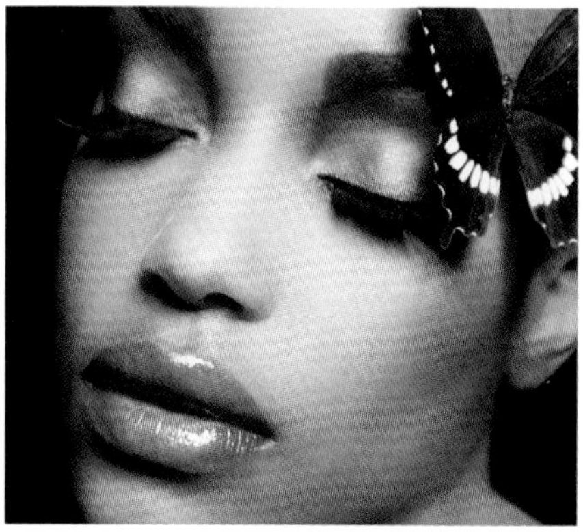

ACTIVITY

Research as many different sources as you can. This will help you decide on what your hair and beauty image will look like. Start to collect and save pictures, sketches and images that are linked to your chosen image and theme.

HANDY HINTS

Remember to always clearly **reference** your work to record where you got the information from. Try to use as many different sources as you can. This will help you to get as many different ideas as possible.

Reference

Where something comes from, for example a website address

HANDY HINTS

There are so many different sources to look at for inspiration: fashion images, the internet, textbooks and magazines, to name just a few!

HANDY HINTS

If you are not sure of a theme yet, you may find it useful looking through these sources of information first to help you decide.

SmartScreen 112 handouts 1 and 2

SmartScreen 112 worksheet 1

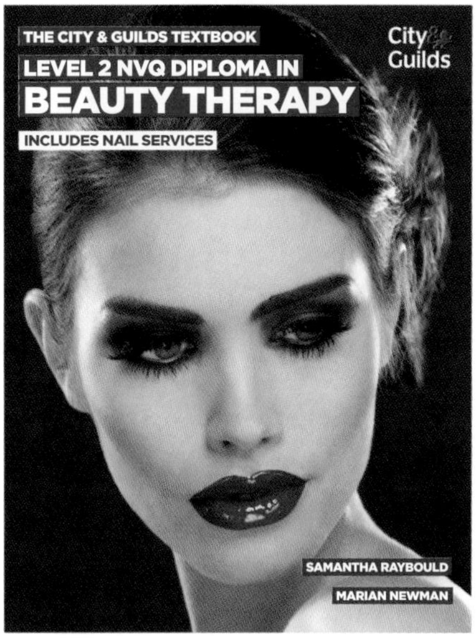

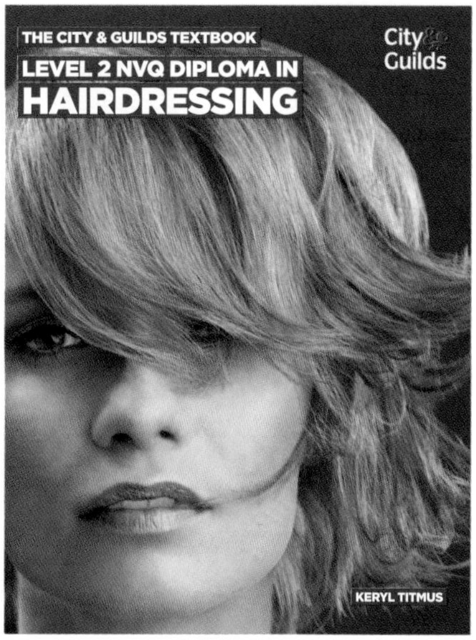

CHOOSING YOUR THEME

In order to create an image, it is important to think about the theme. This will be your starting point, from which your idea can grow. Once you know what you want your theme to be this will help you decide on all the little details that will make up your total look. Use the **sources** mentioned in the previous activity to look for themes and to start getting ideas of what you might like your theme to be.

Sources
Places to go to for information

The following details help to make up a theme:

- the hair colour and style
- the make-up colours used and how they are applied (for example either a more natural-looking make-up or a more dramatic look using darker colours)
- the nail colours used or nail art applied
- the clothes worn and the style and colours used
- the accessories used, for example bags and jewellery, and their colours.

ACTIVITY

To get you started, work on your own, in pairs or in small groups for this activity. Decide on a theme for your hair and beauty image. The following ideas may help you:

- a special occasion – such as a wedding, a party or a prom
- a fantasy look – for example a creative design where you can use your imagination, such as butterflies or fairies
- a historical look – something from the past such as the ancient Egyptians or the 1920s
- a cultured look – for example French
- a futuristic look – such as how you think people will look in the future. Silver might be a good colour for this look.

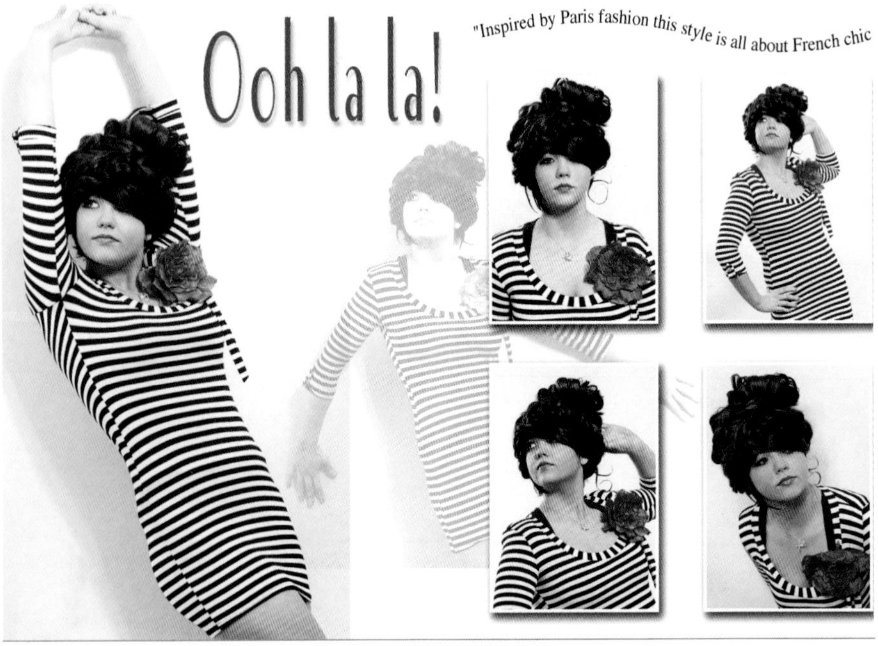
Ooh la la!
"Inspired by Paris fashion this style is all about French chic

Parisian look

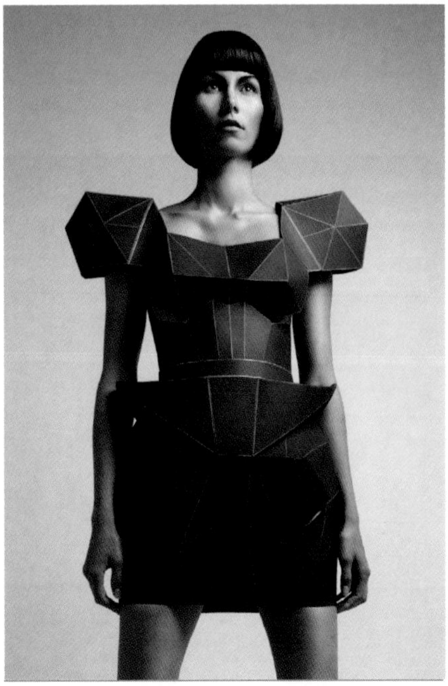

Futuristic look

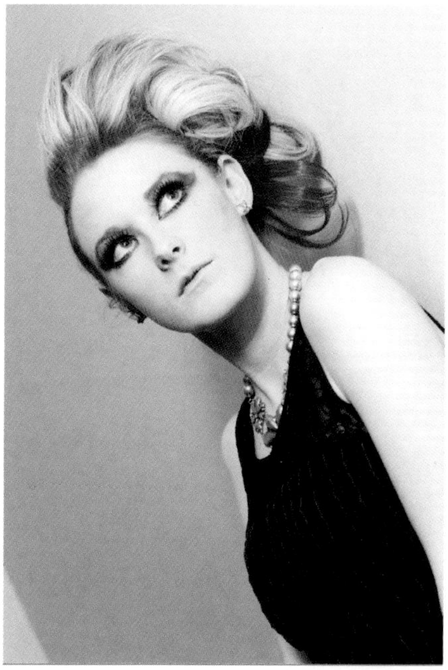

Party look

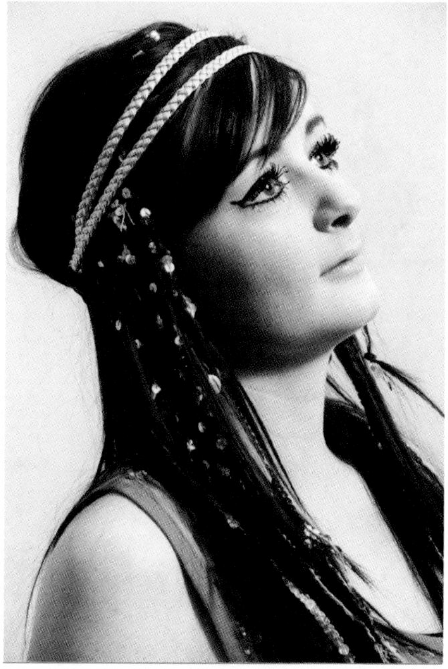

Cleopatra – historical theme

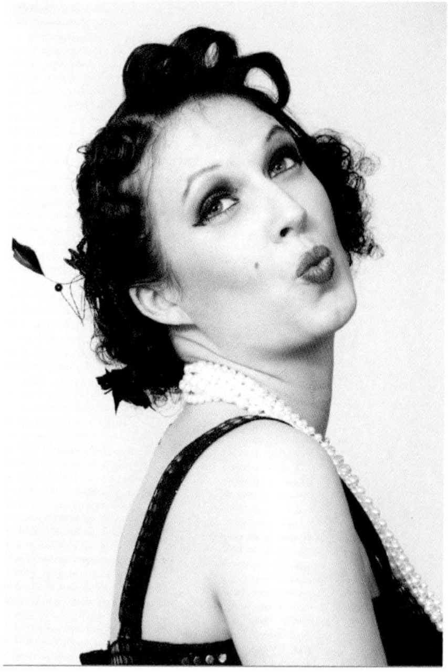

1920s look

PLAN FOR CREATING AN IMAGE

You will now have:

- researched, collected and saved ideas to give you **inspiration** for the final image
- chosen the theme for your image.

Inspiration
Something that gives you ideas

You are now ready to plan for creating the final hair and beauty image. You can do this by putting together a design plan and story board/mood board.

DESIGN PLAN

This will include a breakdown of everything that you will need to create the final image. Examples of what to include in a design plan are:

- a list of all the equipment, products and materials that are needed, for example for the make-up, clothes, hairstyling, accessories, etc
- if you are working in a group, a list of what each person is responsible for, such as: which sources each person is collecting ideas from; which part of the image they are looking for information on (eg hairstyle, make-up look, accessories to be used, etc); who the model is going to be (if a model is to be used to create the image)
- the time that you have to complete this in. This will help to give you a deadline date so that the information can be collected in at a suitable time for the image to be created. Your tutor will help you to set this deadline.

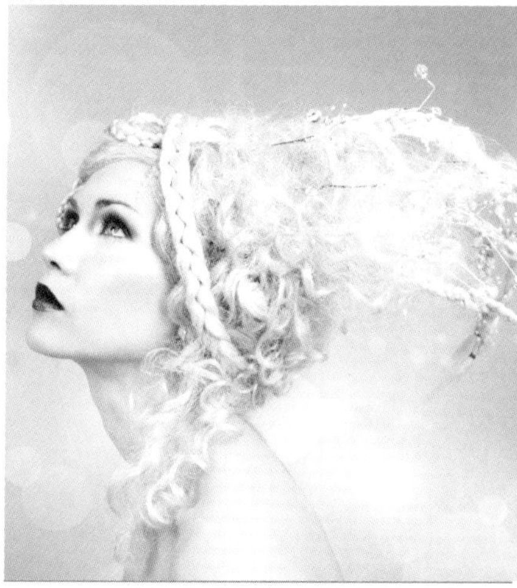

Fantasy look

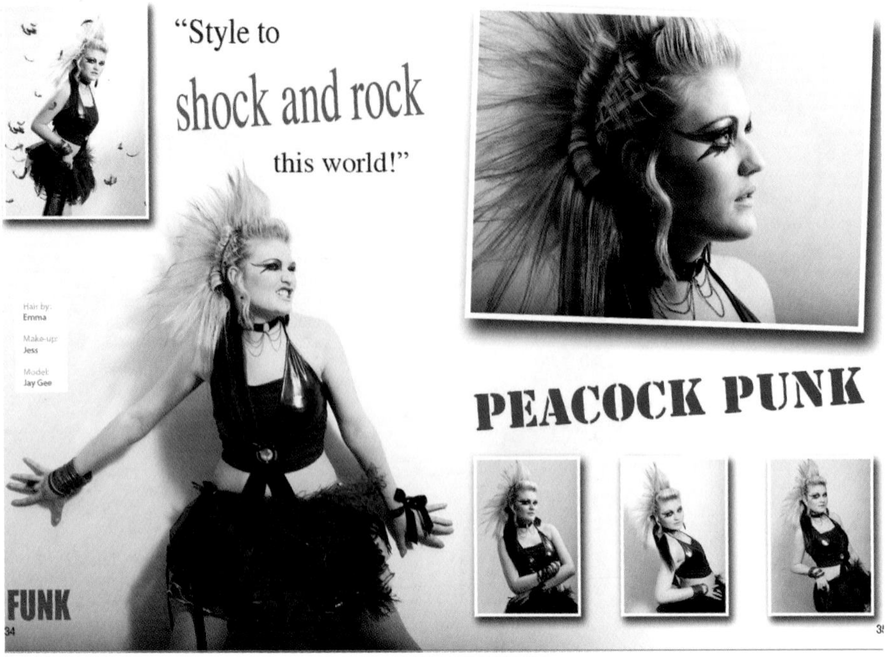

A mood board from Stephensons College, showing a punk theme

ACTIVITY

Look at the above picture showing a punk hair and beauty image. Write down what accessories you think were needed to create this photoshoot image.

STORY BOARD/MOOD BOARD

Collate
Bring together

A mood board is used to **collate** ideas and information from research, and to bring together any materials (such as photos, fabrics, printed images, etc). It could be in the form of a poster or a scrapbook. It can contain anything that has inspired ideas for the image. Mood boards are a good way of bringing all the research ideas together, particularly if you are working in a group.

HANDY HINTS

Go to Chapter 216 The art of photographic make-up and read up on what a mood board is and how to create one.

SmartScreen 112 handout 3

SmartScreen 112 worksheet 1

ACTIVITY

Put together a design plan to include the following:

- what equipment, products and materials are needed to create your chosen hair and beauty image
- a list of what needs to be done/who is responsible/when it has to be done by.

HANDY HINTS

You may find it useful to refer to the following chapters to help you with this:

Chapter 006 Skin care – read up on how to prepare the model's skin

Chapters 106 Basic make-up application and 216 The art of photographic make-up – read up on how to apply make-up

Chapter 103 Styling women's hair – read up on the styling products, tools and equipment needed for different hair techniques

Chapter 107 Themed face painting – read up on face and body painting if this is needed to create your overall theme; make sure that you have all the colours of paints that you will need. Remember that you can mix face paints together to create different colours.

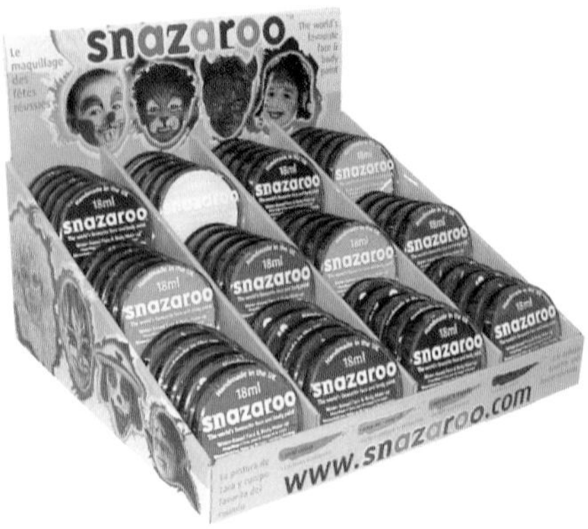

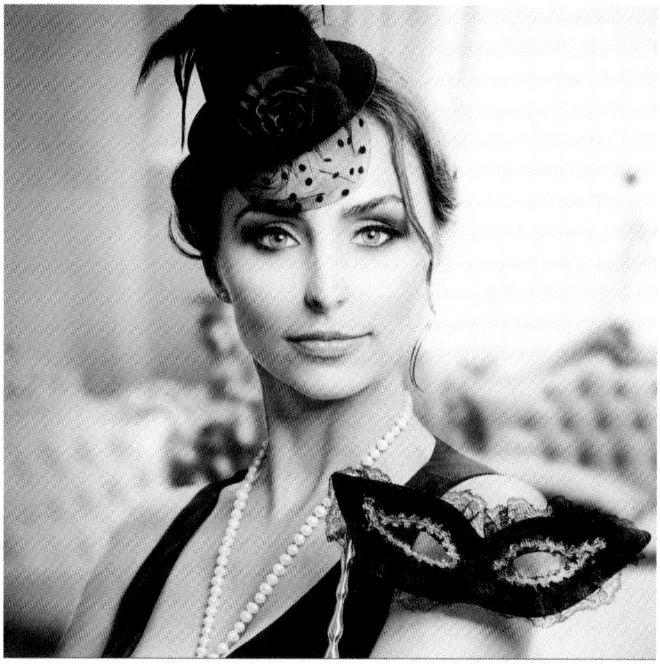

Special occasion

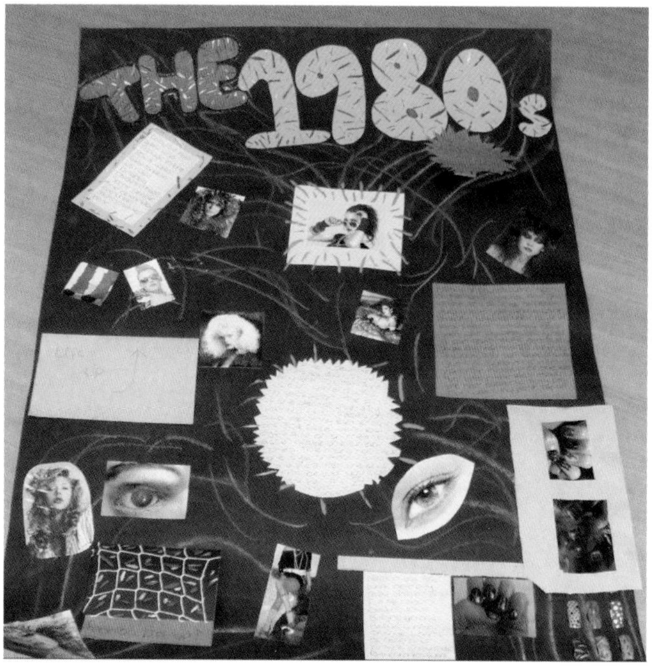

A mood board

ACTIVITY

Plan and prepare a story board/mood board. Include the name of your theme as a heading (eg punk, futuristic, pop star) and include images for the make-up, hairstyles, clothes, accessories and suitable colours.

HANDY HINTS

Include material samples as well as pictures, photographs and brief text on your mood board to bring your ideas to life and to make the theme clear to anyone who looks at it.

HANDY HINTS

Show your story board/mood board to your tutor and/or the rest of the group. This will give you an opportunity to get some feedback on your image plans. If you have more than one idea for an image, why not get the rest of your group to judge which one is the best for you to choose?

HOW TO DEVELOP A PLAN FOR CREATING AN IMAGE

Once you have looked through lots of different sources of information and developed all of these ideas on a mood board, you can then decide on the final image that you would like to create.

HANDY HINTS

It is important that you work safely when creating an image. Examples of safe working practices are:

- using the products, tools and equipment in the correct way and according to manufacturers' instructions
- making sure that suitable PPE is used where necessary, such as wearing protective gloves and putting a gown around the model if a temporary colour is applied (to help create the correct colour for the image)
- taking into account COSHH when using products that come under this legislation, for example correctly using Barbicide when cleaning hair brushes and combs afterwards
- making sure that you are thoroughly prepared and that all of the tools, products and materials are neatly placed in the treatment area when the model is being prepared.

HANDY HINTS

Look at Chapter 113 Following health and safety in the salon to help you with the health and safety laws that you should follow.

CREATE AN IMAGE

Create
To produce from scratch

Once you have decided on the image you want to **create**, you can decide how to present it. Here are some of the ways in which you might present your image:

AS PART OF A SHOW

An example is a hair and beauty show. The theme that you have chosen will form the main basis for the clothes, hair, nails and make-up. By preparing the theme beforehand, you can then follow this theme for the overall look for the show. You will need to work closely with the show organiser (if this is not you) to make sure that you are following the theme for the show correctly.

This is a good way of presenting an image in a more dramatic way and to lots of people.

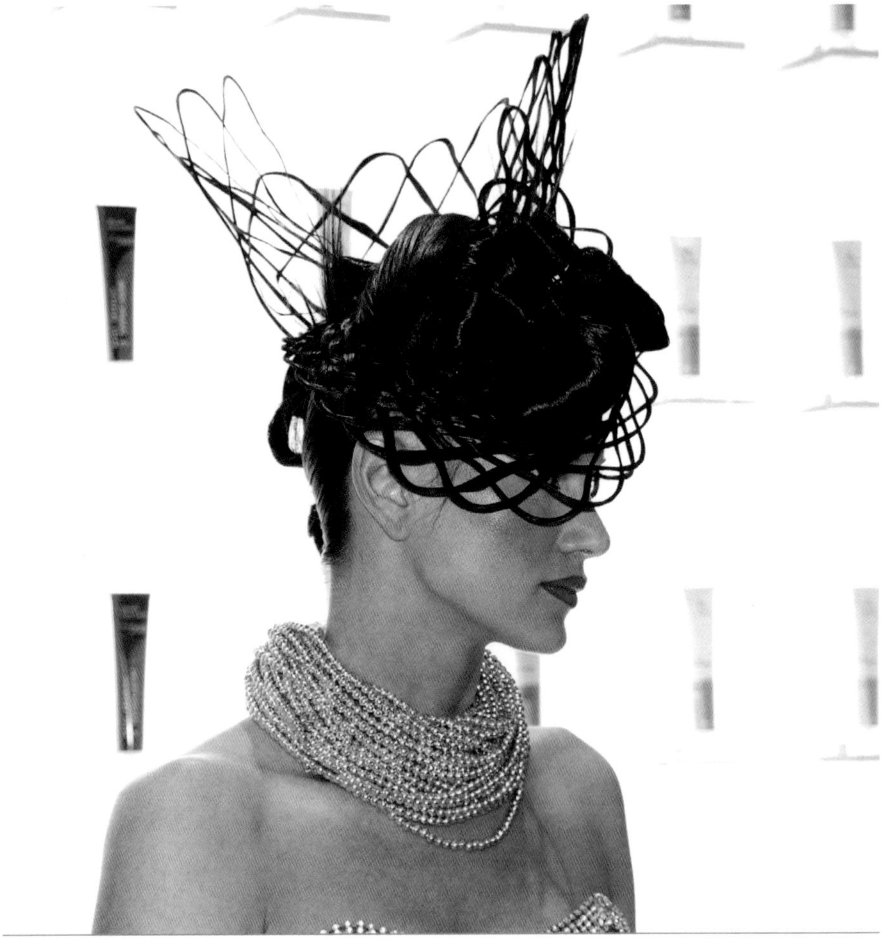

A completed image for a show

HANDY HINTS

It will also be a good idea if the judges give each competitor some feedback on how they scored in the competition. This will then help to develop the skills of the competitors for the future.

IN A COMPETITION

This can be done within your group or across all groups at your college or school. You could even organise a competition and invite other colleges to take part. It may help if you decide on a chosen theme, so that the competition is fair and is the same for all the **competitors**. The purpose of the competition could be to give the students a chance to show off their creative skills.

Competitors
Everyone taking part in a competition

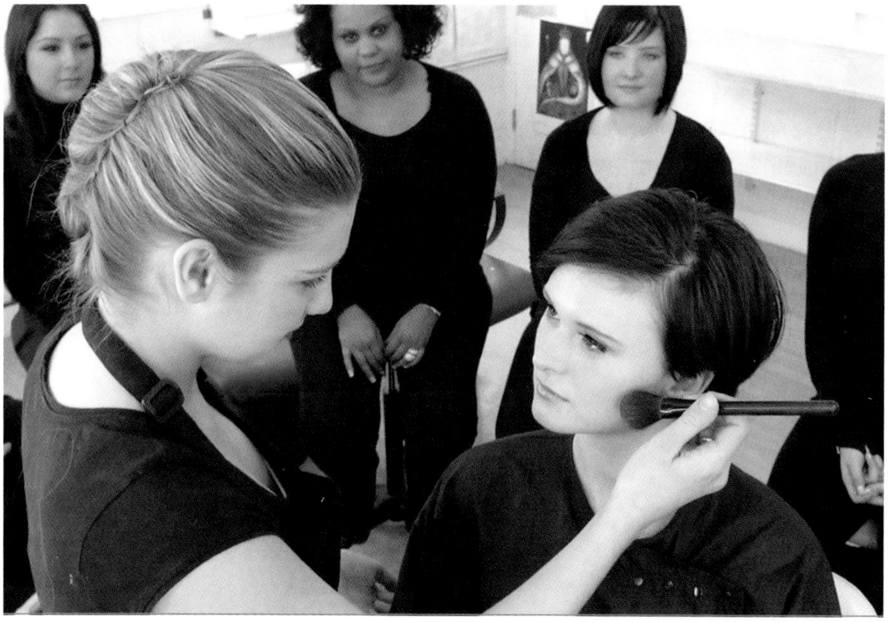

If you have learnt a good way to create your image, show the other students what you've learnt

AS A PRESENTATION

A presentation can be delivered to other students and even clients. The purpose of this may be a team task within the group. The mood board can be used to help to support the final image that is presented.

AS A PHOTOGRAPHIC SHOOT

The image that you create can be presented as a photograph. You will need to take into account the lighting used so that the image is presented in the most effective way. Colours used for make-up may need to be stronger when used for photographic work.

ACTIVITY

Carry out one of the above ways of presenting your hair and beauty image. Try to get feedback from those that you present it to. This will help you know how effective the image was and will also help you develop your skills for the future.

IN A NUTSHELL

You are now at the end of the chapter. Before you test your knowledge with the revision activities, check the following list to see if you feel confident in all the areas covered. If there are still any areas you're unsure of, go back over them in the book and ask your tutor for extra support:

- where to access sources of information
- how to prepare, develop and present an image
- the importance of developing an image
- the safety considerations to take into account.

HANDY HINTS

Go to Chapters 106 Basic make-up application and 216 The art of photographic make-up to read up on how to apply make-up for a photographic shoot.

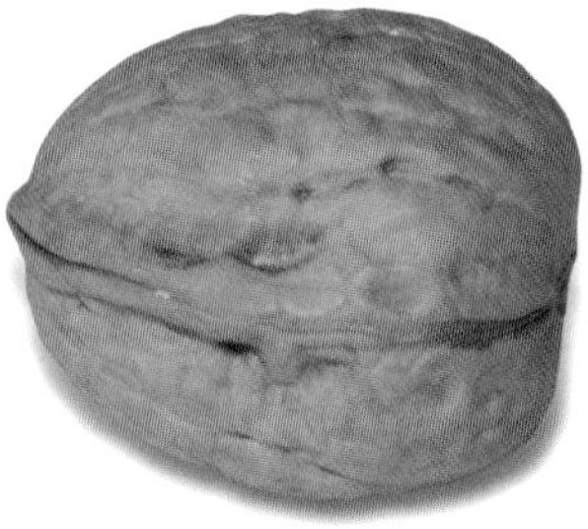

REVISION ACTIVITIES

SmartScreen 112 sample questions

Use the questions below to test your knowledge of Chapter 112 to see just how much information you've gained. This can help you to prepare for your assessments. Turn to pages 483–484 for the answers.

WORDS TO FIND

Copy and complete the sentences below. Use these words to help you fill in the gaps.

image	magazines	make-up	competition
safety	hair	mood board	photoshoot
develop	beauty	design	show
internet	create	plan	presentation

1 You can get ideas for your hair and beauty image from places such as books, films, in ________________, fashion shows, the television and from the ________________ (using search engines such as 'Google').

2 In order to create a ________________ and beauty ________________, it is important to think about what the theme will be.

3 When you have decided on the theme, you will need to be clear about the purpose for the hair and ________________ image.

4 Examples of when a hair and beauty image may be used are for a ________________ (that may be judged), a ________________ for a magazine picture, for a catwalk show or for a mood board.

5 In order to ________________ your overall image, you will also need to take into account the clothing and accessories needed, the make-up colours and the hairstyle.

6 A ________________ is a type of poster that may contain images, text and samples of objects. It is used to ________________ and develop a design idea.

TEST YOUR KNOWLEDGE FURTHER

Now answer these questions:

1 List **three** reasons why a stylist or beauty therapist may need to create an image.

2 When you are deciding on your theme, where can you get information from to help you?

3 What are some of the different ways that you could present the images of your theme?

4 What is a mood board?

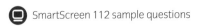

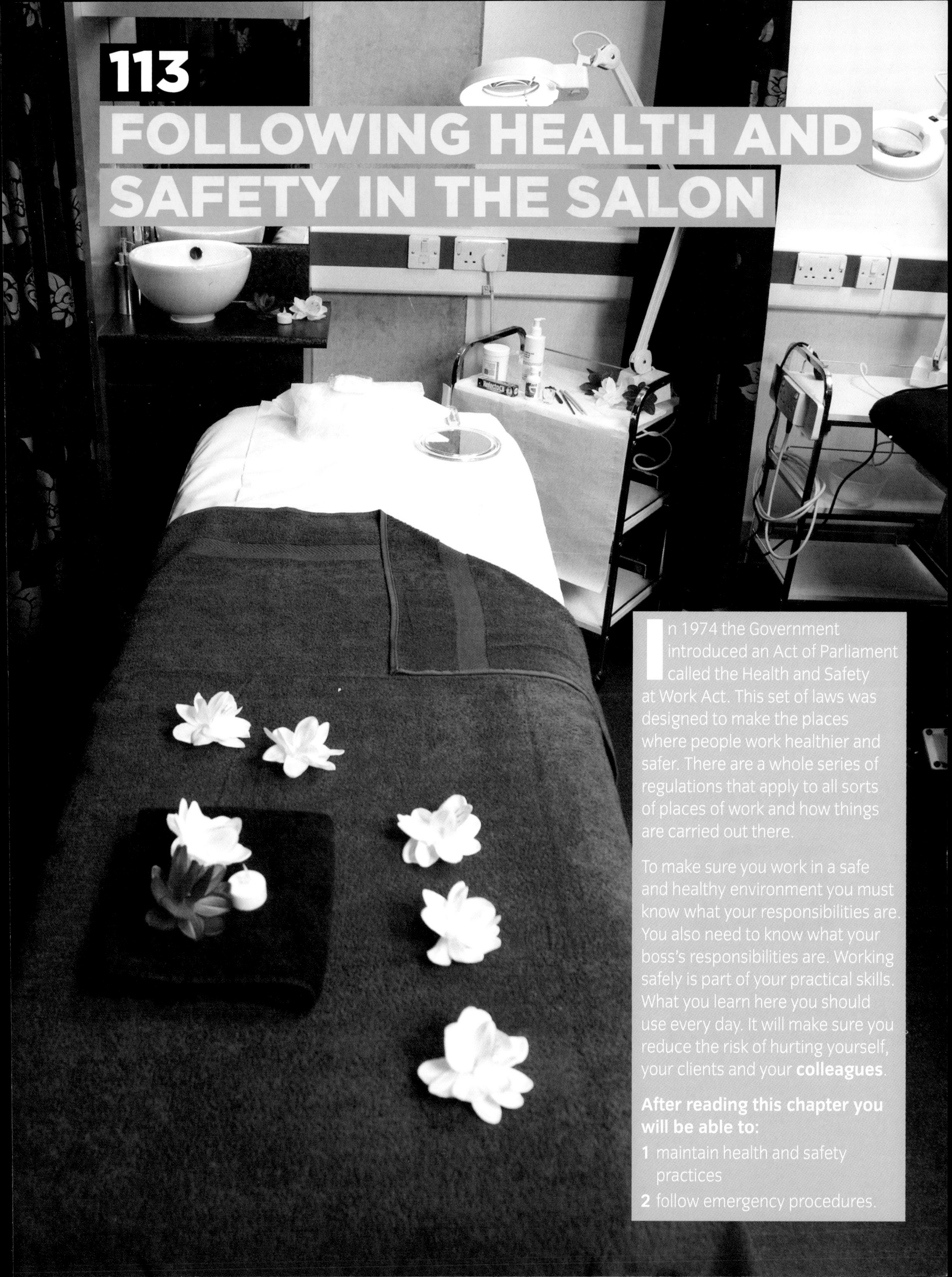

113 FOLLOWING HEALTH AND SAFETY IN THE SALON

In 1974 the Government introduced an Act of Parliament called the Health and Safety at Work Act. This set of laws was designed to make the places where people work healthier and safer. There are a whole series of regulations that apply to all sorts of places of work and how things are carried out there.

To make sure you work in a safe and healthy environment you must know what your responsibilities are. You also need to know what your boss's responsibilities are. Working safely is part of your practical skills. What you learn here you should use every day. It will make sure you reduce the risk of hurting yourself, your clients and your **colleagues**.

After reading this chapter you will be able to:

1 maintain health and safety practices

2 follow emergency procedures.

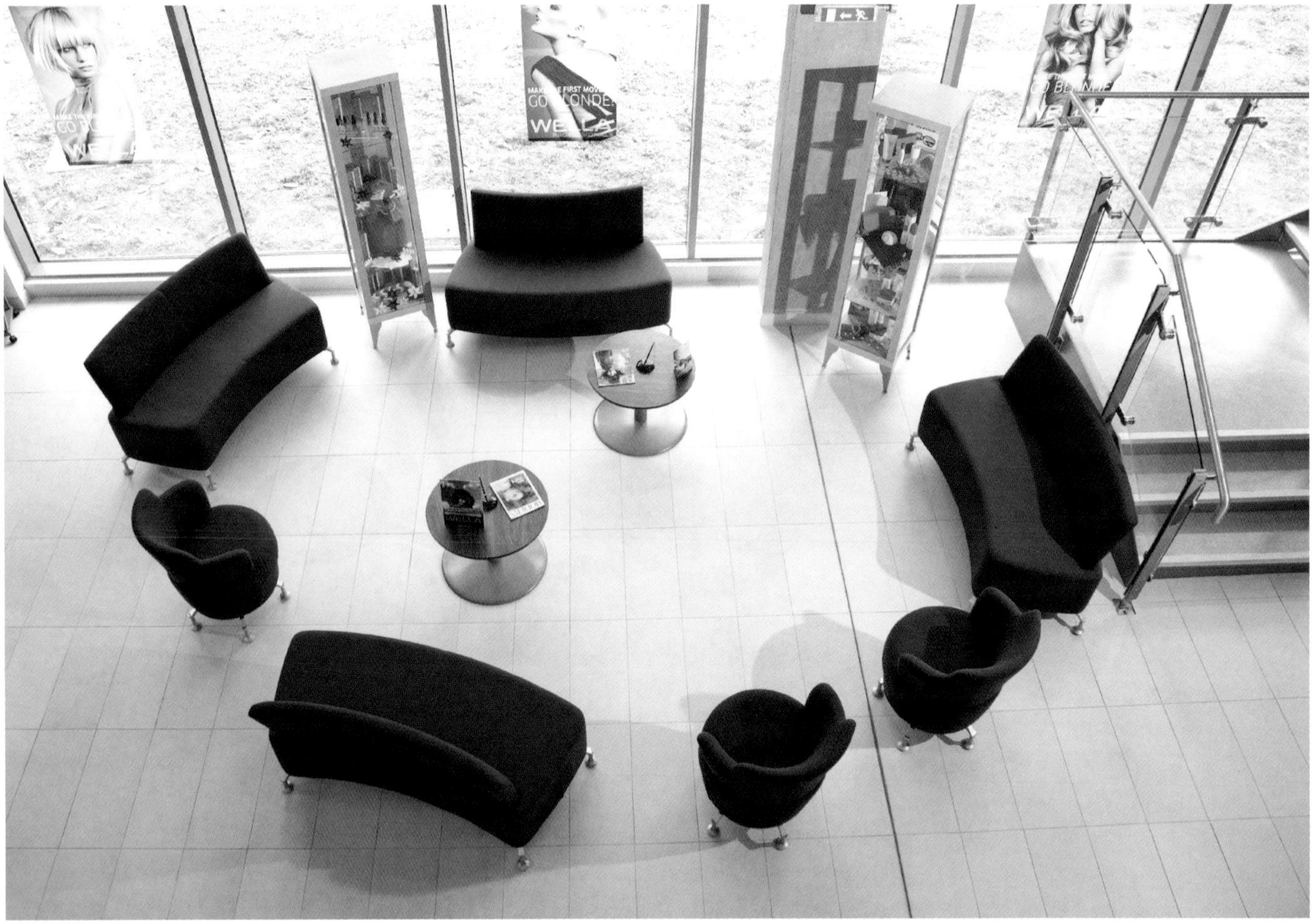

Colleagues
People that you work with

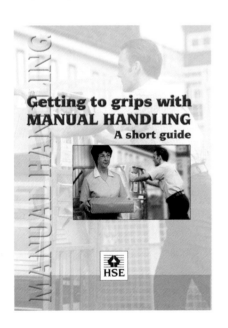

MAINTAIN HEALTH AND SAFETY PRACTICES

In this part of the chapter you will learn about the main provisions of the Health and Safety at Work Act. You will learn the difference between the terms 'hazard' and 'risk'. You will also learn about the employers' responsibilities for the safety of employees and customers in the salon, and details of safe and hygienic working practices.

RESPONSIBILITIES

The Health and Safety at Work Act says that the employer (the boss) must make sure that the workplace is healthy and safe – for the employees, the clients and anyone else who visits the workplace. Health and safety law is enforced by the Health and Safety Executive.

The Act also says that the employees (you) must make sure that they work safely and properly. You must not do anything that is likely to harm yourself or anyone else in the workplace. You must make sure you check for and report anything that might be a risk.

HANDY HINTS

An EMPLOYER has a duty to ensure the health and safety of the employees and any other person who visits the workplace.

HANDY HINTS

An EMPLOYEE has a duty not to do anything that could cause harm to themselves or others while they are at work.

HAZARDS AND RISKS

When we look at things that might cause us harm two words are used to describe them – **hazard** and **risk**.

Hazard
Something that may cause harm

Risk
How likely it is that harm will happen

HAZARD

A hazard can be anything that could be harmful to someone. It could be something quite minor that may just result in a small cut. It could be something serious that could cause a broken arm or leg, or even result in death.

One of your responsibilities is to check for possible hazards while you are at work. For example, a wet floor could cause someone to slip over. It should be reported immediately and dealt with quickly.

There are three types of hazard:

- those to do with the workplace, eg trailing electrical cables and hair clippings on the floor
- those to do with equipment and materials, eg faulty hair dryers and mishandling chemicals
- those to do with people, eg bad posture when applying make-up and lifting objects incorrectly.

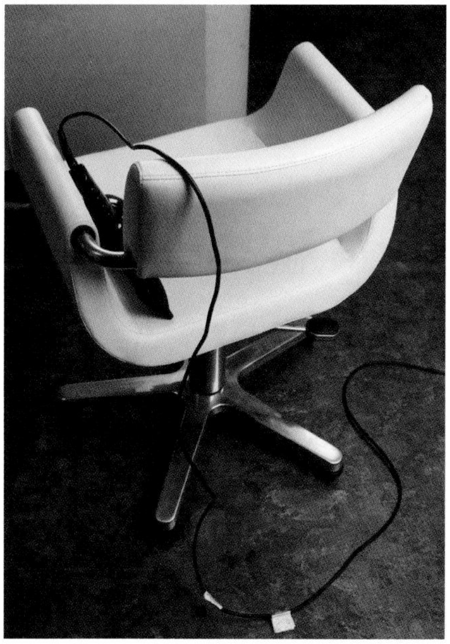

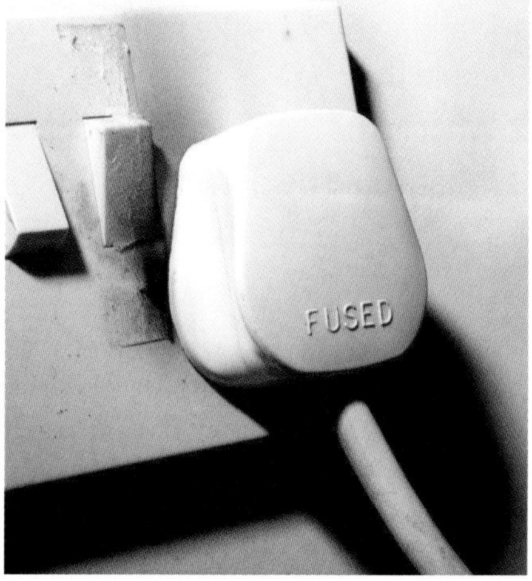

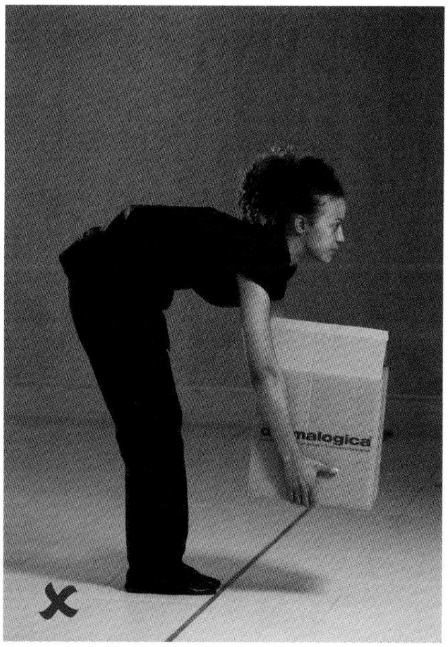

ACTIVITY

Make a list of two more things that could be hazards under each of the three bullet points above.

RISK

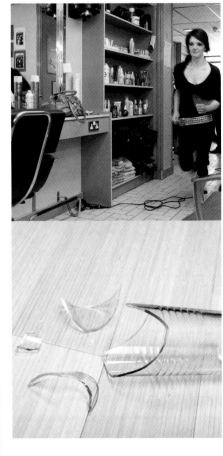

A risk is the chance of someone being injured or affected by the hazard. For example, the risk of someone slipping on the wet floor hazard will depend on where the wet floor is. If it is where lots of people walk then the risk is great. If it is in a corner where hardly anyone walks the risk is very small.

ACTIVITY

In pairs, look round the salon and identify things that could be a hazard. Make a list. Decide how much harm the hazard could cause, eg low, medium or high. Then think about the risk. How likely is it to happen, eg likely, moderately likely or very likely? Compare your hazards and risks with those of other pairs. Did you all agree?

Hairdressing and beauty salons have many possible hazards and lots of risk. The Health and Safety at Work Act requires the boss to identify these hazards and risks. Once they have been identified, the boss has to look at ways they can be reduced. This process is called *risk assessment*.

RISK ASSESSMENT

A risk assessment should be carried out for the salon itself and for each of the services that are carried out. For example, one risk assessment will be done for the reception area and another for a shampoo and blow drying service or a manicure.

How is a risk assessment carried out?

1 Identify the possible hazards – what are they and how harmful could they be?
2 What is the risk – very low, could happen, very likely to happen?
3 What could be done to:
   - take away the hazard – can the procedure be changed so the hazard is removed?
   - reduce the risk – if the hazard can't be removed, what can be done to reduce the chances of it happening?
   - manage the risk – if the hazard can't be removed or the risk reduced how can we manage the risk?

ACTIVITY

Using the list of hazards you identified earlier, look at some of them and discuss with your group how you could:

- take away the hazard completely, or
- reduce the risk by changing something.

Add this information to your original list. This should now contain a list of hazards, the risks and how the hazard and risk can be removed, reduced or controlled.

Well done! You have completed a simple risk assessment.

EMPLOYER'S RESPONSIBILITY

As well as risk assessment, the Health and Safety at Work Act requires your boss to do much more to protect you and others while you are at work.

Employer's responsibility	What does it cover in the salon?	Which set of regulations does it come under?
A safe workplace	A reasonable working temperature (the salon should not be too hot or too cold to work in) Good **ventilation** (windows/air conditioning or extractor fans) Suitable lighting Washing facilities Toilets First aid	Workplace Health, Safety and Welfare Regulations
To provide personal protective equipment	Protective clothing, eg aprons, gloves	Personal Protective Equipment at Work Regulations (PPE)
Safe methods of handling, storing and identification of potentially hazardous substances	The chemicals that are used in the salon	Control of Substances Hazardous to Health Regulations (COSHH)
Safe tools and equipment	All the tools and equipment used in the salon All the electrical equipment	Provision and Use of Work Equipment Regulations Electricity at Work Regulations
Reporting of accidents and the accident register	Reporting serious accidents or incidents Recording all accidents that happen in the salon	Reporting of Injuries, Diseases and Dangerous Occurences Regulations (RIDDOR) Workplace Health, Safety and Welfare Regulations
Provide proper training	Train staff to carry out services to the appropriate standard How to check for hazards How to deal with hazards What to do in an emergency To keep staff up to date in health and safety	Health and Safety at Work Act
Have a health and safety policy	This will contain details of how the salon fulfils its duty of health and safety It will give details of rules and procedures for things like dealing with a fire or other emergency	Health and Safety at Work Act

Ventilation

Provision of fresh air in place of air that has been used

EMPLOYEE'S RESPONSIBILITIES

Properly
In the correct way

Hygienic
Healthy and clean

Your responsibilities when you are at work are:

- Carry out your work properly. Always pay attention to what you are doing. Always use the step-by-step instructions that the salon has.
- Always use the equipment provided **properly**. Make sure you follow the salon procedures.
- Report any hazards that you find to the proper person.
- Make sure your activities do not put others at risk.
- Work with your colleagues and your boss on health and safety matters.

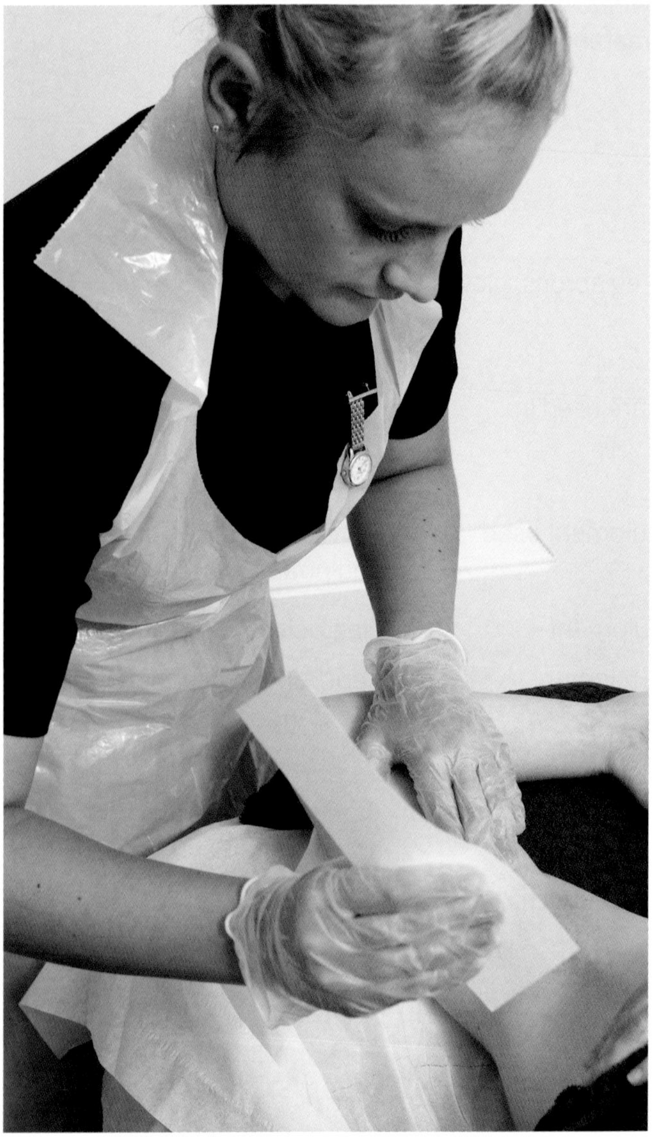

WORKING SAFELY

In everything you do you must follow safe and **hygienic** working practices. For each of the skills you learn you must know how to do them safely and hygienically. Paying attention to this will protect you, your client, your colleagues and the salon.

In each of the chapters that cover a practical skill there will be a section on following safe and hygienic working practices. This will involve:

- personal protective equipment (PPE)
- safe use of chemicals (COSHH)
- methods of sterilising tools
- other health and safety regulations.

These are the important bits for you to do so that you work safely and hygienically:

- Make sure you carry out the task properly; don't cut corners. Pay attention to what you are doing. Think about those parts of the job that might cause harm to you or the client if you do not do them properly.
- Get all the personal protective equipment (PPE) you will need for the job ready before you start the task. You may need a gown and towels for the client if you are doing the client's hair.

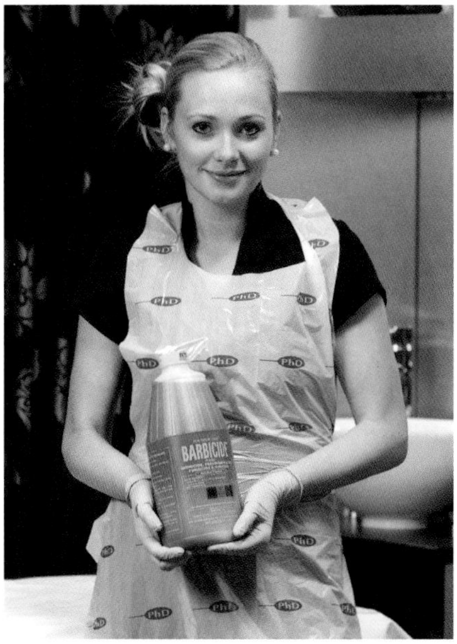

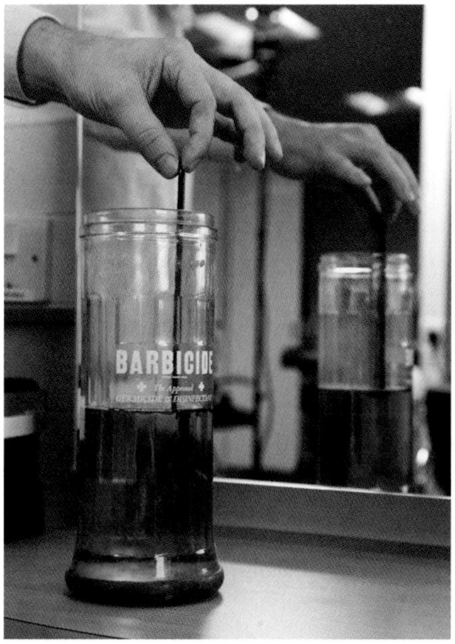

- Learn about the chemicals you will be using for each service and how to handle and use them properly. You need to know how the chemicals should be stored and how they should be disposed of. You should also know what to do if something goes wrong.
- When you prepare the tools and equipment you will need for the service, make sure everything is clean and sterilised. When you have finished the service, remember to clean and sterilise everything. This reduces the risk of cross-infection. The tools and equipment are then safe and ready to use on another client.
- If you are using tools such as dryers or other electrical equipment, make sure you check them before using them. Look for damage to the plug or the cable and cracks or damage to the casing. If there are any, do not use the equipment. Report it straight away. For non-electrical equipment make sure it is not damaged in any way and can be used safely. If not, report it.
- Always check your workstation and the area around for potential hazards. For example, hair on the floor, wet patches. These might cause someone to slip. Take action to deal with them.

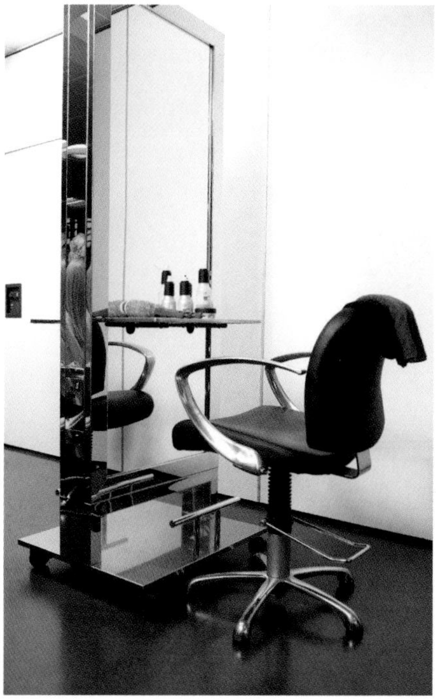

ACTIVITY

Each time you have to carry out a service use the chart on page 49 to check which sets of regulations might be important.

METHODS OF STERILISATION AND DISINFECTION

When you carry out a service or treatment, using clean and sterilised tools and equipment and working in a clean area are essential. Using clean and sterilised tools and equipment will **prevent** the transfer of infection from one person to another. Clean work areas and clean tools will give a better impression to the client.

The work area should be cleaned using normal cleaning materials. Surface cleaner for work areas and glass cleaner for mirrors are examples.

Anything that comes into contact with the client should be cleaned and sterilised before it is used.

There are three principal sterilising methods that are used in the salon using heat, radiation or chemicals.

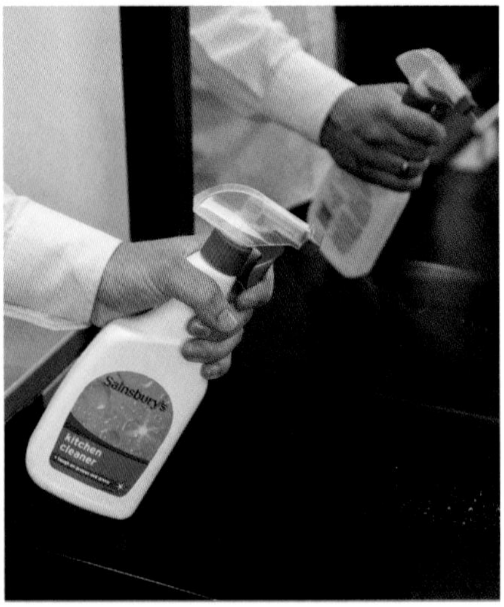

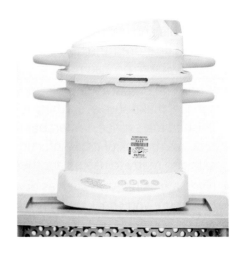

You should always clean work areas with surface cleanser

Prevent

Stop something from taking place

AUTOCLAVE

This works like a pressure cooker and sterilises by using heat. The object is placed inside the autoclave and left in for around ten minutes. Always follow the manufacturer's instructions.

Autoclaves are used for metal and glass tools, for example scissors, and metal cuticle nippers used in beauty therapy. They should not be used for plastic items as they may melt them.

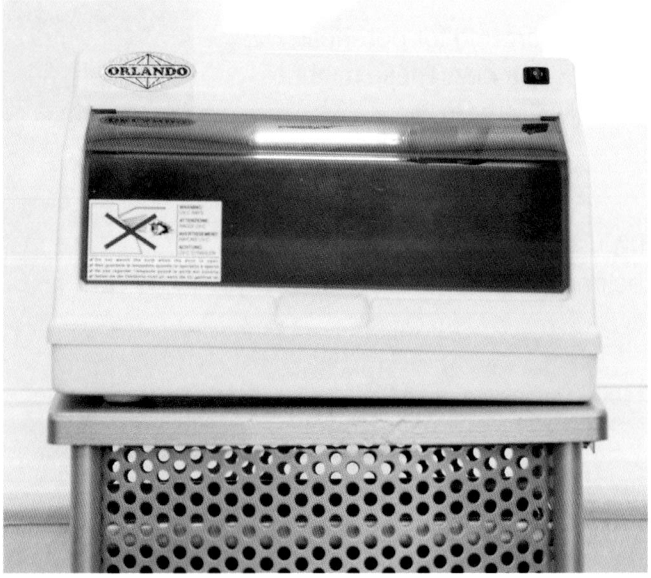

ULTRAVIOLET (UV) CABINET

This **sanitises** by ultraviolet radiation. The object is cleaned and dried and then placed inside the cabinet, where it is exposed to ultraviolet rays. Dirt and grease must be removed first so the radiation can penetrate.

UV cabinets are used for metal, glass and plastic items, eg manicure and pedicure tools. The items should be turned during sanitisation. Always follow the manufacturer's instructions.

Sanitise

Cleansing or washing to stop bacteria growing

CHEMICAL DISINFECTANT

This is a chemical liquid that destroys bacteria. The used object is placed in the chemical in a jar. This will restrict the growth of germs on the surface of the object. Like the UV cabinet, the object must be cleaned and dried before being put in the chemical. The objects should be rinsed when they are taken out of the jar and dried before use. Remember to use PPE when using this method, to protect your hands.

Chemical immersion can be used for metal, glass and plastic, eg scissors, combs and tweezers. Tools should be left in the solution for a short while. Always read the instructions for the solution being used.

Most salons will use this method of disinfecting. It is convenient, simple and efficient. It is often called **Barbicide**, which is the brand name for the solution used.

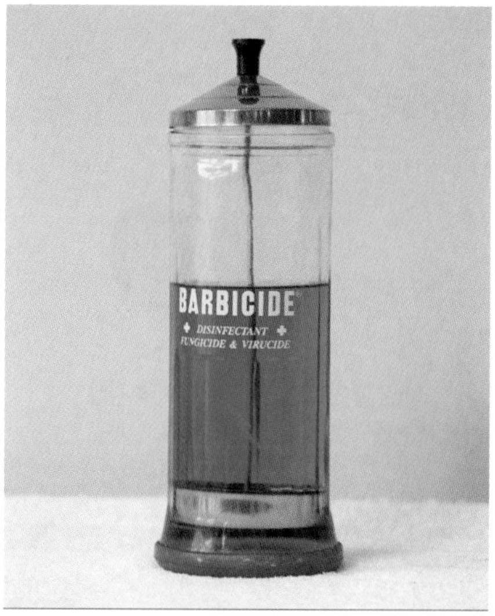

A Barbicide jar with tools

Barbicide
A liquid disinfectant

HEALTH AND SAFETY AT WORK REGULATIONS

There are a number of sets of regulations that are part of the Health and Safety at Work Act. At this level you need to know about four of them. As you make progress in your career you will need to learn more about health and safety at work. Your level of responsibility will grow as you progress.

PERSONAL PROTECTIVE EQUIPMENT AT WORK (PPE) REGULATIONS

These are often referred to as PPE. The regulations require your boss to provide protective equipment to protect you while you work.

Who?	What?	When?	Why?
Staff	Non-latex gloves 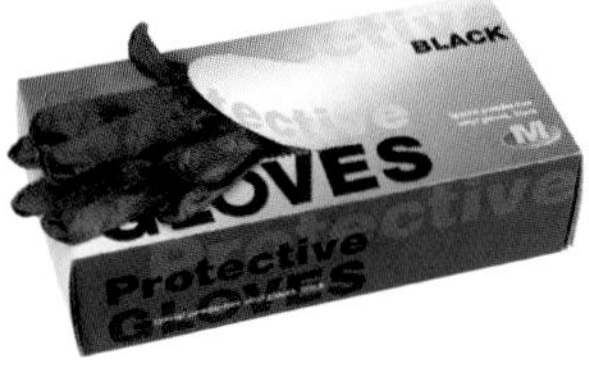	Worn every time colouring, perming or other chemicals are being used or during a Level 2 beauty treatment such as waxing	To protect the hands from damage caused by the chemicals; to help prevent contact dermatitis
	Aprons 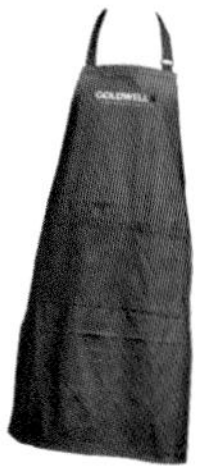	Worn when using chemicals or products such as waxing	To protect the stylist's/therapist's/nail technician's clothes or uniform

PROTECTIVE EQUIPMENT FOR CLIENTS

Who?	What?	When?	Why?
Clients	Gowns 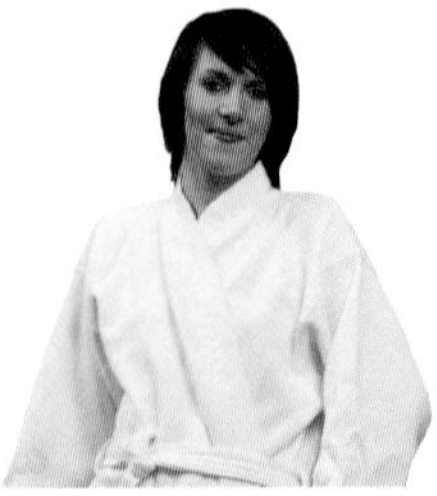	Worn when the client is having a hair or beauty service	To protect the client's clothes from possible damage*
	Towels 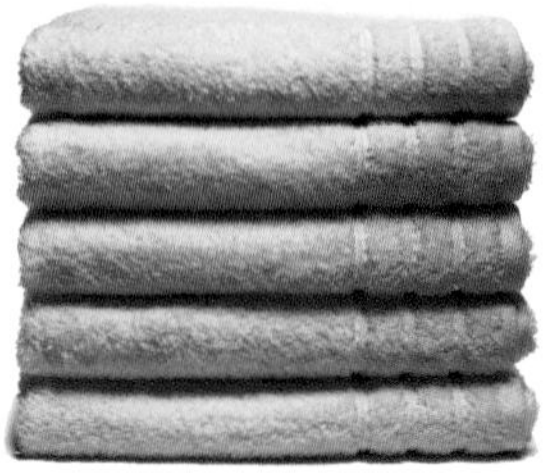	Used when the client is having shampoo services or any service where liquids are used	To prevent the client from getting wet or from the effect of liquids getting on to the client's face or clothes
	Capes 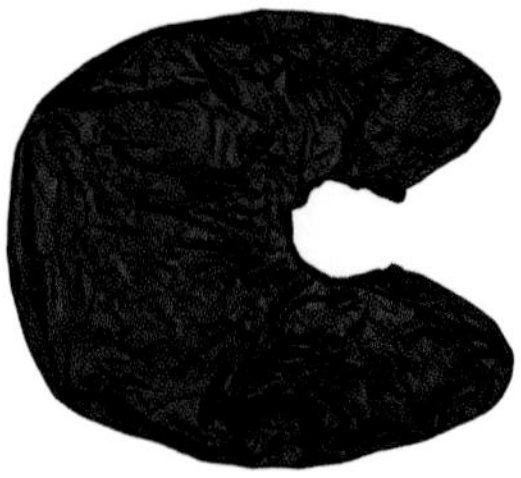	Worn when chemicals such as colour or perm solutions are being used	To stop chemicals from damaging the client's clothes
	Headband 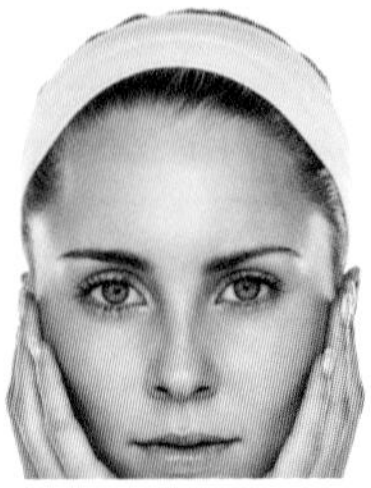	Used when the client is having a facial treatment	To keep the client's hair off the face and protect the hair from the facial or make-up products
	Nail enhancement mask 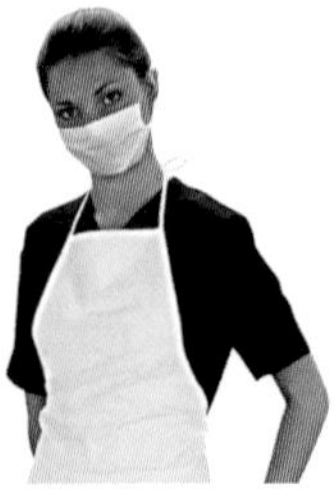	Could be used when completing nail enhancement services	To protect the nail technician from chemical fumes and dust

HANDY HINTS

You must wear the PPE provided whenever the service needs it. This is especially important to protect your hands. Your hands earn you money!

*We have a legal responsibility to look after the clients' property while they are in the salon. If we damage their clothing or belongings the salon can be sued for damages.

CONTROL OF SUBSTANCES HAZARDOUS TO HEALTH REGULATIONS

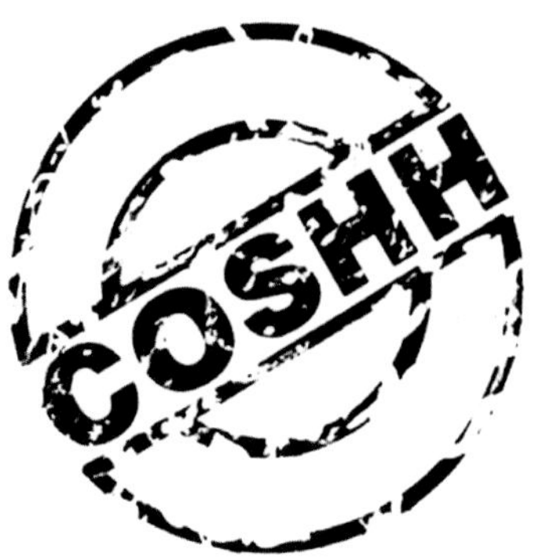

These are often referred to as COSHH. These regulations cover the use of chemicals in the salon that could be harmful to staff and clients. The employer must provide information about all the harmful chemicals that are used.

Always follow SHUD when handling chemicals. They must be:

- **S**tored properly so they are not likely to cause harm
- **H**andled correctly, to prevent harm
- **U**sed properly by following the correct procedure
- **D**isposed of safely to prevent pollution by complying with local bye-laws, the salon policy and the manufacturer's instructions.

ACTIVITY

Choose four products and find out how they should be stored, what precautions should be taken when they are used, and how they should be disposed of safely.

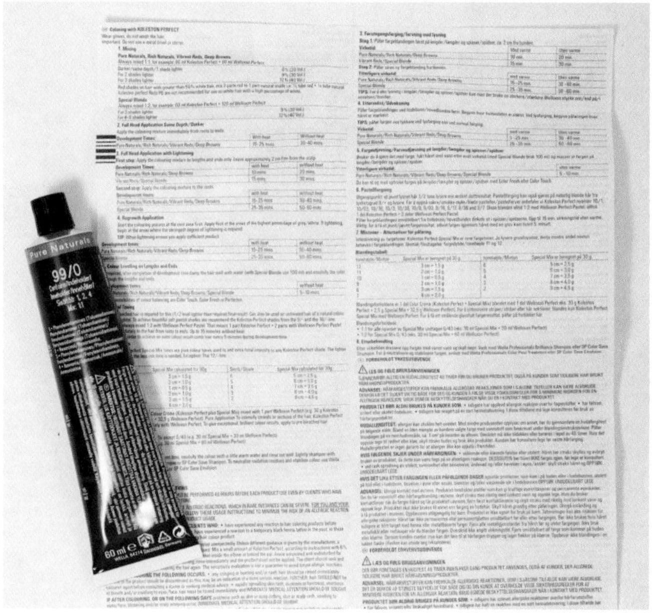

The manufacturer's instructions will give information on how products should be used, stored and disposed of. They also tell you what **precautions** are needed to protect yourself and the client. There will also be information on how to dispose of the product. The salon must follow what the local **bye-laws** say about waste disposal. The salon policy will say where the products should be stored and mixed and where they should be disposed of in the salon.

Precautions
Action taken to prevent danger or damage

Bye-law
Local laws that differ from place to place

Make sure you follow the proper procedures when using products that could be harmful to you or the client.

ACTIVITY

Research more information on COSHH from the HSE website www.hse.gov.uk.

MANUAL HANDLING OPERATIONS REGULATIONS

This set of regulations covers the lifting of objects at work. You may be required to move equipment and stock in the salon. The employer must make sure you are instructed on how to lift objects.

Your responsibility is to only lift things that you feel you can lift. If you do not think you can lift it then you must ask for help.

If you do lift things then you must:

- bend your knees and keep your back straight
- lift with your knees not your back
- keep the object close to your body.

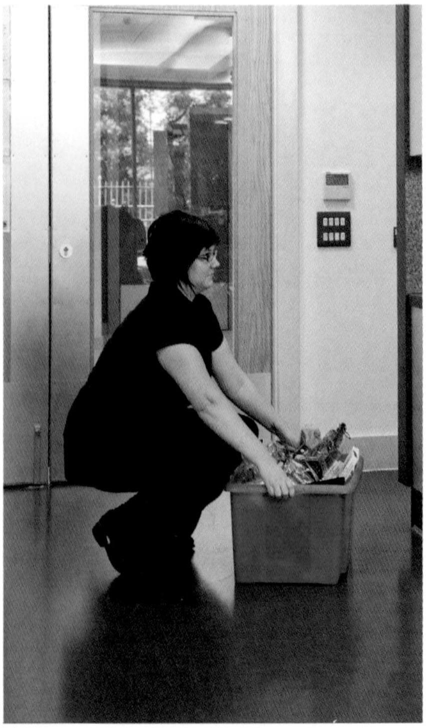

Bend your knees

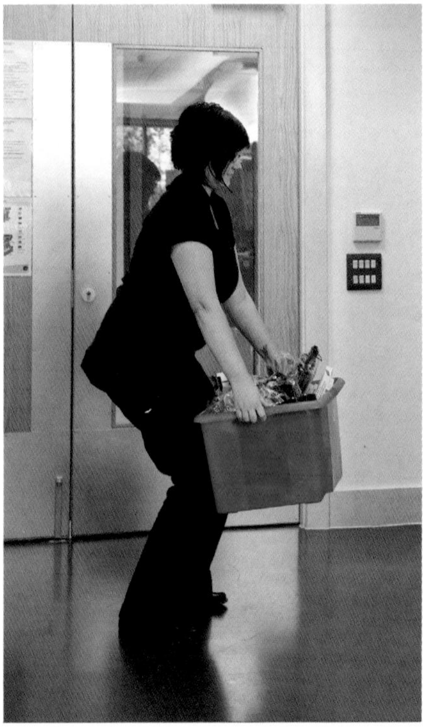

Keep your back straight

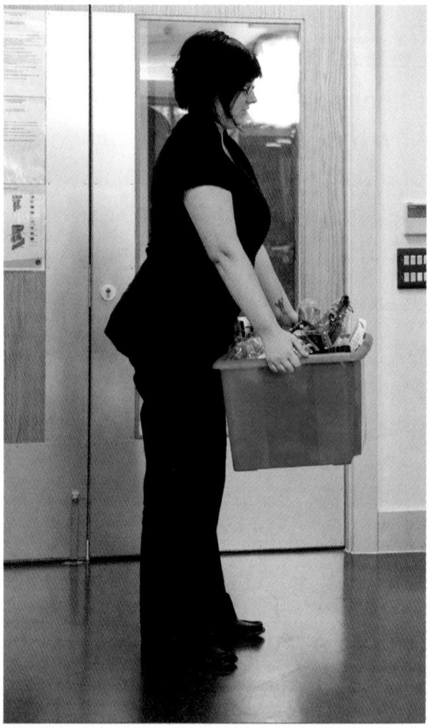

Lift the weight with your legs

ACTIVITY

With a partner, practise lifting objects correctly.

ELECTRICITY AT WORK REGULATIONS

These regulations cover the use of electrical equipment. Hairdressers and therapists use a number of different electrical tools; many are portable. These regulations are designed to prevent injury or possible death from misuse or faulty equipment.

- Always pay attention when using electrical **appliances**.
- Appliances should be checked for faults before use (damaged plugs or cables, damage to the casing for example).
- Faulty equipment must be reported to the relevant person. It should be labelled and, if possible, removed to prevent others from using it.
- Appliances should be switched off after use and properly stored.

Appliances
Pieces of equipment used for specific purposes

The employer is responsible for making sure that all electrical appliances used in the salon are tested regularly. The test is called the portable appliance test or PAT test. This must be done by a qualified PAT tester or electrician at least once a year. A record must be kept of the tests.

Your responsibilities are:

- not to use an appliance that you are not trained to use
- to check an appliance before use
- to know who to report faulty appliances to, and report any that are faulty
- to always use the appliance correctly.

ACTIVITY

Find out your salon's procedure for reporting faulty equipment.

FOLLOW EMERGENCY PROCEDURES

In this part of the chapter you will learn the procedures for dealing with accidents and emergences.

EMERGENCY SITUATIONS

No matter how careful we are when we are at work, accidents and emergencies will happen. These situations include:

- accidents such as slipping, tripping and falling
- a client or colleague being taken ill
- a fire breaking out
- a bomb alert
- a flood.

The salon should have procedures in place to cover such events. You and your colleagues will be trained in what to do in such emergencies.

The Health and Safety at Work Act requires the employer to:

- provide first-aid equipment
- appoint someone to be responsible for dealing with first-aid situations
- provide fire-fighting equipment, such as fire extinguishers
- provide fire exits so that people can escape safely when they need to
- provide assembly points. These are safe places where people go to if the salon needs to be evacuated
- provide a proper procedure that should be followed so that staff know what to do.
- ensure that regular practises of the procedures are held to make sure they work.

ACTIVITY

With your group organise a fire drill. When the drill has been completed, discuss how well it went, and identify anything that needs improvement.

LEVELS OF RESPONSIBILITY

In any emergency situations all the staff will have things to do. They may be responsible for organising the evacuation; they may just be required to do things when asked by someone else. The more senior the member of staff, the more responsibility they will have.

If you do things that you are not supposed to you could make the situation worse. You could cause further injury to someone who has fallen or been taken ill. You could hurt yourself or others in an evacuation.

HANDY HINTS

The first rule for everyone is do not do anything that you have not been told to do, or anything you have not been trained to do.

At this level your first action in any emergency is to tell the person in charge – the boss or the salon manager, or the person responsible. As you become more senior and more qualified, you will take on more responsibility when emergencies occur.

The second rule in an emergency is DO NOT PANIC. Always keep calm and follow the procedure as you have been trained to do. Doing things you are not supposed to do could make the situation much worse.

EMERGENCY PROCEDURES

In all emergency situations, acting quickly, professionally and calmly is essential.

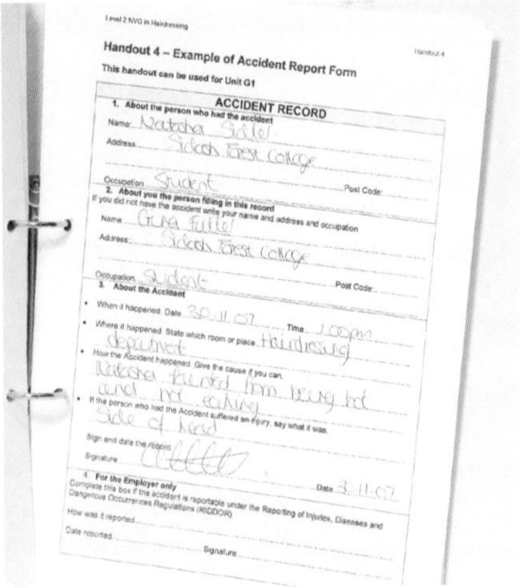

ACCIDENTS OR SOMEONE TAKEN ILL

- Quickly and quietly tell the person responsible for first aid (the first-aider).
- Do not move the person. This may cause further injury.
- Be available to do anything you are asked to do. This might include fetching the first-aid box, looking after other clients, directing ambulance staff.
- The first-aider will determine whether an ambulance is required, or what other action is required.
- Details should be entered into the accident record book. (If it is a serious accident it may have to be reported under the RIDDOR regulations.)

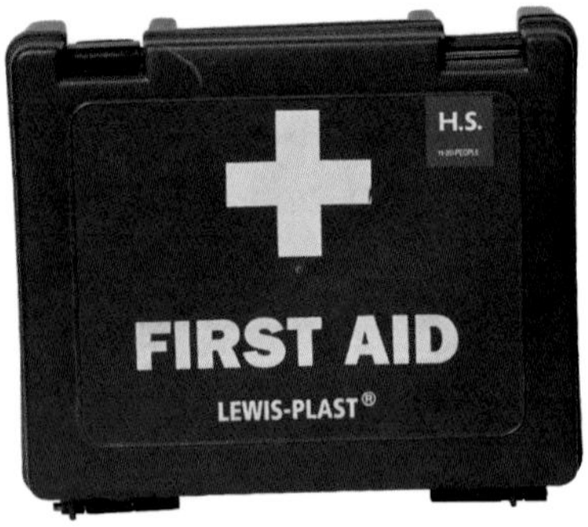

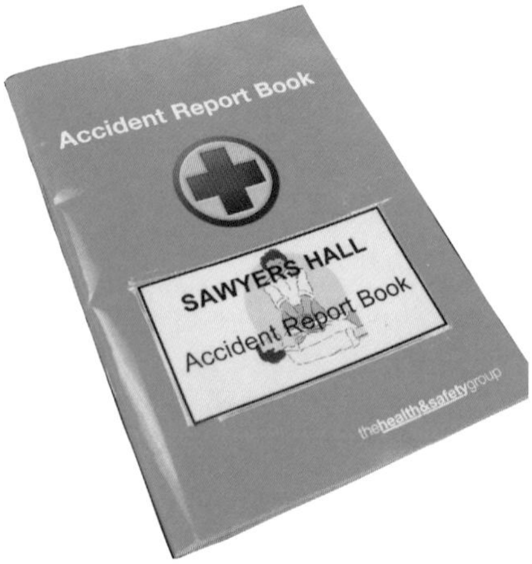

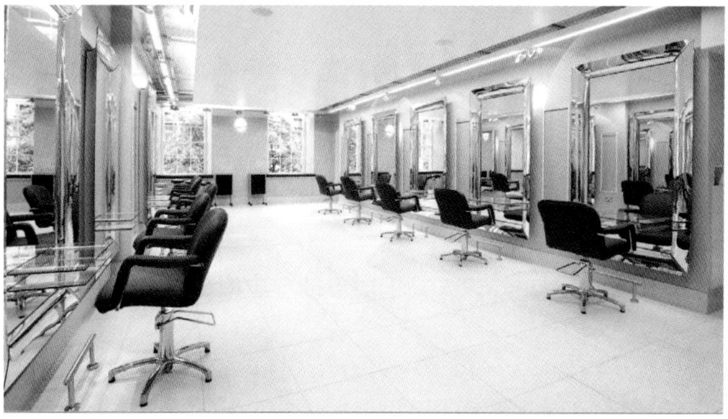

Keep aisles free of objects in case of an emergency

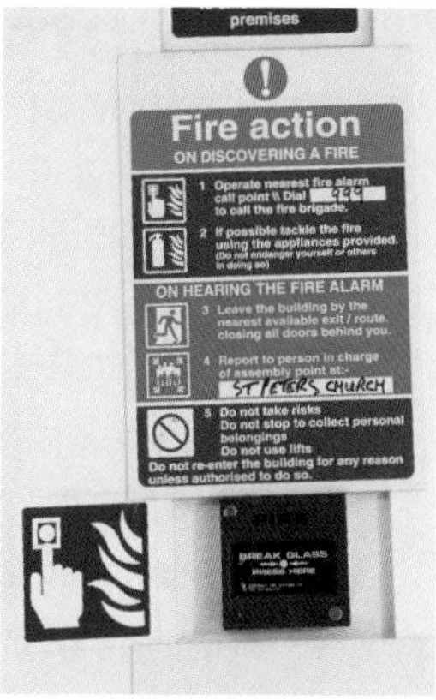

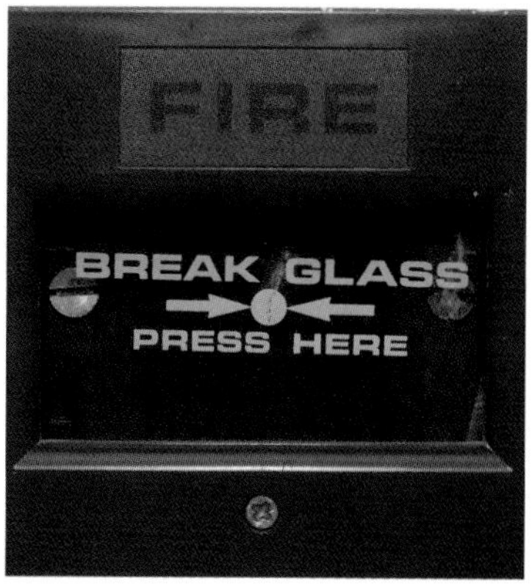

EMERGENCY REQUIRING EVACUATION

In the event of a fire, a flood or a bomb alert the most important thing is saving lives. Getting clients and staff out of the salon is the first priority. The salon, its equipment and people's belongings can be replaced; lives can't.

THINGS YOU MUST KNOW IN EMERGENCY SITUATIONS

- what the accident and emergency procedures are for your salon
- your role and responsibilities
- who is responsible for first aid and evacuation
- where the emergency exits are
- where the first-aid box and accident book are kept
- where the fire extinguishers are.

ACTIVITY

- Find a copy of the accident and emergency procedures for your salon.
- Find out and make a list of your role and your responsibilities in an emergency.
- Make a list of who you should report to in case of accidents and evacuation. You could include who you should report hazards and other health and safety issues to.
- Find out and write down where the first-aid box and the accident book are kept.
- Find out and write down where the emergency exits and the assembly points are.
- Find out and write down where the fire extinguishers are.

This information will be useful for your assignment.

ACTIVITY

You can work with others in your group for this activity.

Find out more about the following:

- what colour the first-aid box should be so you can recognise it
- what colour the fire extinguishers are.

Find out about the different types of fire extinguishers and what they are used for. Find out what sort you have in the salon. Why do we have those sorts?

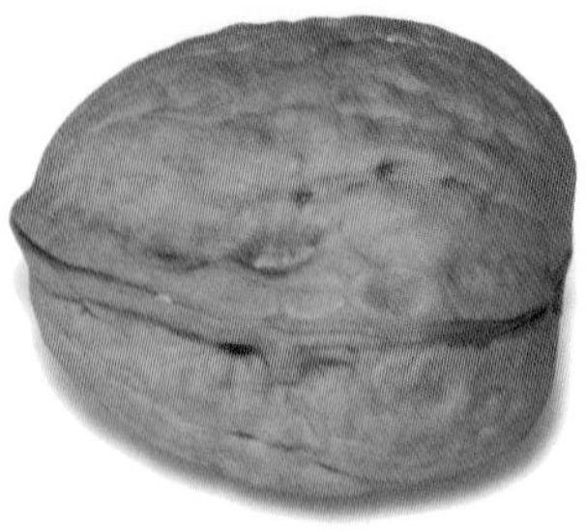

IN A NUTSHELL

You are now at the end of the chapter. Before you test your knowledge with the revision activities, check the following list to see if you feel confident in all the areas covered. If there are still any areas you're unsure of, go back over them in the book and ask your tutor for extra supports:

- what the employee's responsibilities are for health and safety in the salon
- working safely
- methods of sterilisation and disinfection
- important regulations – PPE, COSHH, Electricity at Work Regulations, Manual Handling Operations Regulations
- what sort of emergency situations can occur in the salon
- what the Health and Safety at Work Act requires the employer to do
- levels of responsibility – yours and others'
- what to do if an accident occurs or someone is taken ill
- the procedure in the event of a fire or other incident when evacuation is required
- things you must know in an emergency situation.

Remember all that you have learned. Health and safety is an important part of your work. When you read the other chapters in the book you will find it useful to remind yourself of this chapter.

REVISION ACTIVITIES

Use the questions below to test your knowledge of Chapter 113 to see just how much information you've gained. This can help you prepare for your assessments.

Turn to pages 484–485 for the answers.

WORDS TO FIND

Copy and complete the sentences below. Use these words to help you fill in the gaps.

hazard	ventilation	COSSH	Barbicide
accident book	non-latex gloves	risk assessment	
assembly point	PPE	sterilise	

1 Clothing that is used to protect the stylist when they are working is often called ________________ .

2 Good ________________ will provide a healthy working environment.

3 The ________________ Regulations give information about how to use products safely and how to dispose of them.

4 If the fire alarm goes off you should evacuate the premises and go to the ________________ .

5 Combs can be sterilised in a jar filled with ________________ .

6 ________________ should be used to protect your hands when using chemicals.

7 It is important to ________________ all your tools before they are used on a client.

8 If someone is hurt at work the ________________ must be filled in.

9 Something that could cause injury or hurt someone is called a ________________ .

10 To reduce the possibility of someone being injured in the salon a ________________ is carried out.

TEST YOUR KNOWLEDGE FURTHER

1 Whose responsibility is it to provide personal protective equipment?

2 Describe your duty under the Health and Safety at Work Act.

3 What is a hazard?

4 What is a risk?

5 Name **two** methods of sterilisation.

6 Name **two** things that can be used to protect a client.

7 What is the name of the test required by the Electricity at Work Regulations?

8 Name **two** things that would cause the salon to be evacuated.

9 Why should you not move someone who has slipped over in the salon?

10 What is the first thing you should do if you discover a fire in the salon?

114 SALON RECEPTION DUTIES

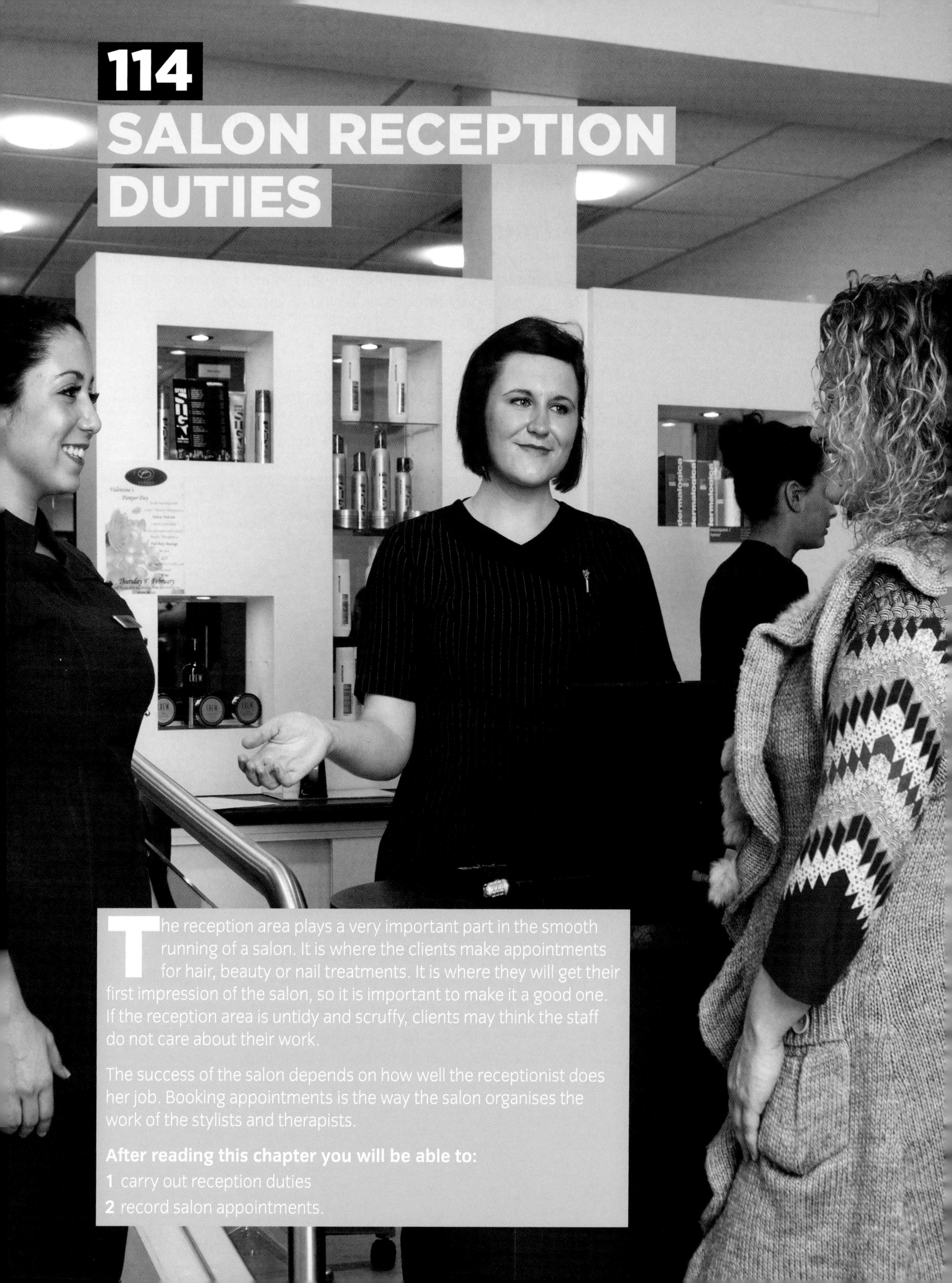

The reception area plays a very important part in the smooth running of a salon. It is where the clients make appointments for hair, beauty or nail treatments. It is where they will get their first impression of the salon, so it is important to make it a good one. If the reception area is untidy and scruffy, clients may think the staff do not care about their work.

The success of the salon depends on how well the receptionist does her job. Booking appointments is the way the salon organises the work of the stylists and therapists.

After reading this chapter you will be able to:

1 carry out reception duties
2 record salon appointments.

CARRY OUT RECEPTION DUTIES

Positive image
Setting a good example

Client confidentiality
Keeping client details private

Receptionists must know how to present a **positive image** of themselves and the salon to the client. They must communicate and behave in a professional manner, record and pass on clear information and keep **client confidentiality**.

PRESENTING A POSITIVE IMAGE

When a client comes into the salon, what they see will give them an idea of the salon and the staff. As receptionist, you should make sure that the client does not get a poor impression of you or your work.

FIRST IMPRESSIONS

A first impression is what you think of somewhere when you go there for the first time. What you see and how you are greeted will give you either a good impression or a bad impression. You want the clients coming in to the salon to have a good impression.

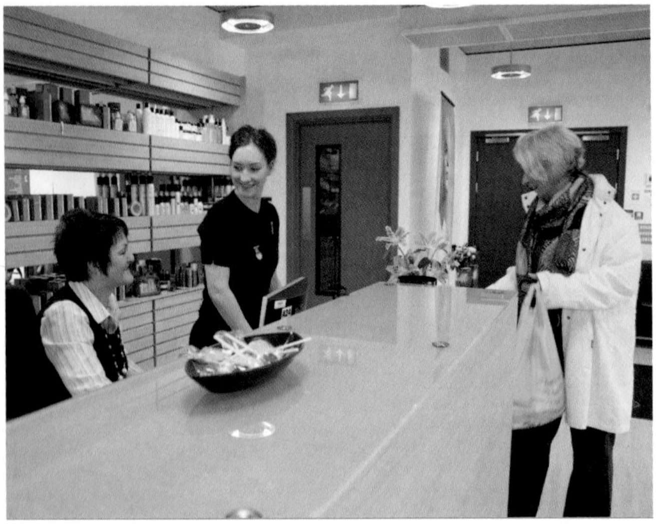

A neat and tidy reception area

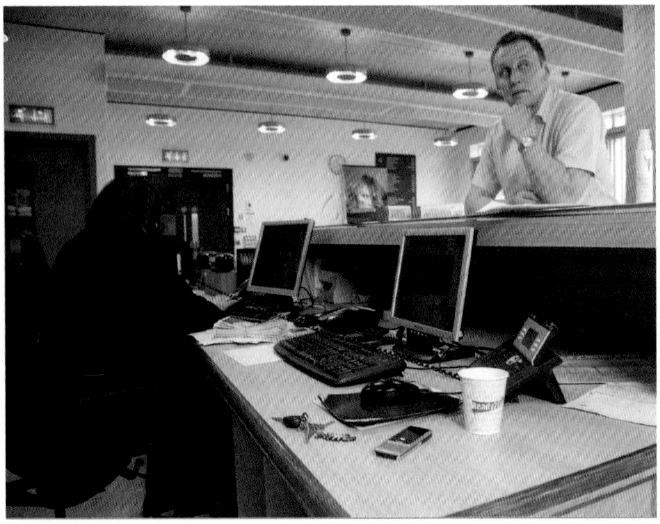

An untidy reception area

ACTIVITY

Think about businesses you have been to, like shops, clubs, cinemas, even salons. Then think about what it was you expected to see when you arrived. How did the staff behave when you arrived? Did what you saw and how the staff treated you give you a good impression or a bad impression? Was there anything else about the place or the staff that you liked or didn't like?

Make some notes of the places and what happened there. Then discuss your experiences with other members of your group.

Make a list of the things your group thinks are important to give a client or customer a good impression. Thinking about these during your work will remind you of what you should and should not be doing.

WHY DON'T YOU...
Read through Chapter 102 again to refresh your memory.

HOW CAN WE CREATE A POSITIVE IMAGE?

In Chapter 102 you learnt how to present a professional image in a salon. Now we can put that into practice for the reception.

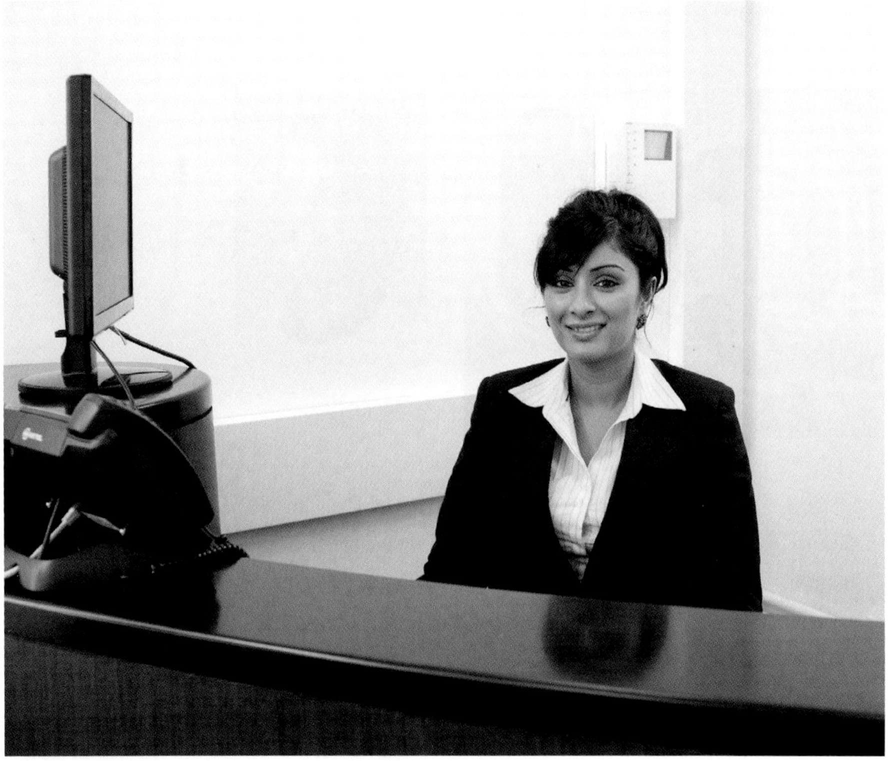

Good personal appearance

- Personal hygiene – wash or shower every day; use deodorant; clean your teeth regularly.
- Dress or uniform – should always be clean and ironed; always look smart; suitable for day wear (not evening).

HANDY HINTS

As a hairdresser, your hair will show clients your salon's standard of work. As a beauty therapist, your make-up and hands will do the same.

HANDY HINTS

Plan a routine that you follow every day to make sure your personal appearance meets your clients' and your boss's expectations.

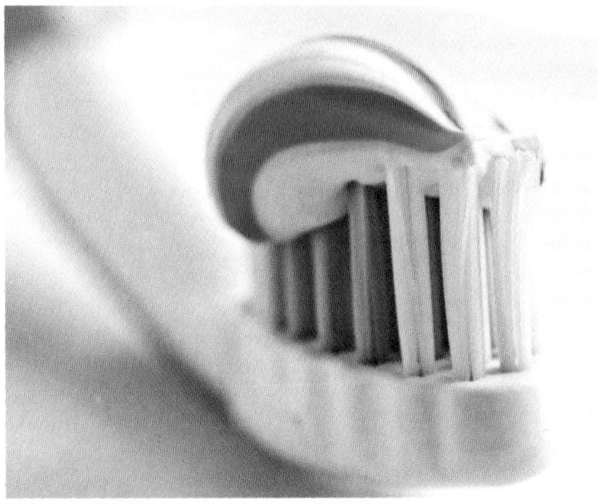

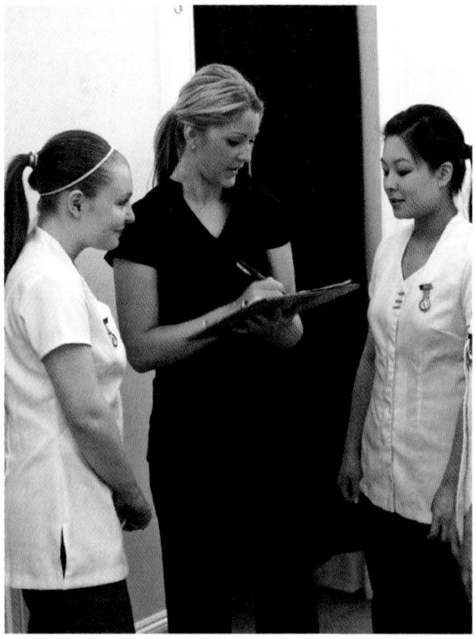

- Hair – your hair is an advert for the salon; it should be cut and styled regularly; always do your hair before you start work. In beauty therapy if your hair is long it must be tied up and off your face and collar.
- Make-up – use day make-up to compliment your skin; make sure it is done before you start work; in a beauty salon your make-up is an advert for the salon's services.
- Hands and nails – should be clean at all times; nails should not be too long; polish should not be chipped or smudged and should not be worn at all by a beauty therapist.

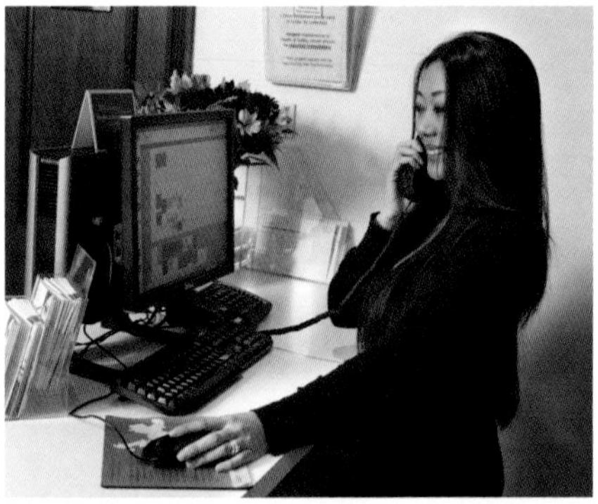

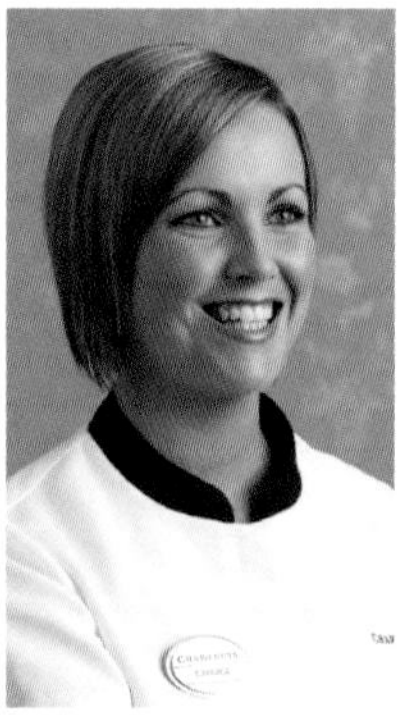

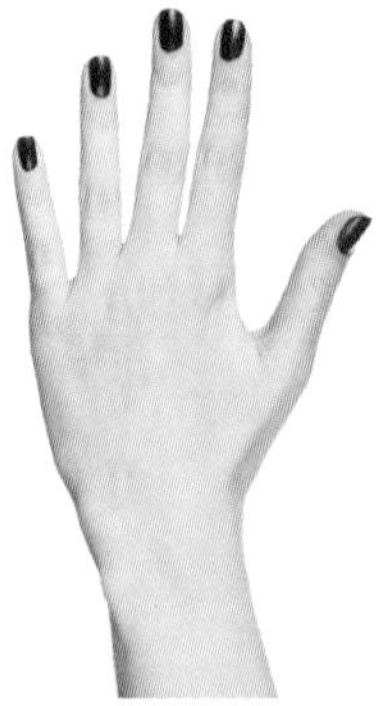

- Shoes – should be clean, comfortable, with low heels and closed toes.
- Jewellery – follow the salon policy for jewellery; don't wear too much – it can be a safety hazard; be aware that rings can increase the risk of dermatitis. For beauty therapy you must not wear any jewellery.

The right behaviour

- Follow instructions.
- Work co-operatively.
- Diversity and equality – treat everyone with respect. Treat everyone equally, whatever their skin colour, sexuality, gender or religion.

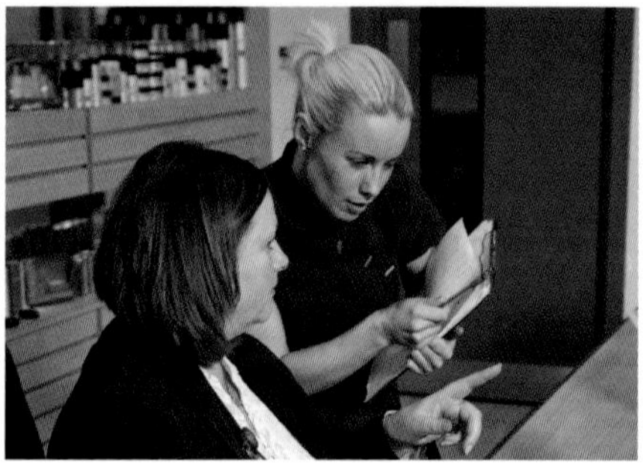

Good communication

- Listening – hearing what others say to you; paying attention to others.
- Speech – verbal communication; what you say to others; how you say it.
- Writing – recording information correctly; writing clearly.
- Body language – non-verbal communication; gestures and expressions; posture and mannerisms; don't forget: 'smile and the world smiles with you'.

Efficient reception service

To provide good reception service you will need to use all of the skills described above in order to perform your duties well.

RECEPTION DUTIES

For Level 1 your duties will include the following:

KEEPING THE RECEPTION AREA CLEAN AND TIDY

The first task of the day is to make sure the reception area is clean and tidy:

- Reception desk – clean the surface with a suitable cleaner; make sure everything is in its proper place; wipe the telephone and any other equipment.
- Stationery – make sure there are enough pens, pencils, paper and appointment cards for the day.

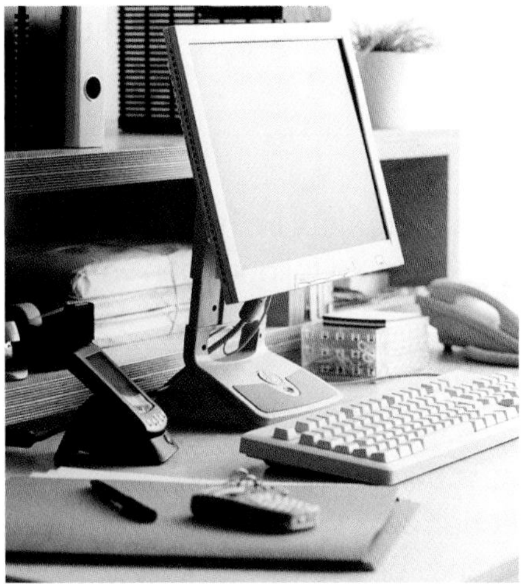

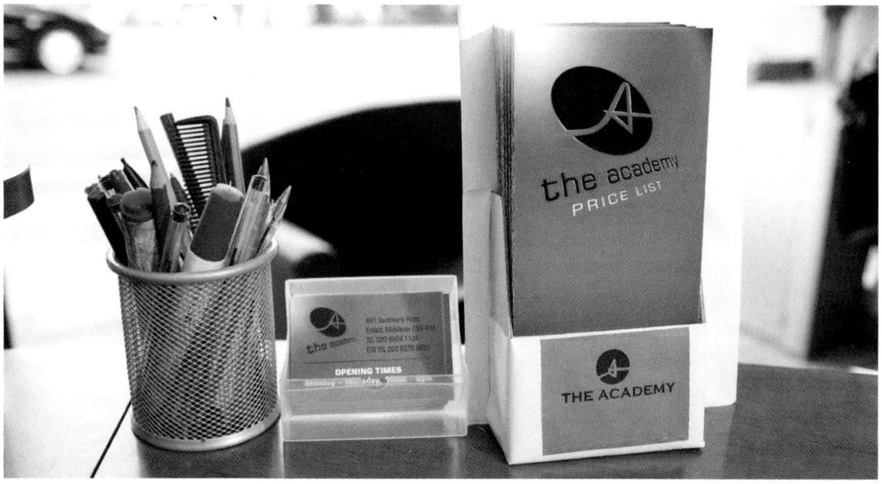

- Chairs and waiting area – check that the chairs are clean. Make sure everything is in its proper place.
- Magazines and newspapers – tidy them up and remove any that are scruffy.

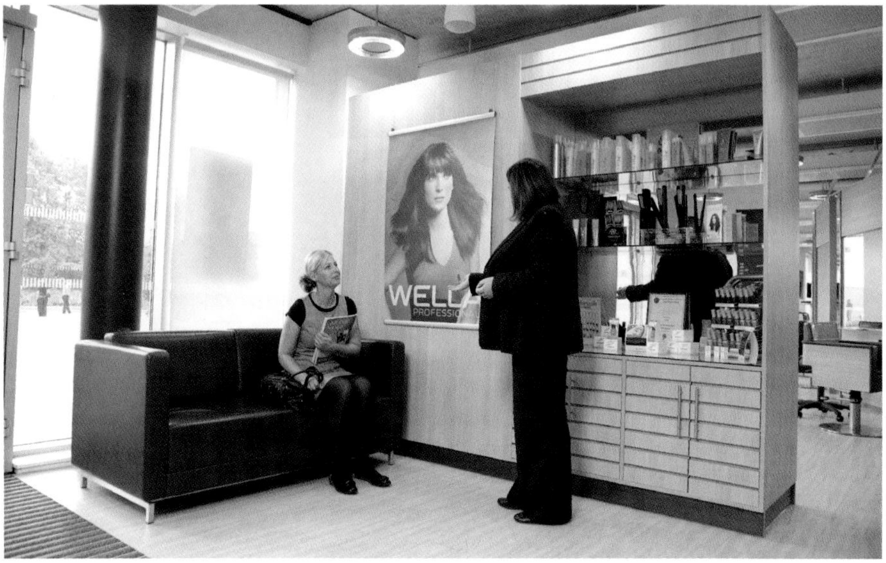

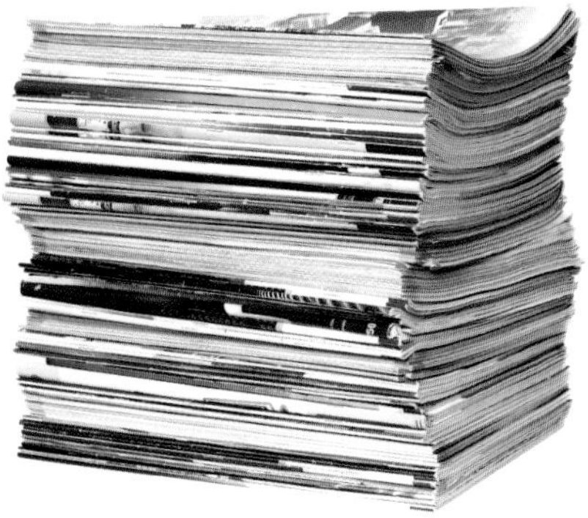

- Cloakroom – make sure coat hangers are tidy and the area is clean.
- Drinks – if the salon provides refreshments, make sure that everything is clean and there are enough supplies for the day.
- Retail display – check that everything is tidy and report any shortages to the salon manager or owner.

ACTIVITY

With the group, make a list of things that should be carried out to give a positive image to the client when they are at reception. Decide when and how often each should be done, to maintain a positive image at reception.

WORKING SAFELY

Always make sure you work safely and keep everything clean and tidy during the day. Check for hazards and report anything you think might cause harm to others.

ACTIVITY

Look back at Chapter 113 Following health and safety in the salon and list all of the health and safety laws that you should follow when working on reception.

ACTIVITY

Together with others in your group, discuss things that could be dangerous to you and others in the reception area. Make a list of them. An example is a wet floor near the salon entrance on a rainy day. Decide what you would do to deal with this and the other dangers you have listed.

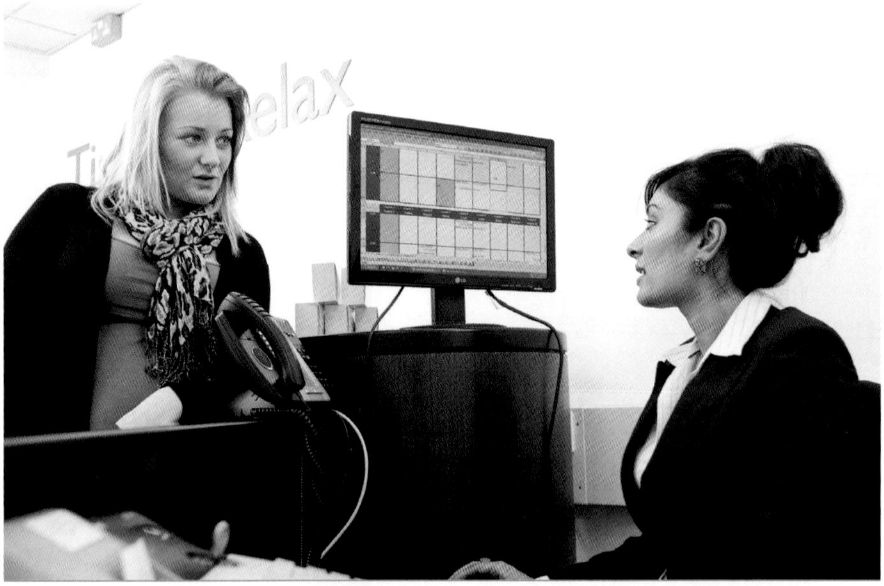

Always be friendly to your clients

MEETING AND GREETING CLIENTS

One of your most important tasks on reception will be to meet and greet the clients as they arrive. Creating a positive first impression may depend on how you greet the clients when they enter the salon. A clean and tidy reception area and a friendly, smiling, welcoming face will create the right impression.

ACTIVITY

Together with others in your group, discuss your experiences when you have visited salons, shops, cinemas, etc. Between you, think of some that gave you a positive impression:

- What was it that you liked?
- Was it clean and tidy?
- Were the staff welcoming, friendly, polite, helpful?

Think of some that gave you a negative impression:

- What was it you didn't like?
- Was it dirty, scruffy?
- Were the staff unhelpful, cold, rude, not interested?
- Were you kept waiting?
- Which ones did you go to again?
- Why?

Make a list of the positive things and the negative things you have discussed.

Greeting the client

When greeting the client:

- Remember to smile.
- Say good morning/afternoon.
- Look interested.
- Be helpful.
- Do not keep them waiting.

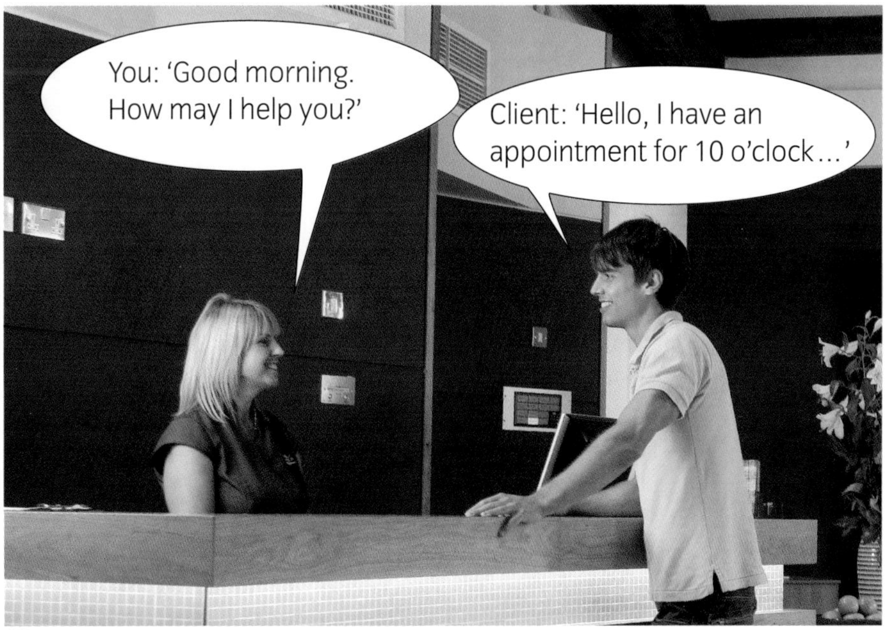
You: 'Good morning. How may I help you?'
Client: 'Hello, I have an appointment for 10 o'clock ...'

HANDY HINTS

Always remember to smile when you greet the client. They are not paying to see a glum, depressing face.

ACTIVITY

In threes, practise welcoming a client. Take turns at being the client and then the receptionist. Use all three situations for greeting the client listed above.

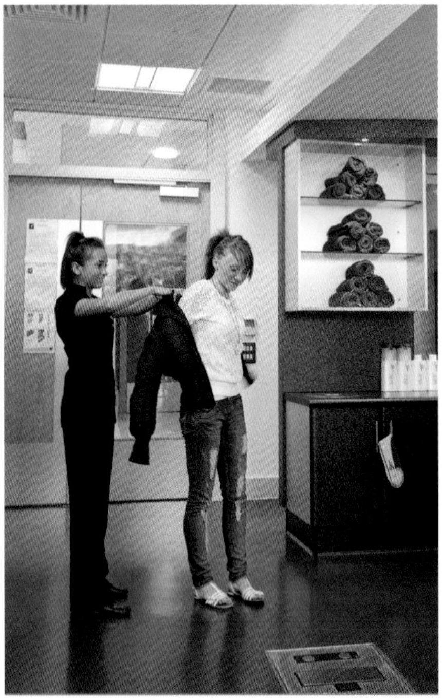

Help the client put on their coat after the service

HANDY HINTS

If the client seems angry or upset when they ask to speak to someone, always be polite and helpful, and quickly report to the stylist/therapist.

DEALING WITH THE CLIENT'S REQUEST

Once you have greeted the client you need to find out what they require. They may have an appointment. They may want to make an appointment. They may wish to speak to one of the staff. Always be polite and helpful. Speak clearly. Deal with their request quickly and efficiently.

Checking their appointments

If they have an appointment, check the appointment system to confirm the time, the stylist/therapist and the service the client is having.

Seating the client and looking after their belongings

If the client is wearing a coat, offer to take it. Then ask them to take a seat in the waiting area. Hang the coat in the cloakroom. If the stylist/therapist is not ready for their client, or the client is early, ask if they would like a magazine.

Informing the stylist/therapist

Next, tell the stylist/therapist that the client has arrived. If they need you to do something then make sure you follow their instructions correctly.

Providing refreshments

If the client has to wait, offer them refreshments – tea or coffee, etc.

If the client wishes to speak to one of the staff, ask them to take a seat. Tell the stylist/therapist that Ms/Mrs/Miss .... wants to speak to them. Make sure you follow the stylist's/therapist's instructions. Make the client tea or coffee if they have to wait and provide them with a magazine.

HANDY HINTS

Always keep up to date with any promotions or special offers that the salon has. Learn about new services so you can confidently inform the clients and answer some of their questions.

PROMOTING THE SALE OF PRODUCTS AND SERVICES

While clients are waiting for their appointments there is an opportunity to promote products and services. For example, special offers on new products or new services, and discounts. Give the client leaflets or other material so they can read about them as they wait. If there aren't any leaflets, point out posters or displays.

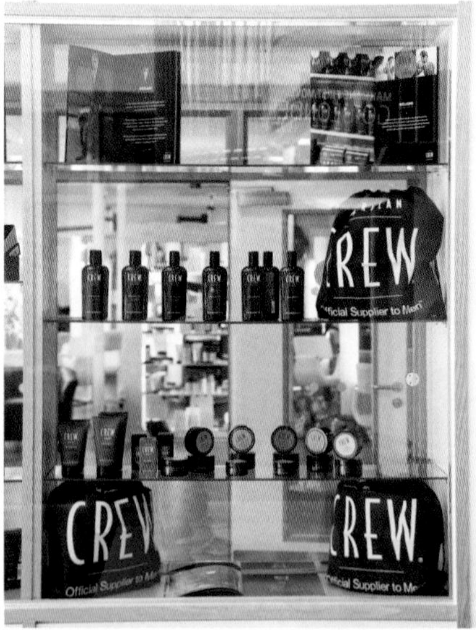

ACTIVITY

In pairs, practise making a client aware of promotions and new products. Take turns at being the client and the receptionist.

TAKING MESSAGES

Another important duty for you will be to take messages for other staff. Make sure you write down all the information needed. Write the information clearly so others can read it. You will need to write down:

- the date and time the message was received
- the name of the stylist/therapist the message is for
- the name of the person the message is from
- the message itself
- your name as the person taking the message.

Always check the details with the person the message is from to make sure you have written it down correctly.

Make sure the person the message is for gets it quickly. Follow any instructions they may give you such as ringing back with a reply.

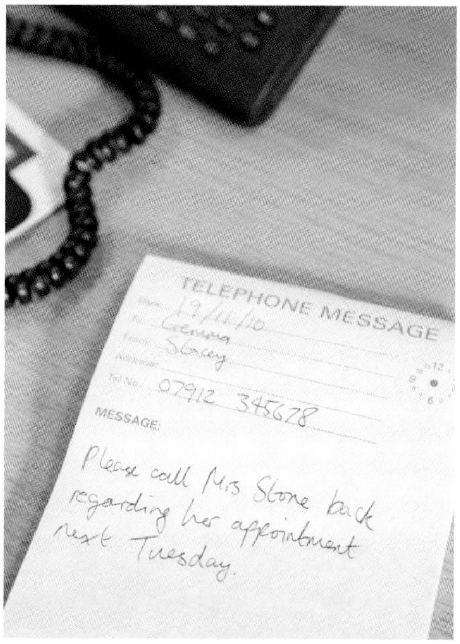

ACTIVITY

With a partner, practise taking messages, taking it in turns to be receptionist and client.

Remember, not everything on reception will be easy or straightforward. If you are not sure about a client's request then seek help. Examples of situations where you should seek help from someone else might include:

- not being able to find a client's appointment in the appointment system
- dealing with a client who wants to complain
- not being able to answer a question from a client
- not being able to understand what a client is saying.

If any of these things happen:

- get the client to take a seat
- go and find someone that can help
- let the client know what is happening.

HANDY HINTS

Always make sure that all the treatments/products the client has had are on the bill. Anything that is left off will lose the salon profit.

ACTIVITY

In pairs, practise handling a client whose request you can't deal with. Take turns at being the client and then the receptionist. Use any of the situations listed above.

METHODS OF PAYMENT

Knowing how the clients will pay for their services and treatment is important. Adding up the bill correctly will make sure the salon gets the income for the work the staff have done. Most salons use a computer-based till. This will calculate the bill for you to tell and show the client.

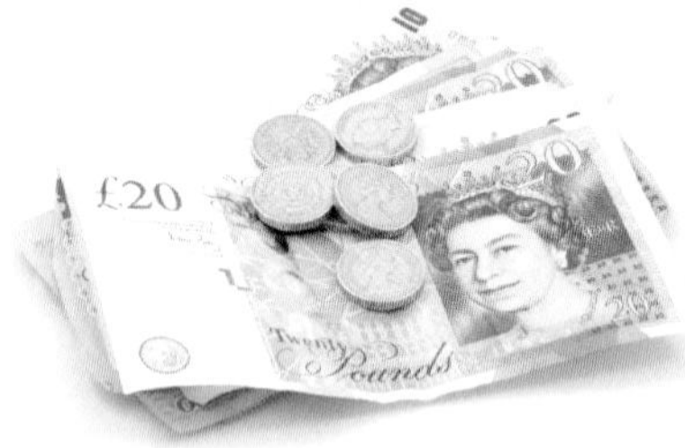

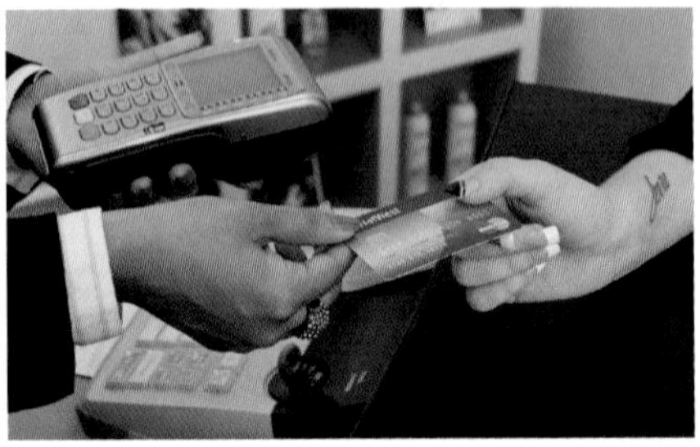

There are several ways by which the client can pay:

- Cash – this is the most commonly used method of payment. The till will tell you how much change is required. Count the change carefully and make sure it is right.
- Credit or debit cards – many clients pay by card. You may receive training on how to use a card machine.
- Cheques – many clients used to pay by cheque. Nowadays they are being used less. The cheque must have:
  - the correct date (day, month and year)
  - the salon/business name
  - the amount in words
  - the amount in figures
  - the client's signature.

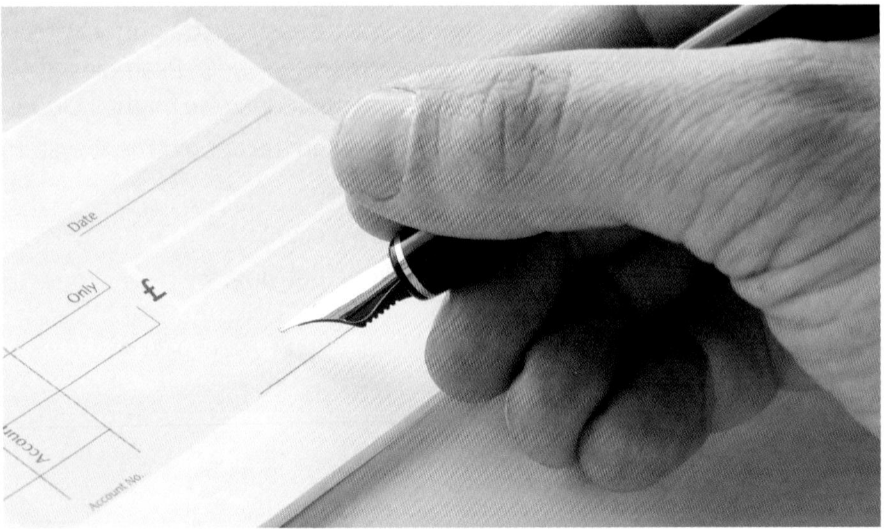

When the client gives you the cheque you must check that:
  - the date is right
  - the amount in words matches the figures
  - they have signed it.

WHY DON'T YOU...
Find out the difference between a debit card and a credit card.

- Cash alternatives – these include gift vouchers, money-off vouchers and special-offer tokens. They can be used by clients to pay for all or part of their bill. Gift vouchers can be given as presents for either individual services or for a certain amount of money.

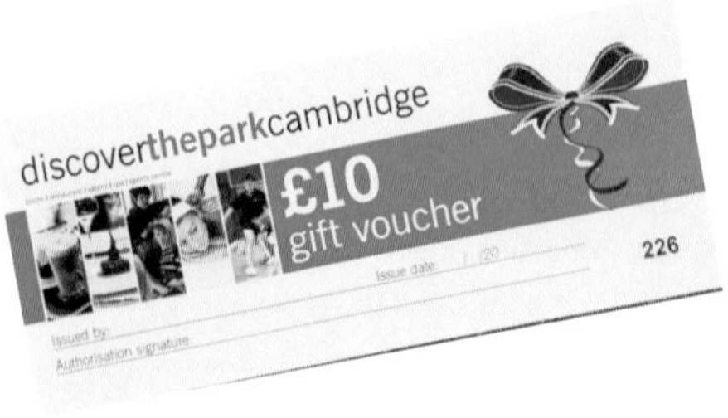

ACTIVITY

Together with others, practise calculating a client's bill and taking their money.

RECORD SALON APPOINTMENTS

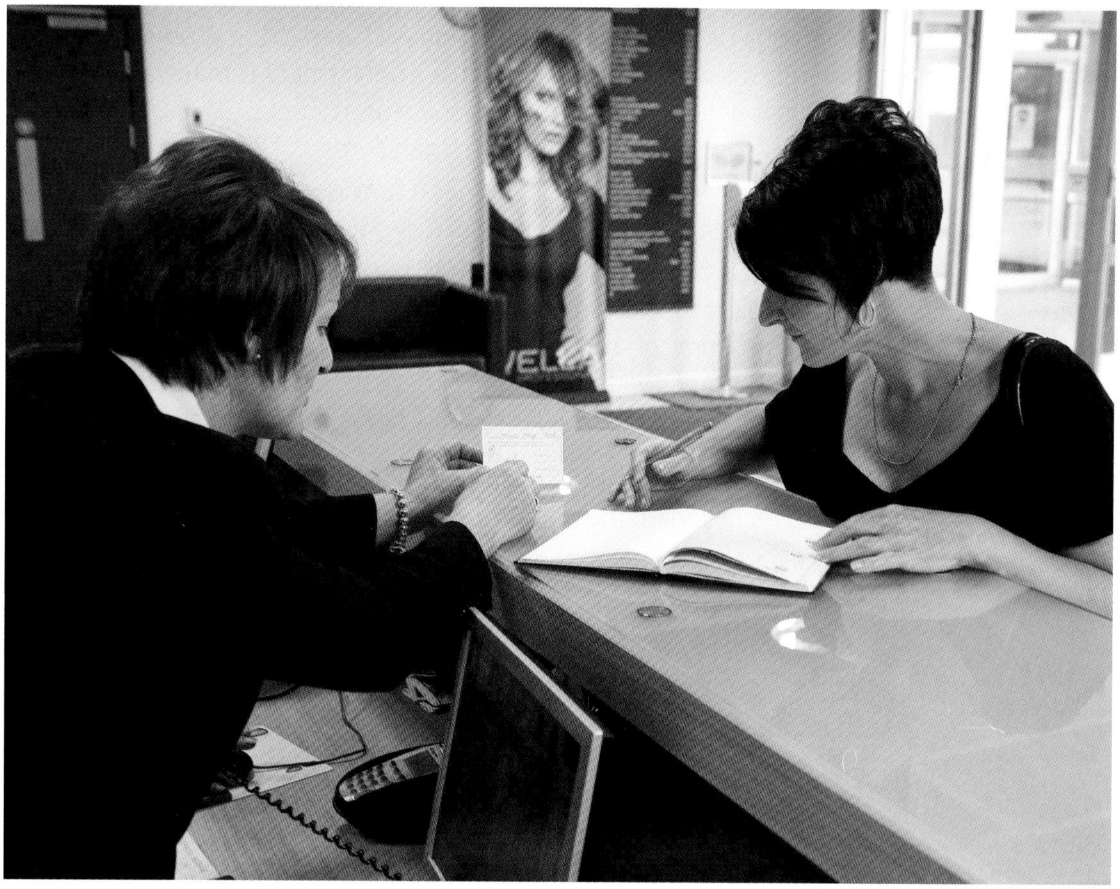

Making appointments correctly is important to the success of the salon operation. The stylists/therapists need to be working on clients as much as possible. Organising the appointments to make the best use of their time will make sure they earn the maximum money for the salon. Careful planning of the appointments means that stylists/therapists do not have to rush each client or keep them waiting. This will improve client satisfaction.

Salons use either a paper-based or computer-based system to organise and record the appointments.

To be able to make an appointment for a client you must know how to use the system that your salon uses.

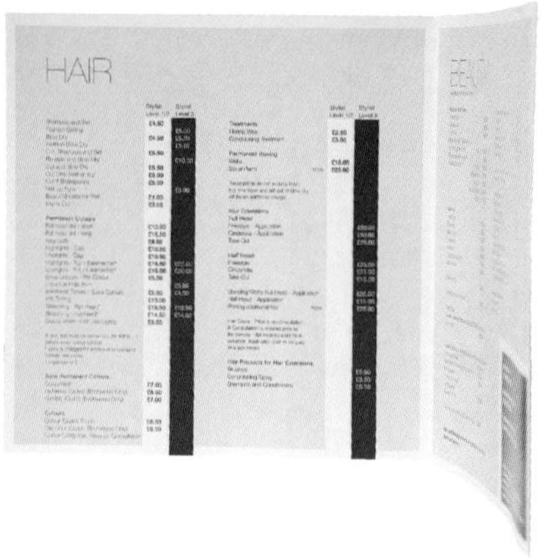

SERVICES OFFERED

Before you can make an appointment for a client you will need to know information about the services offered in the salon:

- The range of services available – you will need to know about the different services offered. When the appointment is made a shorthand system is used to write it in the book. For example, CBD is short for cut and blow dry and man is short for manicure.
- The stylists/therapists – you will need to know the hours and days they work, the services they specialise in and when they have their breaks.
- The time each service takes – you will need to know how long each service takes so you can book an appropriate time for the appointment. For some chemical services, like colour and perm, you may need to make two entries with a gap in between to allow for processing, and then book a finishing service like blow drying.

HANDY HINTS

Not all salons use the same shorthand. Talk to your manager if you're not sure.

The table below gives some examples of hairdressing services, how they are recorded on the appointment sheet and the time they take.

Service	Shorthand	Time to book out
Blow dry	BD	30 mins
Shampoo and set	S/S	30 mins
Cut and blow dry	CBD	45 mins
Wet cut	W/C	30 mins
Restyle	Res	60 mins
Semi-permanent colour	Semi	30 mins
Perm	P/W	45 mins
Highlights	H/L	60 mins

The table below gives details about beauty services.

Service	Shorthand	Time to book out
Cleanse and make-up	C/M/Up	45 mins
Manicure	Man	45 mins
Facial	Fac	60 mins
Full leg wax	FLW	50 mins
Eyebrow tint	EBT	10 mins
Pedicure	Ped	45 mins

WHY DON'T YOU...

Add extra rows to your chart. Find the details for other services offered in your salon and add the details to the chart.

ACTIVITY

Copy one of the charts.

Complete the chart by finding the cost of the service in your salon, and whether a gap is needed before another service is booked. Ask your tutor for help.

PAPER-BASED APPOINTMENT SYSTEMS

These systems have a page for each day of the week. The page will be divided into time slots (usually 15 minutes) and columns for each stylist/therapist.

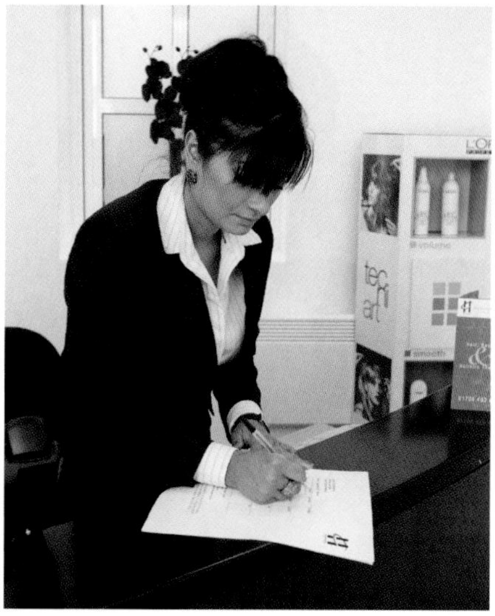

BEAUTY APPOINTMENT PAGE

Time	Jo	Mary	Steve	Clare
8.30	Mrs Brown			
8.45	FLW		Mrs Gibson	Mrs Owen
9.00		Mrs Fuller	Fac	Man
9.15		Ped		
9.30				
9.45				
10.00				

HAIRDRESSING APPOINTMENT PAGE

Time	Melanie	Leanne	Rod	Natalie
8.30	Mrs Smith			
8.45	CBD			
9.00		Mrs Patel	Mrs Rossi	
9.15		S/S	½ H/L	
9.30				
9.45				
10.00				

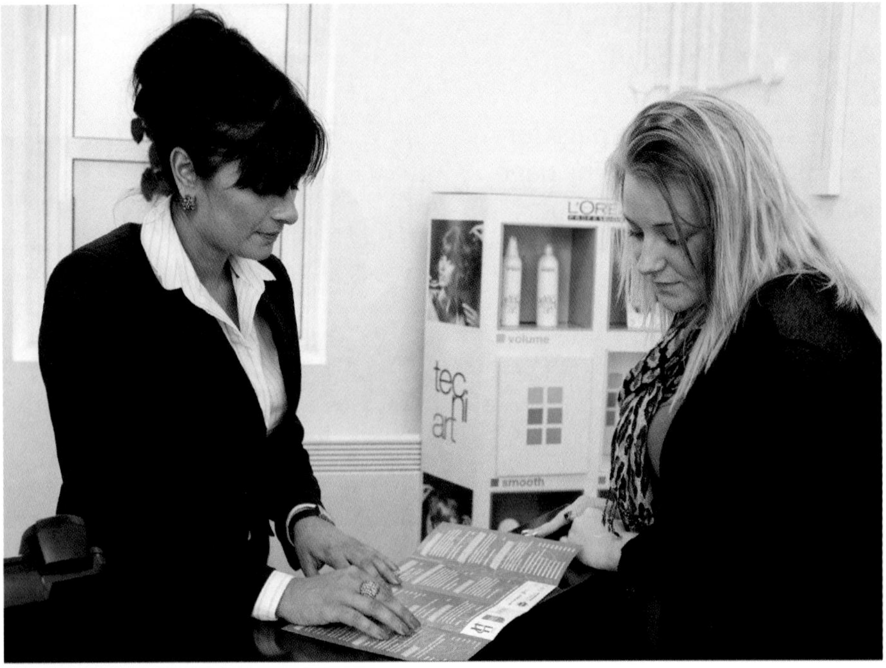

Discuss the services your salon offers with your client

MAKING THE APPOINTMENT

Once you have greeted the client and they ask to make an appointment, you will need to ask some open questions to find out their needs. Here are some examples:

- 'What service or treatment would you like?'
- 'When would you like to have it done?'
- 'Who usually looks after you?'
- 'If the day and time are not available, are there any other days you could make?'

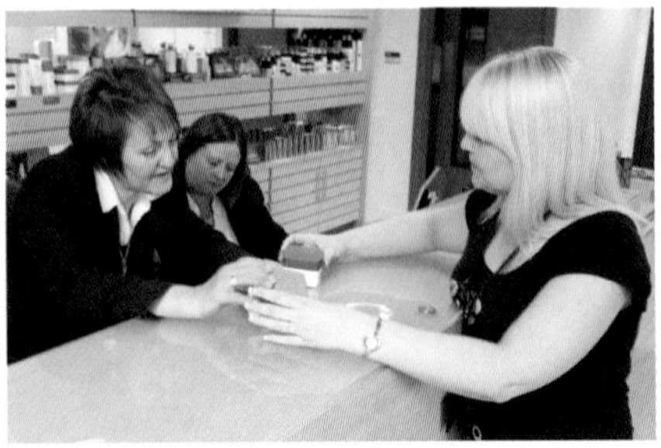

Now you have the client's requirements. Next, see if the stylist/therapist is available at the time requested and has enough time to complete the service required. If they are then you can tell the client that they can have the service when they wanted it. For example, you can say 'Yes Mrs Smith, Melanie is able to give you a blow dry on Thursday at 2 o'clock. Would you like me to book that for you?' When the client says 'Yes please', you can then record the details clearly in Melanie's column at 2 o'clock. Don't forget to book out the required time.

You will need one more piece of information – a contact telephone number for the client. This is necessary in case you need to contact the client about any changes to her appointment. For example, Melanie may be ill and not able to work on that day.

The last thing to do is to write the date, the time and the service on an appointment card and use closed questions to confirm that everything is OK with the client. You can say 'I have booked you for a blow dry with Melanie on Thursday the 16th at 2 o'clock. Is that OK for you?' If it is OK the client should reply 'Yes, thank you very much'.

Finish by asking 'Is there anything else I can do for you today Mrs Smith?' If she says 'No thank you' then you could reply 'Thank you for booking with us and I look forward to seeing you on Thursday, goodbye'.

ACTIVITY

Make a chart for one day's appointments. You will need enough spaces down the page for the time slots to cover from 8.30 am to 5.30 pm. You will need two columns for staff.

- Melanie works full time from 8.30 to 5.30 and has a break for lunch at 1.00pm.
- Leanne works part time from 10am to 3pm and has a 20-minute break around 12.30 but is flexible.

Fill in your sheet so it shows when the staff are at work and when they have their breaks.

HAIR EXAMPLE

If you would like to do the activity for hair services then use these appointments:

- Mrs Smith wants a cut and blow dry with Melanie at 9.15.
- Shona Jones would like cap highlights with Leanne at 10.30.
- Ms Brown would like a blow dry with Melanie as late as possible in the morning. What is the latest time you can book for her?
- Rory Watson would like his hair cut with Leanne at 3pm.

BEAUTY EXAMPLE

If you would like to do the activity for beauty treatments then use these appointments:

- Mrs Smith wants a facial with Melanie at 9.15.
- Shona Jones would like a full leg wax with Leanne at 10.30.
- Ms Brown would like a manicure with Melanie as late as possible in the morning. What is the latest time you can book for her?
- Ruby Watson would like a pedicure with Leanne at 3pm.

WHY DON'T YOU...
In a group, practise making appointments by taking turns in being clients and receptionist.

COMPUTER-BASED APPOINTMENT SYSTEMS

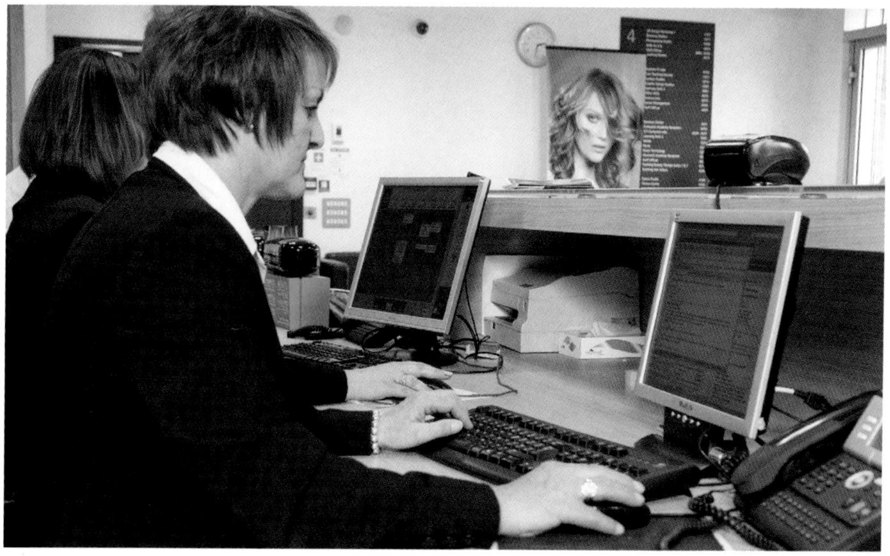

WHY DON'T YOU...
Fnd out more about computer-based appointment systems.

There are many computer-based appointment systems that salons can use. They are based on software that will automatically make appointments when you enter the information. If your salon uses a computer-based system the salon will train you to use it correctly.

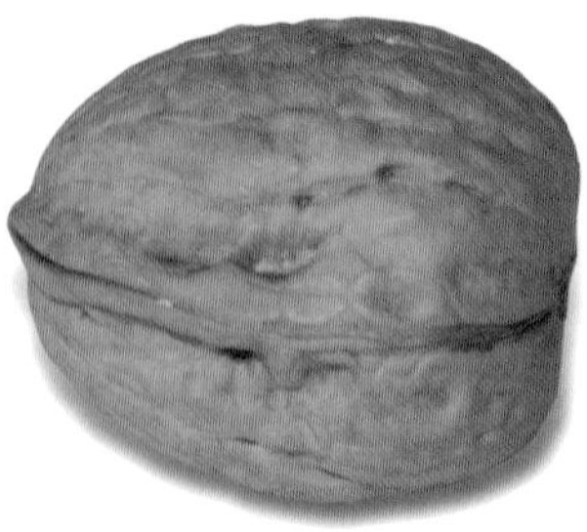

IN A NUTSHELL

You are now at the end of the chapter. Before you test your knowledge with the revision activities, check the following list to see if you feel confident in all the areas covered. If there are still any areas you're unsure of, go back over them in the book and ask your tutor for extra support:

- the importance of presenting a professional image in a salon
- how important first impressions are when you working on reception. (Did you find your own experiences helpful when you learnt this?)
- how important a positive image is on reception
- how personal appearance, behaviour and good communication help you to carry out your reception duties efficiently
- why having your hair and make-up looking good are important to the salon
- how keeping the reception area clean and tidy will give the client a good impression and will make it easier to work safely
- how to greet the client and deal with their request, look after their belongings, make them comfortable and make them drinks
- inform the stylist that the client has arrived
- why it is important that messages are accurate and delivered quickly
- methods of payment – cash, credit and debit cards, cheques and vouchers
- the importance of the appointment system
- how paper-based systems work
- how to make an appointment for a client
- how computer-based systems need training to learn how to use them.

REVISION ACTIVITIES

Use the questions below to test your knowledge of Chapter 114 to see just how much information you've gained. This can help you to prepare for your assessments. Turn to pages 485–486 for the answers.

WORDS TO FIND

Copy and complete the sentences below. Use these words to help you fill in the gaps.

telephone	meet and greet	retail display
appointment book	messages	credit cards
follow instructions	magazines	cheques
positive image	first impression	

1. A junior should always ________________ given to them by the stylist.
2. The reception area should always be clean and tidy to create the right ________________ when a client enters the salon.
3. ________________ and ________________ are methods the client may use to pay their bill.
4. The receptionist should always present a ________________ to the client.
5. ________________ can be offered to a client if they have to wait for their appointment.
6. A good ________________ can help sell products to the client.
7. It is important that the ________________ is filled in correctly so that the stylists know when their clients are expected.
8. Always ________________ the client as soon as they enter the salon.
9. Accurately recording ________________ will make sure the right information is given to the stylist.
10. The receptionist should always speak clearly and use the right tone when answering the ________________ .

TEST YOUR KNOWLEDGE FURTHER

1 Name the four things that will provide a positive image when you are working on reception.

2 Why is it important to have your hair and make-up looking good when you are working?

3 Name **four** things that you should do to keep the reception area clean and tidy.

4 When should you greet a client that has just arrived at the salon?
   a After you have finished your tea.
   b As soon as possible.
   c When you have finished dealing with another client.
   d When the stylist arrives.

5 List **three** things you should do when a client arrives for their appointment.

6 Why is important to write clearly when taking a message?

7 What should you do if you cannot deal with a client's request?

8 List **three** methods of payment that a client could use to pay their bill.

9 When making an appointment for a client, what information do you need from them?

10 Why do you need to know how long a service takes when making an appointment?

115 WORKING WITH OTHERS IN THE HAIR AND BEAUTY SECTOR

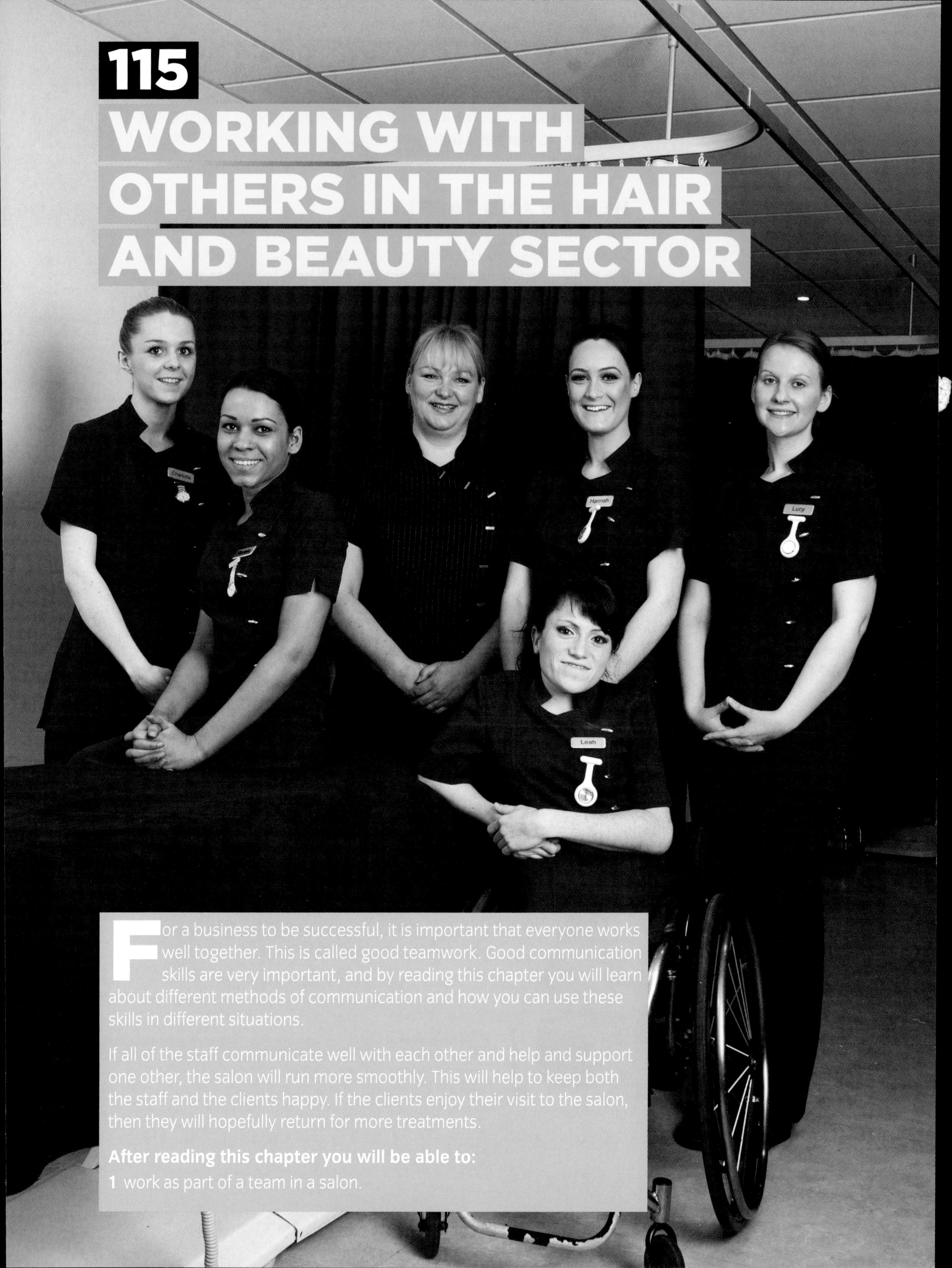

For a business to be successful, it is important that everyone works well together. This is called good teamwork. Good communication skills are very important, and by reading this chapter you will learn about different methods of communication and how you can use these skills in different situations.

If all of the staff communicate well with each other and help and support one other, the salon will run more smoothly. This will help to keep both the staff and the clients happy. If the clients enjoy their visit to the salon, then they will hopefully return for more treatments.

After reading this chapter you will be able to:

1 work as part of a team in a salon.

WORK AS PART OF A TEAM IN A SALON

Health and safety will be important for all areas of your learning. It is important to work as a team in giving your clients a safe environment to come to.

HEALTH AND SAFETY

It is important that you work in a safe and clean way in the salon and treatment areas. You should always keep your work area tidy and only use hygienic tools and equipment. This will help to reduce the risk of harm to you and your clients and help to prevent cross-infection. The client will also have more confidence in you and you will look more professional. When you are working in a salon, every member of staff is responsible for working in a healthy and safe way, for example tidying away after their clients.

HANDY HINTS

Have a look in Chapter 113 to help you with the activity.

ACTIVITY

In small groups, discuss ways in which you can help and support each other to work in a healthy and safe way in the salon. Share your ideas with the rest of the group and then devise a 'group contract' that you all agree to follow using these ideas.

WAYS OF COMMUNICATING

Communication can be described as passing information, ideas or feelings from one person to another. There are many different ways to do this and by using these different methods, hopefully the message will be clearly understood.

Verbal communication
Communicating through spoken language

Non-verbal communication
Communicating through body language

Communication comes in different forms, such as **verbal communication** and **non-verbal communication**.

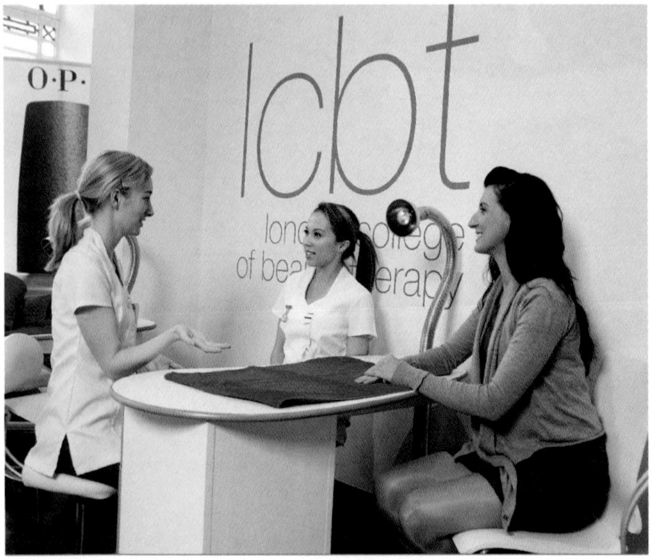

Good communication between therapists and clients is important

VERBAL COMMUNICATION

Verbal communication is when people speak to each other face to face or on the phone. This method of communication uses speaking, language, words and sound.

Verbal communication is important in the hair and beauty industry as you need to be able to talk to your colleagues and also clients.

HANDY HINTS

The more practice you have at talking to different people, the more confident you will become.

The following simple steps will help your verbal communication skills when speaking to your colleagues and clients:

- Speak slowly and clearly – this will help the person that you are talking to understand what you are saying.
- Speak in a friendly manner – this is important as it will help to make the other person feel comfortable and relax.
- Use simple language – make sure that you use words that the client will understand. If you use technical words, such as 'temporary colours' or 'manicure', you may need to explain what these mean to the client.
- Try to vary the **tone** of your voice – this means changing the level of your voice as you speak. If you speak in the same tone all the time it sounds very boring to the person who is listening.
- Speak in a professional way – you should always speak in an appropriate way to both clients and colleagues. Examples include not swearing, speaking softly and not shouting across the salon. Try to speak slowly and calmly so that the client can hear what you are saying to them.

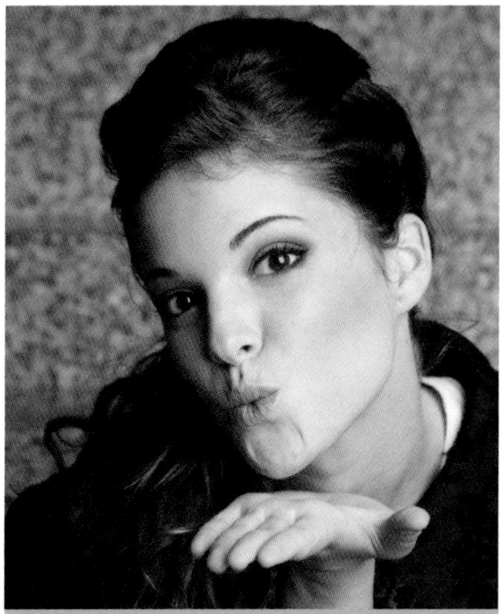

HANDY HINTS

When communicating verbally, remember the acronym 'KISS' – Keep It Short and Simple.

Tone

The level of your voice, for example high or low

ACTIVITY

Write down more examples of how you could speak in a professional way. Then discuss your answers with the rest of the group.

- Smile when you talk – even when you may not feel like smiling, it will help to give a positive impression to the person that you are talking to. This will help to make the communication you have with them more positive.
- Do not chew gum whilst speaking to a client – this looks very unprofessional.

HANDY HINTS

When you smile at someone, they will more than likely smile back at you!

HANDY HINTS

Try smiling, even when you are talking on the phone. Even though the other person cannot see you smiling, your voice will sound happier!

ACTIVITY

Working in pairs, choose a card that has an emotion written on it (but do not show your partner). Examples of emotions on the cards could be:

- angry
- sad
- happy
- not interested
- nervous
- preoccupied

HANDY HINTS

Remember, it is not just what we say, it is how we say it.

HANDY HINTS

Good communication is needed for a relationship to be successful.

Have a conversation with each other for a few minutes about any topic. Take it in turns to talk in a way that matches the emotion that you have picked. Continue the conversation until the other person guesses the emotion. Afterwards, make a note of the following:

- How did your voice change?
- Did you use any words to help you communicate the emotion?
- Were there any other changes that you noticed?

Then discuss your findings with the rest of the group.

NON-VERBAL COMMUNICATION

We communicate with more than just spoken words. In fact, research shows that we communicate more with our body language, known as non-verbal communication, than we do with what we actually say. It is important that you learn to understand the different non-verbal signals that other people are communicating. This will help you to know how to react to them and also make the people feel more comfortable.

Here are some examples of how we communicate non-verbally.

LISTENING

You probably spend more time using your listening skills than any other kind of skill. Like other skills, listening takes practice. It is important that people know that you are listening to them and that they are being understood. This will help to promote good communication.

What does it mean to really listen? Real listening has three basic steps:

1. Hearing – listening enough to hear what the other person is saying.
2. Understanding – taking in what you have heard and understanding what has been said.
3. Making a decision – after you have understood what has been said, you can then either answer them back or ask them a question.

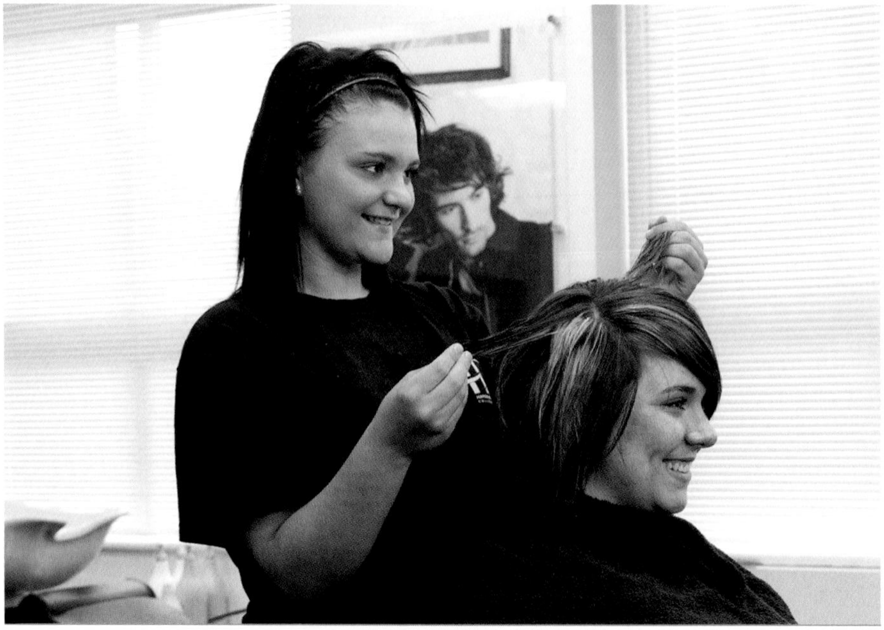

Good communication includes good listening skills

ACTIVITY

Are you a good listener? Tick either A, B or C for the following statements:

		Most of the time A	Sometimes B	Almost never C
1	When listening to someone, I make eye contact.			
2	I nod my head when I agree with what someone is saying.			
3	If I'm not sure whether I've understood what someone is saying I will ask them, to make sure that I've got it right.			
4	I keep still and do not fidget (play with my hair, watch, pen, etc) whilst listening to someone else.			
5	If I lose interest in what they are saying, I can still listen to them.			
6	I give my full attention if someone is talking to me.			
7	When background noise makes it difficult for me to listen I can block it out and still focus on what someone is saying to me.			
8	I wait for someone to finish speaking before I respond to them.			
9	I pause a moment to think over what someone has said before offering my feedback.			
10	I find it easy to wait until a person has finished speaking before I talk.			

Now look at your scores to find out how good you are at listening:

Mainly As – you have excellent listening skills.

Mainly Bs – you have good listening skills, although you could improve on some skills. See the 'tips for being a good listener' below to help you.

Mainly Cs – you need to try to improve your listening skills. This will then help you with your communication with other people. The following 'tips for being a good listener' will help you.

Tips for being a good listener

- Give the client your full attention.
- Let them finish before you begin to talk.
- Let the client finish talking before you begin to speak! You can't really listen if you are busy thinking about what you want say next.
- Ask questions. If you are not sure you understand what they have said, just ask.
- Sit up straight and look directly at the speaker.
- Now and then, nod to show that you understand.
- You may also smile, frown, laugh or be silent where appropriate. These are all ways to let the speaker know that you are really listening.

HANDY HINTS

Practise these tips on your family, friends and with other students in your group. The more you practise, the more you will develop these skills and be more confident in using them.

WRITING

Written communication means passing information from one person to another in a form that is written down. It might be written communication carried out in the form of a treatment plan. This is where the details of a client's treatment are noted down, for example the products that were used and the colours that were chosen.

The client may also make a comment about how they found the treatment. This will help you to improve your skills. You can discuss this with your tutor afterwards and make a plan of ways that you can improve how you carry out the treatment next time.

Another reason why written communication is important is that another therapist or stylist may work on the same client and they may need the information from the previous treatment. For example, if the client wants the same hair colour or nail polish colour, if it is written down they will know exactly which product to use.

RESPONDING CORRECTLY

Whether you are responding to a client or a colleague at work, it is important that you communicate with them in a warm, thoughtful and caring way. An example of this is smiling and nodding your head when they are talking to you to show that you understand what they have said.

At all times, try to put the other person at ease. This can be done by having an open posture, ie arms and shoulders relaxed, and by speaking in a slow, clear manner. If you ask them a question, give them time to think of the answer.

ACTIVITY

When we communicate:

- 50 per cent is through our body language
- 40 per cent is through our tone of voice
- 10 per cent is through the words that we say.

So it is not always what we say, but how we say it!

Design a mood board on communication showing the percentages above. You may decide to show these in a chart. Include examples of pictures showing each of the communication methods mentioned.

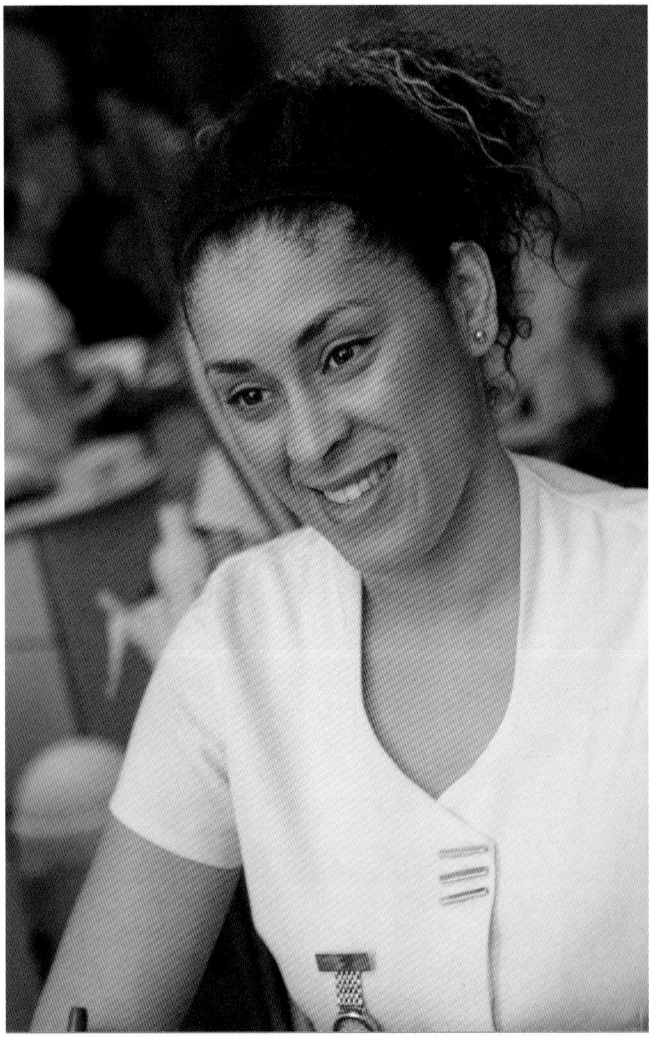

Smiling is one way of responding to a client well

ACTIVITY

Write down how you communicate differently with the following people:

- your family
- your friends
- your tutor
- someone who you have not met before.

Discuss how you communicate with them – this may be different with each one.

FACIAL EXPRESSIONS

Examples of facial expressions are smiling when you are happy and frowning when you are not! Sometimes someone may not have to say anything to you, but you know how they are feeling from the look on their face.

ACTIVITY

Write down some emotions on cards, such as:

- happy
- sad
- angry
- surprised
- frightened
- tired
- nervous.

In pairs, choose one of these cards, and without talking or showing your partner the card, show this emotion using your facial expressions only. See if they can guess which emotion it is.

Discuss your findings with the rest of the group.

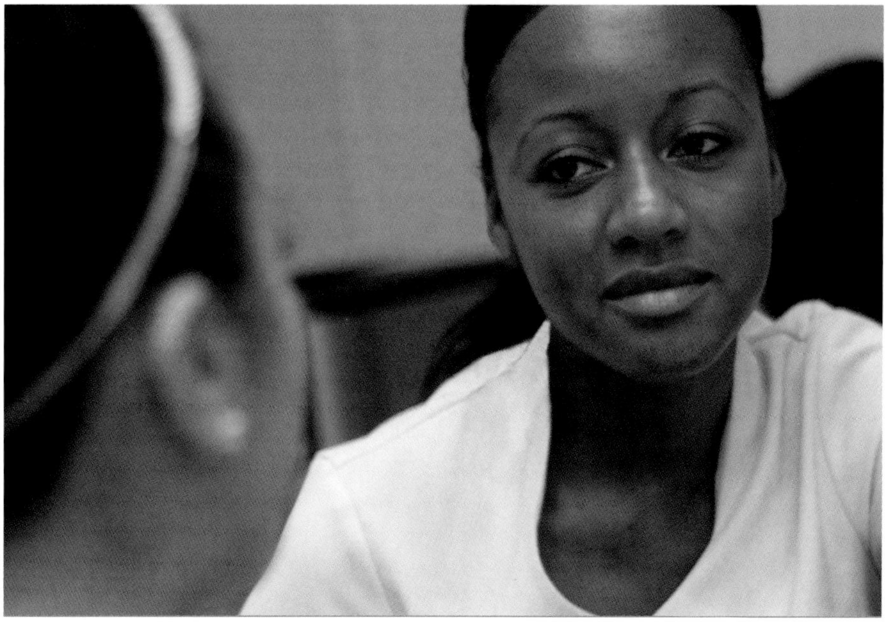

Talking clearly and slowly will help communication between you and your client

HANDY HINTS

It is not just what we say that helps in communicating with other people, but also the tone and sound of our voice. This can let the other person know what our true feelings are and also what we really mean. For example, we may talk more quickly when we are excited about something or we may speak more slowly when we are trying hard to be understood.

HANDY HINTS

How you hold your body when you are talking to people will give the other person an idea of how you are feeling. An example of this is smiling and standing upright when you are happy, and crossing your arms and frowning when you are not happy.

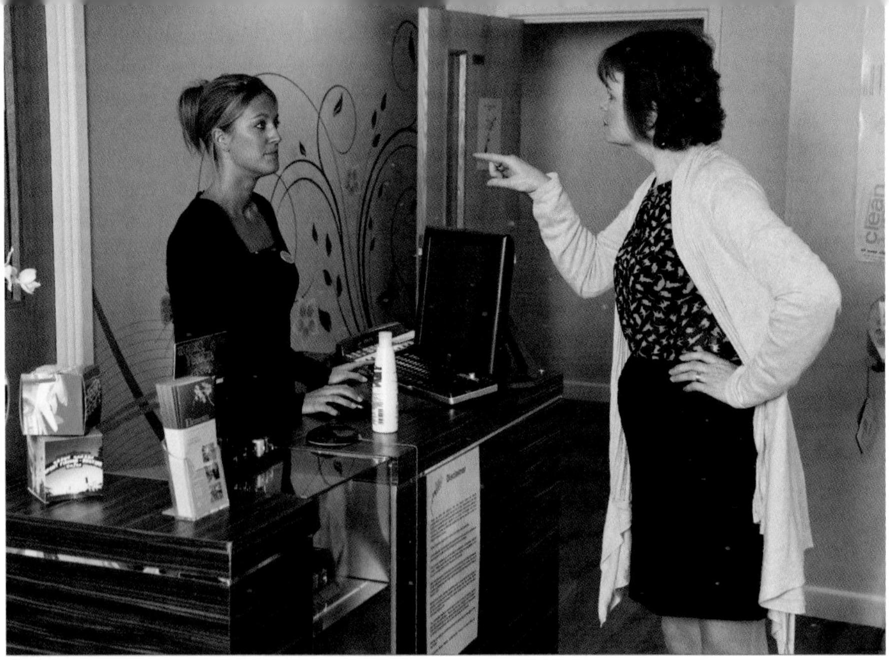

You know your client is angry if they point their finger at your

Gestures

Movements of the body to help communicate what you are saying, such as pointing a finger when you are angry

GESTURES

Gestures are when you use your body to support what you are trying to say. Examples of gestures are:

- nodding your head when you agree with what someone is saying
- shaking your head when you disagree with something
- pointing your finger at someone when you are cross
- waving your hand to say goodbye to a client
- straightening your arm to show the client where to go for the treatment
- moving your hands when you are talking to help get your point across.

However, the meaning of gestures can be very different across cultures and regions, so it's important to be careful to avoid confusion.

HANDY HINTS

If eye contact is made with someone for too long, it can make the other person feel uncomfortable. So although it is important to help you communicate with someone, do not overdo it!

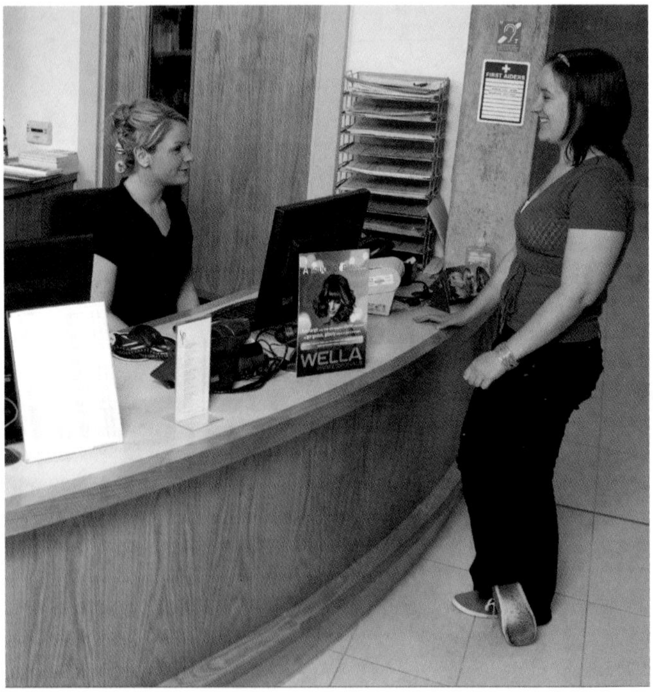

You must use good eye contact when talking to your clients

EYE CONTACT

Eye contact is a very important type of non-verbal communication. The way you look at someone can communicate many things. For example, the other person will feel that they are being listened to if you are looking at them. Good eye contact will not only help the flow of communication, but it can also help you to see their facial expressions and body language. This will tell you a lot about how they are feeling.

ACTIVITY

In pairs, have a conversation with each other for a few minutes. Take it in turns with one of you not giving any eye contact at all. Afterwards, write down your thoughts using the following questions as a guide:

- How does it make each of you feel when you are not giving any eye contact to your partner?
- How does it make each of you feel when your partner is not giving you any eye contact?
- How does this affect the conversation?

HANDY HINTS

A person who is shy may not feel comfortable looking at someone when they are talking. If you have a shy client, you can make them feel more relaxed by smiling at them and talking to them clearly and calmly.

BODY LANGUAGE

This type of non-verbal communication is all to do with how you hold yourself, for example the way you stand and move your body. The way that you sit and stand is called your 'posture'. If you have a good posture, it will help to stop backache and it will also communicate a more positive impression to your client. Examples of good posture are:

- sitting or standing upright, with your shoulders back
- holding your arms in an open or relaxed way, for example not crossed
- keeping your head up, not bent forwards.

If you sit or stand with your shoulders down and your back bent, this will not only give you backache after a short while, but will also make you look like you are not interested in what you are doing. This is not a positive body language to communicate to a client.

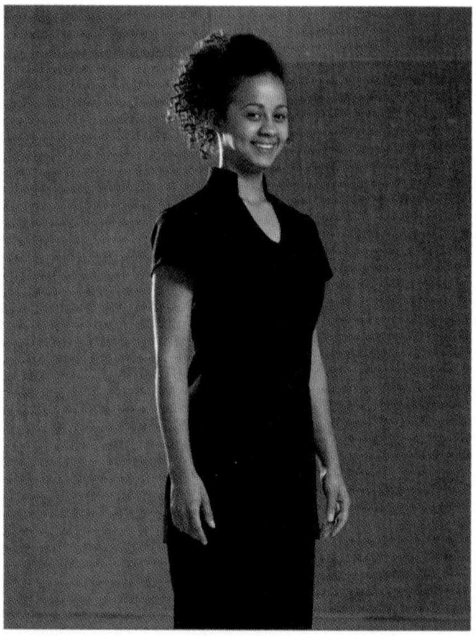

Good posture

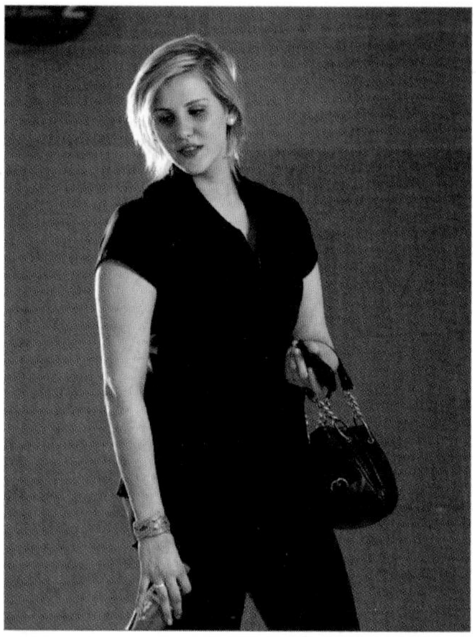

Bad posture

ACTIVITY

This activity involves you watching the people around you. You can do this in the reception area of a salon or in the cafeteria when you go on a break. Make a note of the different body-language signals that you see and how people are communicating with each other (such as yawning or making good eye contact). Ask yourself the following questions about what you see:

- What is their body language saying about how they are feeling?
- What is their body language saying about what they are talking about?

Discuss your answers with the rest of the group.

ACTIVITY

Working in small groups, design a poster illustrating examples of poor communication on one side and good communication on the other side. Try to use a variety of different resources such as magazines, the internet, books, photos of each other, etc.

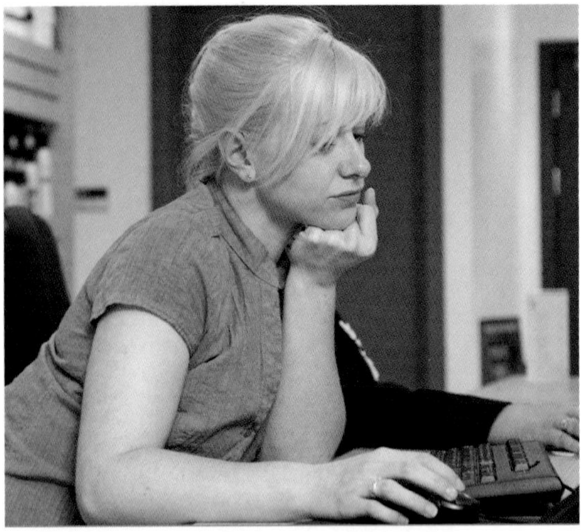

Closed body language

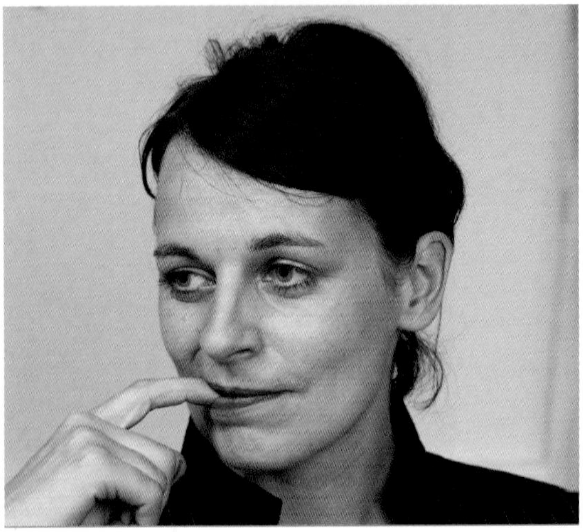

Biting the nails

ACTIVITY

For each of the following examples of poor body language, state what you think the person is telling you about how they are feeling:

- sitting with legs crossed, shaking their foot
- arms crossed on chest
- walking with hands in pockets and head down
- talking with their hand over their mouth
- biting their nails.

TOUCH

We communicate a great deal through touch. Whether it is hairdressing or beauty therapy, both industries involve some form of touch, e.g. shampooing a client's hair or massaging their arms in a manicure. It is important that you are aware that everyone has their own personal space (see below). This means that some people can feel very uncomfortable when someone else stands or sits too close to them. It is important to be aware of this as a hairdresser or beauty therapist, so that you can work in a professional and confident way. If you feel that the client is feeling nervous, then you can reassure them by lightly putting a hand on their arm or shoulder to reassure them. When you are treating the client, for example massaging conditioner into the hair or massaging the arm in a manicure treatment, it is important that you check with the client that the pressure you are applying is comfortable for them. This will help to make sure that the client is happy with the treatment.

HANDY HINTS

If you are unsure about how much pressure to apply with your massage, a good question to ask the client is: 'Would you like the pressure lighter, deeper or to remain the same?'

ACTIVITY

Think about and discuss what messages are being given by the following forms of non-verbal communication:

- a firm handshake
- a gentle tap on the shoulder
- a hug
- a gentle pat on the back
- a pat on the head
- a firm grip on your arm.

Discuss your answers with your tutor.

SPACE

Personal space
An area around the human body that people see as their own

Have you ever felt uncomfortable during a conversation because the other person was standing too close? We all have a need for our own **personal space**. This will differ depending on culture, the situation and the closeness of the relationship. In the hair and beauty industry, you will have to touch people. This can be very difficult when you first start working on clients. As you grow more confident, it will get easier.

HOW TO ADAPT COMMUNICATION

TONE AND CLARITY

How we sound when we speak does make a difference. If you talk in a voice that has the same tone throughout, your voice can sound very boring and dull. If you vary the **pitch** and **pace** of your voice, it will sound much more interesting to listen to. An example of this is speaking slowly when you are discussing the treatment with your client so that they can understand what is being said; also speaking in a higher pitch if you are excited about what you are talking about.

Pitch
How high or low the sound of your voice is

Pace
Speed

ACTIVITY

A good way of practising how to change the **tone**, **clarity**, pitch and pace of your voice is to talk to someone. Read out the following passage to a partner and repeat the passage by changing the following:

- Speak very quickly and quietly (pace and clarity) and in a deep voice. Do not change the tone of your voice.
- Now speak more slowly and in a louder voice. Use a different tone to the words you speak.

'Good communication is important for a hairdresser and beauty therapist. Good communication skills include smiling, being polite, having good eye contact and a relaxed posture. This will make the client feel comfortable and relaxed.'

Discuss with your tutor how it felt to be the one doing the talking and also what it was like to be on the one listening to what was being said.

Ways to improve the tone and clarity of your voice:

- Try slowing your voice down; don't talk so quickly.
- Take a few more breaths in between talking and lower your voice.
- Talk in a strong, steady voice, not shouting nor mumbling.

Tone
The level of the sound of your voice

Clarity
How clearly the words are spoken

ACTIVITY

Think about how you talk to someone in the following situations:

- someone who is ill
- greeting a friend across the street
- stopping a child from running out into the traffic
- telling someone you are not happy about something.

How does the tone of your voice change for each one? Discuss your answers with the rest of the group.

USING SIMPLE WORDS

When you communicate with your clients, it is important to remember that the client may not be aware of the technical terms that you use in the industry. It is therefore important that you use language that they will understand. Therefore, if you want your message to be understood, you must be careful of the words you use.

ACTIVITY

Write down some technical words that are used in either hairdressing or beauty therapy, such as manicure, temporary colour, disinfectant, conditioner, etc. (Use your log books to find other words that you might use.)

For each of these words, write down how you would explain what they mean (in more simple terms) to a client. Discuss this with the group.

HOW TO WORK AS A TEAM

It is very important to use your communication skills with your clients, but it is also important to create a good relationship with your colleagues too. You can improve **teamwork** between staff by:

- being friendly to each other
- by helping each other out, for example, helping a colleague tidy away after the client has gone
- being professional at all times, for example speaking politely to each other
- working together – two employees can get more work done in a shorter time if they work together
- by sharing each other's skills – each person has different skills and abilities and by working together, ideas can be shared
- supporting each other – the members of a team can offer support to each other, particularly during busy times. If there are lots of clients booked in for a treatment, then helping each other prepare for the treatments can save time.

HANDY HINTS

Good teamwork will make for a more enjoyable place of work.

Teamwork

Everyone working together for the good of the salon

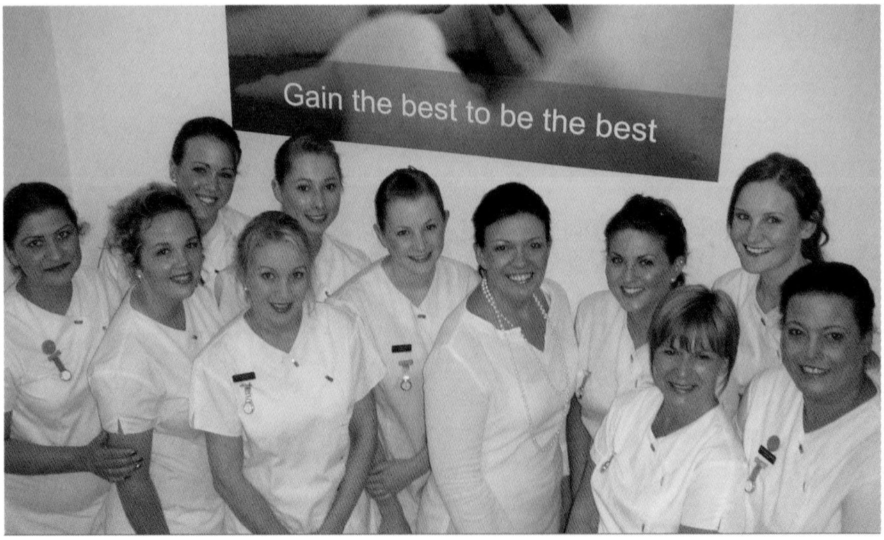

It's great to be in a team

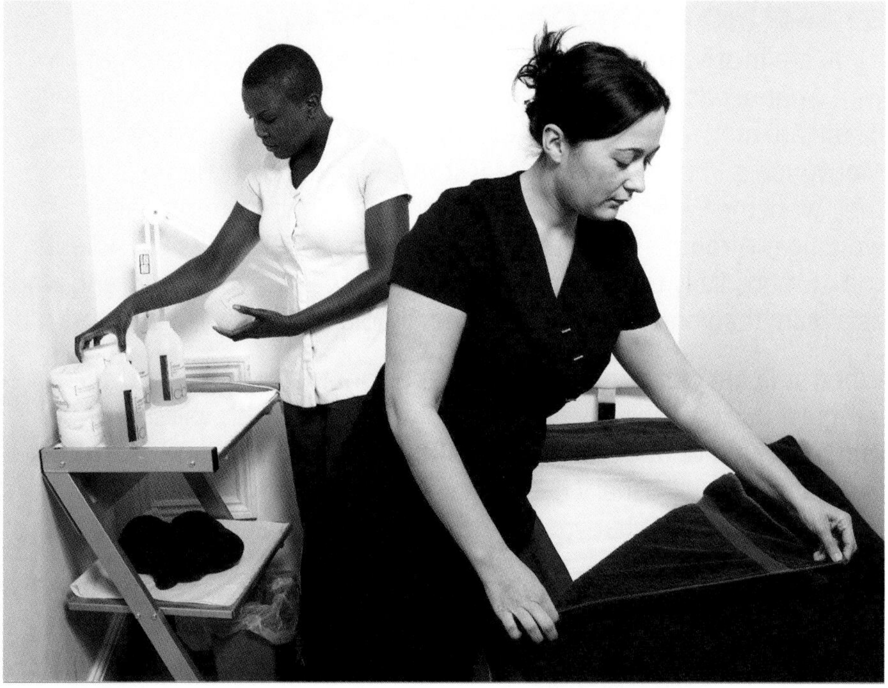

An example of good teamwork

THE BENEFITS OF GOOD TEAMWORK

There are many benefits to working as a team – here are a few of them.

HARMONY IN THE WORKPLACE

Having a **harmonious** workplace will create a positive working atmosphere and will make the salon a great place for staff to work, but will also help to encourage clients to the salon too!

Harmonious
Peaceful and calm; working well together

Harmony can be developed by making sure that there is good communication between all of the staff. You may not always get on with everyone that you work with, but if you behave in a professional way at all times, for example being polite and helpful, then the salon will be a more enjoyable place to work.

HANDY HINTS
It is important to look after both new and existing clients.

CLIENT SATISFACTION

If you have given a good service to your clients, they may **recommend** you to their friends and family. A happy client may recommend you to five friends who in turn have five friends who then recommend you. This will result in building your business. The best way to build a loyal client base is by having good communication and listening skills, being professional and by giving honest advice. If you give a bad service and act unprofessionally your clients may also relate this to their friends and family. This could have a negative effect on the business.

Recommend
Put forward or suggest someone

HANDY HINTS
Remember the acronym 'TEAM' – Together Everyone Achieves More.

STAFF MOTIVATION AND MORALE

Motivated
Feeling keen to do your work

If you are **motivated** at work, this means that you enjoy it and get on with what needs to be done, such as working on clients or tidying away. If staff are motivated, they will be happy and enthusiastic in their work. Motivation is important because if staff feel needed and respected in their work they will be happy. This will not only help to improve the working environment for other staff but also for the clients too. Clients will be more likely to come to a salon where the staff are happy and work as a team than one where they are miserable and not willing to work.

Morale
Confidence levels. Can be positive or negative

Appraisal
A meeting between an employee and their manager to discuss the progress of the employee

When staff are performing well it is important that they are told so on a regular basis, usually by their boss or supervisor. This will show how much they are valued and will improve their confidence and **morale**. In a salon, you will usually have regular **appraisals** with your supervisor or tutor to find out what you are doing well and what could be improved.

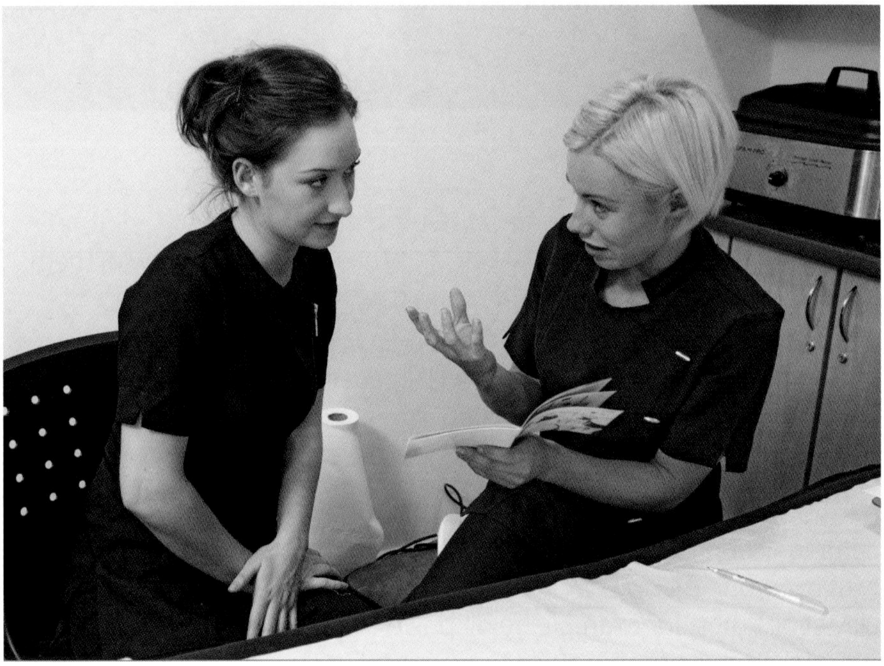

A therapist having an appraisal

POSSIBLE REWARDS

Some salons motivate staff by offering some kind of reward for hard work, such as selling the most products in a month. The following are examples of possible rewards:

- a prize, such as hair or beauty products
- a bonus in your wages
- time off work
- a promotion, eg from a junior to a senior stylist.

These rewards are there to give staff something to work towards and should help to motivate you. If you work well both on your own and as part of a team you will be rewarded.

OPPORTUNITIES FOR PROGRESSION

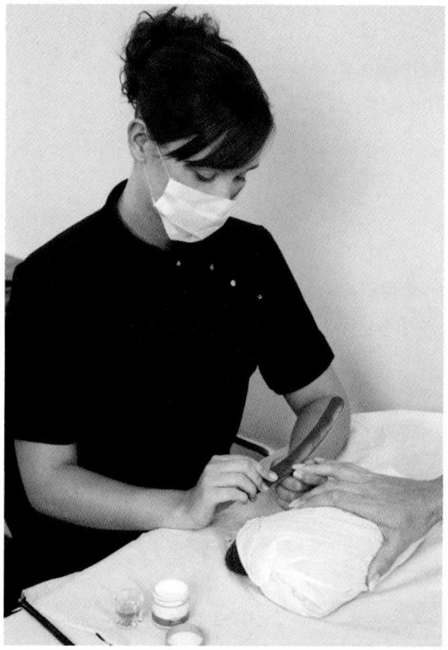

Training and personal development

Staff are important. If a salon owner makes sure that their staff are fully trained in all the latest techniques and products, this will not only help to motivate them, but will also make sure that the salon is kept up to date. The clients will also benefit from the updated knowledge and skills of the staff.

A good salon owner will:

- set aside money to spend on training courses for their staff
- make sure the courses that the staff go on will benefit the salon and the clients
- get feedback from staff as to how useful the training was. This will help them assess how useful it was sending them on the course.

If you behave professionally, are keen and work well in a team your tutor is more likely to let you go on training courses.

Personal and team achievement

In the hair and beauty industry there are many different roles that you may have in a salon. As you develop your skills you may move up to a more senior role. Here are of some of the roles available:

- salon junior
- hair stylist
- barber
- beauty therapist
- make-up artist
- nail technician
- salon manager
- receptionist
- salon owner.

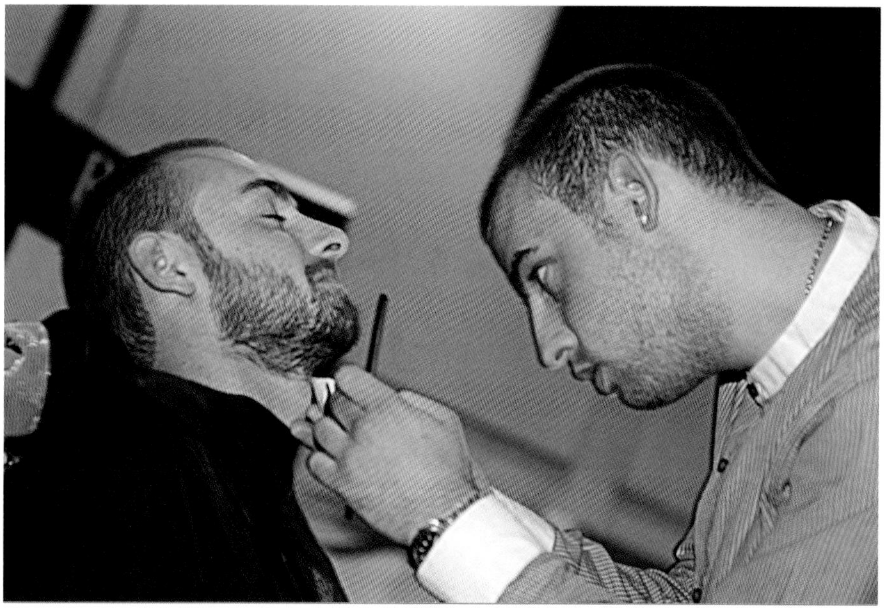

Some of the roles you may progress to during your career

ACTIVITY

For each of the above-mentioned roles, write down what someone in that role may be responsible for and what treatments they may be able to carry out. Check your answers with your tutor.

Each person in the salon has their job to do. In order for the salon to run well, every member of staff needs to carry out their job role properly. If everyone helps and supports each other, the salon will run more smoothly. It will also give the client a positive impression and encourage them to come back for more treatments.

HANDY HINTS

Look at Chapter 101 Introduction to the hairdressing and beauty sector, and read up on the above job roles.

HANDY HINTS

Many hands make light work. If everyone helps, jobs will get done more quickly.

ATTITUDE AND BEHAVIOUR

It is important to behave in a professional manner at all times. The following are ways that your **behaviour** can be more positive:

- Follow instructions given by your tutor, such as working with products and equipment in a hygienic and safe way. This will make sure that treatments are carried out professionally and correctly.
- Work co-operatively with others; this means treating your work **colleagues** and tutor with respect. This will help to make the workplace a more enjoyable place to be.
- Follow salon requirements; your salon may have certain rules that you will need to follow such as a dress code, for example a uniform, and being on time for your lessons and your clients.

Behaviour
The way you act

Colleagues
People that you work with

ACTIVITY

Refer to Chapter 102 Presenting a professional image in the salon, for more detailed information on communication and behaviour.

HANDY HINTS

Good impressions bring clients back. Good impressions lead to good business.

The following are all examples of negative attitudes and behaviour. You may come across people in a salon who behave in this way. If you do, then you may need some support from your salon manager to help you deal with them.

- Rudeness – examples of rude behaviour are using swear words, saying personal things about someone (eg they have a large nose), saying nasty things about another person, not listening to someone, gossiping about someone, talking when someone else is talking and telling lies or spreading rumours.
- Having a bad temper – this may create tension between staff and also put clients off from coming for treatment.
- **Indifference** – if someone is indifferent it means that they don't care. Working with someone who is not bothered about their work can be frustrating for other staff and does not develop good teamwork.
- **Arrogance** – arrogant people brag about themselves and tend to put other people down. Someone who is arrogant is very full of themselves. They feel they can do whatever they want. This kind of behaviour is not positive and can make people feel uncomfortable. It would be very unprofessional in a salon to behave in this way to either your colleagues or clients.
- Poor time keeping – being late to work will mean that you will be late for your clients. Unhappy clients will not be good for business and it may result in them not returning. If you are continually late, you will get into trouble with your boss and may even lose your job.

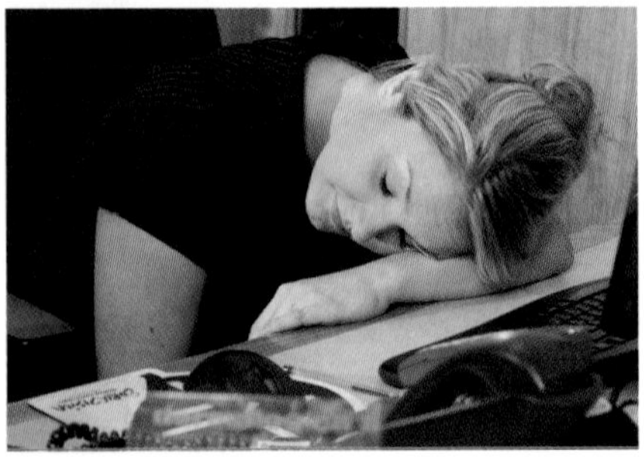

This receptionist is showing her clients a bad image

Indifference
Not caring about something

Arrogance
Pride; self-importance

ACTIVITY

Can you think of any more examples of rude behaviour that you may come across in a salon environment?

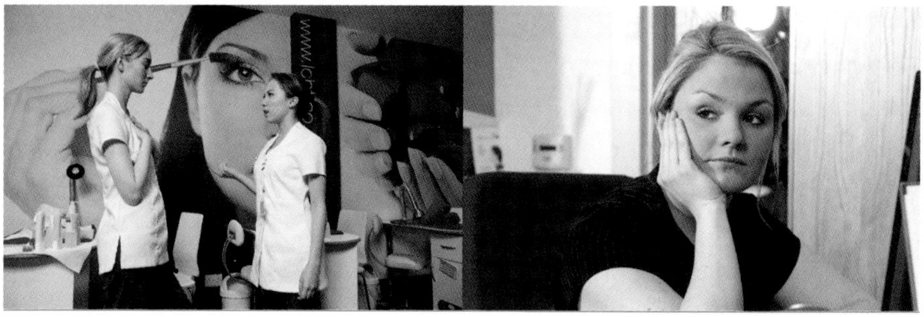

Having a bad temper and acting with indifference can damage the salon's image

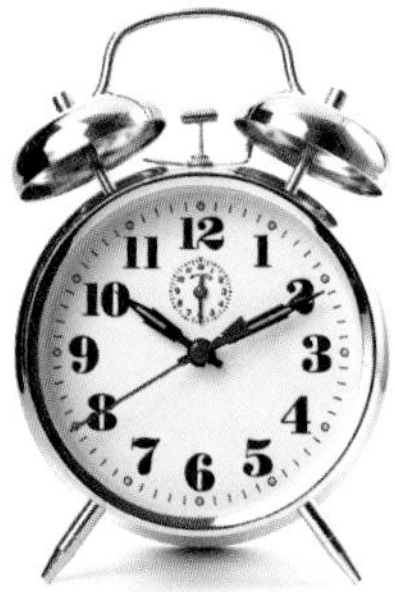

Good time keeping is important

ACTIVITY

Read the following case study and answer the questions that follow. Discuss your answers with the rest of your group.

Manjit has always wanted to be a hairdresser and is really pleased when she gets a job as a trainee hairdresser in a city-centre salon. She settles into her new job very quickly. When she arrives, she has to check how many clients are booked in. She also has to check the laundry to make sure that there are enough clean towels for the day. Manjit really enjoys her job and she is very reliable. She always arrives on time and completes her work very well. She is a friendly, popular person and the customers really like her. Manjit always says 'hello' to the other people she works with (Tom and Helen) before getting on with her work.

Manjit notices that Tom and Helen spend about half an hour chatting to each other before they get on with any work. Sometimes they also take long breaks and don't seem to tidy up properly at the end of the evening. It bothers Manjit as she works very hard to make sure that the jobs she is asked to do have been done properly and completely.

Manjit does not like to stand around with nothing to do. When she has finished her jobs, she helps Tom and Helen with their work. Tom and Helen are grateful for her help. Manjit is always happy and friendly. They begin to feel a bit guilty that Manjit is always helping them out. They don't say anything, but they do start to work a bit harder and sometimes help Manjit out.

The owner of the salon notices how hard they are all working and decides to give them all more money per hour.

Questions

1 Describe Manjit's attitude to her job.

2 What did Manjit do that helped Tom and Helen improve their work?

3 What might have happened if Manjit only focused on her own work?

4 How would you describe Tom and Helen's attitude towards their job before Manjit arrived?

5 What might have happened to Tom and Helen if Manjit had not started work at the salon?

When you have answered these questions, discuss them with the rest of the group to see what lessons you can learn from this case study.

WHEN TO REFER PROBLEMS

There may be times when you have to ask someone else for help. Examples of when this might happen include:

- when it is outside your level of responsibility – for example, if there is a query over an order of products and the person who deals with this is your employer
- when assistance is required – for example, if you are dealing with a query over a product and you are not fully trained in its use you may need to ask another colleague to help
- potential risk or hazard identified – for example, if you notice that there is a piece of broken equipment you will need to inform your supervisor
- in line with salon policy – for example, if the salon policy states who you should refer any queries to.

ACTIVITY

Think of some more examples for each of the situations described above. Write them down.

IN A NUTSHELL

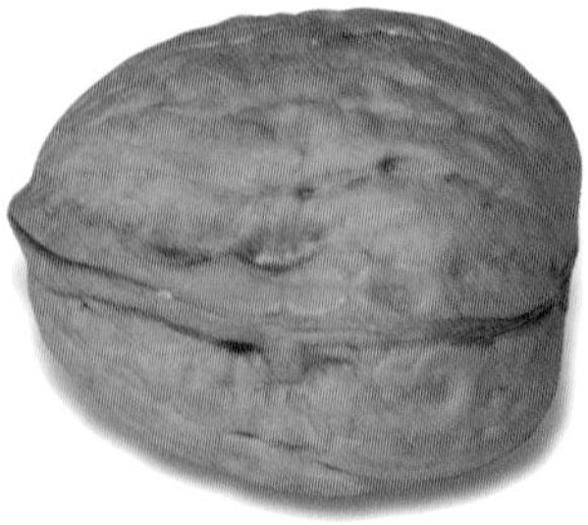

You are now at the end of the chapter. Before you test your knowledge with the revision activities, check the following list to see if you feel confident in all the areas covered. If there are still any areas you're unsure of, go back over them in the book and ask your tutor for extra support:

- how to communicate clearly and effectively
- how to support others to resolve problems
- how to follow safe and hygienic working practices
- the different ways to communicate
- how to adapt communication for different situations
- the benefits of effective teamwork
- the effects of negative attitude and behaviour
- the roles and responsibilities of team members
- when to refer problems.

REVISION ACTIVITIES

Using the questions below, test your knowledge of Chapter 115 to see just how much information you've gained. This can help you to prepare for your assessments.

Turn to page 487 for the answers.

WORDS TO FIND

Copy and complete the sentences below. Use these words to help you fill in the gaps.

verbal	rudeness	harmony	tone
non-verbal	teamwork	morale	body language
listening	communication	motivated	hygiene

1 Talking is a form of ______________ communication.

2 When we communicate, 50 per cent is through our ______________, 40 per cent is through our tone of voice and 10 per cent is through the words that we say.

3 Ways that you can show good ______________ skills include smiling, being polite, making good eye contact and having a relaxed posture.

4 An example of good ______________ is everyone working together.

5 If you speak with the same ______________ to your voice, it will sound very boring.

6 Smiling, nodding your head and having good eye contact are all examples of ______________ communication.

7 It is important for a hairdresser or beauty therapist to have good ______________ skills so that they understand what their clients are saying to them.

8 If staff are happy in their work then they will feel ______________ to do their job well.

TEST YOUR KNOWLEDGE FURTHER

Read the sentences below. State whether they are true or false.

1 When staff get along and help each other to get work done, everybody benefits. True or false?

2 An example of good teamwork is when everyone completes their own jobs. True or false?

3 Sharing ideas is not good teamwork. True or false?

4 Smiling is an example of verbal communication. True or false?

5 Rudeness is an example of negative behaviour. True or false?

6 Listening is an example of positive communication. True or false?

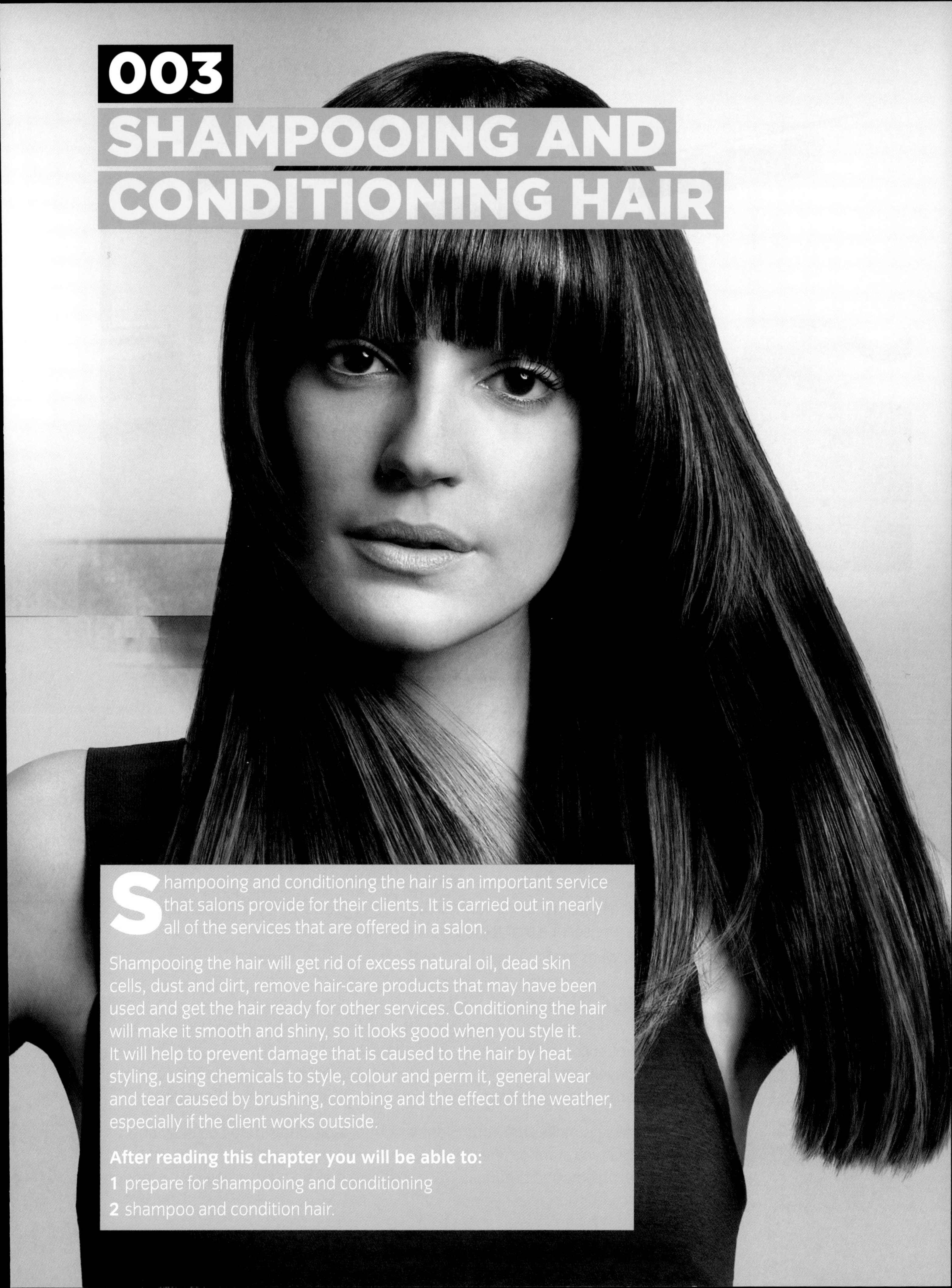

003 SHAMPOOING AND CONDITIONING HAIR

Shampooing and conditioning the hair is an important service that salons provide for their clients. It is carried out in nearly all of the services that are offered in a salon.

Shampooing the hair will get rid of excess natural oil, dead skin cells, dust and dirt, remove hair-care products that may have been used and get the hair ready for other services. Conditioning the hair will make it smooth and shiny, so it looks good when you style it. It will help to prevent damage that is caused to the hair by heat styling, using chemicals to style, colour and perm it, general wear and tear caused by brushing, combing and the effect of the weather, especially if the client works outside.

After reading this chapter you will be able to:

1 prepare for shampooing and conditioning

2 shampoo and condition hair.

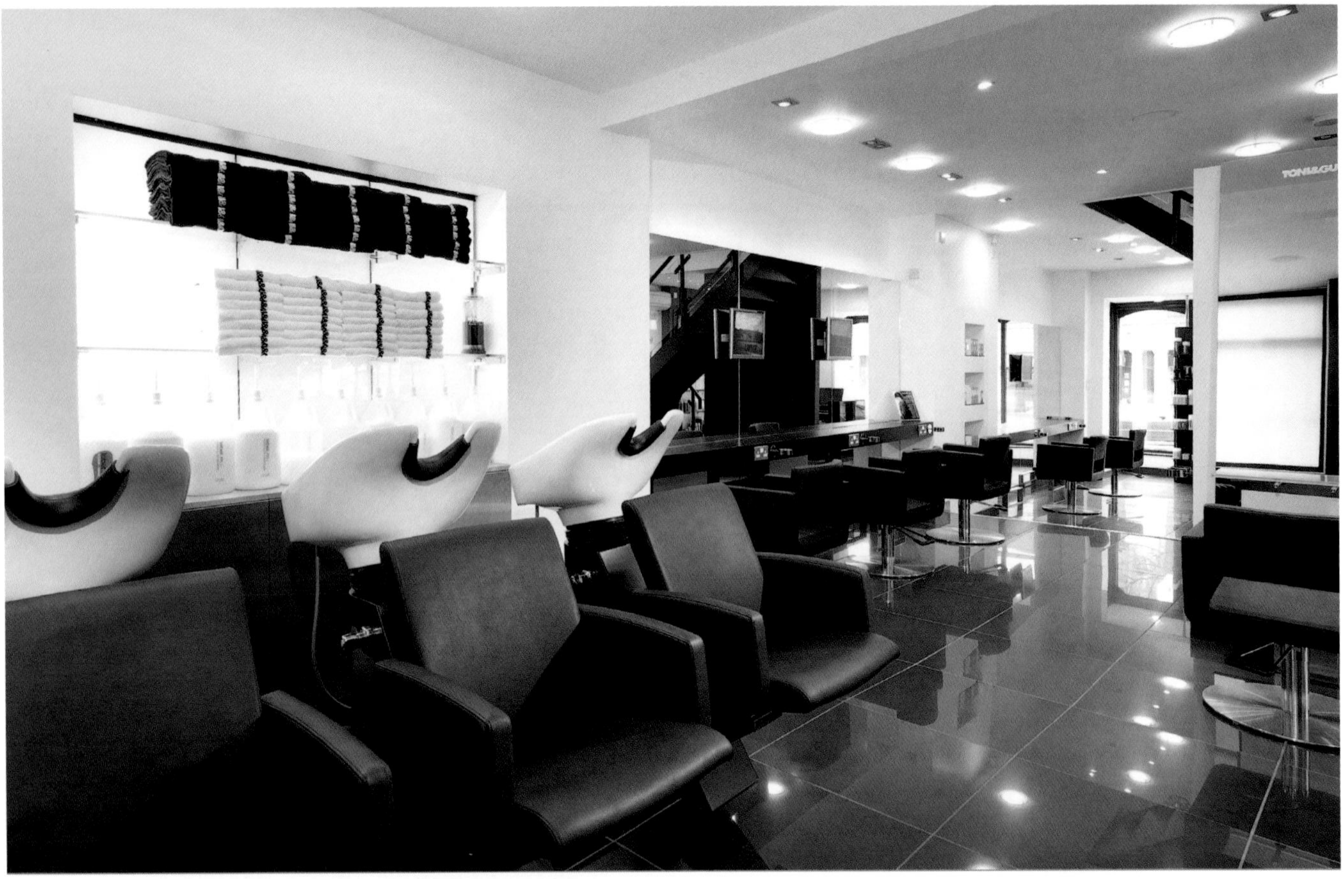

Shampooing and conditioning hair is an important part of hair styling

PREPARE FOR SHAMPOOING AND CONDITIONING

Experienced
Skilled; through doing a job for a long time

Experienced hairdressers will tell you that the shampoo part of the service is very important. It:

- cleanses the hair
- improves the condition of the hair
- relaxes the client
- prepares the hair for the service the client is having
- makes it easier to work with
- assists in making sure the hair looks good when you have finished the service that the client is having
- gives a good impression of the quality of your work.

WORKING SAFELY

Hygienically
In a way that keeps you healthy and clean

Colleagues
People that you work with

Working safely and **hygienically** is very important. You must make sure you follow salon procedures and the instructions from the stylist. Always pay attention to what you are doing and make sure you do not cause any injury or damage to yourself, your clients or your **colleagues**.

Always make sure your client is comfortable and sitting correctly and that you stand properly with your weight evenly spread to prevent back problems and tiredness. You must also make sure that you pay attention to your personal hygiene.

HANDY HINTS

Read Chapter 113 for more information on health and safety.

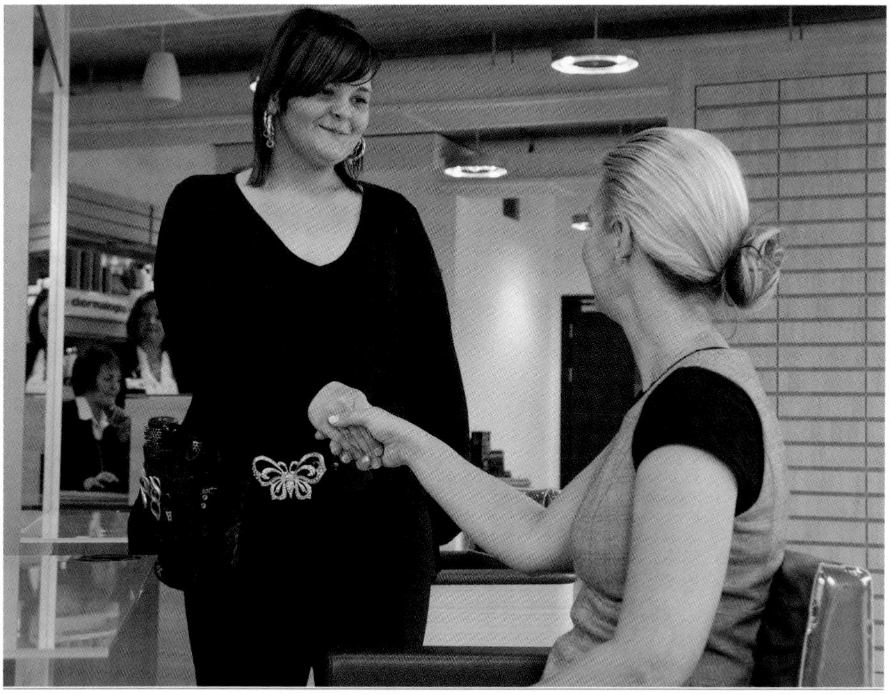

Introduce yourself to the client before shampooing their hair

HANDY HINTS

Read Chapter 102 to find out more about personal appearance and personal hygiene.

HANDY HINTS

Find out more about personal protective equipment from Chapter 113 Following health and safety in the salon.

HANDY HINTS

Poor personal hygiene can offend your clients and colleagues and presents a poor image of the salon.

For shampooing and conditioning, you must:

- know how to keep the work area clean and tidy
- make sure all the tools and equipment you need to use are hygienically clean and in good working order
- know the dangers and risks to yourself, your client and colleagues, and take all necessary steps to keep everyone safe
- know what personal protective equipment (PPE) you may need, eg gloves to protect your hands
- know how to carry out the shampooing and conditioning service.

PREPARING THE WORK AREA

There are three reasons why you should prepare your work area ready for work:

- to help you work safely and hygienically
- to give the client the right impression.
- to help you work efficiently.

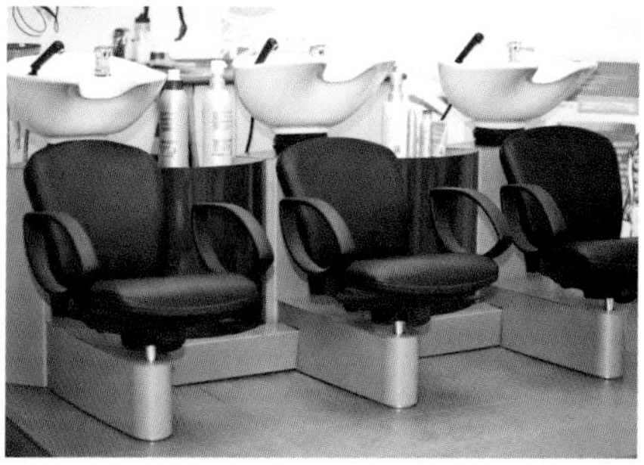

Keep work surfaces clean by wiping regularly with a suitable cleaner. Mirrors should be cleaned to remove smears and smudges. Tools and equipment should be in their proper places and always cleaned and sterilised after use to help prevent passing an infection from one client to another.

Sweep and clean the floor when necessary. Make sure the chair is clean. Clean the basin ready for the next client.

All the tools and equipment you use must be kept hygienically clean, in good working order and **sterilised** where necessary. All the items that come into direct contact with the client, such as combs, brushes, clips, towels, gowns and rollers, should be washed and sterilised after use to reduce the risk of **cross-infection**.

Sterilised
Made free from germs and viruses

Cross-infection
When an infection (like a cold) or an infestation (like head lice) is passed from one person to another

METHODS OF STERILISATION AND DISINFECTION

SmartScreen 003 worksheet 2

STERILISATION

Autoclave

This is a very effective way of sterilising. It is the method used in hospitals and dentists. The items to be sterilised are placed inside the container and water is heated to a temperature of 125° Centigrade. The items are left for ten minutes. This method is only suitable for metal or glass objects, as soft, plastic items will melt under the extreme heat.

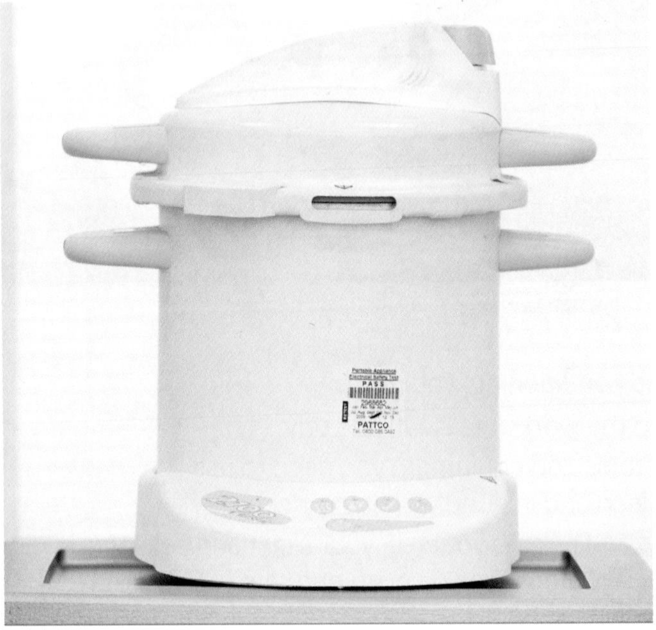

An autoclave

DISINFECTION

Ultraviolet (UV) radiation

A form of energy that prevents germs from growing

Ultraviolet radiation

This method uses **ultraviolet (UV) radiation** to disinfect items. The items should be washed first to remove grease, which can block the effect of the radiation. Items should be exposed to the radiation for at least 15 minutes. This method can be used for plastic items because the radiation will not affect them.

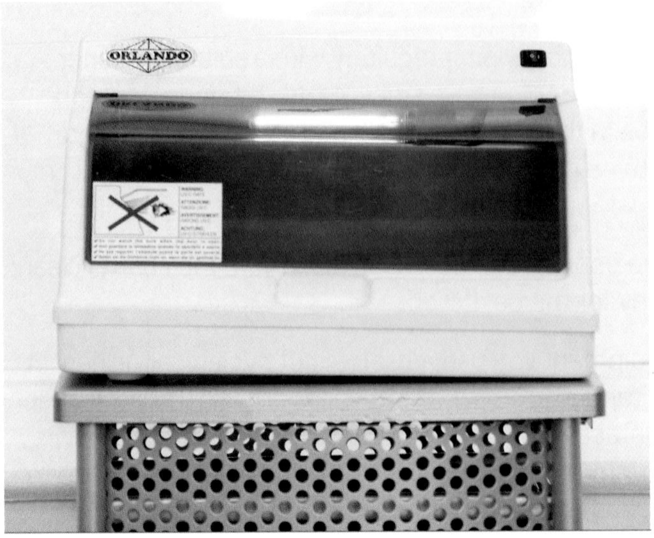

A UV cabinet

Chemical disinfection

This method is the one most commonly used in salons. The items are placed in a container filled with a chemical disinfectant. It can be used for most of the tools you use. The items should be washed first to remove dirt and grease, then totally **immersed** in the fluid. It is wise to use personal protective equipment (PPE) supplied by the salon such as suitable gloves because the fluids could damage your skin. Many salons use a brand called Barbicide for this method.

Immersed
Completely covered by a fluid

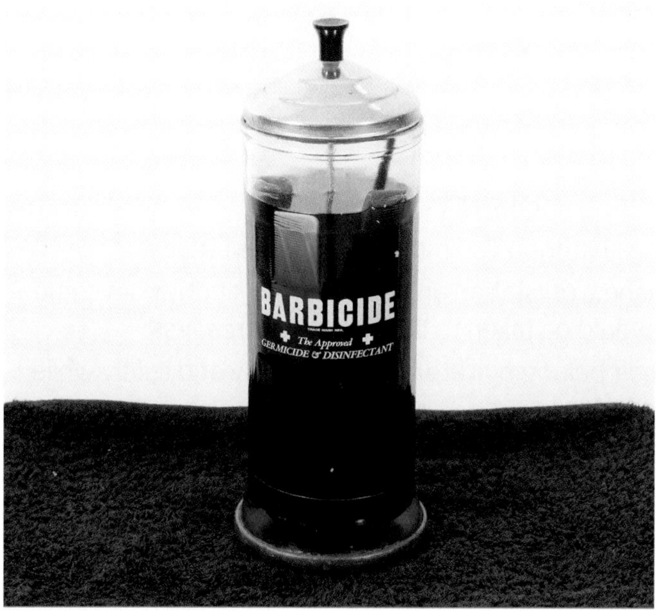

Barbicide

As well as sterilising/disinfecting all the tools you use on the clients, you need to make sure you keep all the work areas clean to stop **bacteria** from growing on them. Work surfaces should be cleaned thoroughly with a suitable cleaner and wiped regularly during the working day. This will help prevent the transfer of infection.

Bacteria
Germs that can cause an infection

The floors should be swept regularly to remove loose hair cuttings and other material that could cause you, your colleagues or clients to slip and injure themselves.

TOOLS AND EQUIPMENT

To carry out the shampoo you will need:

- a clean gown
- clean towels
- a wide-toothed comb (sometimes called a basin comb or a rake)
- a bristle brush
- shampoo (this will need to be selected after the client's hair has been assessed)
- conditioner if it is necessary.

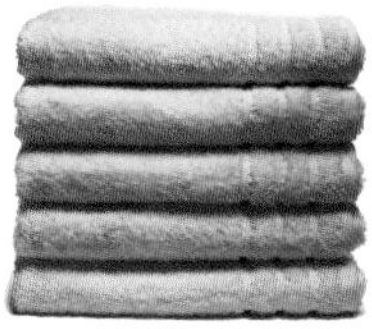

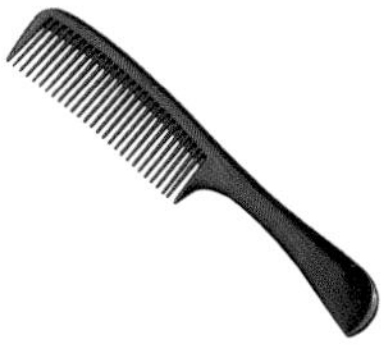

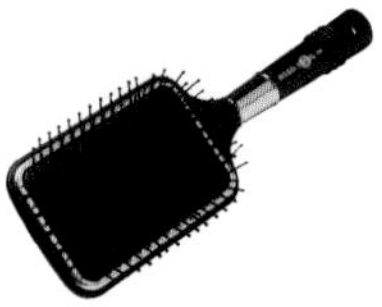

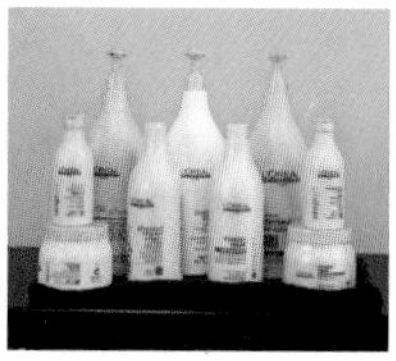

ACTIVITY

In pairs look around the salon to see what methods of sterilisation and disinfection are used.

SmartScreen 003 worksheet 1

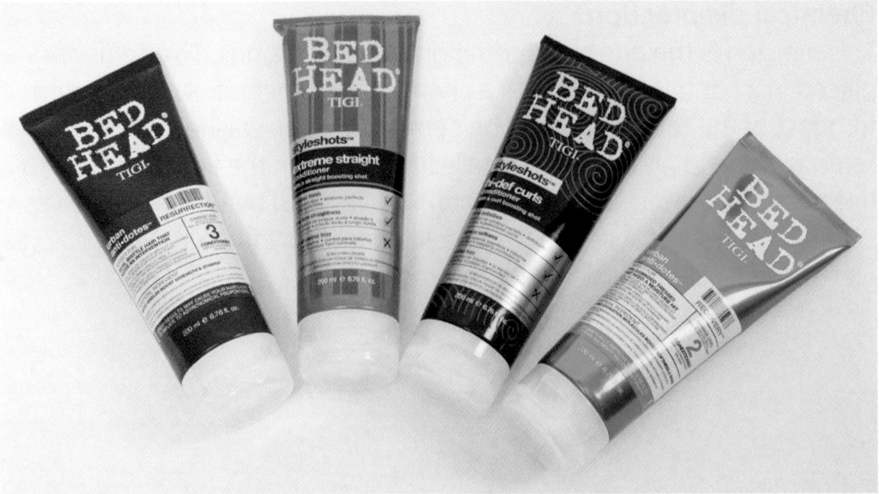

PREPARING THE CLIENT

Before you begin the shampoo you must get the client ready:

- Take the client to the workstation and ask them to sit down (in some salons the client would be taken to the shampoo area first).
- Make sure that their belongings are stored carefully and safely while they're in the salon.
- Place the gown around the client to protect their clothes while they're having their service.
- A clean towel should then be put round the shoulders.
- Some salons will use a strip of tissue or cotton wool around the neck to stop loose hair from going down the client's neck.

HANDY HINTS

Make sure the client is comfortable and sitting correctly.

HANDY HINTS

Remember – the salon is responsible for clients' clothes and belongings while they are in the salon and if they are damaged the salon may have to replace them.

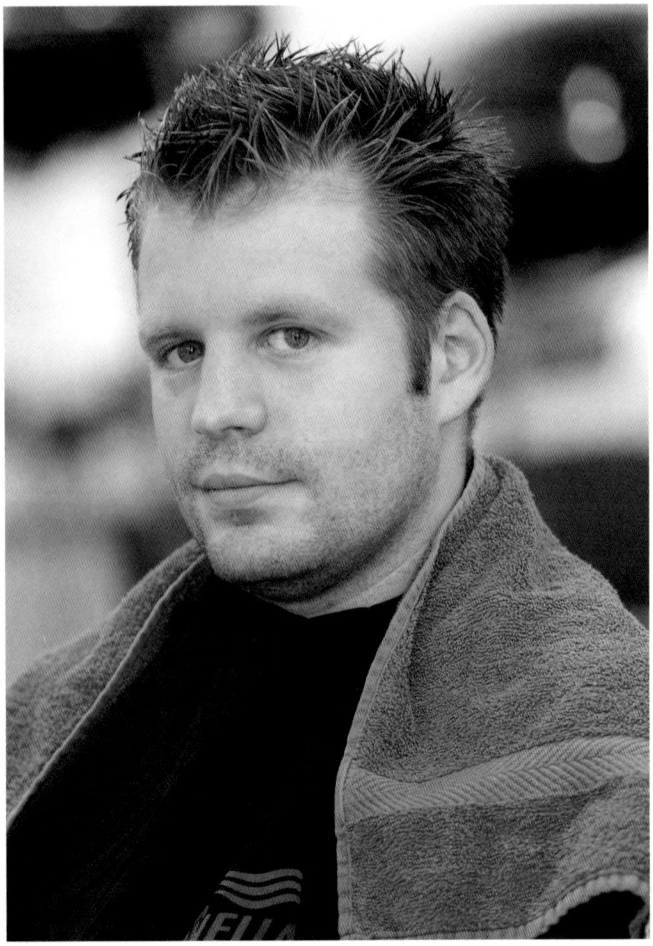

- Always make sure that client preparation is done properly.
- Before shampooing, brush the hair with a bristle brush to remove tangles (detangling), loose hair and dirt particles.
- Always start in the nape area (neck) at the points (ends) of the hair.
- Place one hand on the hair – this reduces any pulling on the scalp, which may be uncomfortable for the client.
- If the hair is mid-length to long, divide the hair into sections and do each section separately, again starting at the nape.
- Combing and brushing can be done before or during the consultation.

ACTIVITY

Read the text and fill in the blanks below:

Take the client to the ______________________.

Make sure that their ______________________ are stored carefully.

A towel should then be put round the ____________.

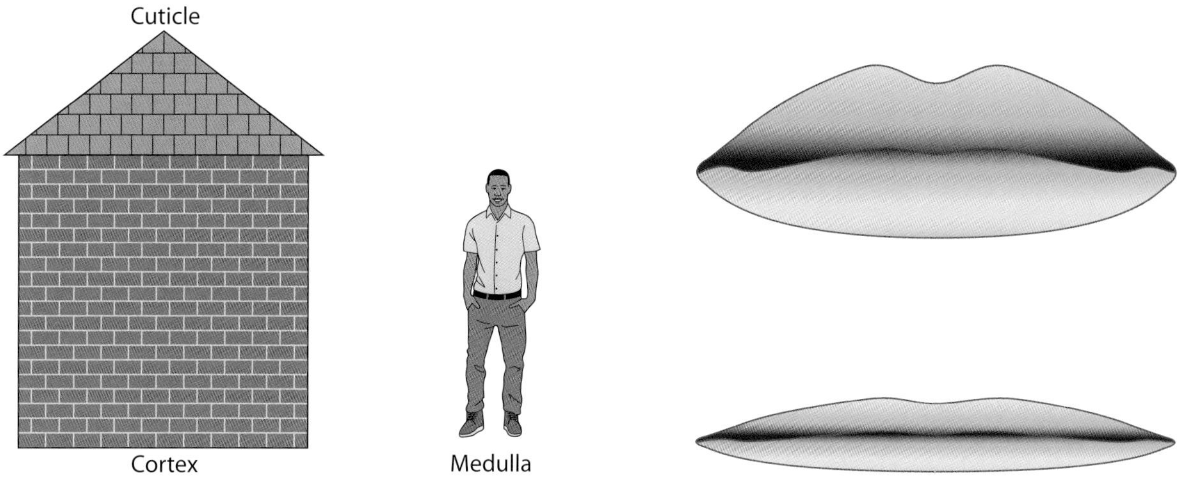

A cuticle is like the roof tiles on a house – they protect the structure of the house. The cortex is like the main structure of the house. The medulla is like a person – it has no real effect on the main structure of the house – sometimes they are at home and sometimes not!

THE STRUCTURE OF THE HAIR

Learning about the structure of the hair is important. It will help you understand what happens when you carry out all the services the client wants. Knowing how things work and the way they are carried out is important.

A single hair has three parts. The outside of the hair is called the **cuticle**. It is made up of scales or tiles that are 'see-through' and look like the scales you find on a fish. The scales overlap each other from the '**root**' to the 'point' of the hair. The cuticle protects the hair and when it is in good condition makes the hair shine. It is easily damaged by heat, chemicals, the weather and rough treatment.

Between the cuticle and the centre of the hair is a layer called the **cortex**. This layer gives the hair its shape so it is important to you when you style the hair. This layer contains the pigments that give the hair its colour and also gives the hair its strength. The cortex can be damaged if you use chemicals on the hair.

The centre or core of the hair is called the **medulla**. This layer attracts water and some colour pigments are found here. Some hair types do not have this layer.

The client is now ready for the consultation part of the service.

ACTIVITY

Use the internet to find out more about the structure of the hair. Share what you find out with the rest of your group.

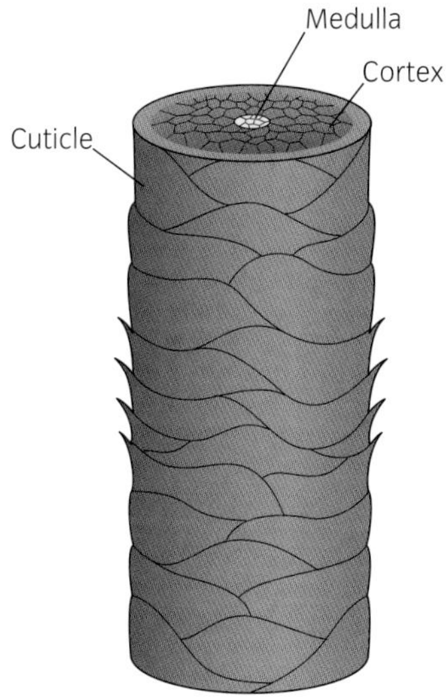

The structure of the hair

SmartScreen 003 handout 1

Cuticle
The outer layer of the hair; protects the hair and gives the hair its shine

Root
The part nearest to the scalp

Cortex
The middle layer; gives the hair its strength and contains the colour

Medulla
The centre or core of the hair; attracts water and contains some colour pigments

Experience
Knowledge gained from working

CLIENT CONSULTATION

This will probably be carried out by the stylist who is carrying out the other services that the client is having. As you gain **experience** you will be able to carry out the consultation yourself.

The consultation helps you to find out what the client wants done and for the stylist to decide how it will be done.

To decide on how you are going to carry out the shampoo and conditioning service you need to find out quite a bit of information. Use the following activity to help you.

ACTIVITY

Working in pairs, ask the following questions and discuss the advice you would give:

- What has the client had done to their hair recently?
- What hair type does the client have?
- What is the texture of the hair?
- What products has the client used on their hair?
- Are there any hair and scalp conditions that might affect the services you have to give?

When you have found out all this information you can make your decisions:

- what shampoo you are going to use
- how you will carry out the shampoo
- whether you need to condition the hair, and if so, which conditioner you will use
- how you will carry out the conditioning treatment.

The stylist will also make lots of other decisions about the other services that the client is going to have.

You will find out what you need to know by:

- talking to the client
- asking them questions about their hair, eg what products they use, how often they shampoo their hair and why, what chemical treatments they've had (colour or perm for example).

Looking at the hair will tell you about the texture and the condition of the hair. Does it look greasy, or dry and straw-like? It may look shiny, or it may look dull and the ends of hair may be rough-looking. You can also see how thick the hair is and how long it is.

Feeling the hair will tell you more about the condition of the hair and its texture. The hair might feel rough or greasy; it might feel fine and delicate or thick and coarse.

COMMUNICATION AND BEHAVIOUR

Communication and **behaviour** are very important when shampooing and conditioning. You may have great hairdressing skills but if you can't communicate with clients then they will not feel comfortable enough to visit the salon again. In order for clients to feel happy about coming to you for shampooing and conditioning, you need to feel comfortable with them, even if you haven't met them before. This starts with being confident about what you're doing, and thinking about the types of question you're asking.

Communication
The way you talk to your clients

Behaviour
The way you act

HANDY HINTS
Refer to Chapter 102 for more detail about communication and behaviour.

PROFESSIONAL IMAGE

To show a truly professional image to the clients you must always:

- treat them with politeness and respect
- give them your full attention when working on them
- make sure they have everything they need during their visit
- communicate with them clearly
- make sure your body language is positive and gives the right messages
- make sure your appearance and behaviour are up to standard
- respect client confidentiality (don't tell others what the client tells you)
- talk to the client while you are working on them.

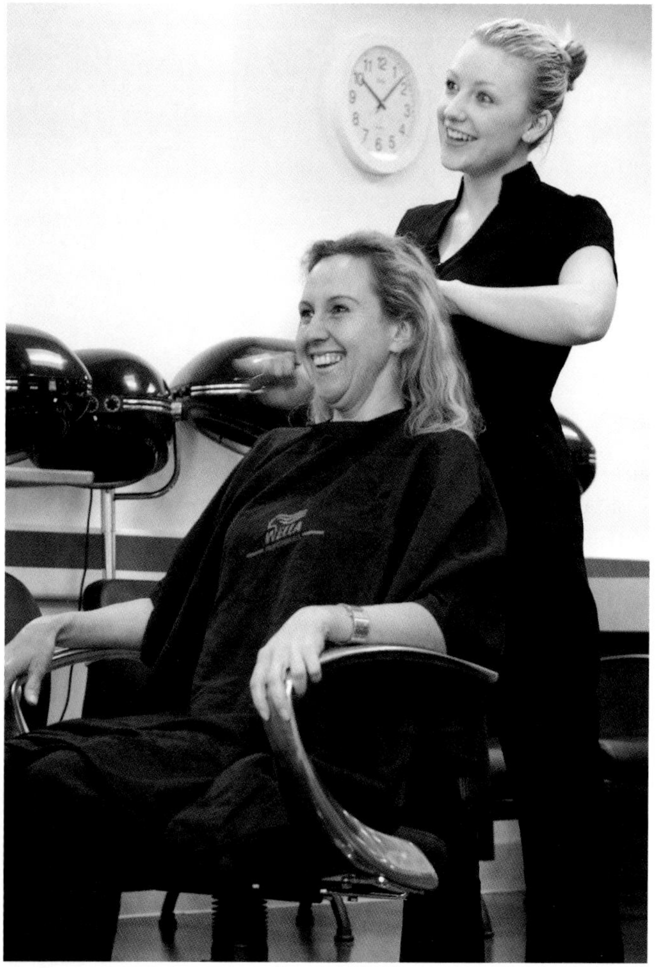

Let's go through a consultation for the shampoo and conditioning service.

Begin by talking to the client and asking the following questions to find out how they treat their own hair:

- what shampoo they use
- if they use conditioner
- what styling products they use and how they style their hair (eg do they use tongs, etc).

While you are talking to the client, look at and feel the hair to feel the hair's natural condition. This will help you decide what hair type the client has:

- Normal – the hair shines and looks good; it feels smooth.
- Oily – the hair looks greasy and dull; it feels sticky.
- Dry – the hair looks dull and straw-like; it feels rough to the touch.
- Dandruff – the hair has white flecks in it; these might also be on the client's clothes around the shoulders; the scalp looks scaly and rough.
- Damaged – the hair looks similar to dry hair but is rougher to the touch.

It may sometimes be difficult to make your choice because of a build-up of products that the client has used. These can sometimes hide the condition of the hair. They must be removed during the shampoo because they may affect other services that the client is going to have.

CONDITIONS TO LOOK OUT FOR

At this stage of the consultation you should look at the hair and scalp to see if the client has any infections or conditions that might prevent you from carrying out the service. Look for:

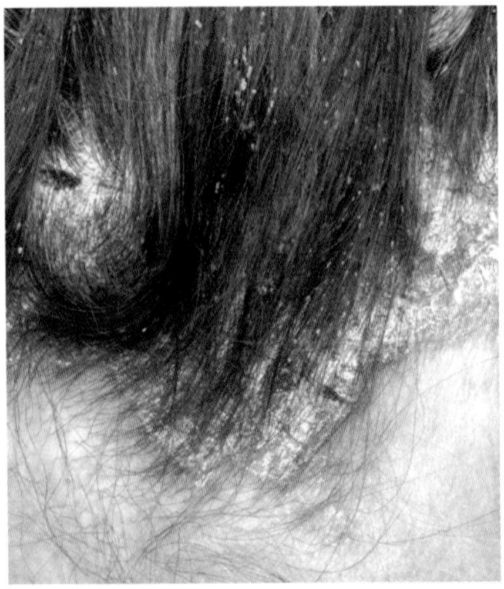

- scaly patches or rough areas on the scalp

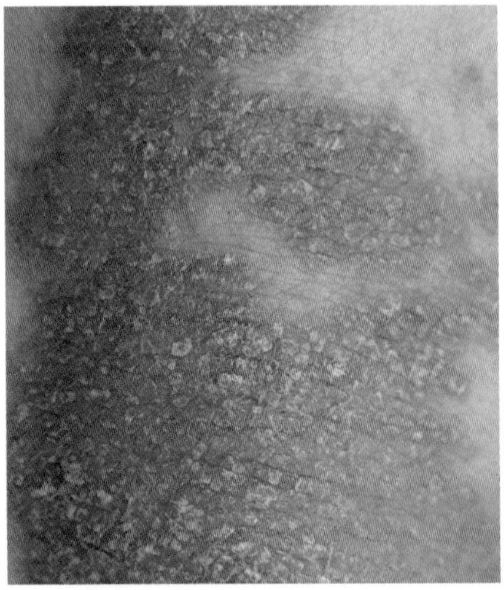

- red, inflamed patches

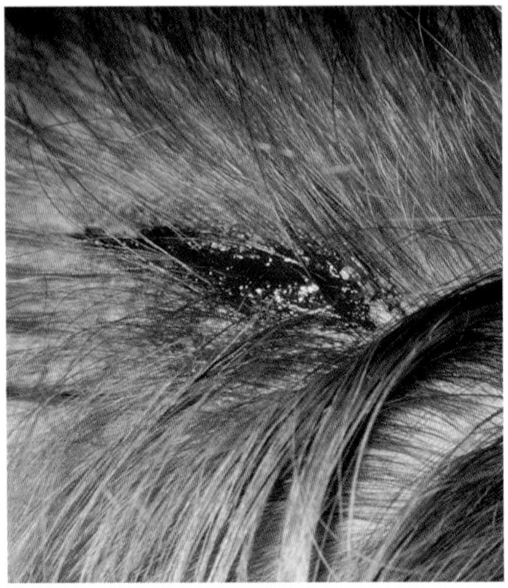

- cuts and abrasions on the skin

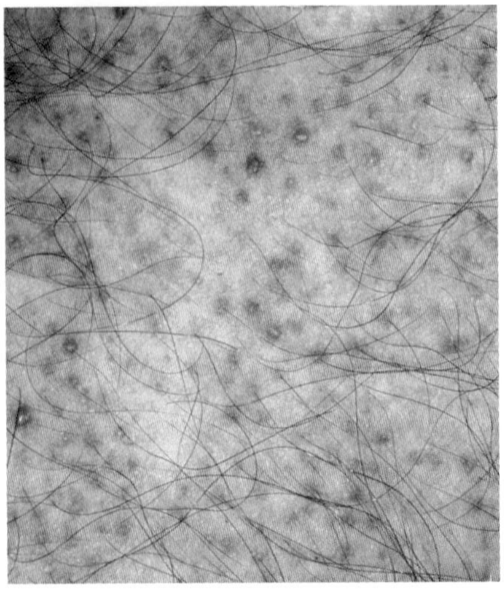

- lumps and bumps or raised areas

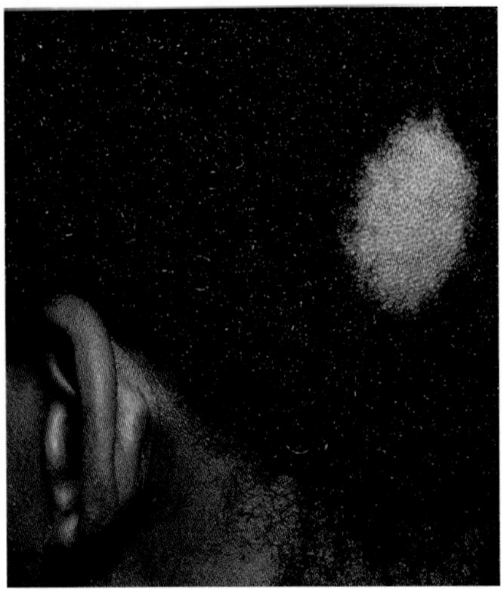

- bald patches

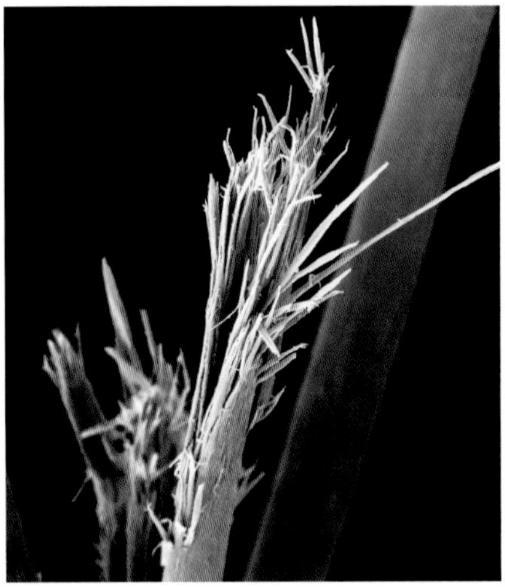

- hair breakage.

ACTIVITY

See if you can find out what may cause these six conditions.

Head lice

It is also important to look for things like head lice. This is an infestation of parasites that cement their eggs on the hair. The eggs are called nits and look like dandruff but do not move. This condition is very **contagious** and the lice can be easily passed from person to person by sharing combs and brushes and close contact. If a client is found to have head lice, action must be taken quickly. The salon will have its own procedure that should be followed if a client is found to have head lice. Everything that has come into contact with the client should be washed and sterilised as soon as possible. The lice and eggs can be killed using a suitable medicated lotion. It is important not to embarrass the client. Always be tactful and helpful. As you progress in your career you will learn more about hair and scalp disorders.

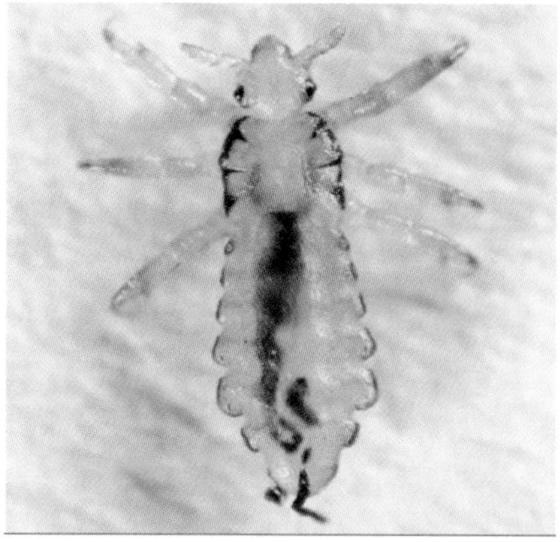

A head louse

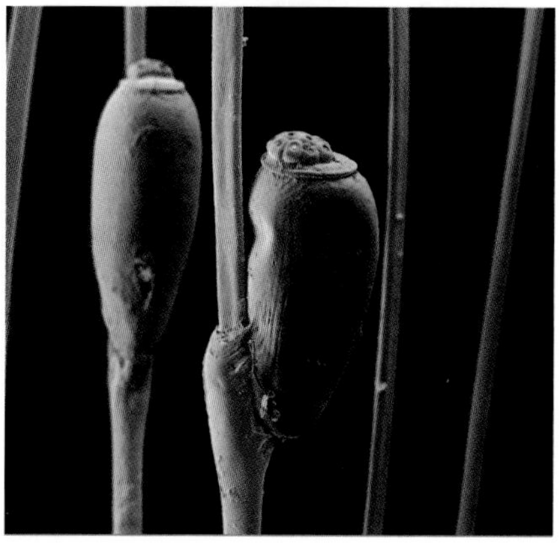

Eggs/nits

SmartScreen 003 handout 2

Contagious
Describes a condition that can be passed from one person to another, for example by using unclean tools or the same tool for two clients

ACTIVITY

Find out what your salon's procedure is if you suspect that a client has head lice. With a partner, practise carrying out that procedure. Pretend that one of you is the client and the other one is the stylist.

SELECTING THE SHAMPOO AND CONDITIONER

The last part of the consultation is to select the shampoo you will use and how you will shampoo the client's hair. You will also do the same if you need to condition the hair.

SHAMPOO

Shampoos come in many forms – gels, creams, liquids and pastes. Each manufacturer will produce a range of shampoos for use on all the hair types you looked at earlier. For example:

- mild shampoos that can be used every day
- medicated shampoos such as anti-dandruff or greasy hair shampoo
- conditioning shampoos for dry or damaged hair
- colour-saving shampoos for coloured hair.

ACTIVITY

- Make a list of all the shampoos that are used in the salon. Read the manufacturer's instructions to find out what type of hair they are suitable for and how they should be used. Complete the table below.
- Find out about the safety precautions that you need be aware of when you use the shampoo and what to do if something goes wrong during use.

Hair type	Shampooing product
Normal	
Greasy	
Dry	
Dandruff	
Coloured	

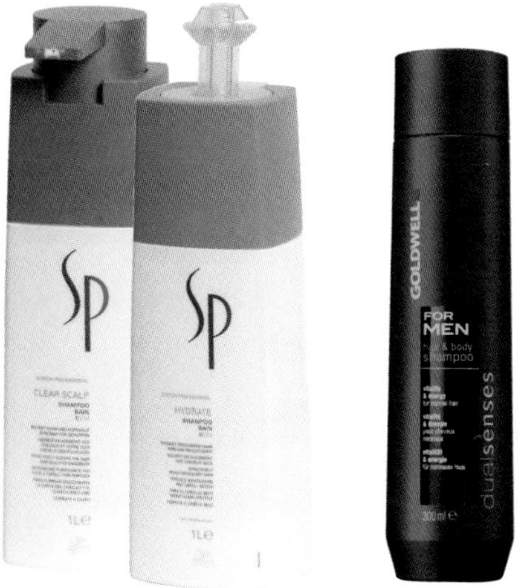

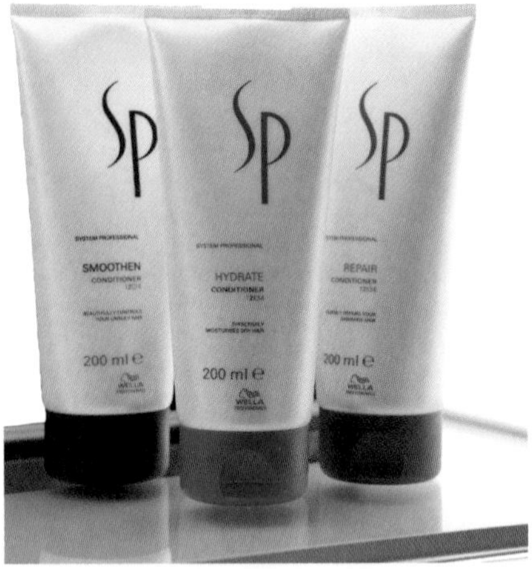

CONDITIONERS

There are conditioners to suit all hair types. For example:

- Surface conditioners – these will help to improve the condition of the cuticle layer of the hair. They soften and flatten the cuticle scales.
- Penetrating conditioners – these are used if the cortex has been damaged by the use of chemicals.
- Treatment conditioners – these are used where the hair is badly damaged and in very poor condition.

At this stage we will look at the use of surface conditioners and how they help improve the look of the client's hair.

HANDY HINTS

Read about the COSHH regulations for chemicals you use in the salon in Chapter 113.

HANDY HINTS

Clients with fine or thin hair often prefer the water cooler than those with thick, coarse hair.

ACTIVITY

As you did with shampoos, make a list of the surface conditioners available in the salon. Read the manufacturer's instructions and make notes on what they tell you. Complete the table below.

Hair type	Conditioning product
Normal	
Greasy	
Dry	
Dandruff	
Coloured	

MASSAGE MOVEMENTS

There are four massage movements that are used for shampooing, conditioning and giving a scalp massage. Each has a different effect on the hair and scalp.

EFFLEURAGE

This is a soft stroking movement made by gently rubbing the palms of the hands over the scalp.

It is used to spread the shampoo or conditioner over the hair and scalp and has a relaxing effect on the client. It can be used on greasy hair as you do not want to rub the scalp too vigorously which would make the hair greasier by stimulating the sebaceous glands.

ROTARY

This is given by making the hand like a claw and then rubbing the pads of the fingers in circular movements over the hair and scalp. This will cleanse the hair and it will relax the muscles of the scalp and improve the blood flow in the skin. This will help to produce healthy hair. It should be given for at least a minute.

FRICTION

This technique is the same as rotary but is carried our out faster and with more pressure. Friction will stimulate the sebaceous glands so is useful if the hair is dry.

PETRISSAGE

Petrissage is a kneading movement used when conditioning or giving a scalp massage. The fingers are spread out and used in a slow circular deep kneading movement. It stimulates the sebaceous glands, relaxes the muscles and improves the blood flow through the skin. It is a very relaxing massage movement.

DECIDING WHAT YOU ARE GOING TO DO

In deciding how you are going to carry out the shampoo you must follow the manufacturer's instructions for the shampoo you have selected and what you found out in the consultation. This will include:

- the temperature of the water – this will be decided by the client's preference and the hair type
- what massage movements you will use
- whether you need to shampoo once or twice
- how much product is needed.

You will do the same for the conditioner if you are going to use one.

You should now be ready to carry out the shampoo and conditioning service.

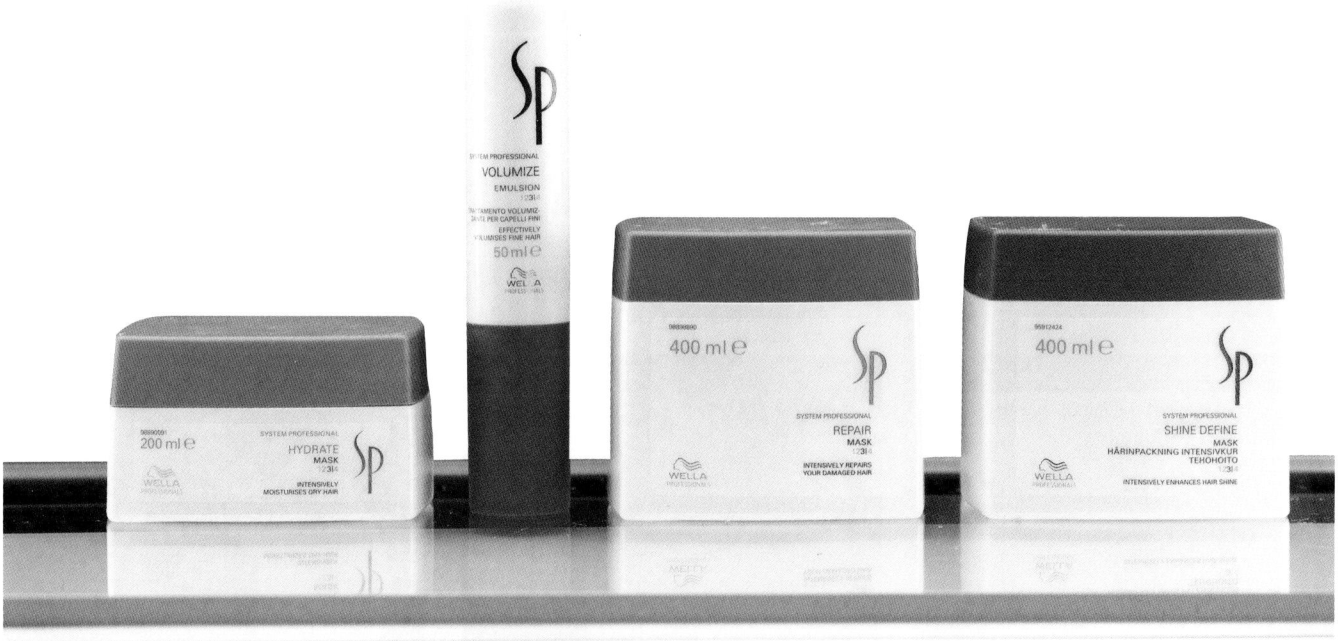

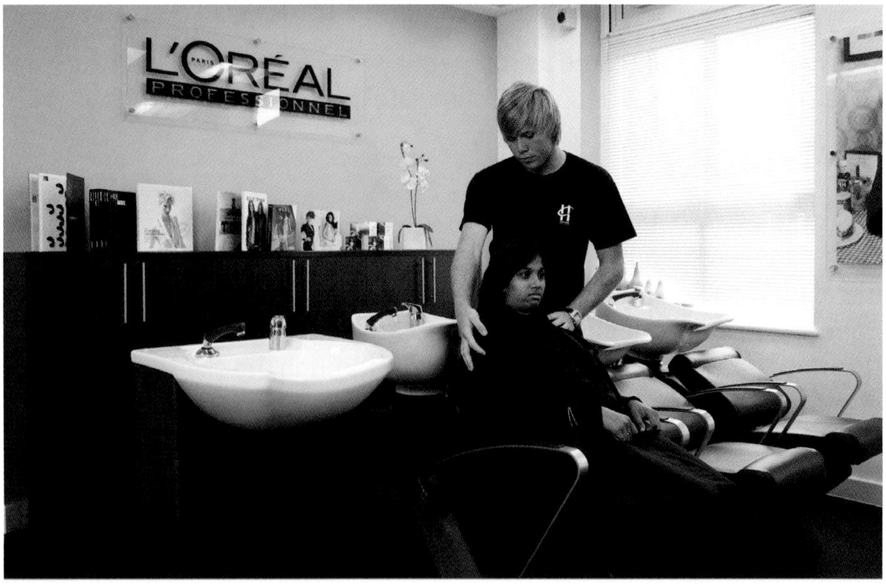

Seating a client at the shampoo area

HOW TO CARRY OUT THE SHAMPOO AND CONDITIONING SERVICE

In this part of the chapter you will learn how to shampoo and condition the hair, and how to towel dry and detangle it ready for the next part of the service.

SHAMPOOING THE HAIR

Take the client to the shampoo area and seat them at the basin. Many salons have both front-wash and backwash basins. Which you use is determined by the client's preference; if they have a back or neck problem they may need a front-wash.

Make sure the client is comfortable, and if you are using the backwash basin that their neck is in the correct position as it may hurt them or cause injury.

Turn on the water and adjust to the required temperature. Test it on the inside of your wrist or the back of your hand.

With a backwash, wet the hair starting at the front, using one hand to stop the water going onto the face.

HANDY HINTS

Check regularly with the client that the water temperature is OK for them.

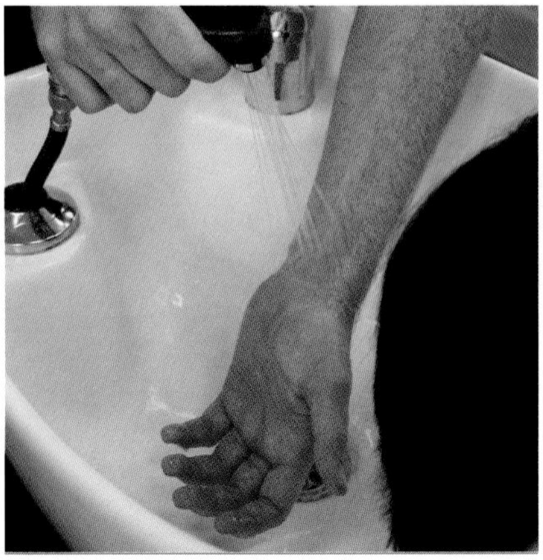

Make sure the water isn't too hot or cold

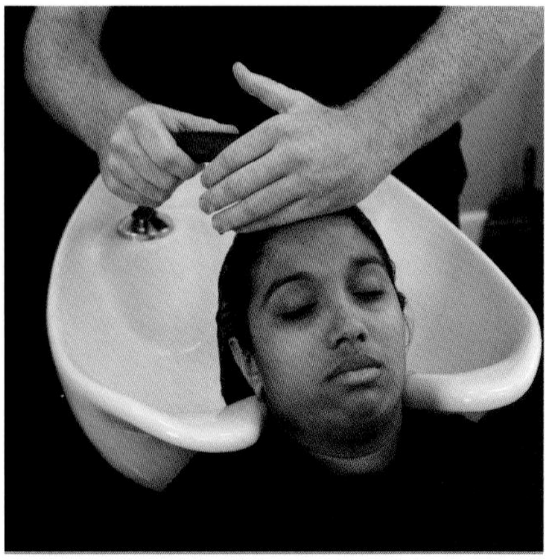

Make sure the water doesn't go in the client's eyes

When the hair is wet turn off the water; do not leave it running as this is wasteful and costs money.

Pour the required amount of shampoo into the palm of your hand (how much will depend on what the manufacturer recommends, the length of the hair and whether the hair is greasy or dirty). Do not use more than you need to.

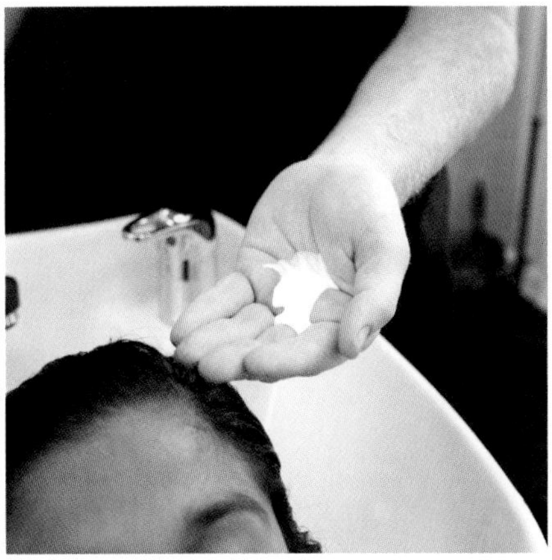

MASSAGE MOVEMENTS

Rub the hands together and use a effleurage movement to spread the shampoo over the hair with the hands flat to the head.

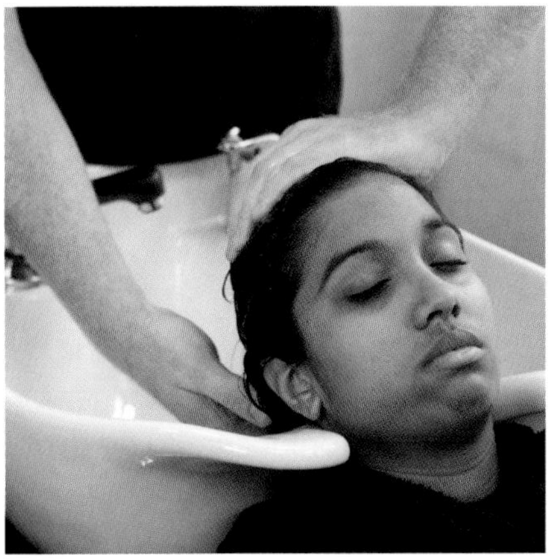

When the shampoo is well spread through the hair, use the next massage movement called rotary to cleanse the hair.

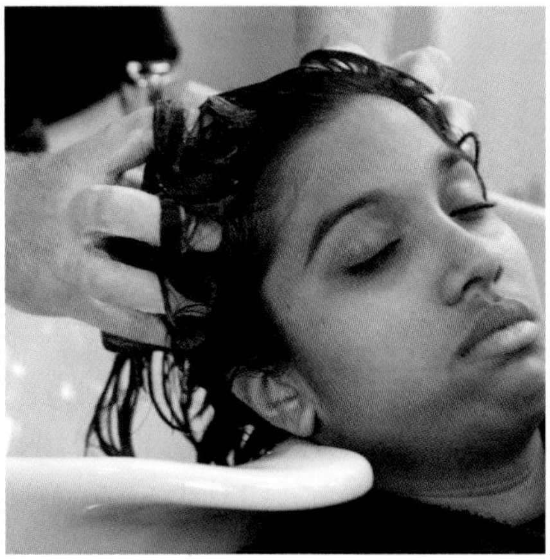

This will work the shampoo into a lather, causing it to break up the grease and loosen the dirt particles sticking to it. The lather will collect the bits of dirt that are on the hair. When you rinse the hair the dirt and the grease will be washed from the hair.

This massage should be given for at least a minute. With long hair you need to rub the hair in the hands to work up the lather and spread the shampoo. Be careful not to tangle the hair too much as you do this.

Always ask the client if the massage is firm enough for them and rub harder or more gently if you need to.

HANDY HINTS

Using more shampoo than you need is wasteful and costs money.

HANDY HINTS

Always make sure you have worked up a lather throughout the hair so it can clean the hair properly.

HANDY HINTS

Remember – client preference as well as the hair type will determine which type of massage is used and how firmly or gently you carry it out.

RINSING THE HAIR

Contact dermatitis
A serious skin condition that can affect the hands

When the massage is complete, the hair needs to be rinsed thoroughly to remove the shampoo together with the grease and dirt. Turn on the water and test the temperature on the inside of your wrist or the back of your hand. Always rinse your hands well, especially between the fingers, before you rinse the hair to help prevent **contact dermatitis**.

Ask your client if the temperature is OK for them. Rinse the hair thoroughly to make sure all the shampoo is removed. This may take several minutes depending on the length and thickness of the hair.

If the stylist has said that the client's hair should be shampooed twice then repeat the process. You will need less shampoo for the second shampoo than for the first.

When you have rinsed all the shampoo from the hair you should make sure your hands are rinsed well also.

HANDY HINTS

If you leave some shampoo in the hair it may affect other services the client is having. It will also make the hair dull and perhaps tacky when it is dried. Make sure you rinse the hair properly.

HANDY HINTS

If you towel dry the hair too much it will be more difficult to achieve the finish you need when the hair is styled.

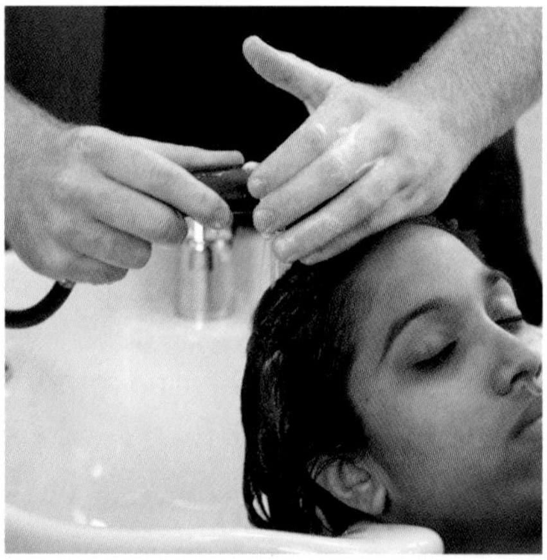

Sometimes, if the hair is very greasy, very dirty or has a product build-up on it then a third shampoo might be required.

FINISHING THE SERVICE

Gently squeeze the excess water from the hair (particularly where the hair is long) and then blot the hair with a towel to remove the excess water. You must be careful not to over dry the hair, but it should be dry enough so as not to drip down the client's neck or her face. Detangle the hair with a wide-toothed comb.

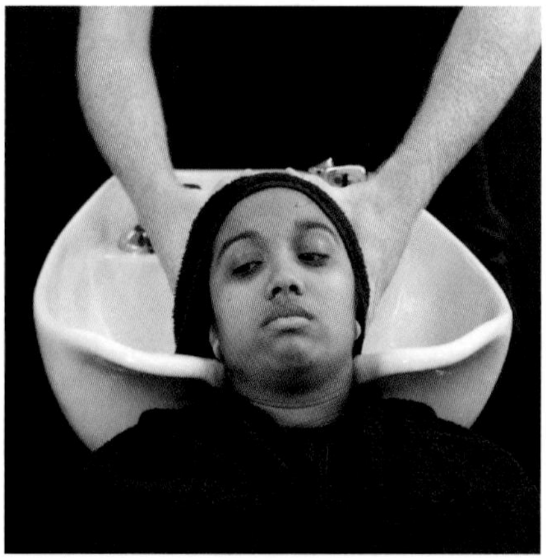

Comb the hair carefully starting at the nape, ready for the stylist to do the next part of the service.

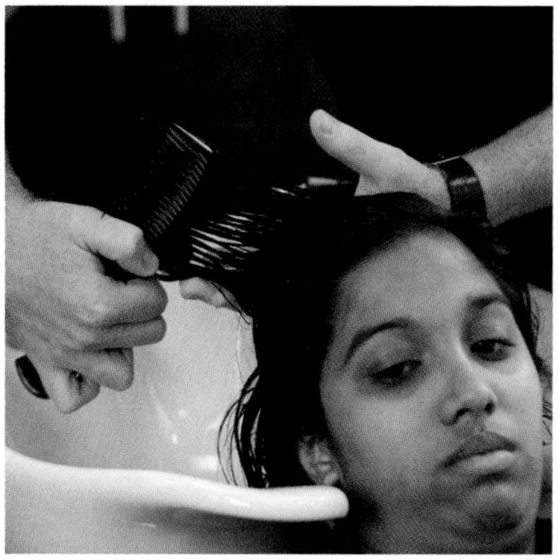

Make sure the towel around the client's shoulders is dry before you move them to the work area. If it is not, change it.

When the client is seated at the workstation, make sure the basin is cleaned and any waste is disposed of so the area is ready for the next client.

Dry your hands thoroughly, especially between the fingers when you have finished the shampoo and apply some moisturiser.

CHECKLIST

Earlier in the chapter you learned about working safely and hygienically. Here is a list of the things you need to think about during the shampoo that could affect yourself and your client:

- ☐ Make sure the client is properly protected with the gown and the towel.
- ☐ Check the water temperature.
- ☐ Check you have the right products.
- ☐ Check you are using the right massage movement and at the right pressure.
- ☐ Make sure your hands are rinsed, and when you have finished the shampoo, dried thoroughly.
- ☐ Use the product correctly and safely. Remember you looked at COSHH regulations that tell you how to use, store and dispose of the product, what could go wrong and what to do if it does.
- ☐ Make sure all empty containers are disposed of correctly.
- ☐ Place dirty towels in the bin ready for washing.
- ☐ Wash and sterilise combs and brushes ready to be used on the next client.

ACTIVITY

For each of the points above, make a list of what could happen if you forget to do any of them when you are shampooing.

HANDY HINTS

COSHH stands for Control of Substances Hazardous to Health. Don't forget:
S – store
H – handle
U – use
D – dispose
according to manufacturer's instructions.

CONDITIONING THE HAIR

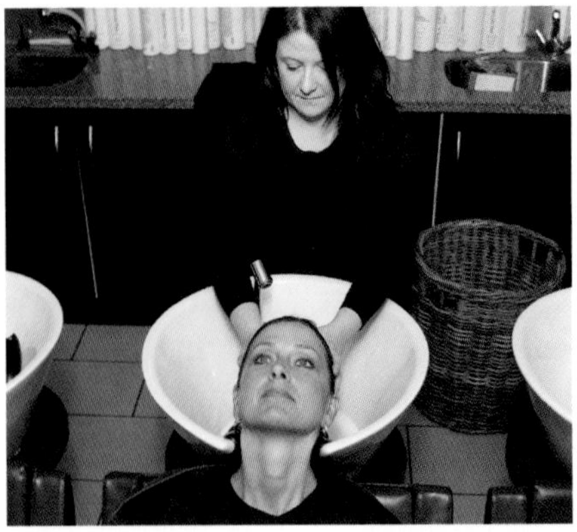

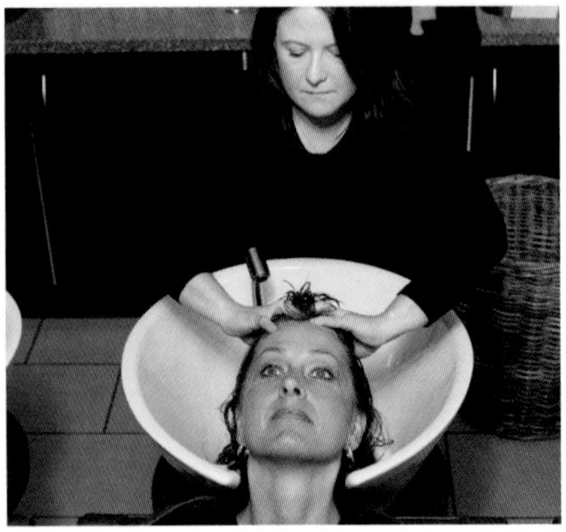

When you have completed the final rinse of the shampoo you should squeeze out the excess water ready to apply the conditioner. At this stage you will look at using a surface conditioner which will smoothe down the cuticle scales, add moisture to the hair and give it shine, making it look and feel better.

As you did with the shampoo, place the required amount of product onto the palm of the hand, rub the hands together and using the effleurage massage movement, massage the product through the hair and relax the client.

You then use the petrissage massage movement. This is a kneading movement similar to rotary but slower and with more pressure. It relaxes the muscles and improves the blood supply.

Remember with long hair to make sure to work the conditioner right through to the ends of the hair. After the petrissage, use some more effleurage just to relax the client.

Once the massage is complete, turn on the water, remembering to check the temperature and rinse the product from the hair. You must make sure that you rinse the hair thoroughly. Remember to rinse and dry your hands at the end of the service.

Remove the excess moisture by blotting with a towel but not too much. Comb the hair starting at the nape, ready for the stylist to do the next part of the service.

The client is now ready to have their hair styled.

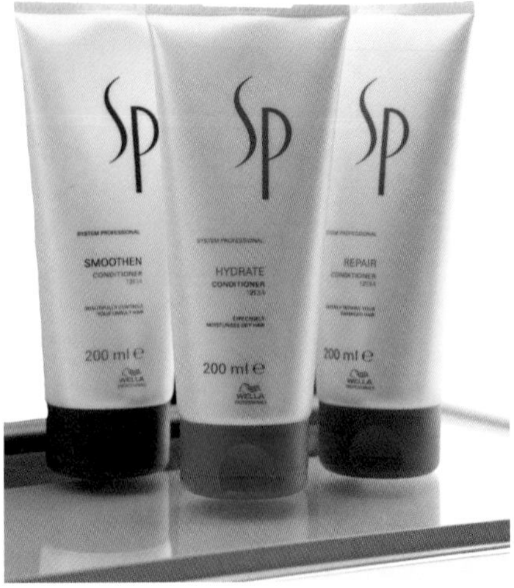

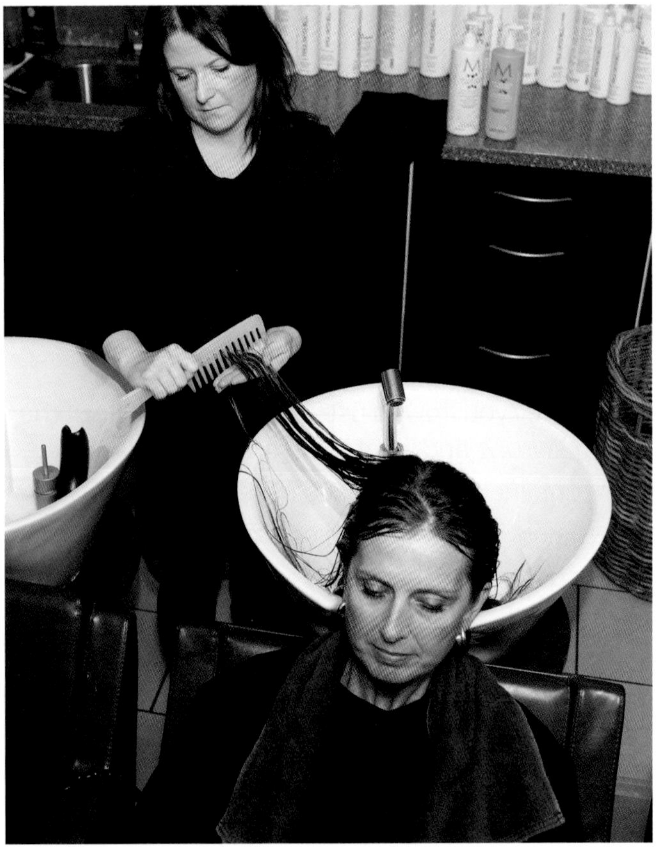

DERMATITIS

Not only do you have to make sure you look after the client and reduce the risk of injury to them, but you must also do the same for yourself. Your biggest asset as a hairdresser is your hands so it is vital that you look after them. When you shampoo there is a risk of developing contact dermatitis as a result of the hands being wet and using chemicals during the **process**.

You can reduce the risk of developing dermatitis by making sure you rinse all of the product from your hands, particularly after the last shampoo or conditioner. Dry your hands thoroughly, especially between the fingers, every time the hands get wet, and use a good hand cream regularly during the day.

If the skin of your hands is dry or you have sensitive skin, then the use of protective gloves is essential. If your hands do develop the symptoms of contact dermatitis, which include redness, cracking of the skin and soreness, then you must consult your doctor as soon as possible.

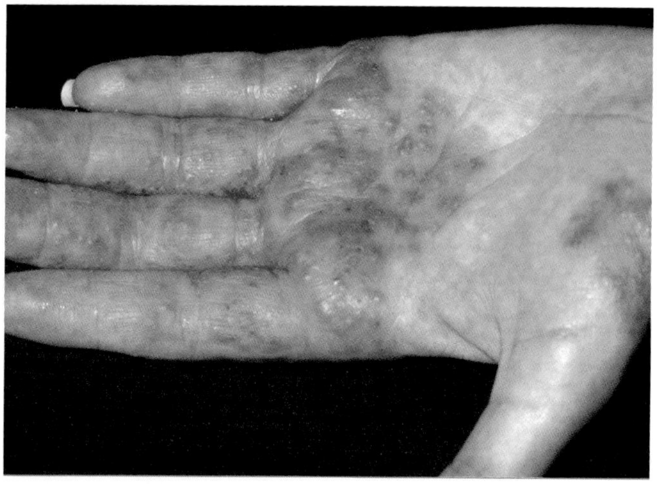

Dermatitis

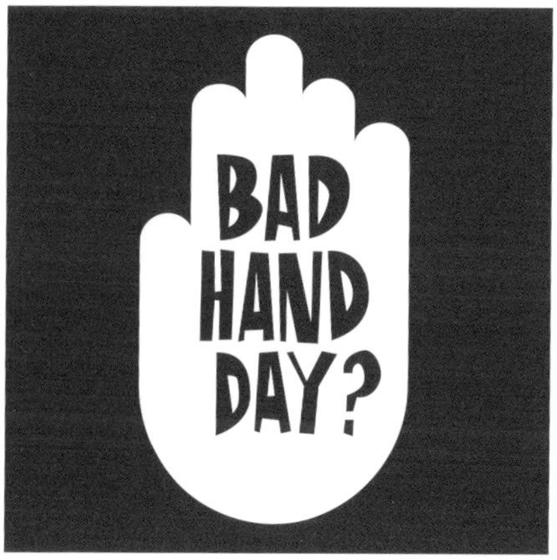

Process

A series of actions taken to achieve something

ACTIVITY

Find out more about contact dermatitis and what you need to do to reduce the risks of developing it. Have a look at the HSE's website www.hse.gov.uk/hairdressing/bad-hand.htm. Discuss your findings with the group.

IN A NUTSHELL

You are now at the end of the chapter. Before you test your knowledge with the revision activities, check the following list to see if you feel confident in all the areas covered. If there are still any areas you're unsure of, go back over them in the book and ask your tutor for extra support:

- preparing for shampooing and conditioning
- working safely
- preparing the work area
- methods of sterilisation
- tools and equipment used in shampooing and conditioning
- preparing the client
- the structure of the hair
- consulting with the client
- professional image
- types of shampoo and conditioner
- how to shampoo and condition the hair
- types of massage and when to use them
- preparing the client for the next part of their treatment.

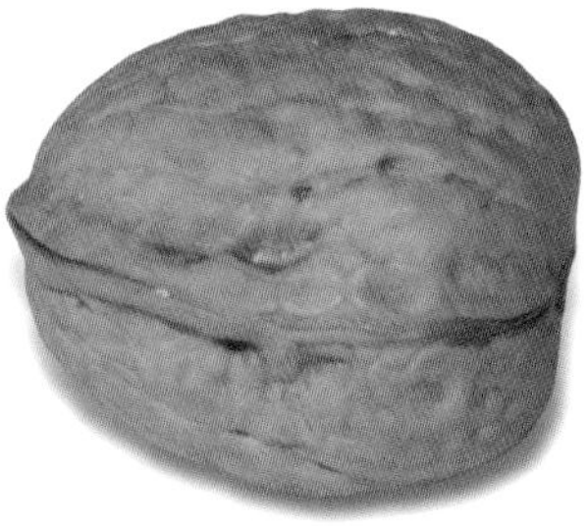

REVISION ACTIVITIES

Use the questions below to test your knowledge of Chapter 003 to see just how much information you've gained. This can help you to prepare for your assessments. Turn to pages 488–489 for the answers.

CROSSWORD

See if you can answer the questions and write in the answers.

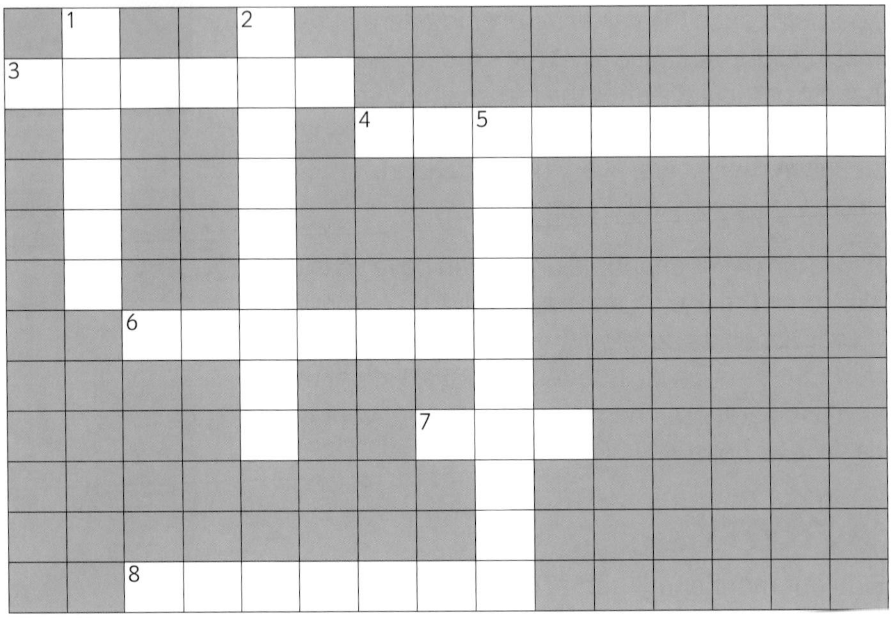

Across

3 The part of the hair shaft that gives the hair its strength and elasticity

4 A type of conditioner for hair in very bad condition

6 The outer layer of the hair shaft

7 A hair type that feels straw-like

8 A type of conditioner to help soften and flatten the cuticle

Down

1 A massage movement used during shampooing to cleanse the hair

2 A shampoo used for dandruff

5 A massage movement used to spread the shampoo or conditioner

WORDS TO FIND

Copy and complete the sentences below. Use these words to help you fill in the gaps.

towels	liquid	cortex	water temperature
cuticle	cream	consultation	dermatitis
rotary	rinsed	surface conditioner	friction
medulla	gown	effleurage	wide-toothed comb

1 ______________, ______________, and ______________ are the massage movements used in shampooing and conditioning.

2 It is important to test the ______________ before using it on the hair.

3 A ______________ is used to remove tangles from the hair before shampooing.

4 The three parts of the hair shaft are called the ______________, ______________ and ______________.

5 The cuticle of the hair can be smoothed using a ______________.

6 Drying the hands and using hand cream will help prevent ______________.

7 ______________ and ______________ are types of shampoo used to clean the hair.

8 To protect the client's clothing a ______________ and ______________ are used.

9 The type of shampoo that will be used on the client will be decided during the ______________.

10 The hair should be ______________ thoroughly to remove all traces of the shampoo.

TEST YOUR KNOWLEDGE FURTHER

See if you can find out how important a good shampoo is to a client. Ask some friends and relations how they like their hair shampooed and why.

Write down the answers you get. You can use them to link to what you have learned about shampooing and conditioning. It will help you understand the important parts of the service and why you need to do them this way.

Now answer these questions.

1. Name **two** reasons for shampooing and conditioning the hair.
2. Why is it important to stand properly when shampooing?
3. Why should floors be swept regularly?
4. Name the three parts of the hair shaft.
5. Name **three** things you need to find out when consulting with your client before shampooing.
6. Why is it important to rinse your hands thoroughly during the shampooing service?
7. List **three** things that will help you present a professional image.
8. Name the three massage movements used in shampooing.
9. What effect do surface conditioners have on the hair?
10. Name the massage movement used in conditioning.

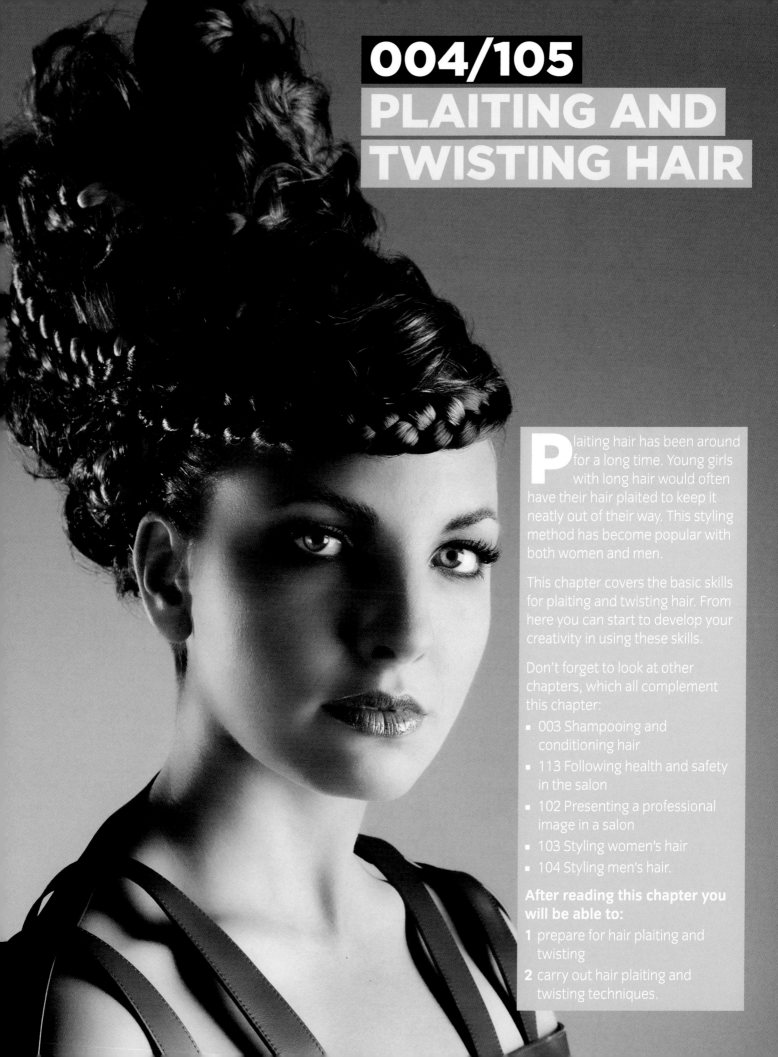

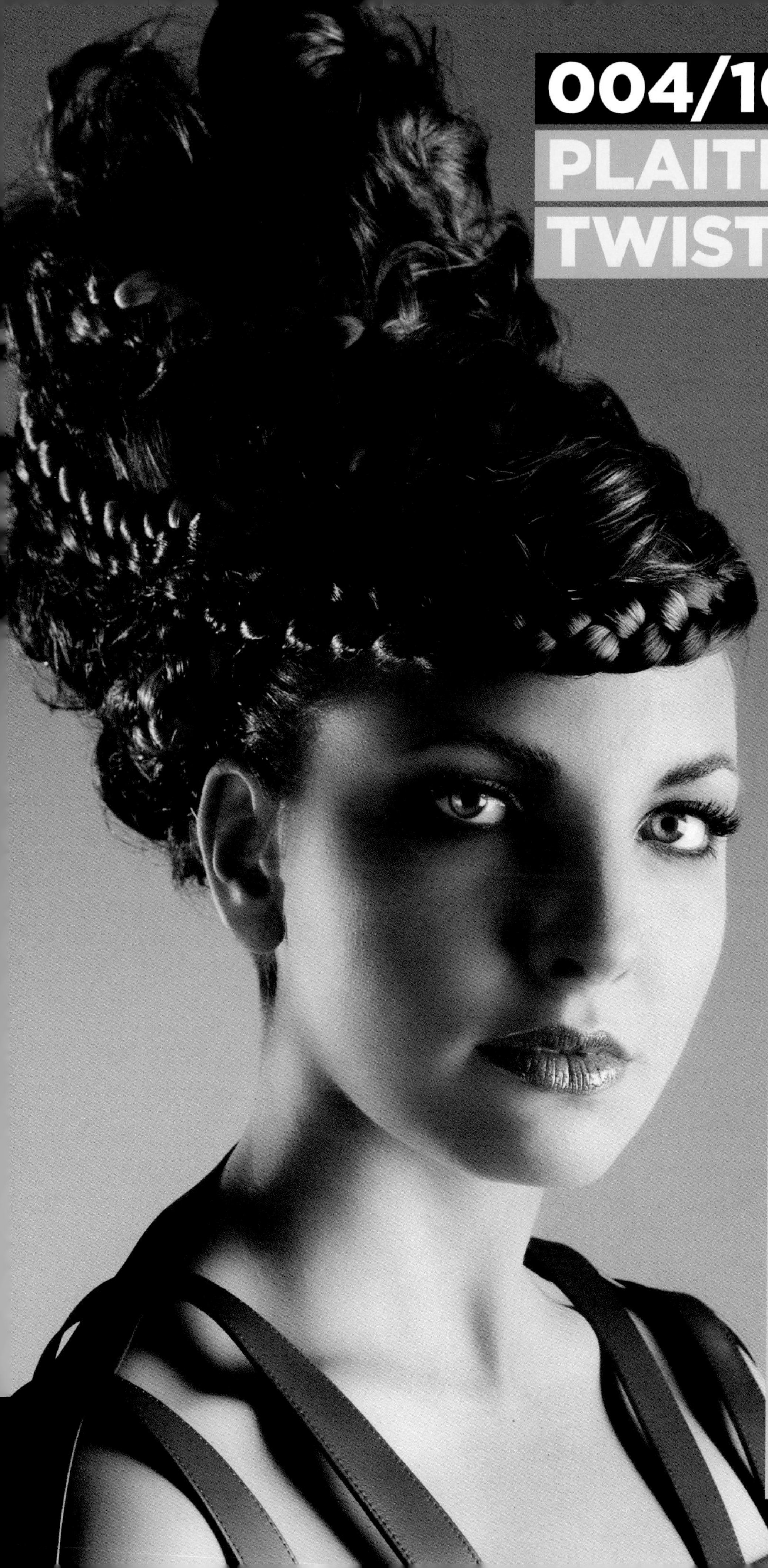

004/105 PLAITING AND TWISTING HAIR

Plaiting hair has been around for a long time. Young girls with long hair would often have their hair plaited to keep it neatly out of their way. This styling method has become popular with both women and men.

This chapter covers the basic skills for plaiting and twisting hair. From here you can start to develop your creativity in using these skills.

Don't forget to look at other chapters, which all complement this chapter:

- 003 Shampooing and conditioning hair
- 113 Following health and safety in the salon
- 102 Presenting a professional image in a salon
- 103 Styling women's hair
- 104 Styling men's hair.

After reading this chapter you will be able to:

1. prepare for hair plaiting and twisting
2. carry out hair plaiting and twisting techniques.

PREPARE FOR HAIR PLAITING AND TWISTING

This part of the chapter shows you how to select products and tools and prepare for basic plaiting and twisting techniques.

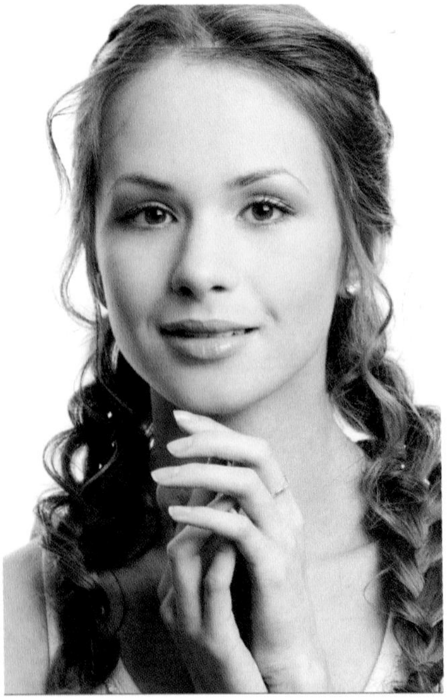

An off scalp plait

THE TECHNIQUES FOR PLAITING AND TWISTING HAIR

There is a huge range of finished looks that use plaiting and twisting techniques. These are achieved using the various techniques described here.

LOOSE PLAIT

Loose plaiting is an 'off scalp' method of plaiting the hair. It is a method of combining sections of hair and can be done with three or more strands. Loose plaits are designed to last a few days.

- A three-strand plait is a simple practical method.
- It is a neat style that keeps the hair off the face.
- It is a practical style for clients who want long hair but have to keep it off their face for their work.
- It can also be used for special occasions using multiple strands and ornamentation, eg flowers, beads, jewellery, etc.
- It is often used as part of a more dressy style for weddings or parties.

'CORNROW' OR 'CANEROW' PLAITING

Cornrow plaiting is an 'on scalp' form of plaiting. This is another form of three-strand plaiting where the hair is plaited close to the scalp and forms patterns on the scalp. This technique originated in Africa. It was used to indicate status in tribes. Cornrow plaiting will last for up to a month or two. The hair can be shampooed and conditioned with the cornrows in place. However, this will not clean the hair as well as normal shampooing because you cannot massage the shampoo through the hair.

The hair is sectioned into small rows or channels. Starting at the front, three sections are made which are plaited close to the root. More hair is added to each section as you work back to the end of the row.

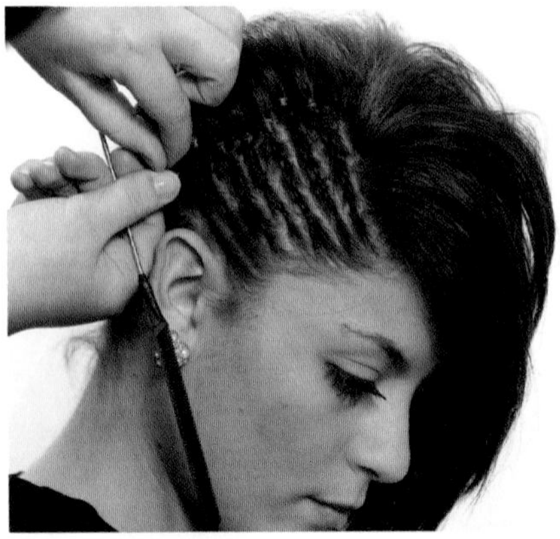

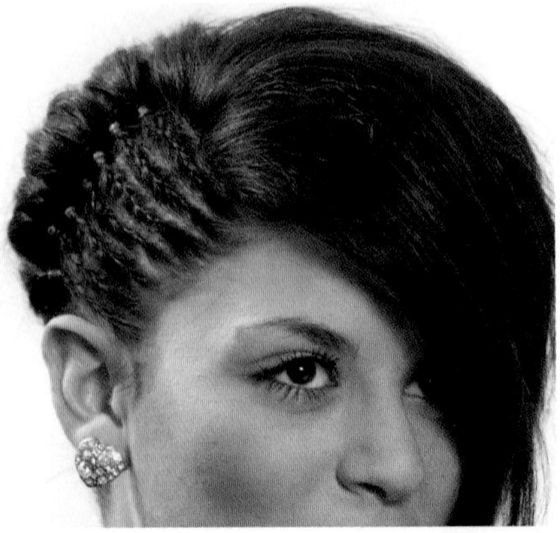

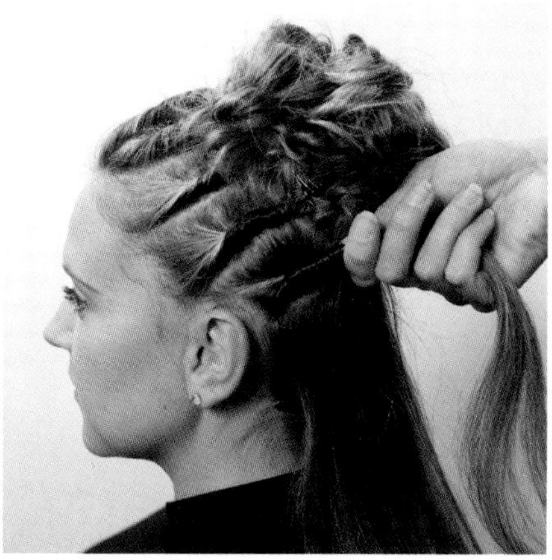

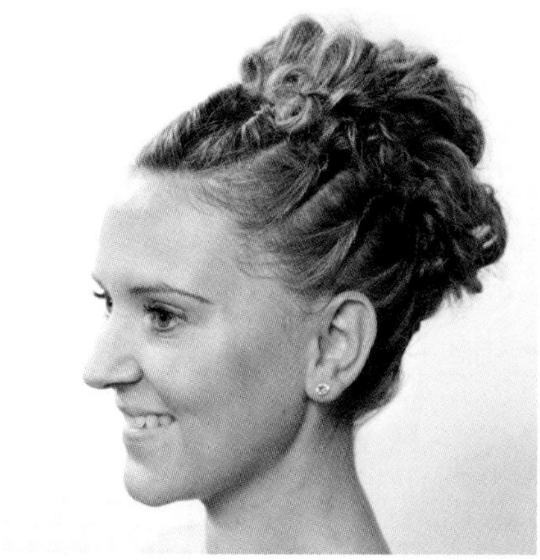

TWISTING

Twisting is another 'on scalp' technique. Small sections of hair are taken, keeping the hair flat to the scalp. The hair is held at the points, twisted into a roll-like shape down to the scalp and secured with grips and hair pins. The points of the hair can then be curled using tongs or dressed out using a comb.

HANDY HINTS

Read Chapter 103 Styling women's hair or Chapter 104 Styling men's hair to learn more about the factors that may influence your choice of styling technique.

ACTIVITY

Using the internet, research the origins of the different types of plaiting in different cultures such as Africa.

FACTORS THAT CAN AFFECT YOUR CHOICE OF STYLING TECHNIQUES

Like the other methods of styling hair, there are many **factors** that you will need to take into account when choosing a technique to style the client's hair. These factors will help you decide how to use the selected technique on both male and female clients.

Factors
Things to consider about a subject

FACE SHAPE

People have different shaped faces. Here are five of the more common ones.

ACTIVITY

Look at photographs of people who have plaits and twists in magazines and on the internet. Try to work out what face shape they have. Collect examples of those you find.

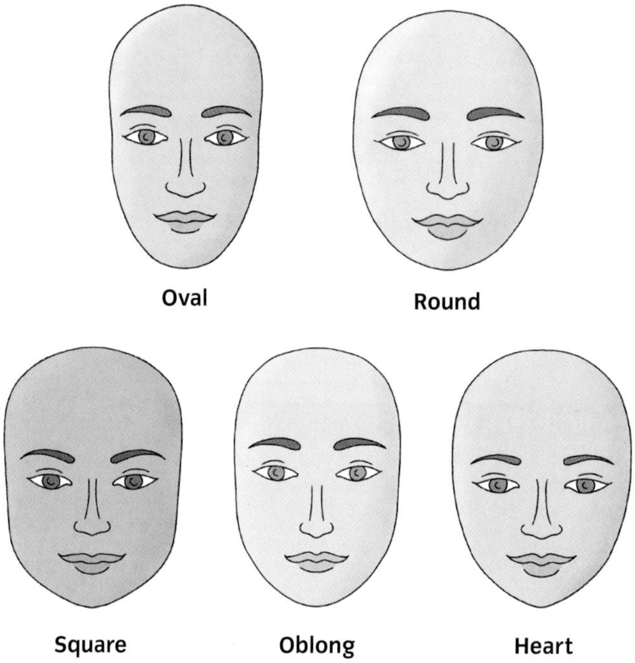

HEAD SHAPE

Head shapes will affect whether you can use plaits or twists alone or combined with other styling techniques. Plaits and twists will often sit close to the scalp and will not add height or width to the style or create a softening effect. You may need to use a combination of styling techniques to achieve a suitable style.

LIFESTYLE

The client's lifestyle is a very important factor in the styling process. You need to decide whether plaiting or twisting will go with:

- the type of clothes they wear
- their age
- their job
- their personality.

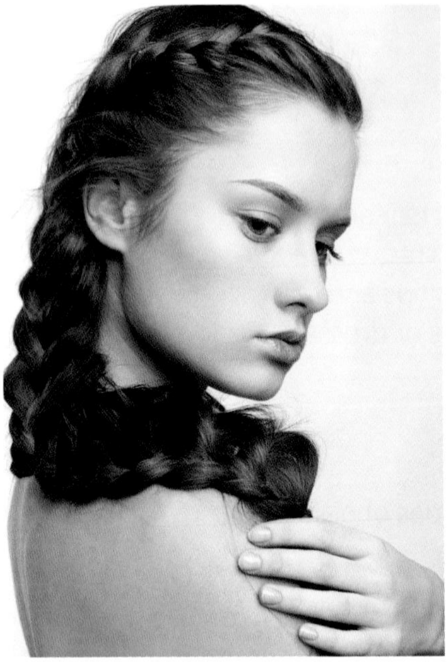

HAIR TEXTURE

Hair texture is about the thickness of each individual hair. This can prevent the client from having some types of plaits or twists.

Coarse Hair
There may be too much hair for fine cornrows or twists.

Medium Hair
This texture works well for most plaiting and twisting styles.

Fine Hair
The client's hair may not be strong enough to have cornrows or twists. There may not be enough hair for the client to have a French plait.

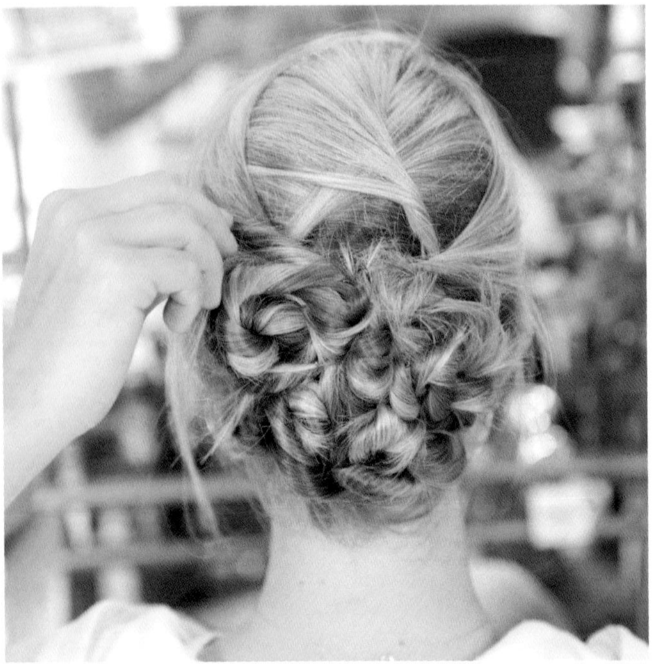

ACTIVITY

With other members of your group, look and feel each other's hair and decide what texture the hair is. Compare your **analysis** with the rest of the group.

HAIR DENSITY

Density describes the number of hairs on the head. Lots of hair may create chunky plaits that the client may not be happy with. Sparse hair may produce plaits that look too thin and show too much scalp.

HAIR ELASTICITY

The hair's elasticity is important for plaiting and twisting. Hair is naturally elastic; it can stretch and go back to its original shape. If the hair has been damaged by chemical treatments like colouring, or is very fine, it may not be very elastic. The tension needed for cornrows and twists may cause more damage to the hair and result in breakage. Loose plaiting like a French plait does not put too much pressure on the hair.

HANDY HINTS
The density can be determined by looking at the scalp. The more scalp you can see the less hair the client has.

Analysis
The result of looking at something carefully

HAIR CONDITION

The condition of the hair can affect your choice of plaiting and twisting. Cornrows and twists can last for perhaps several weeks before they are taken out. The condition of the hair can affect how they look over that time. The condition may prevent you plaiting or twisting the hair.

Hair type	How it may affect the styling service
Normal	This hair type will not present any major problems when plaiting or twisting.
Oily/greasy	If the hair is very greasy it can cause some problems if cornrow plaiting is carried out. The hair is washed with the plaits in place, so the shampoo may not get all the grease out of the hair, causing the plaits to become dull.
Dry	The hair will need regular conditioning to help achieve a smooth finish. Avoid using too much heat.
Damaged	If the hair is damaged as a result of previous services like perming or colouring the hair may be weak. Treat the hair carefully. Avoid using too much heat or too much tension.

Deciding on hair condition is done by looking at and feeling the hair. You may also need to ask the client some questions.

ACTIVITY

Work in pairs to discuss how you would suggest plaiting and twisting styles to a client who hasn't had them before.

HAIR TYPE

The client's hair will be straight, curly or wavy. If the hair is very curly or has a strong natural wave, loose plaiting may not be very successful. Cornrowing and twisting can be used on very curly hair with super results.

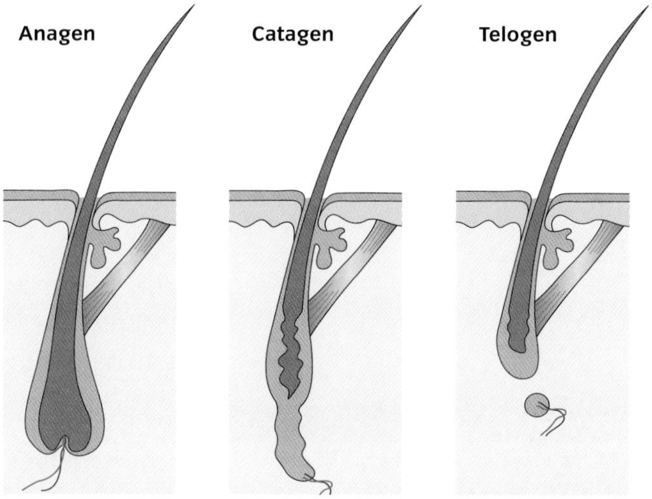

HAIR LENGTH

Longer hair is needed for plaiting and twisting. You must make sure that there is enough hair for you to do what the client wants.

HAIR GROWTH CYCLE

A hair does not grow continuously. A single hair has a life of between 18 months and seven years. At the end of its life it will fall out and after a short while another hair will grow in its place.

There are three stages in the growth cycle:

- Anagen – Active or growing period – lasts for 18 months to seven years. This is the anagen stage of hair growth.
- Catagen – Breaking down stage – lasts about two weeks. This is the catagen stage of hair growth.
- Telogen – Resting – lasts about a month. This is the telogen stage of hair growth.

This can affect the type of plaiting or twisting the client is able to have. If he/she wants a long hairstyle but the hair life cycle is short, the hair may not grow long enough.

ADVERSE SKIN, SCALP AND HAIR CONDITIONS

Like all styling techniques you must check the hair and scalp for any diseases or conditions. Remember, some diseases and conditions may be **contagious**. This may prevent you from carrying out any service on the client.

Contagious
Describing disease that can be spread from person to person

HANDY HINTS
Look at Chapters 103 or 104 for more information and pictures of what to look for when examining the hair and scalp.

When you are consulting with your client you should look at the hair and scalp for:

- scaly patches or rough areas on the scalp
- red, inflamed patches
- cuts and abrasions on the skin
- lumps and bumps or raised areas
- bald patches
- hair breakage.

SmartScreen 105 handout 2

If you see anything unusual, then you should ask a stylist to look and advise you. If you are unable to give the service then you may need to explain to the client that the treatment cannot go ahead. Remember that you are not medically trained. You should not name the condition in case you are wrong. Ask your client to go to their doctor who can treat them properly.

HANDY HINTS
Remember to look for head lice when you are checking the scalp.

HAIR GROWTH PATTERNS

Hair growth patterns are areas where the hair grows in a particular direction or directions. This may affect how the hair is styled – you may need to design your plaits to work with the growth pattern. As the hair is long and the plaits and twists are secured with bands there are generally no major problems.

HANDY HINTS
Read Chapters 103 or 104 to find out about hair growth patterns.

CULTURAL AND FASHION TRENDS

Your client may want a hairstyle worn by their favourite pop star or celebrity. They may want a style that is worn by different cultures. Keep up to date with these trends so you know what your client is asking for.

Doing what your client wants is not always easy. The client may not have:

- the right type of hair. It may be too short.
- she/he may not have a suitable face shape or even a suitable body shape.

HANDY HINTS
Remember, you must be very tactful and polite when you discuss face shape and lifestyle with your client.

You may need to explain to the client that it might be necessary to change the style because of the hair type, face shape, etc.

ACTIVITY

Keep your eye on which plaiting and twisting styles are popular at the moment. Keep up to date for your clients. Magazines and the internet are good places to find examples. Make your own style book.

HANDY HINTS
Remember to make sure your appearance and your personal hygiene are up to standard. Read Chapter 102 to refresh your knowledge.

PREPARE THE WORK AREA

There are three reasons why you should prepare your work area ready to work:

1 It helps you to work safely and hygienically.
2 It looks good and gives the client the right impression.
3 It helps you to work efficiently.

Make sure you keep work surfaces clean by wiping them regularly with a suitable cleaner. Mirrors should be cleaned to remove smears and smudges. Tools and equipment should be in their proper places and always cleaned and sterilised ready for use to help prevent the passing of infection from one client to another. Sweep and clean the floor when necessary. Make sure the chair is clean.

You may not be able to get all the things you need ready before the client arrives. When you have completed your consultation with the client, get the rest of the products and tools you need.

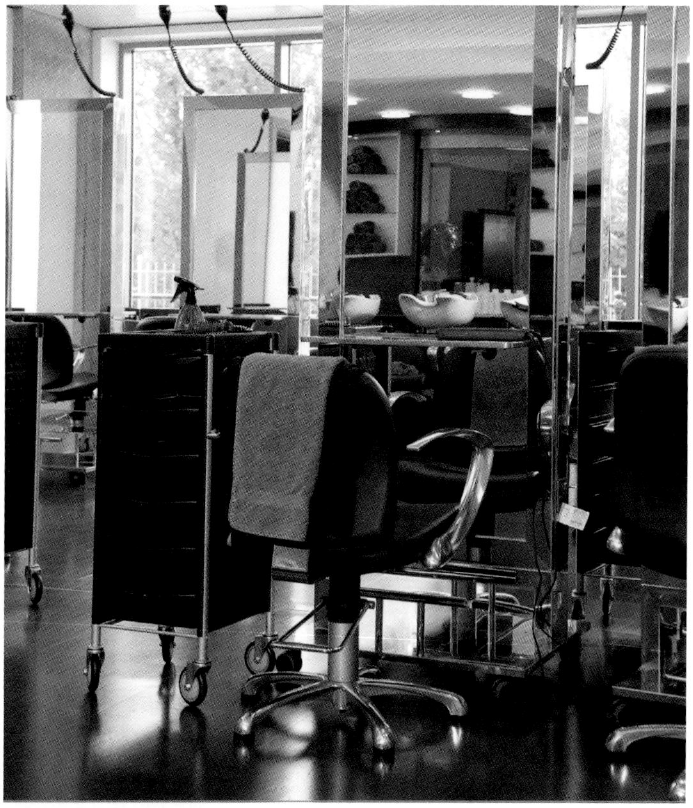

A work area for plaiting services

SAFE AND HYGIENIC WORKING PRACTICES

Working safely and hygienically is very important. It is part of every practical skill you learn; it is part of every service you give to a client; it is part of the whole of your working day.

You should keep your work area tidy and use only **hygienic** tools and equipment. This will help to reduce the risk of harm to you and your clients and help to prevent **cross-infection**. The client will also have more confidence in you and you will look more professional.

Hygienic
Clean and germ free

Cross-infection
Passing germs from one person to another

ACTIVITY

Go to Chapter 113 Following health and safety in the salon and list all of the health and safety laws that you should follow when carrying out a plaiting and twisting service.

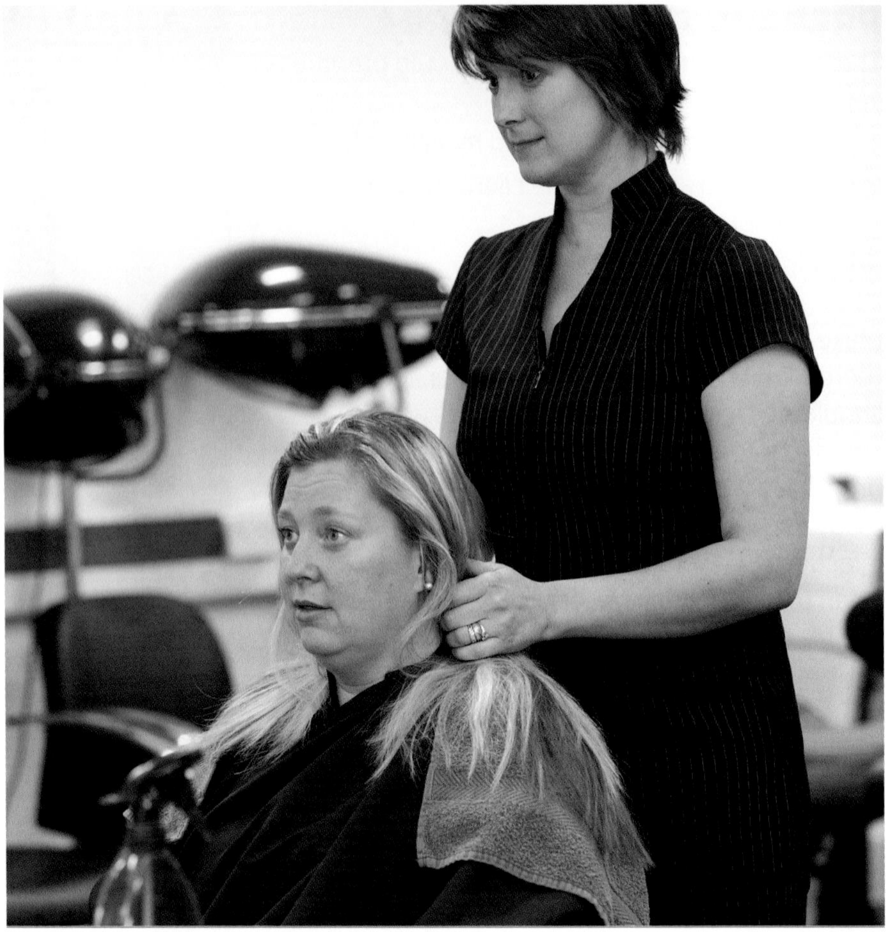

Position your client comfortably for the service

HANDY HINTS

Go to Chapter 113 Following health and safety in the salon and read more about methods of sterilisation.

SmartScreen 105 handout 3

SmartScreen 105 worksheet 1

HYGIENE WHEN PLAITING AND TWISTING HAIR

The following is a guide for keeping your tools and equipment ready for use.

Towels and gowns	Machine wash on a high temperature to destroy harmful germs.
Combs	Wash in warm, soapy water. Place in the sterilising jar.
Clips	Wash in warm soapy water and dry. Then place in the sterilising jar or the UV cabinet.
Disposable gloves	Throw away after use. Use a new pair for each client.
Bands	Throw away after use. Use new bands on each client.

PREPARE THE CLIENT

Preparing the client for plaiting and twisting services is the same as for styling services. It will involve the following:

- gowning the client to protect their clothes
- carrying out a consultation with the client
- choosing the tools, equipment and products to be used
- shampooing and, if needed, conditioning the client's hair.

GOWNING THE CLIENT

Place a gown around the client to protect their clothes, and a clean towel around their shoulders.

CONSULTATION

Consulting with the client is a way of finding out what the client wants. It is how you decide what you are going to do. Chapter 003 Shampooing and conditioning hair describes how to consult with your client to find out what shampoo and conditioner you will use, and how you will carry out the service.

If you are going to style the client's hair, then you need to find out more information from the client:

- The first thing you must find out is what the client wants the finished look to be. This will help you decide which technique you need to consider using.
- The next thing to do is to look at all the factors that can influence your choice of technique.
- When you have looked at the factors you need to decide if you can achieve what the client has asked for. If you cannot then you will need to suggest other options.
- Next select any styling products to use, such as mousse or setting lotion, etc.
- Last of all decide how you will carry out the technique and the tools and equipment you need to use.

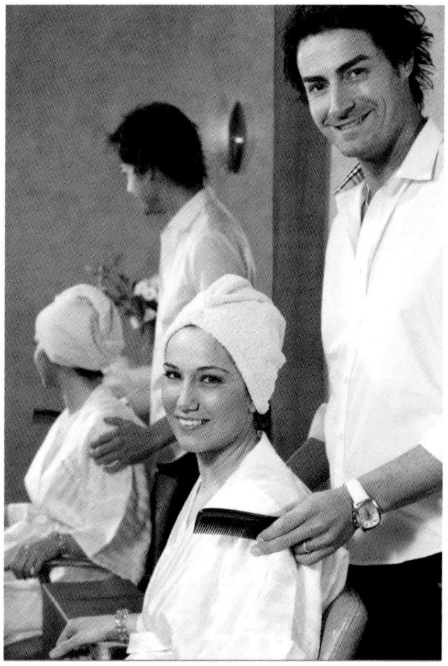

A gowned client

HANDY HINTS

Read more about preparing your client in Chapter 003 Shampooing and conditioning hair.

HANDY HINTS

Check regularly that the gown is still in place and the towels are not too wet. Change the towels if you need to.

HANDY HINTS

Make sure you check the hair and scalp for diseases and conditions. If the client has a contagious disease you may not be able to carry out the service.

SmartScreen 105 handout 1

COMMUNICATION AND BEHAVIOUR

Communication and behaviour are very important when plaiting and twisting. Whether clients feel happy about coming to you for the service depends on how you communicate and behave. Refer to Chapter 102 for more details about communication and behaviour.

SHAMPOO AND CONDITION THE CLIENT'S HAIR

When you have finished your consultation, the next step is to shampoo the hair ready for the plaiting service. Chapter 003 Shampooing and conditioning hair describes the method of shampooing and conditioning the hair ready for other services.

Don't forget to use conditioner if the hair needs it. Make sure the client agrees to have it.

The hair may need to be dried ready for the plaiting or twisting service. Make sure the hair is as smooth as possible.

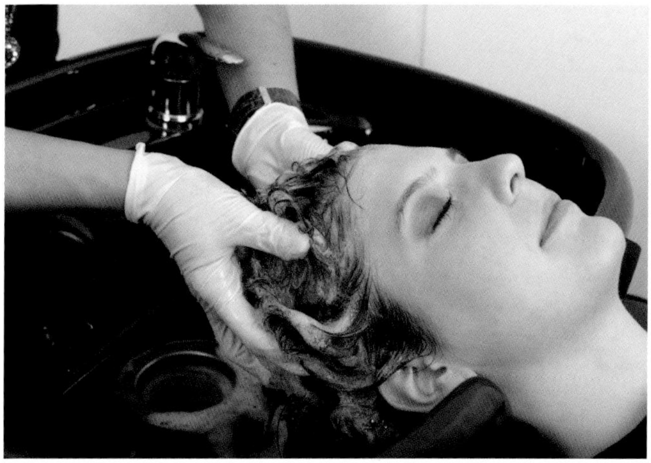

HANDY HINTS

Read Chapter 003 Shampooing and conditioning hair to refresh your knowledge of the procedure.

TOOLS AND EQUIPMENT USED IN PLAITING AND TWISTING

Tools and equipment	Use
Wide-toothed comb 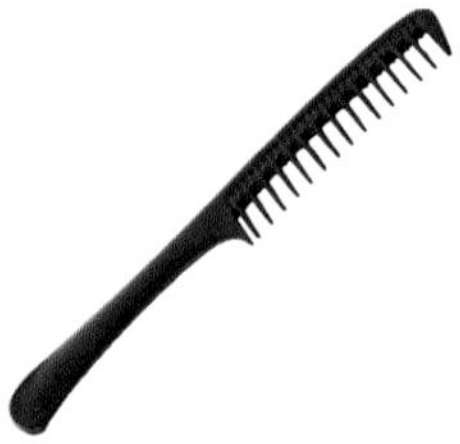	Used to detangle wet hair after shampooing and conditioning.
Tail comb 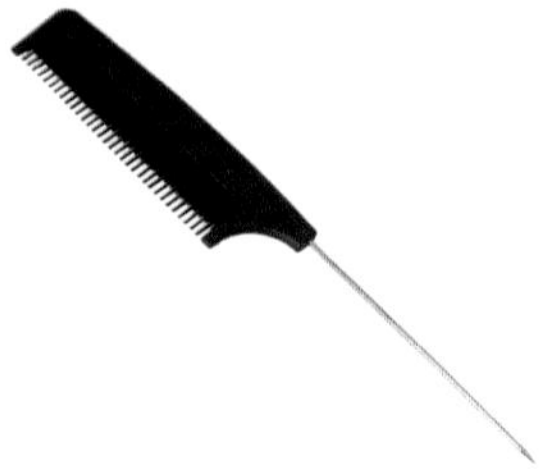	Can be used to make partings and split sections into strands ready to plait.
Sectioning clips 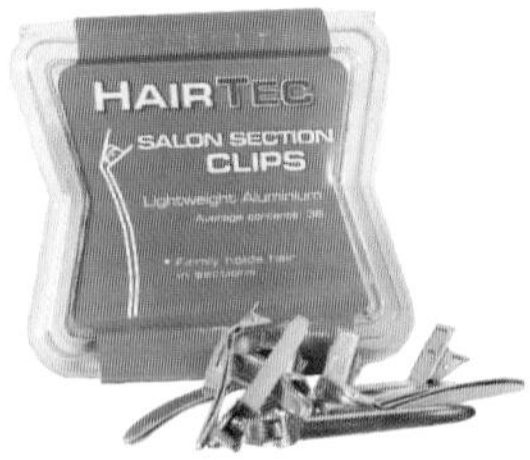	Used to secure the hair as you work.
Bristle brush 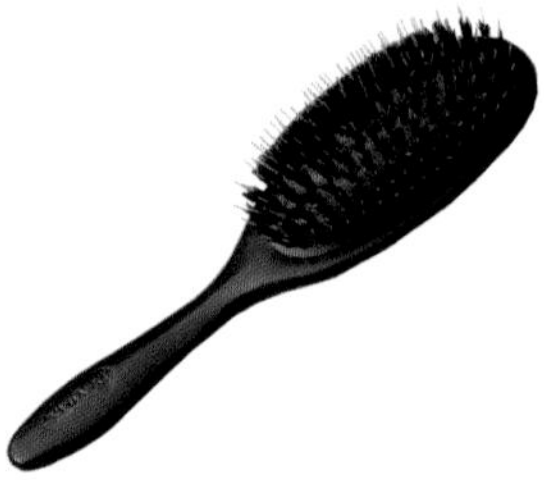	This is a soft bristle brush used for general brushing.
Denman brush 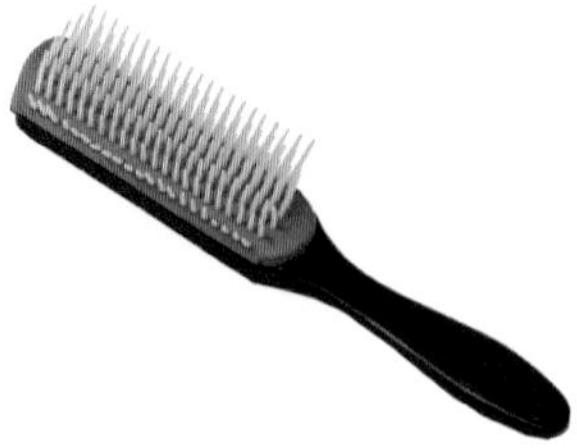	Used in blow drying to create a smooth, straight finish such as a 'bob' style.

Tools and equipment	Use
Grips 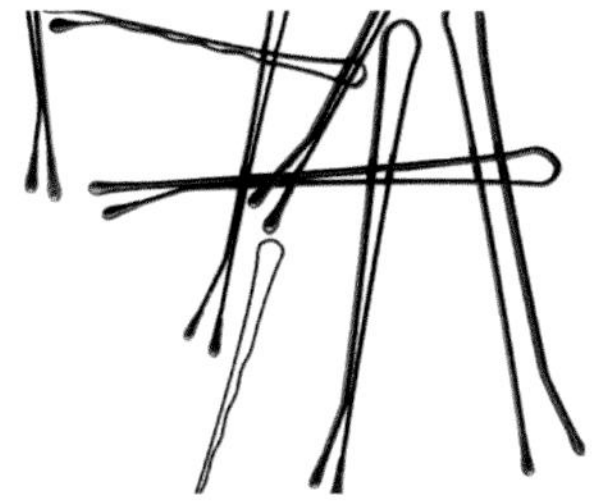	Sometimes called 'kirby' grips. They are used to secure twists in position.
Pins 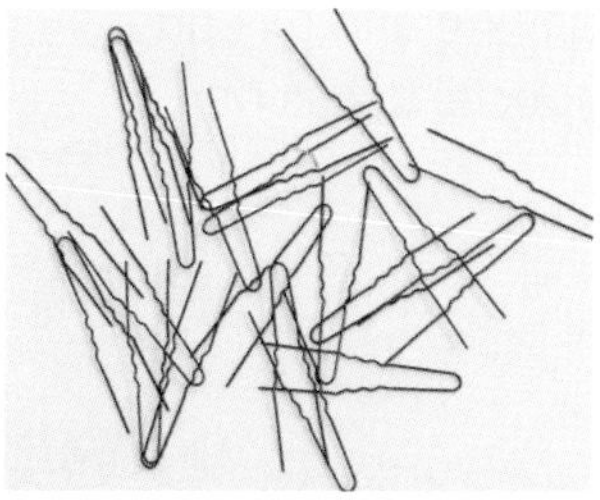	Fine hair pins are used to hold and secure twists and plaits.
Hand-held dryer 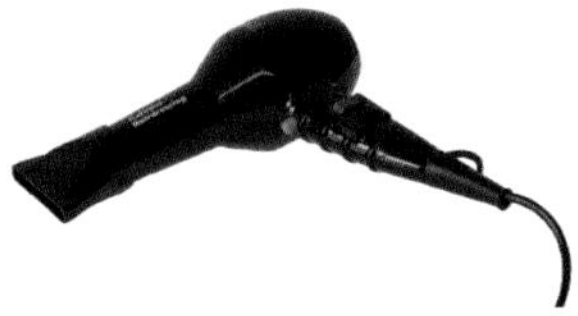	Used to dry the hair before plaiting and twisting.
Straightening irons 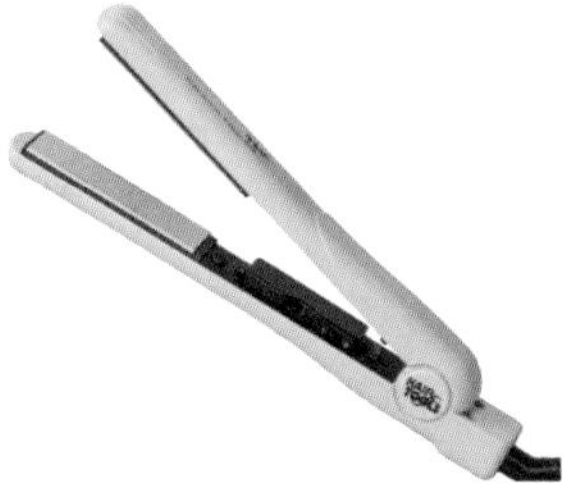	Used to smooth the hair before plaiting.
Tongs 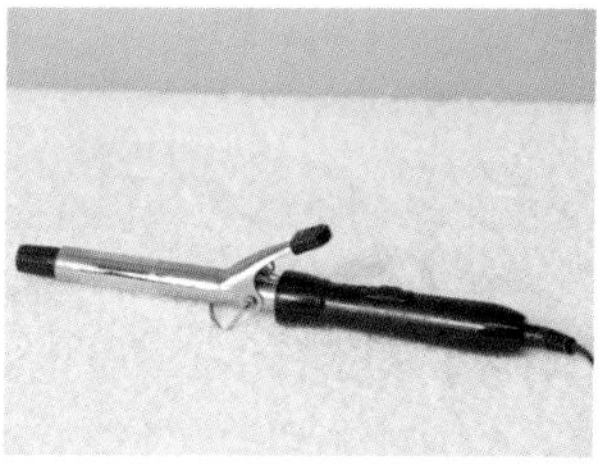	These are used to curl hair when plaiting and twisting is part of a more complex style.
Bands 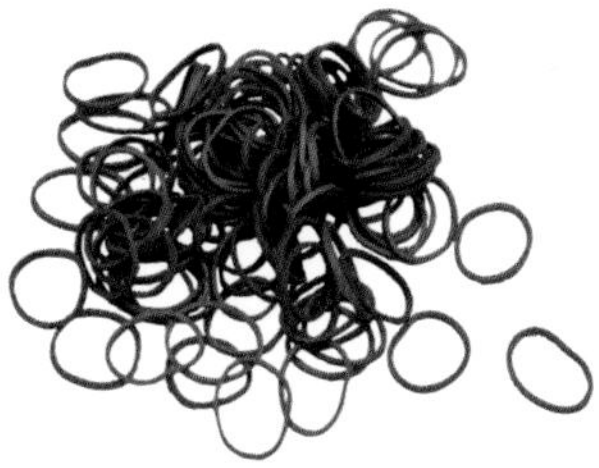	These are used to secure the plait. Professional bands should always be used.

Tools and equipment	Use
Accessories 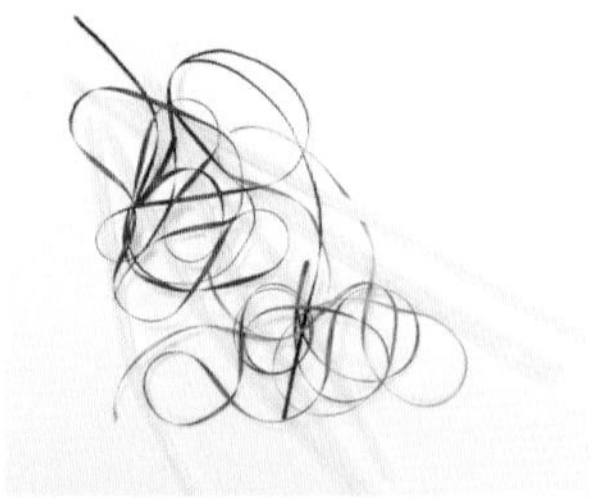	Ribbons, strips of fabric, coloured threads, pipe cleaners, etc can be used to enhance the style.
Decorations 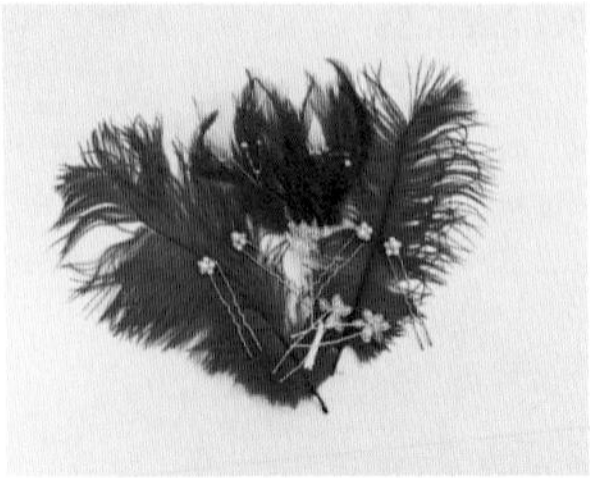	Jewellery, flowers and added hair can be used when plaiting and twisting styles are for a special occasion.
Gown 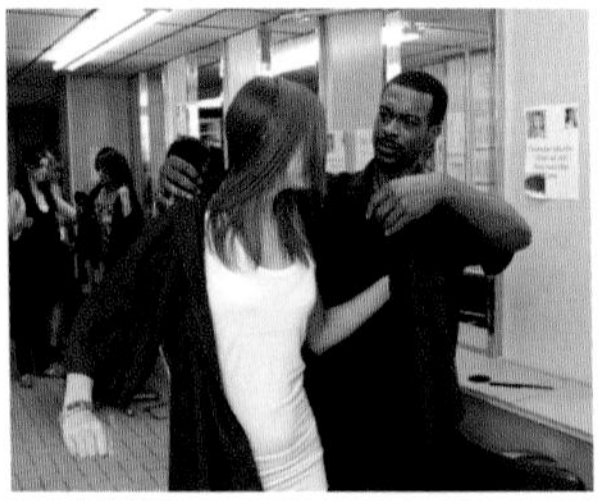	This will cover the client and help to prevent any products getting onto their clothes.
Towels 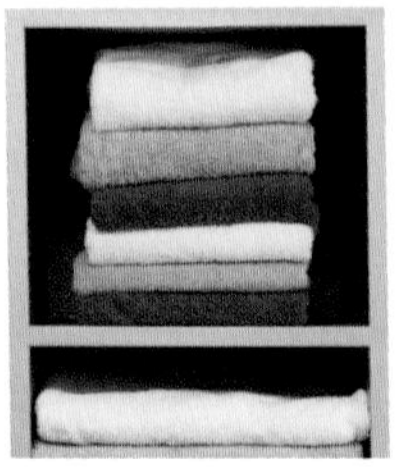	Used when shampooing and styling to prevent the client's clothing from getting wet.
Hand mirror 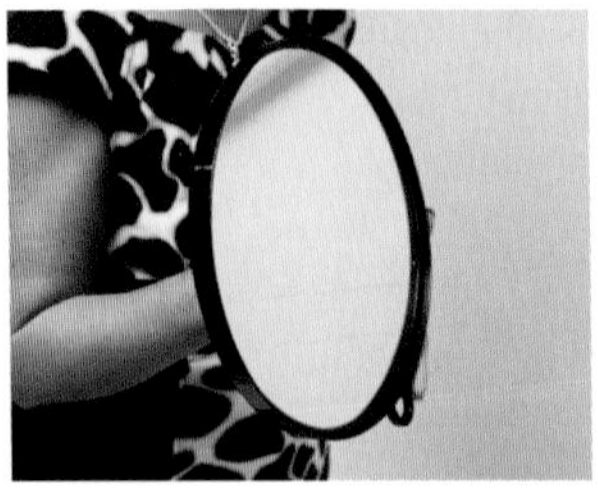	Used to show the client the back of their head so they can see the finished result.

SmartScreen 105 worksheet 2

PRODUCTS USED IN PLAITING AND TWISTING

Gel 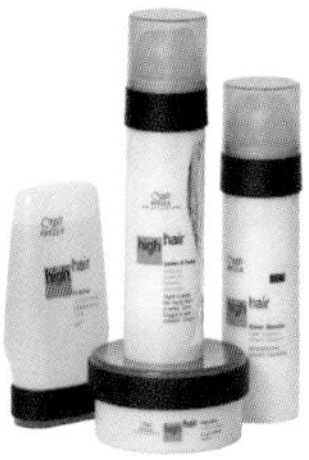	Used on wet or dry hair to provide volume and texture.
Serum 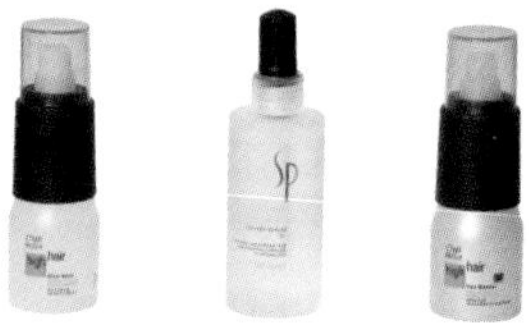	These are oil-based products. They help smooth the hair and prevent it from tangling when you are sectioning.
Blow dry/setting lotion 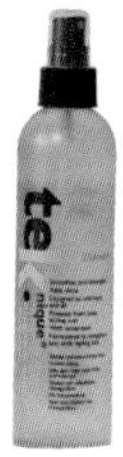	Used on wet hair before blow drying. Gives volume, lift and support for fine hair.
Hairspray 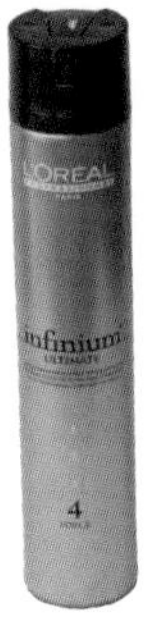	Used on dry hair. The hair is sprayed lightly when plaiting is finished. It holds the hair in place and gives it shine.
Spray moisturisers 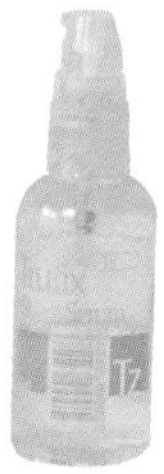	Used on dry hair to add shine. Be careful not to use too much.

SmartScreen 105 worksheet 3

ACTIVITY

Look on the internet for products that are currently available to use when plaiting the client's hair.

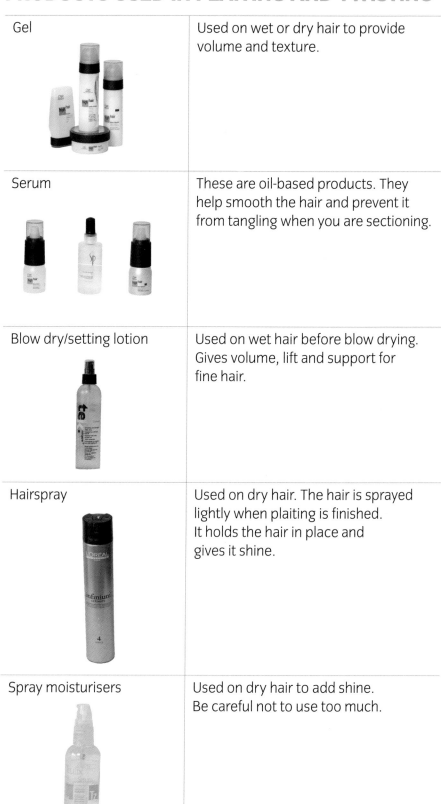

HANDY HINTS

Remember to work safely and concentrate on what you are doing.

CARRY OUT HAIR PLAITING AND TWISTING TECHNIQUES

Traction alopecia
A condition where the hair is pulled out at the root when too much tension is used

Like blow drying and other styling techniques, it is important to have the hair under control. If the hair is not under control you will not get the shape and finish you want.

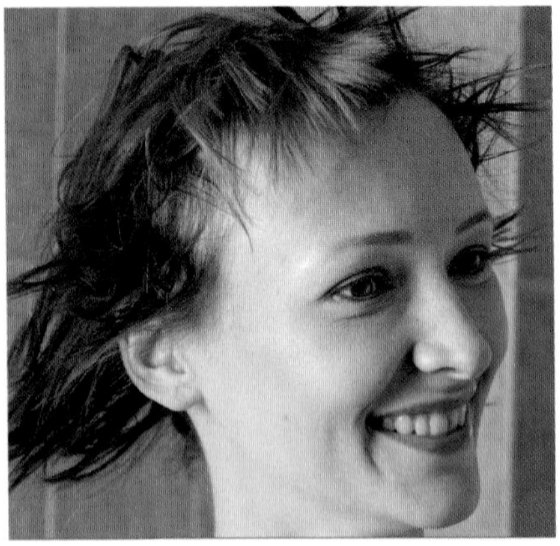

Traction alopecia

THE EFFECT OF TENSION

When you section the hair and make the plait or twist you will need to apply even tension. For cornrows and twists the tension stops the plait or twist from becoming baggy or loose.

Using too much tension can be very uncomfortable for the client. It can also cause **traction alopecia**. This is a condition where the hair is pulled out where it is tightest. This will cause bald patches to occur. It will often be seen around the hairline where the hair is fine. Make sure you do not use too much tension when you make your plait or twist. Ask your client often if the tension is comfortable for them.

STEP-BY-STEP THREE-STEM LOOSE PLAIT

A simple three-stem loose plait is an 'off scalp' plait and can be achieved by following these steps:

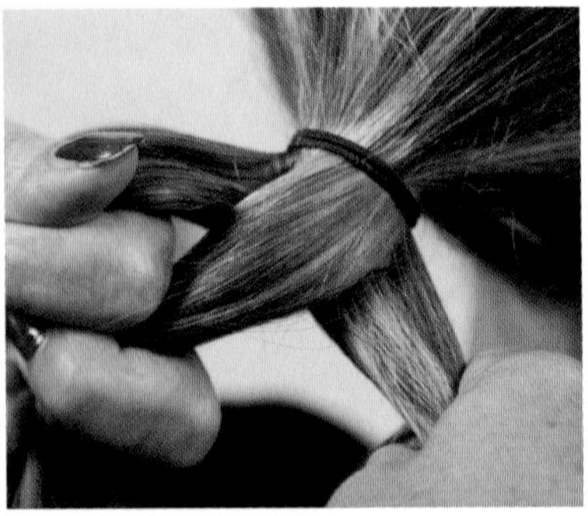

STEP 1 – Secure the hair with a professional band. Divide the hair into three equal sections. Hold sections in one hand and one section in the other.

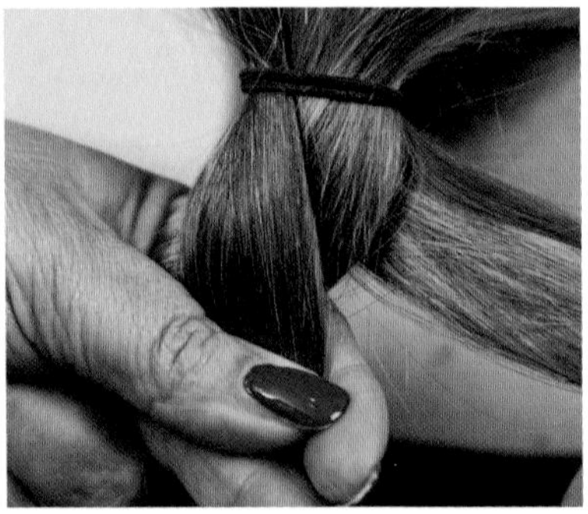

STEP 2 – Pass the left section over the middle section. This will become the new middle section. You can start with the right hand section if you wish as well.

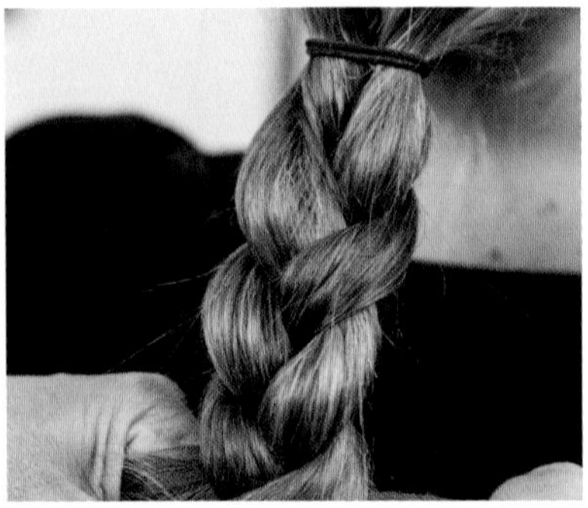

STEP 3 – Now pass the right hand section over the middle so it becomes the new middle section. Repeat these steps till the points of the hair are reached.

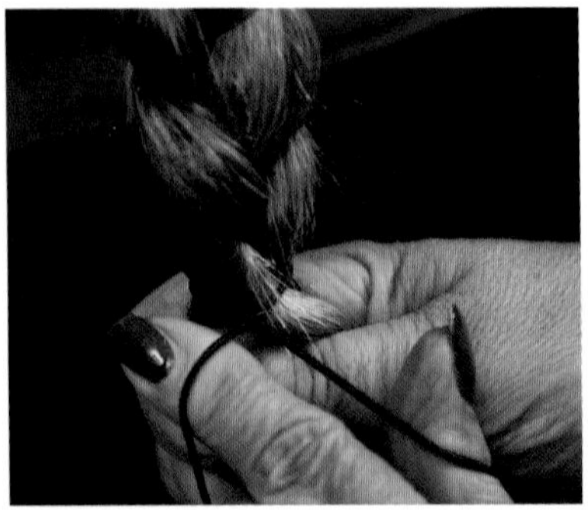

STEP 4 – Secure the points with a professional band.

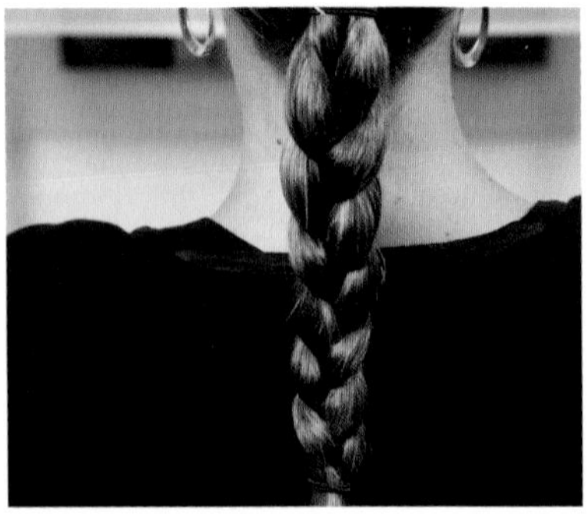

STEP 5 – The finished three-stem loose plait.

STEP-BY-STEP THREE-STEM FRENCH PLAIT

A three-stem French plait is an 'on scalp' plait and is made using the same technique as you used for a simple three-stem plait. To achieve this effect you add sections of hair to the outer sections of your plait as you work from the front of the head to the back. Do not put too much tension on the hair as you work.

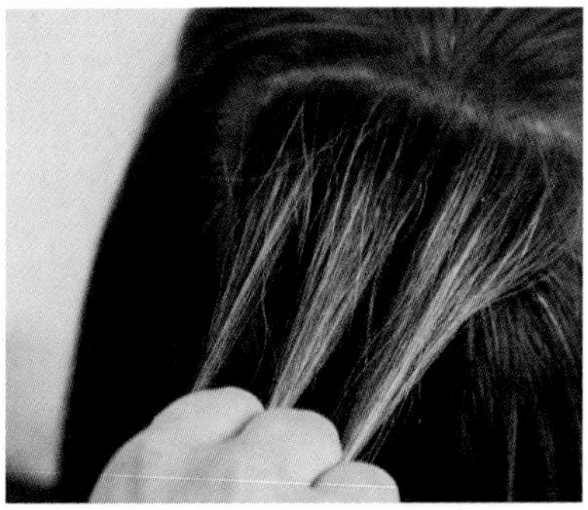

STEP 1 – Determine where you want the plait to start and make three sections.

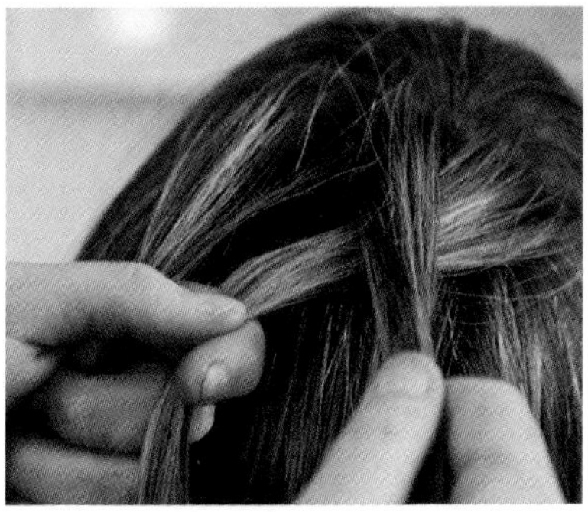

STEP 2 – Cross the right section under the middle section so it becomes the new middle section.

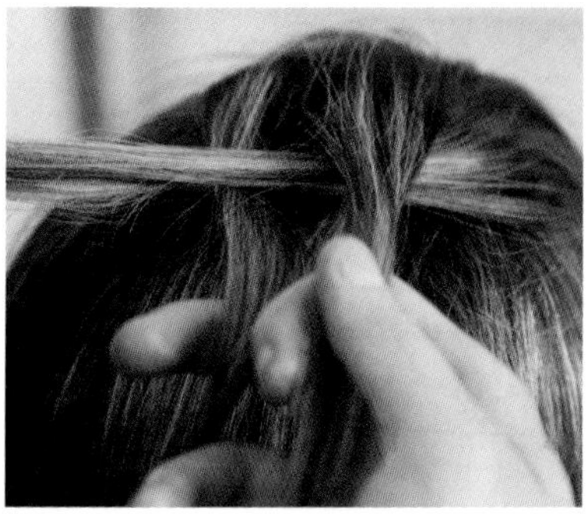

STEP 3 – Now cross the left section under the middle section.

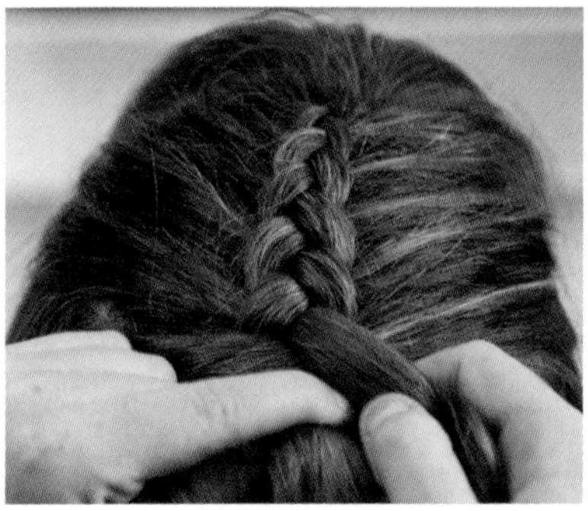

STEP 4 – Add smaller sections of hair to each outer section and intertwine as before.

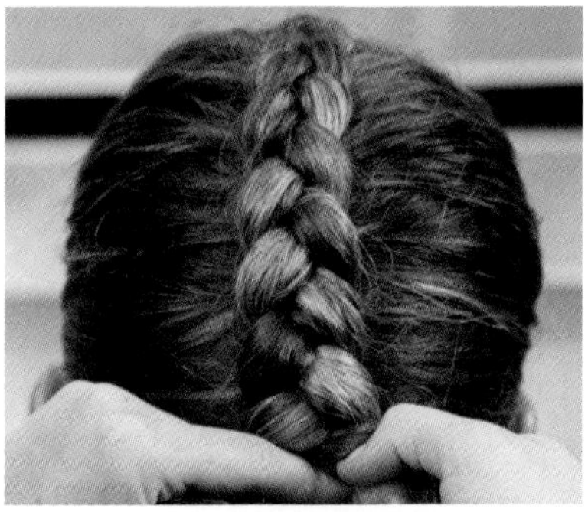

STEP 5 – Keep the tension even as you work down the head.

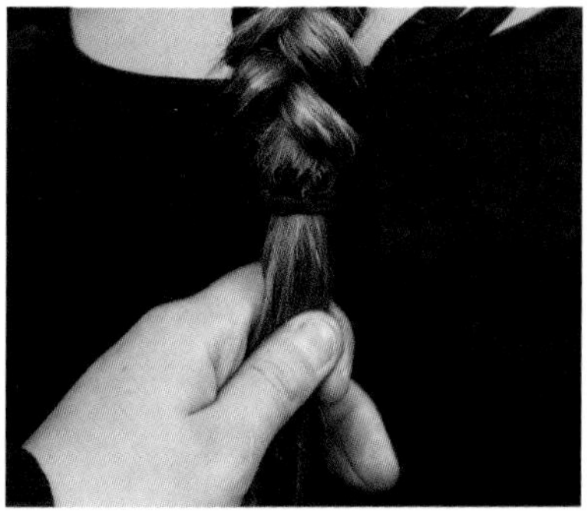

STEP 6 – Secure with a professional band.

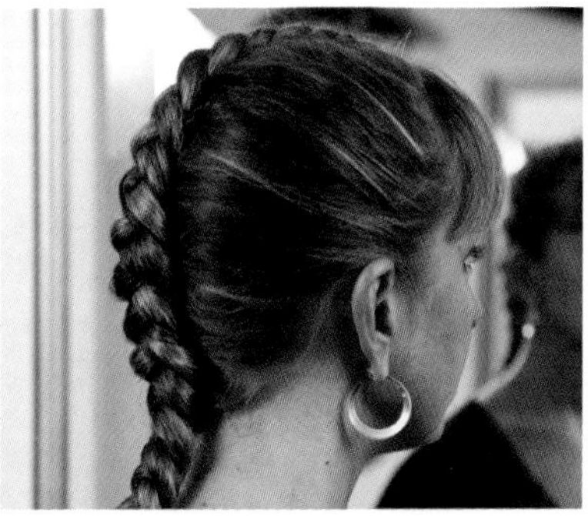

STEP 7 – Check that the client is happy with the finished result.

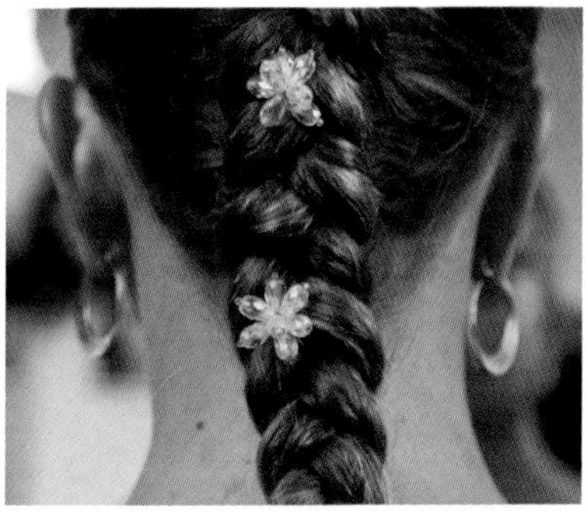

STEP 8 – You can add decorations to the plait to create a party style.

CORNROW PLAITING

The key to this technique is planning. You need to plan the design of the finished look. The plan should include the direction and size of the 'channels' (the sections you use). You need to decide where you are going to start working. This will usually be at the front of the head, or the sides if you are not plaiting the whole head. Once you have your plan clear in your mind you can begin.

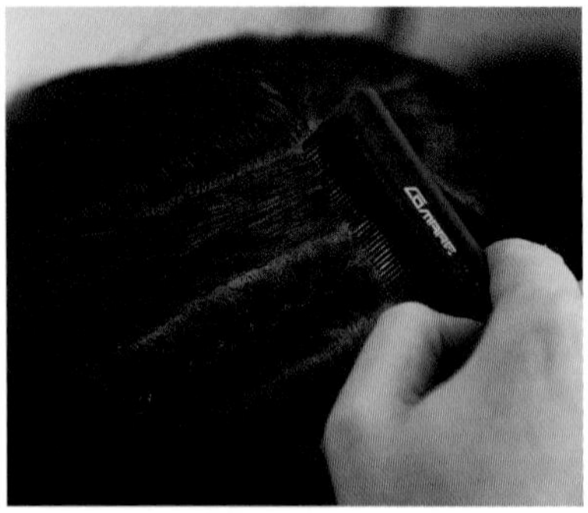

STEP 1 – Make clean neat channels for your cornrow.

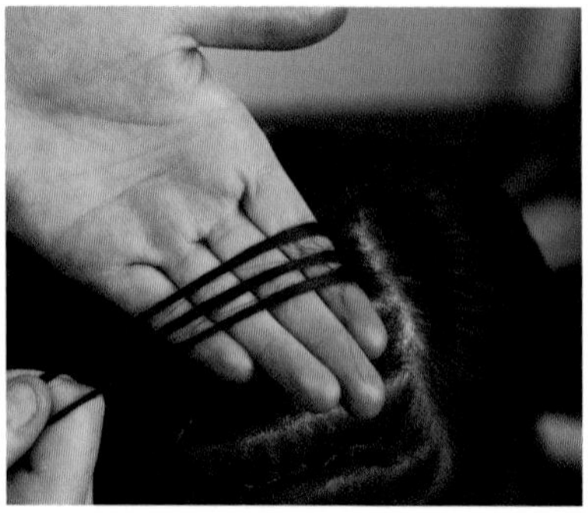

STEP 2 – Make three even sections where you want to start the cornrow.

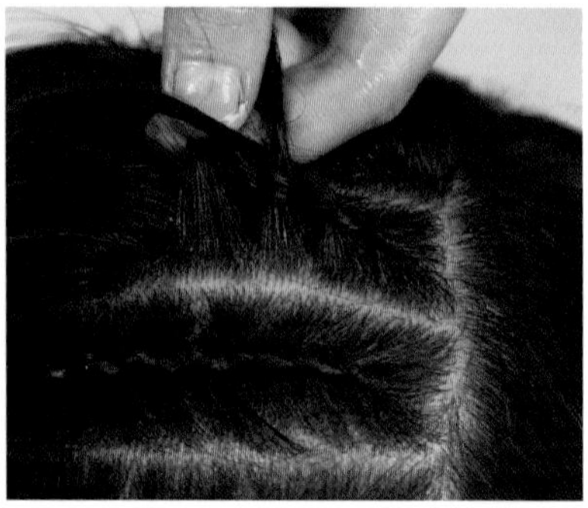

STEP 3 – Move the right section over the middle section and then the left section over the new middle section.

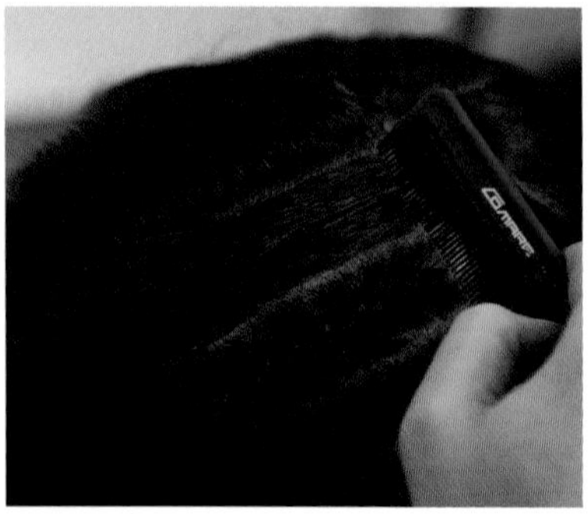

STEP 4 – Make a new channel next to the first.

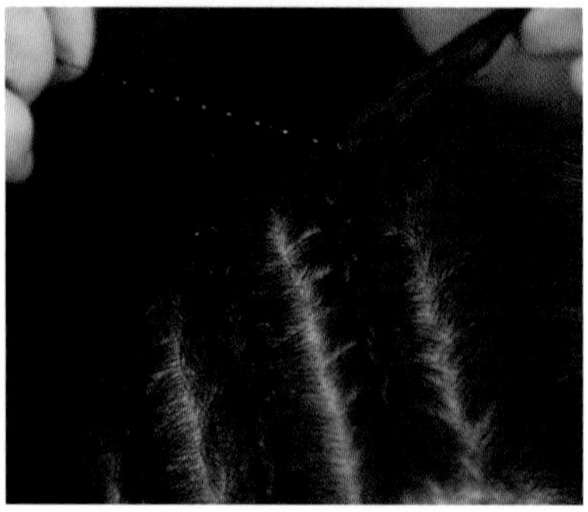

STEP 5 – Add small sections of hair to each outer section as you work down the channel.

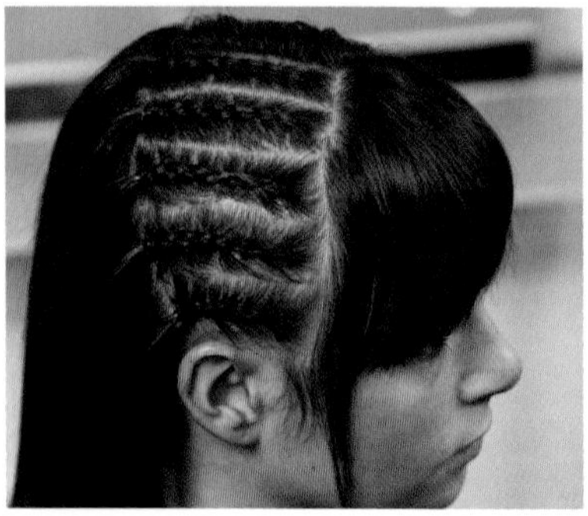

STEP 6 – Continue to add channels following your planned style.

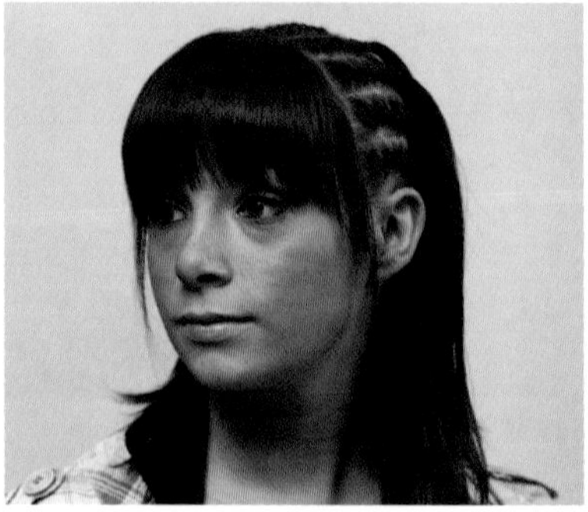

STEP 7 – The finished result.

HANDY HINTS

Don't forget the products that you agreed to use at the consultation. Remember not to overload the hair with product.

HANDY HINTS

Be careful not to use too much tension when cornrowing. Traction alopecia can occur if the tension is high and the cornrows are left in for several weeks.

TWISTS

Twists are an alternative to cornrow plaits. The hair is 'rolled' instead of intertwined. Like cornrows planning is important and should include the direction and size of the channels. Make sure you apply enough tension to give a neat finish. Too much tension can cause traction alopecia.

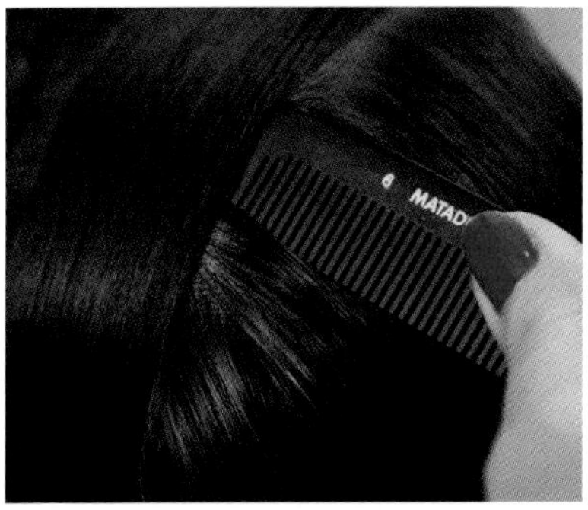

STEP 1 – Using the tail comb, make a clean neat channel where you want the twist. Use sectioning clips to secure the rest of the hair and keep it out of your way.

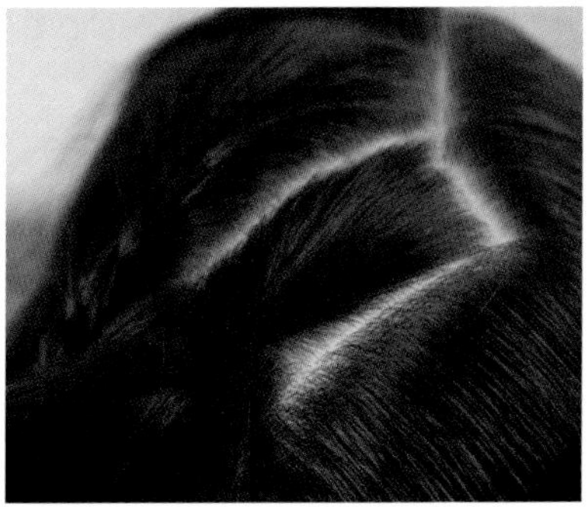

STEP 2 – Start twisting the hair from the front of the channel, keeping the hair flat to the head.

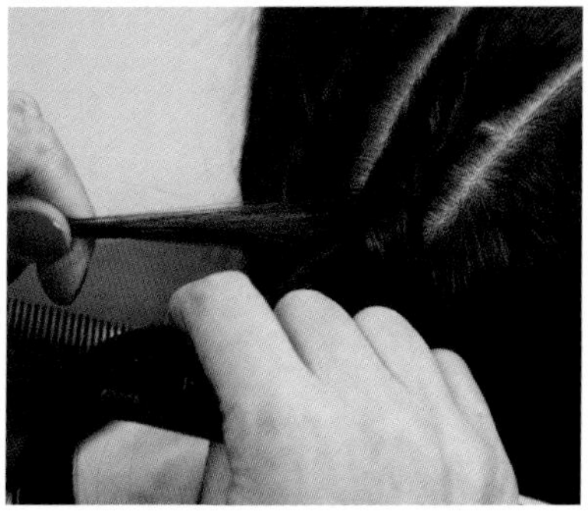

STEP 3 – Start twisting the front part of the channel and add sections of hair as you work towards the end of the channel.

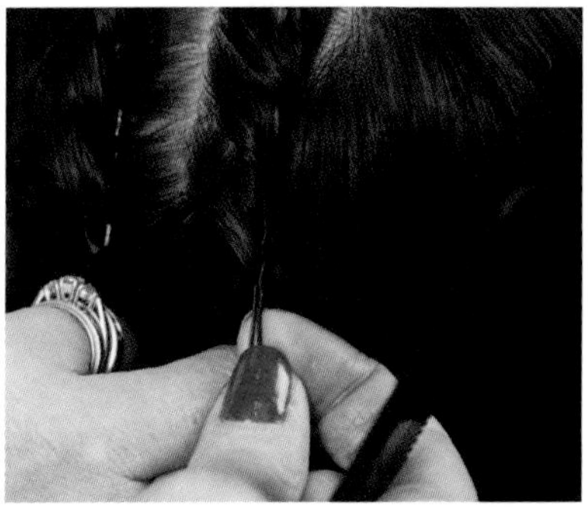

STEP 4 – When you reach the end of the twist secure with a grip. Continue until you have achieved your finished look.

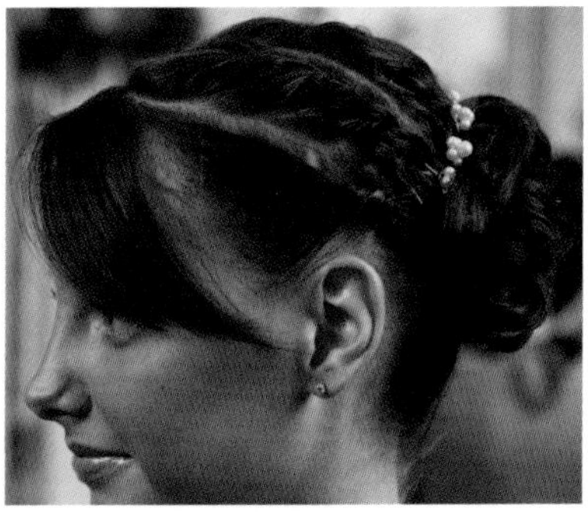

STEP 5 – The finished look.

AFTERCARE ADVICE

Giving the client information about how to look after their hair at home is an important part of the service. Plaits and twists can be left in the hair for several weeks. Keeping them looking nice will be important to the client.

The client will also need to know how to unwind the plaits or twists without damaging their hair. Don't wait until you have finished the service to give the client advice on how to look after the style at home.

- Talk about what they need to do as you work.
- Tell them not to rub the hair as this will cause stray hairs to come away, making the style untidy. If they need to shampoo the hair with the plaits in place they should not massage the hair. A conditioner should be used to keep the hair shining. Make sure the client knows the importance of rinsing all the shampoo out of the hair.
- Remind them not to use too much aftercare product so as not to cause overload. This may make the hair dull.

HANDY HINTS

Remember not to use technical jargon when talking to the client. Keep it simple so they understand. Show them how to do things.

HANDY HINTS

This is your chance to sell the client products to use at home.

Explain how to remove the bands or grips carefully so as not to cause damage to the hair. You cannot just pull them out:

1. Using a tail comb, gently unpick the plait starting at the points, or unwind the twist from the point.
2. Brush the hair with a bristle brush to remove tangles after unpicking.
3. Use a good cleansing shampoo to remove product build-up.
4. Use a conditioner to restore the condition of the hair.

ACTIVITY

In a small group, make a list of all the things that you need to tell the client when giving aftercare advice after you have plaited their hair.

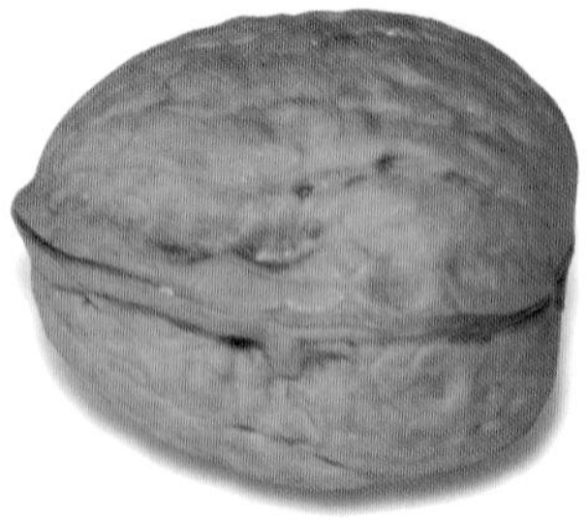

IN A NUTSHELL

You are now at the end of the chapter. Before you test your knowledge with the revision activities, check the following list to see if you feel confident in all the areas covered. If there are still any areas you're unsure of, go back over them in the book and ask your tutor for extra support:

- the basic techniques for plaiting and twisting the hair
- the factors that can influence your choice of techniques
- the tools, equipment and products that are used in styling women's hair and selecting them
- how to prepare for plaiting and twisting hair
- following safe and hygienic working practices
- the importance of good communication, behaviour and attitude when styling women's hair
- carry out plaiting and twisting services
- giving the client aftercare advice.

SmartScreen 105 revision cards

SmartScreen 105 activity assignment

REVISION ACTIVITIES

Use the questions below to test your knowledge of Chapter 004/105 to see just how much information you've gained. This can help you to prepare for your assessments. Turn to pages 490–491 for the answers.

WORDS TO FIND

Copy and complete the sentences below. Use these words to help you fill in the gaps.

tail comb	elasticity	three-stem
channel	twists	professional bands
cornrows	traction alopecia	serum
cross-infection	face shape	French

1 Twists and plaits should be secured using ______________ .

2 The client's ______________ will determine whether plaits or twists will suit them.

3 The ______________ of the hair describes how the hair will stretch.

4 If there are bald areas just inside the hairline it could be a sign of ______________ .

5 The section taken for 'on scalp' plaits is called a ______________ .

6 ______________ is the term used to describe the transfer of a disease from one client to another.

7 ______________ is a product that can be used when plaiting.

8 ______________ and ______________ are examples of 'on scalp' plaiting.

9 A ______________ is used to make partings and split sections.

10 A ______________ plait and a ______________ plait are 'off scalp' plaits.

TEST YOUR KNOWLEDGE FURTHER

1 French plaiting is an 'on scalp' method of plaiting. True or false?

2 Name **four** factors that can influence your choice of plaiting or twisting technique.

3 Why is it important to prepare your work area before you start work on the client?

4 Name **three** styling products that can be used during plaiting or twisting and state what they are used for.

5 Name **four** tools or pieces of equipment that can be used for plaiting or twisting.

6 What can happen if too much tension is used in plaiting or twisting?

7 What face shape is ideal for plaiting and twisting styles?

8 What should be used to secure a cornrow plait?

9 Name **two** things that can be used to enhance plaiting and twisting styles.

10 Name **two** things that you should tell the client when giving aftercare advice.

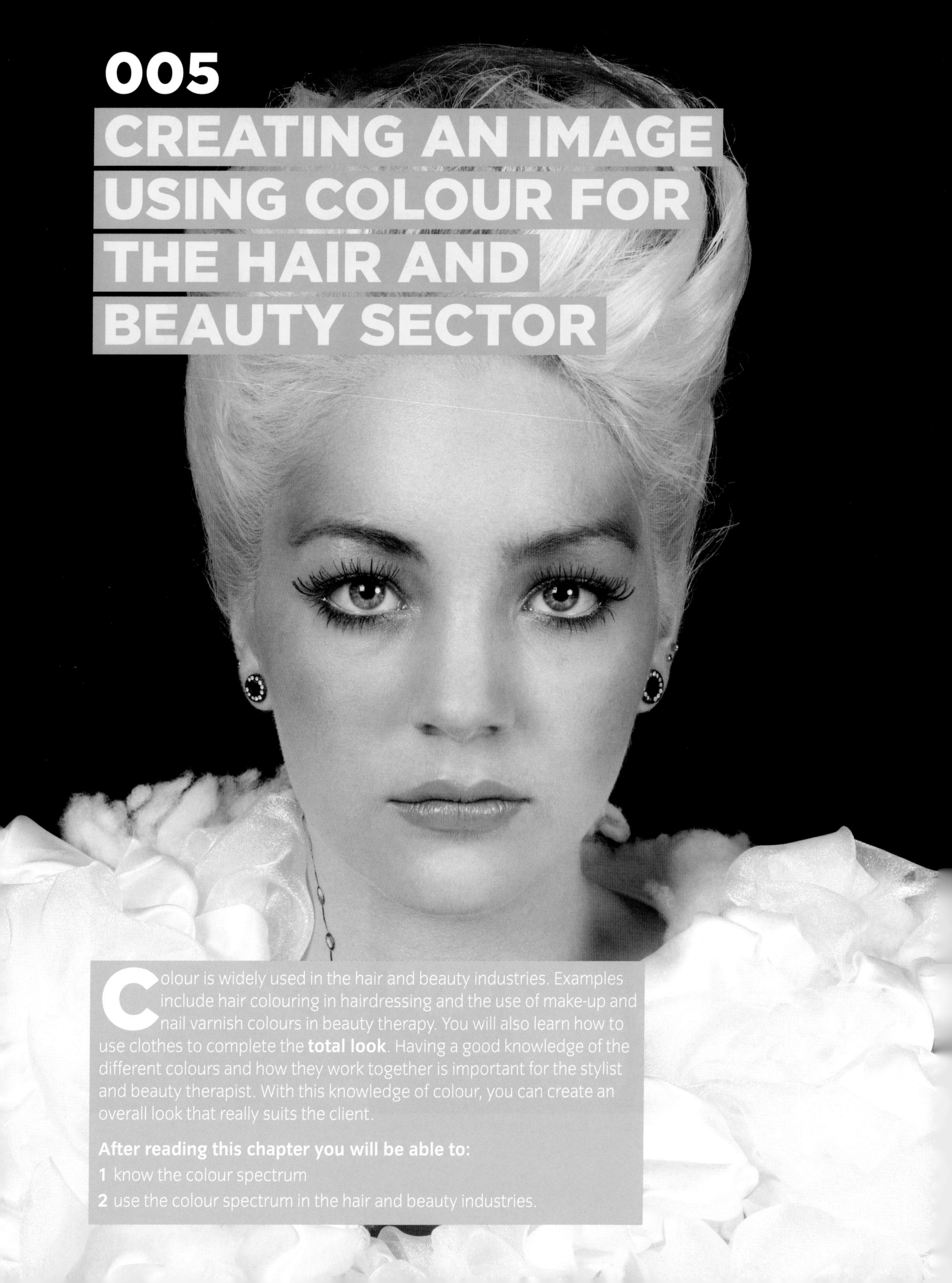

005 CREATING AN IMAGE USING COLOUR FOR THE HAIR AND BEAUTY SECTOR

Colour is widely used in the hair and beauty industries. Examples include hair colouring in hairdressing and the use of make-up and nail varnish colours in beauty therapy. You will also learn how to use clothes to complete the **total look**. Having a good knowledge of the different colours and how they work together is important for the stylist and beauty therapist. With this knowledge of colour, you can create an overall look that really suits the client.

After reading this chapter you will be able to:

1 know the colour spectrum

2 use the colour spectrum in the hair and beauty industries.

Total look
The complete image, made up of hair colour, make-up tones, nails and clothes

KNOW THE COLOUR SPECTRUM

In order to understand how colours are made and used, we need to know about the colour spectrum. These are the colours that can be seen naturally in a rainbow – red, orange, yellow, green, blue, indigo and violet.

HANDY HINTS

The colours of the spectrum can be easily remembered by using the first letter of each word in this sentence:

Richard – Red
Of – Orange
York – Yellow
Gave – Green
Battle – Blue
In – Indigo
Vain – Violet

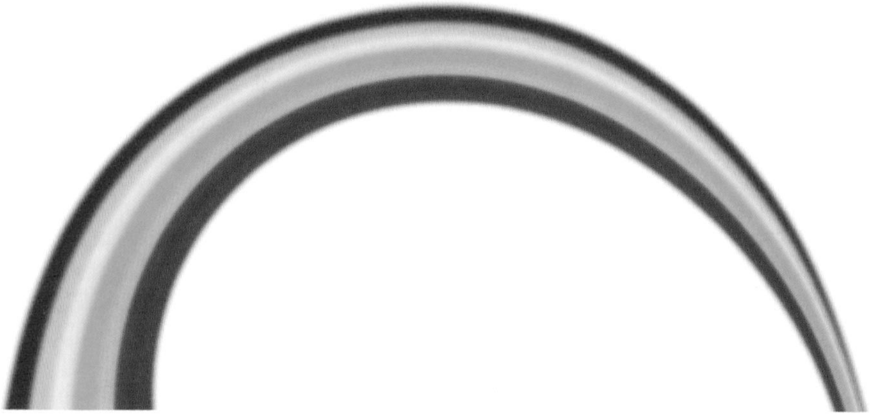

ACTIVITY

Learn the handy hint to help you remember the colours of the spectrum.

Colour plays an important role in the hair and beauty sector. The most obvious use of colour in these industries is:

- hair colours
- nail enamel colours
- make-up colours.

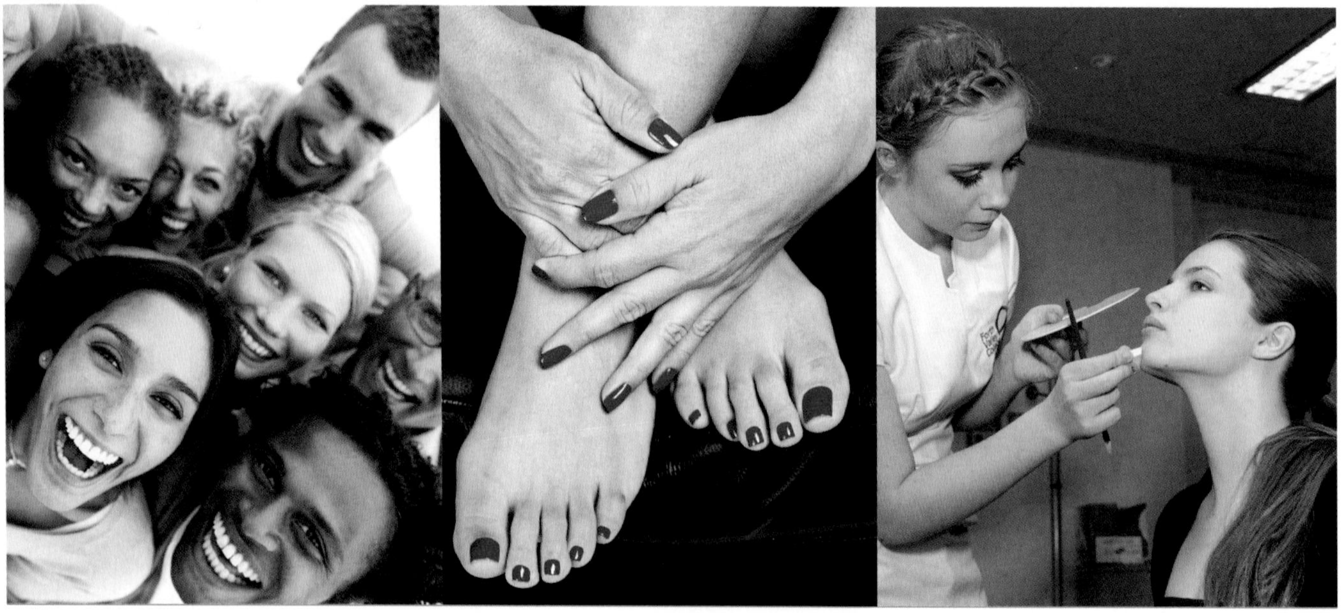

Hair colours, nail colours and make-up colours all help to make up an exciting hair and beauty image

Natural light is sometimes called 'white light'. All the colours of the spectrum are found in natural light. To be able to see them, the natural light has to pass through a different object, such as a glass **prism**. This will make the colours separate to form the different colours of the rainbow.

Prism
A piece of glass that has five triangular surfaces. When white light is passed through it, it creates the colours of the spectrum

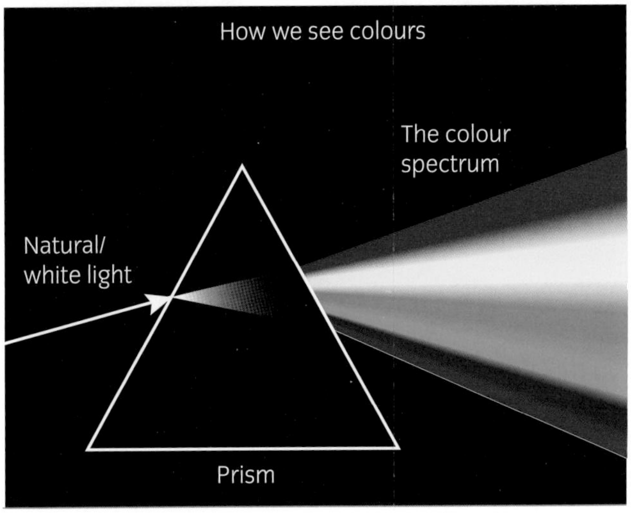

White light passing through a prism to create the colour spectrum

HANDY HINTS
When it rains and the sun is shining at the same time, the sunlight shines through the raindrops and this causes a rainbow in the sky (just like the example of the prism).

It is important to know about these colours and which ones may suit your client. You will learn more about this later on in the chapter.

HANDY HINTS
It is important for a salon to take into account the type of lighting that it uses, as different lights will make colours look different.

The colours that are used when colouring hair, in make-up and also nail enamels are all colours that use a mixture of primary and secondary colours.

PRIMARY COLOURS

These are colours that cannot be created by mixing other colours together. The three primary colours are:

- red
- yellow
- blue.

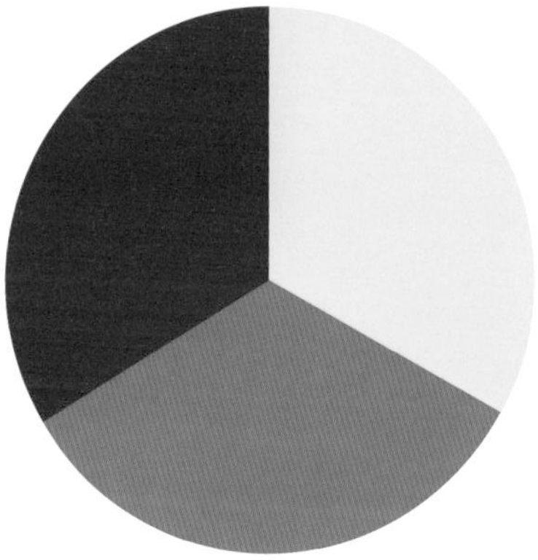

ACTIVITY

Working in pairs find two red things, two yellow things and two blue things.

SECONDARY COLOURS

These are colours that are created when the primary colours are mixed together. They are:

- green
- orange
- violet.

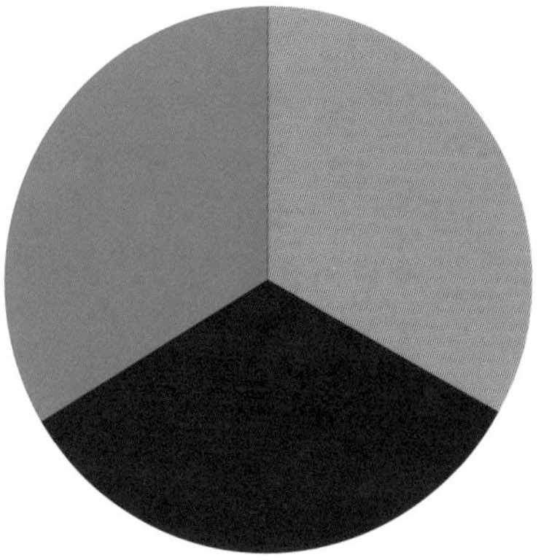

ACTIVITY

Working in pairs find two green things, two orange things and two violet things.

Combination
Mixture (of colours)

HANDY HINTS
Sometimes violet is referred to as purple.

The table below shows which **combination** of primary colours are needed to produce the secondary colours.

yellow	+	blue	=	green
blue	+	red	=	violet
red	+	yellow	=	orange

ACTIVITY

Using red, yellow and blue paints, mix these primary colours together in pairs to see what secondary colours are made.

ACTIVITY

See what happens if you mix different amounts of each primary colour together. Make a note of your findings and discuss them with your group.

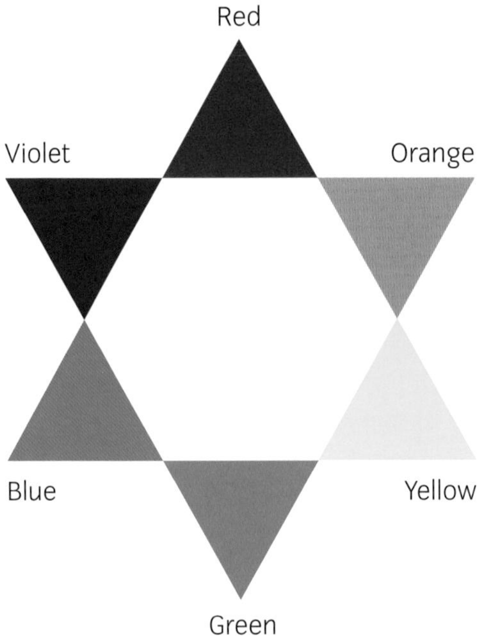

A colour star

Colour star
A picture made up of the three primary colours and the three secondary colours

This knowledge about the colour spectrum is used to create a **colour star**.

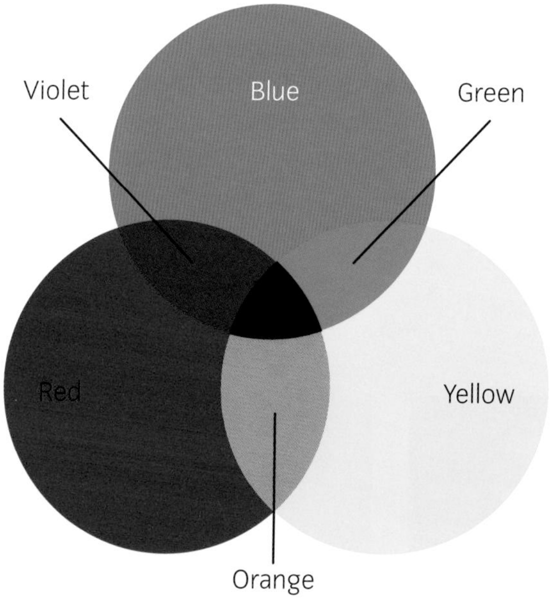

How primary and secondary colours are connected

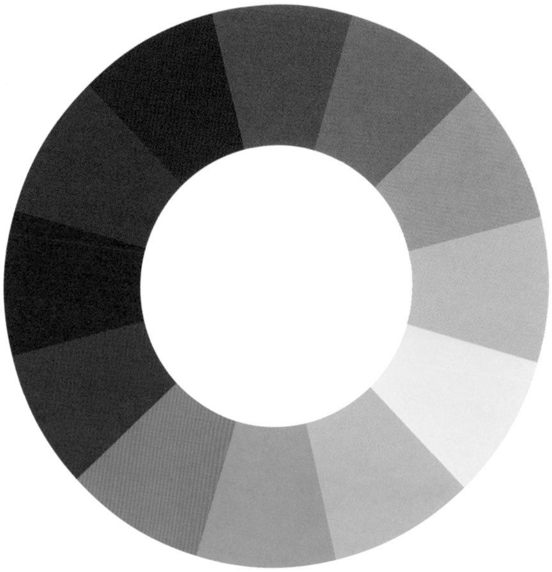
Colour circle showing different shades of secondary colours created by mixing together different amounts of the primary colours

COMPLEMENTARY COLOURS

Complementary colours are secondary colours and primary colours that are opposite each other on the colour star.

HANDY HINTS

The colour star is sometimes referred to as a colour wheel.

ACTIVITY

Draw a copy of the six-pointed colour star on a plain piece of paper. Use paints or pens to fill in the primary and secondary colours.

The complementary colours for the three primary colours (red, blue and yellow) are found by mixing the two other primary colours together, for example:

- The complementary colour for red is green (made by mixing blue and yellow together).

ACTIVITY

Work out what the complementary colours are for yellow and blue. Copy and complete the sentences below, filling in the gaps with the correct colours.

- The complementary colour for yellow is ____________ (made by mixing ____________ and ____________ together).
- The complementary colour for blue is ____________ (made by mixing ____________ and ____________ together).

Check that your answers are correct with your tutor.

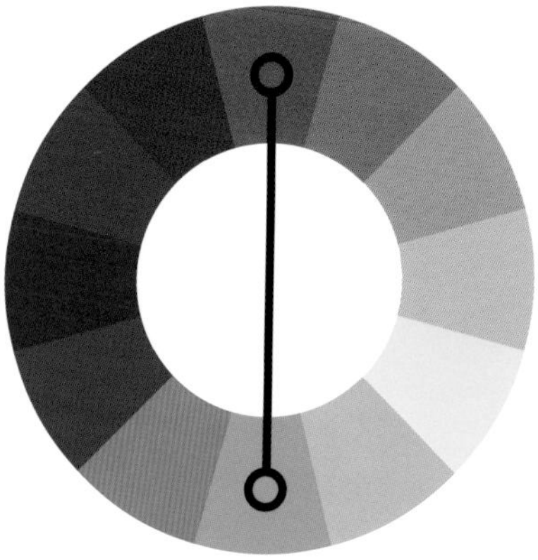
Red and green are complementary colours as they are opposite each other on the colour wheel

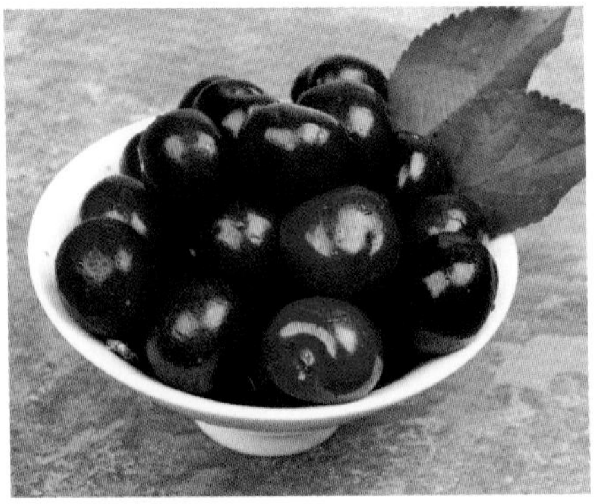

When placed next to each other, complementary colours can make each other appear brighter. The use of complementary colours works well when you want something to stand out. Look at the photo of the bowl of red cherries with green mint leaves. Can you see how bright these two complementary colours look when they are together?

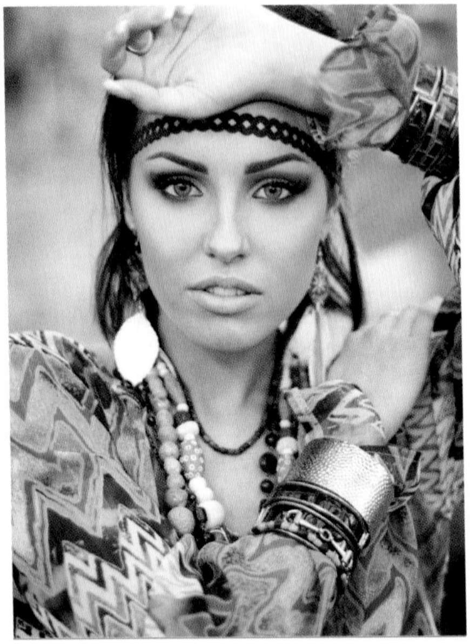

Complementary colours are used in product advertising to make things stand out more

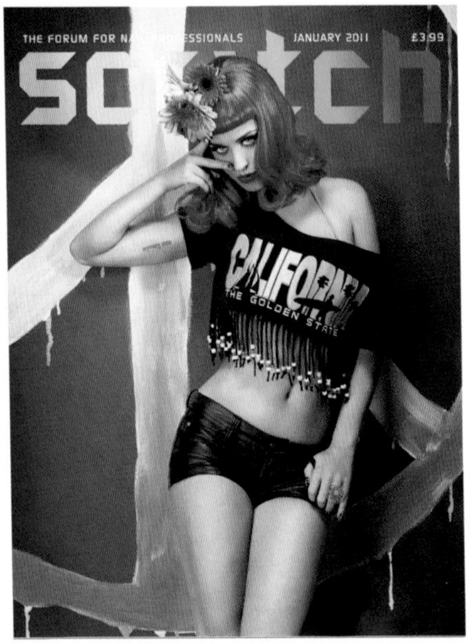

Complementary colours are used in fashion to create an image that will be noticed

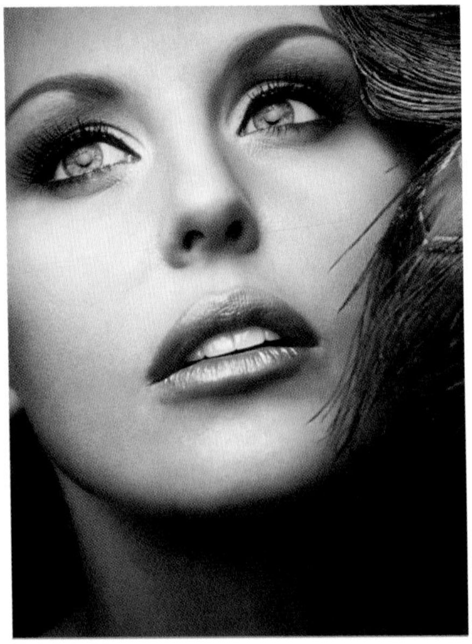

Complementary colours can be used in hair and make-up to create an image that will look more dramatic

Mood board
A type of design (often a poster) that may consist of images, text and samples of objects; used to develop design ideas and to show the image to other team members or clients

ACTIVITY

You may choose to work in pairs or groups for this activity.

In order to help you fully understand complementary colours, create three **mood boards** for each of the following complementary colours:

- red and green colours
- blue and orange colours
- yellow and purple colours.

Use images from the internet or from magazines that show these colours being used together. Use coloured paper and materials as well to make your mood boards look even more exciting.

Once you have created your mood boards, display them to other groups and discuss what you have learnt about complementary colours and how these colours might be used in hairdressing and beauty therapy.

HANDY HINTS

For more information on mood boards, go to Chapter 216 The art of photographic make-up.

WARM AND COOL TONES

The primary and secondary colours can be put into two groups:

- Warm **tones** – these are colours that make you think of heat. Examples are yellow, orange and red.
- Cool tones – these are colours that make you think of the cold. Examples are blue, violet and green.

Tones
Shades of colour

ACTIVITY

- Look at the colour star. Can you see the difference between a warm and cool tone?
- Discuss with the rest of the group why it is important that a hairdresser or beauty therapist knows about warm and cool tones.

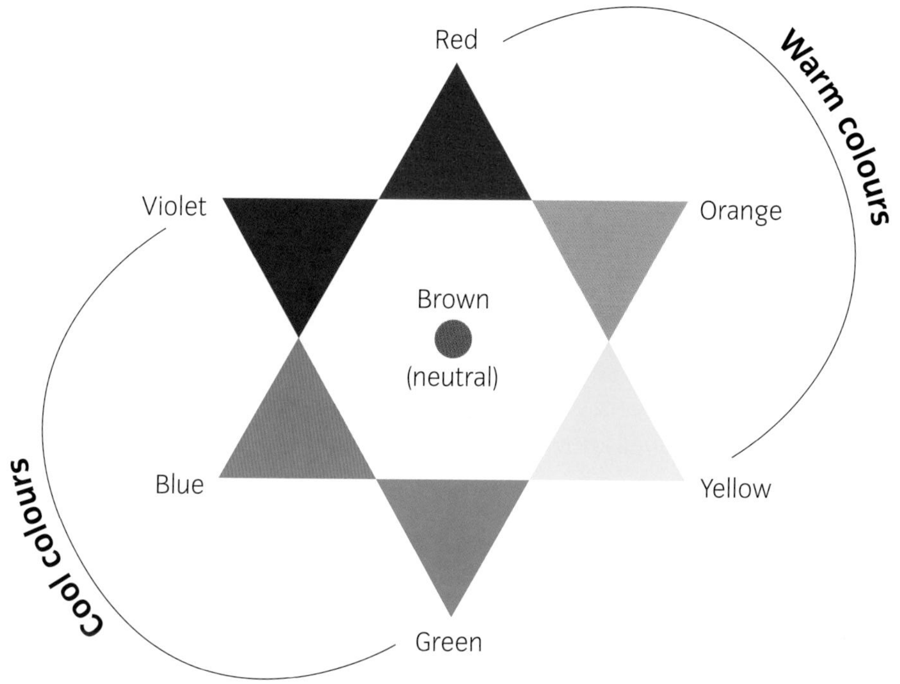

SmartScreen 005 worksheet 3

USE THE COLOUR SPECTRUM IN THE HAIR AND BEAUTY INDUSTRIES

COLOUR TONES IN HAIRDRESSING

Hairdressers need to be aware of the different tones of colour. Some people will suit warm tones and others will suit cool tones.

A hairdresser is often asked to change their clients' hair colour. There are many different hair colour services that hairdressers can offer such as:

- temporary colours
- quasi-permanent colours
- semi-permanent colours
- permanent colours
- highlights
- lowlights.

ACTIVITY

- Research on the internet to find out the hair-colour products that professional retail companies offer (eg Wella and Goldwell). Present your findings in a chart and discuss them with the rest of the group.
- If you had your own salon, which product company would you choose and why? (Reasons may include price, variety of products available, packaging, how well known the company is.)

HANDY HINTS

Refer to Chapter 111 Colouring hair using temporary colour for more information on colour services used in hairdressing.

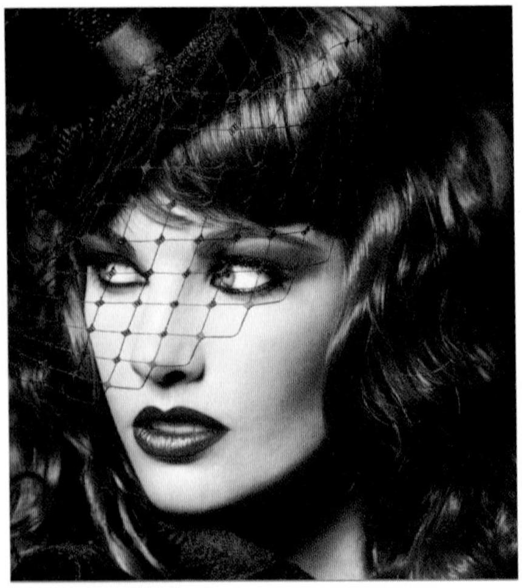

Red hair has warm tones...

WARM HAIR TONES

Warm hair colours include those with red and orange tones, for example golden brown, chestnut, mahogany and copper colours.

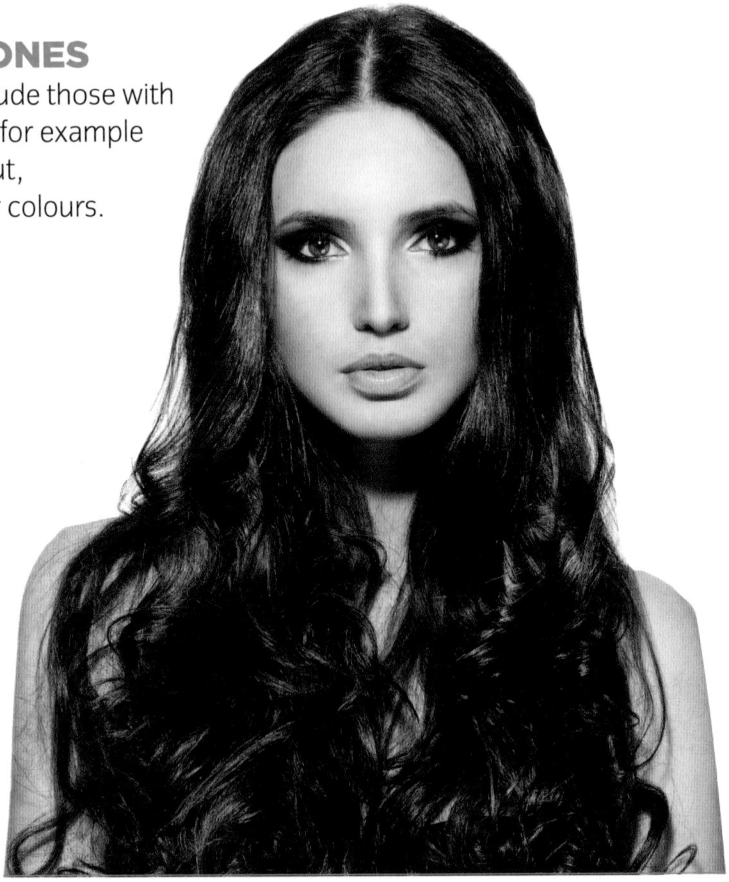

... and so does chestnut

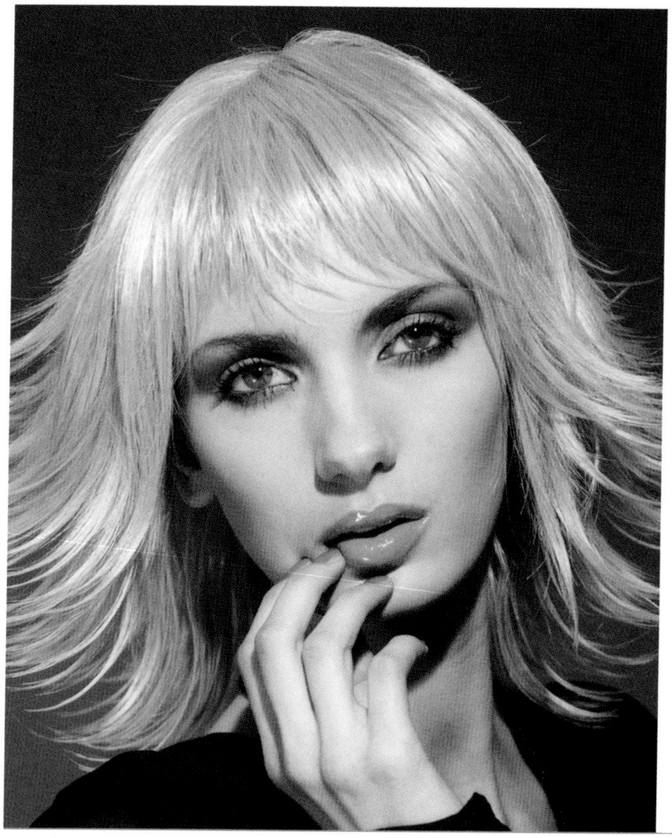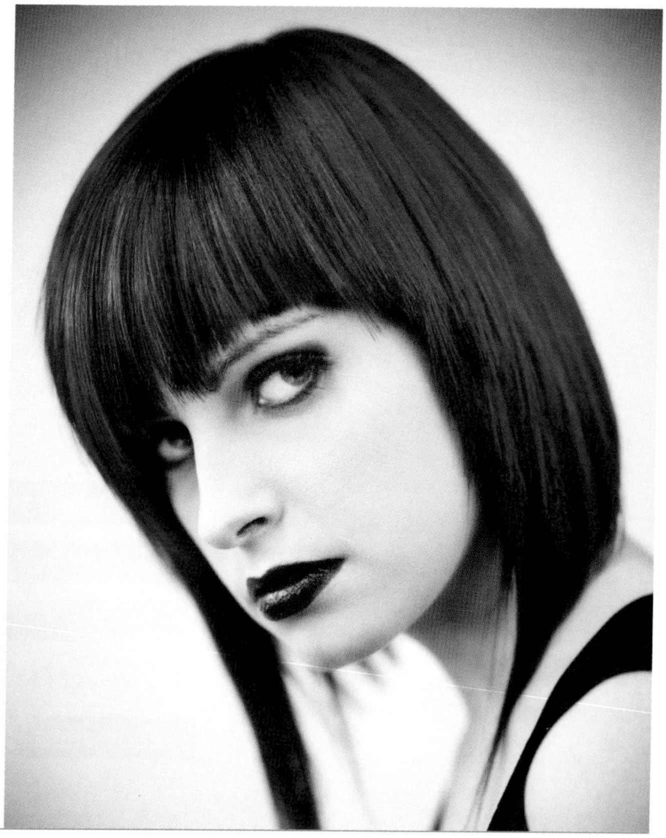

Blond and purple hair with cool hair tones

COOL HAIR TONES

Cool hair colours include those with purple and blue tones, for example platinum blond, dark browns and black.

ACTIVITY

Research different hair colours on the internet and in magazines. Build up a portfolio of images and separate them into cool and warm colours.

ACTIVITY

Look at the colour charts in the hairdressing salon. Can you work out which ones are the cool tones and which are the warm tones?

CORRECTING HAIR COLOURS

The colour star is also used when hair colour needs to be corrected. This may be needed if the hair colour is not the shade of colour that the client wants. This is known as **neutralising colours**.

When we mix colours from opposite sides of the colour star, we create a brown or **neutral tone**.

Some clients may want to change their natural hair tone, so their hair tone is neutralised by using the opposite colour on the colour star.

Neutralising colours
Unwanted colour on the hair can be changed by adding another colour. This is usually the complementary colour (opposite colour on the colour star)

Neutral tone
Colour that is neither too warm nor too cool

HANDY HINTS

A hairdresser needs to understand the colour star in order to know which colours to use to correct hair colour.

Usually, the opposite colour on the colour star is used to correct the hair tone.

- Too much red tone in the hair can be corrected by adding a green tone.
- Too much orange tone in the hair can be corrected by adding a blue tone.

In hairdressing, however, the names of the colours are changed when referring to colour correction, to make them seem softer and more natural. The following words are used in hairdressing to describe colour tones to the client.

blue = ash

violet = silver/burgundy

red = mahogany

orange = copper

yellow = gold

green = matt

HANDY HINTS

A hairdresser will not tell the client that they are putting orange or blue colours on their hair; instead they will use words such as 'copper' or 'ash'.

ACTIVITY

To help your understanding of how colours are used in hairdressing to neutralise tones, see if you can work out which colour will be used to correct the following hair tones. Remember to use the correct hairdressing colour tone (mentioned above). Use the colour star to help you.

Which tone will you use to neutralise:

- highlights that are too golden
- strong natural copper tones
- strong red tones?

Check your answers with your tutor.

HANDY HINTS

Refer to Chapter 111 Colouring hair using temporary colour for more information on colouring hair.

COLOUR TONES IN BEAUTY THERAPY

Beauty therapists also need to be aware of colour tones. In beauty therapy, colours are taken into account when applying make-up or in face painting. In a make-up treatment, the colours chosen must suit the client's natural skin and eye colour. For nail services nail polish must suit the client's skin, eg red nail polish won't work on a reddish skin tone.

WARM SKIN TONES

A warm skin tone has more yellow and red tones in it. People with a warm skin tone will usually have hazel or brown eyes.

HANDY HINTS

Look at the make-up that you use. Try and work out if they are cool or warm tones and whether they work with your skin tone.

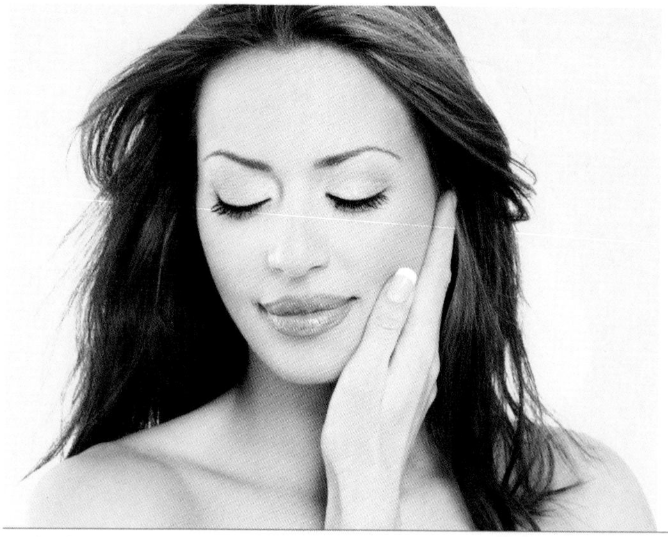

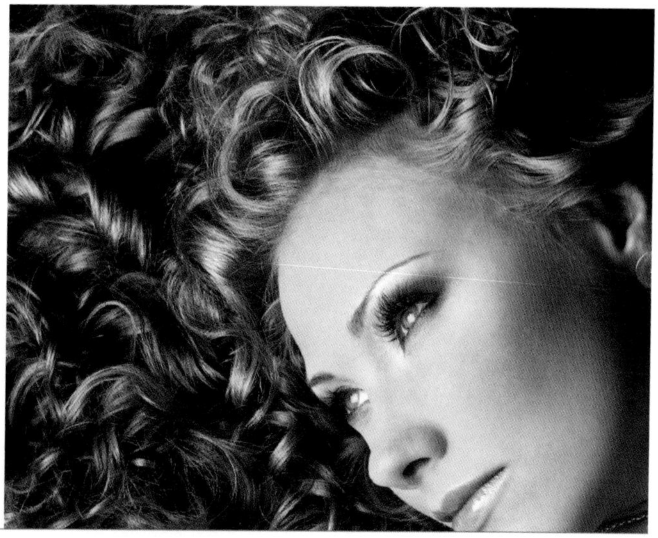

Both of these models have warm skin tones

COOL SKIN TONES

A cool skin tone has more beige tones in it. People with a cool skin tone will usually have blue, green or very dark eyes.

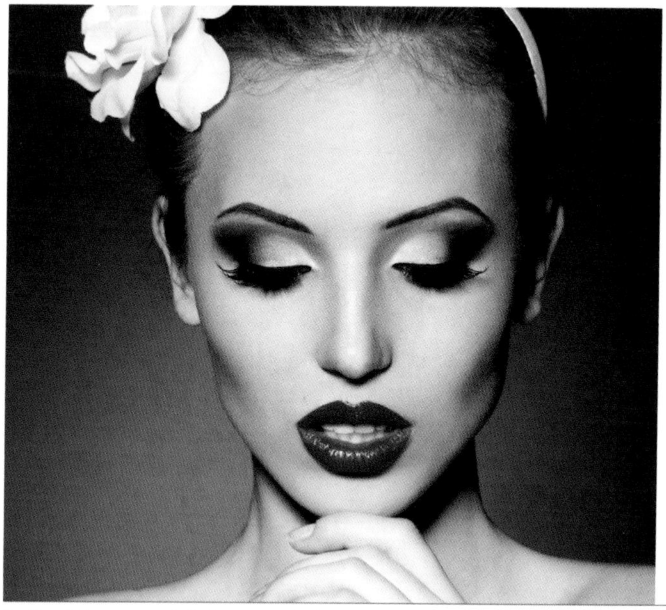

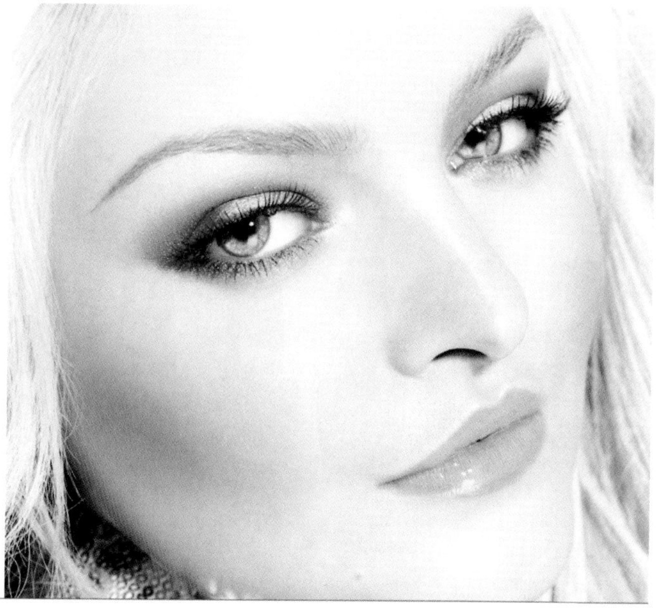

Both of these models have cool skin tones

ACTIVITY

Research different make-up looks on the internet and in magazines. Build up a portfolio of images and separate them into cool and warm colours.

HANDY HINTS

Refer to Chapter 106 Basic make-up application for more information on how colour is used in make-up.

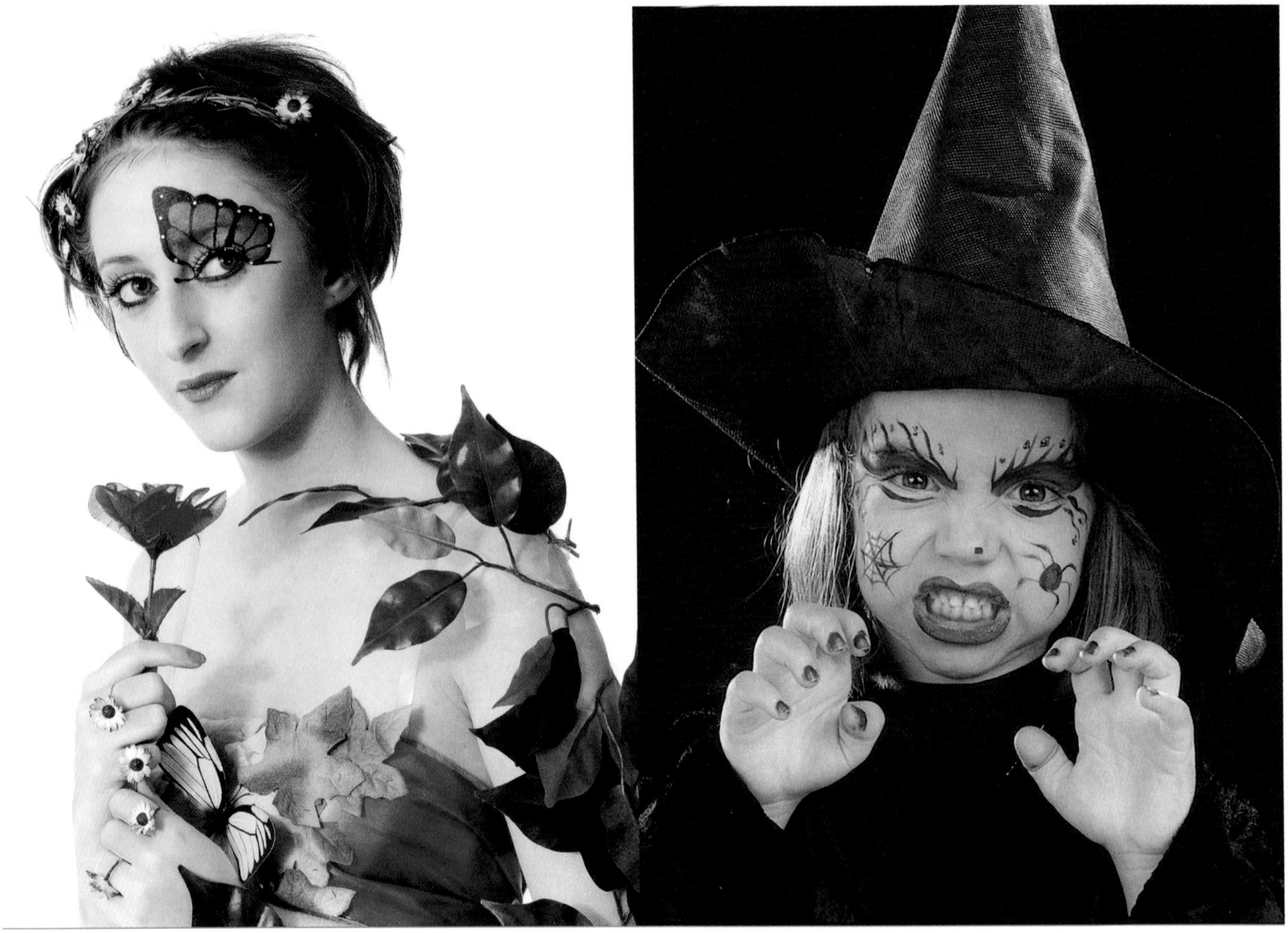

In face painting, the colours used can be bolder and stand out more

Manicure
Treatment for the hands and nails

HANDY HINTS

Refer to Chapter 107 Themed face painting for more information on how colour is used in face painting.

COLOUR FOR THE NAILS

Colour is also used in beauty therapy during a **manicure** or nail art treatment. The nail enamel and nail art that are applied to the nails come in many different colours.

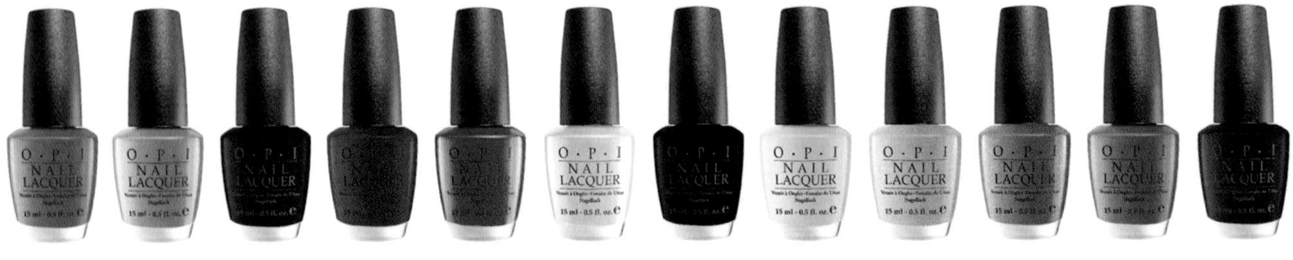

Examples of nail emamel colours

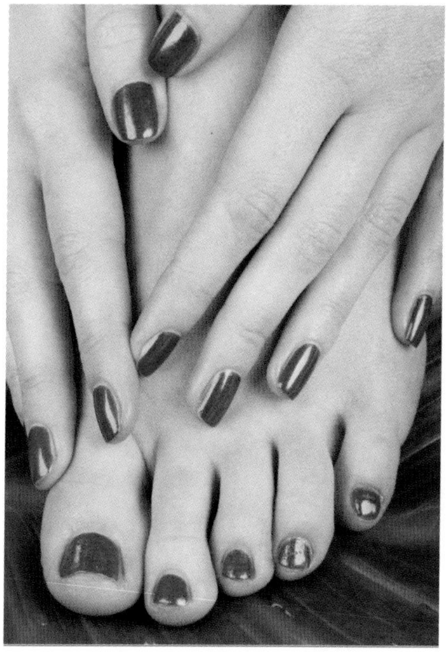

A warm-coloured nail enamel

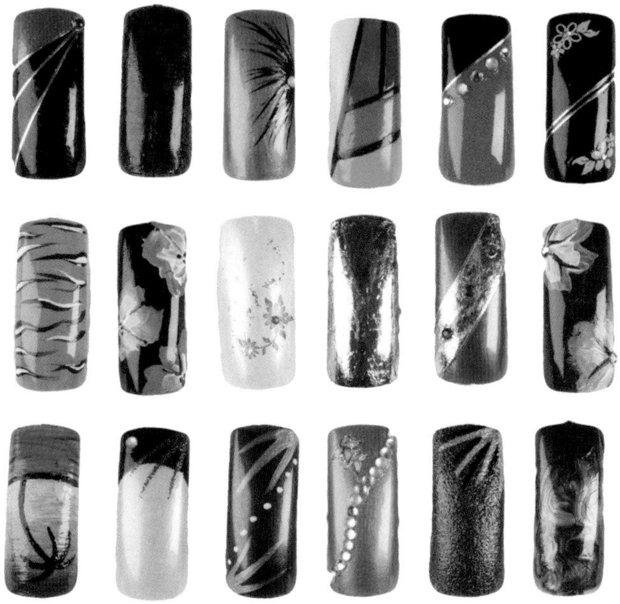

Colour used in nail art

ACTIVITY

Bring a selection of different colours of nail enamel to your class. Your tutor will make sure that there is a selection of all the colours of the spectrum available. Working in small groups, put these varnishes into a circle to show the colour star.

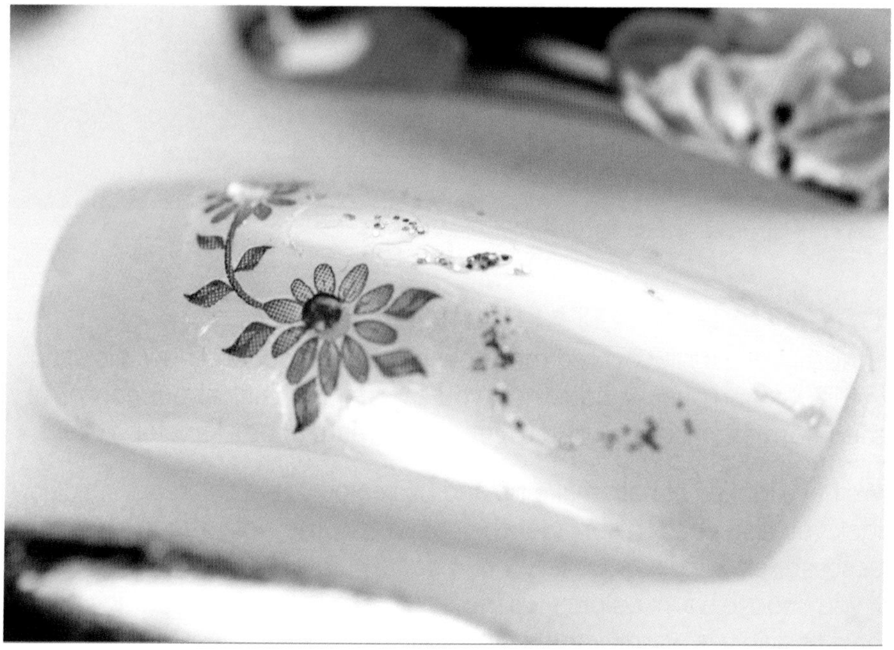

Warm colours used in nail art

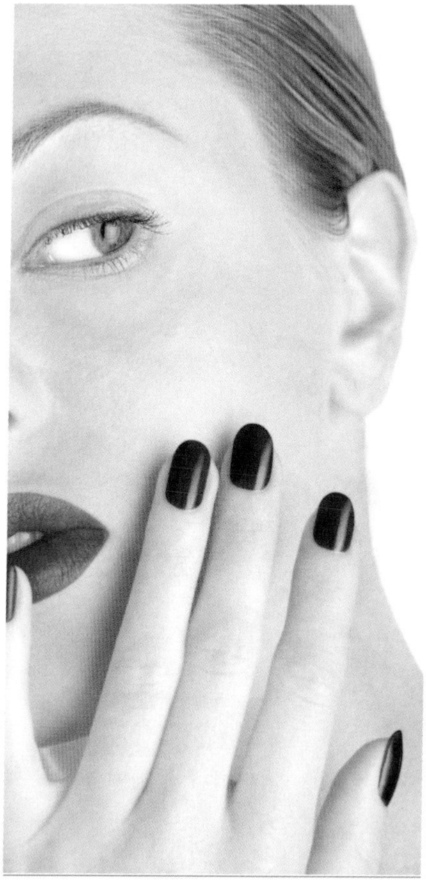

A cool-coloured nail enamel

HANDY HINTS

A person with a warm skin tone (yellow toned) may look better with warm-toned nail enamel or nail art, for example brown, cream, yellow, red and orange colours.

HANDY HINTS

A person with a cool skin tone (beige toned) may look better with cool-toned nail enamel or nail art, for example black, white, blue, green and purple colours.

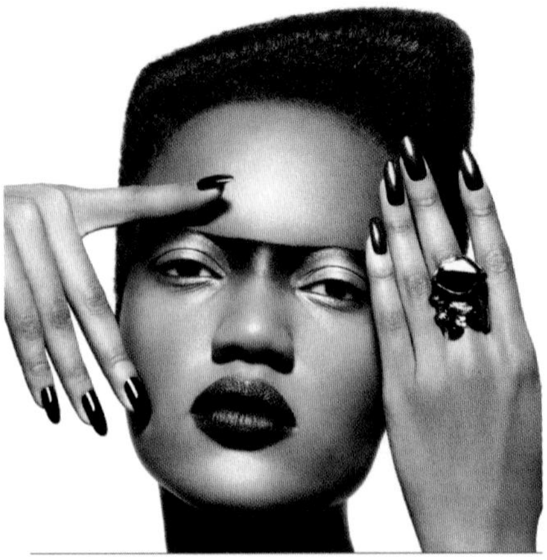

Cool make-up colours

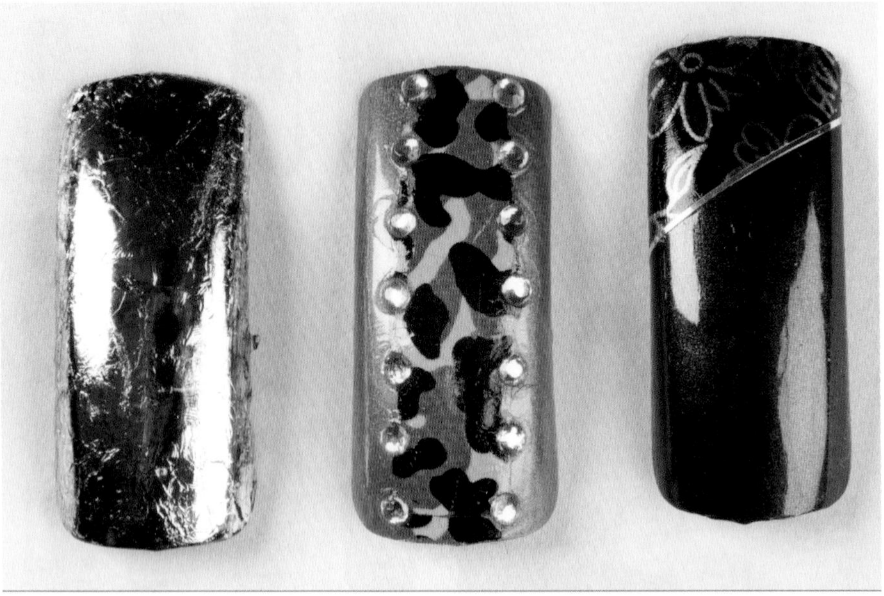

Cool colours used in nail art

HANDY HINTS

For a more dramatic nail look, complementary colours may be used on the nails, such as red and green, blue and orange, and yellow and purple.

HANDY HINTS

Refer to Chapter 007/109/110 Hand care and providing basic manicure and pedicure treatments for more information on how colour is used on the nails.

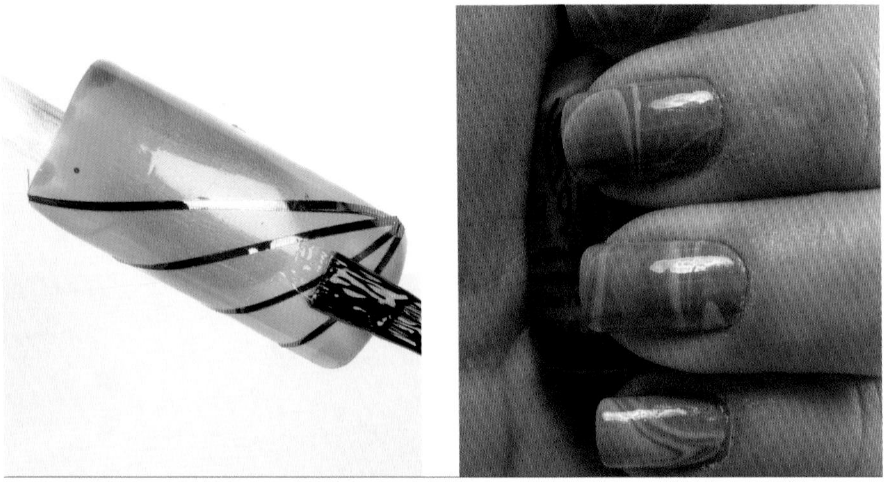

Some examples of nail art using complementary colours

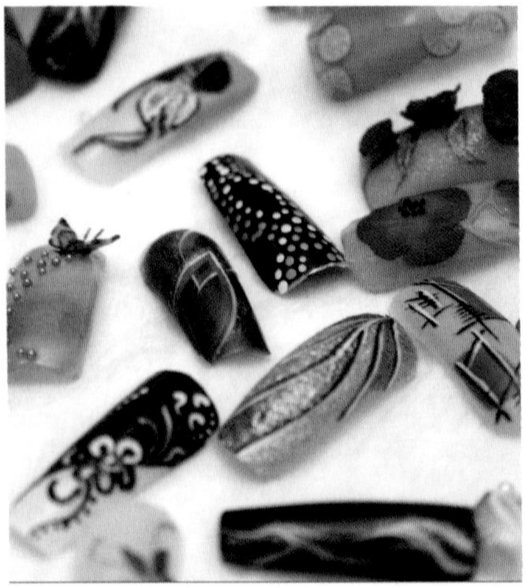

Choose nails to go with your total look

CREATING A TOTAL LOOK

Now that you have covered the knowledge of colour and how it is used in the hair and beauty industries, you can start to think about how all of this information can be used together to create a total look for a client.

We have looked at hair, make-up and nail colours, but to create a total look you also need to consider the colours for the clothes and also accessories, such as jewellery, hand bags, hair clips, etc. For example, if you choose warm colours for the hair, make-up and nail colours, it is best to also use warm colours with the clothes. Gold would be a better colour for jewellery as this complements the warm colours better.

On the other hand, if you choose cool colours for the hair, make-up and nail colours, it is best to also use cool colours with the clothes. Silver would be a better colour for jewellery as this complements the cool colours better.

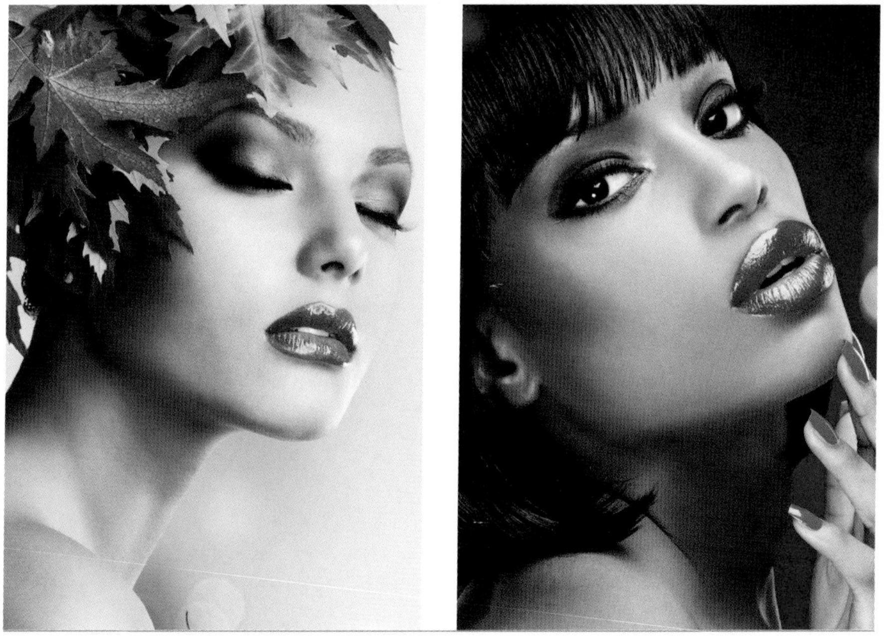

Look at these photos of warm and cool colours. Can you see how the colours of the hair and make-up complement the clothes and the accessories?

HANDY HINTS

It is best to have lights that are as near to natural daylight as possible, such as warm/white lights. This will mean that the colours used, in hair colouring, make-up or nail enamels, will be as near to how they appear in natural daylight as possible.

ACTIVITY

Have a go at this activity to check your understanding of warm and cool tones and also primary and secondary colours. Produce a mood board for each of the following:

1 warm colours

2 cool colours.

For each mood board, cut up different pictures to make a collage of a whole person, for example use the head from one picture and add it to the body of another picture. The aim is create a colourful picture of a total look – one using warm colours and one using cool colours. You will need to include the following colours in your picture:

- make-up
- nails (nail enamel and nail art)
- hair
- accessories (such as a handbag, shoes, jewellery)
- clothes.

It is an opportunity for you to be creative!

IN A NUTSHELL

You are now at the end of the chapter. Before you test your knowledge with the revision activities, check the following list to see if you feel confident in all the areas covered. If there are still any areas you're unsure of, go back over them in the book and ask your tutor for extra support:

- the primary colours
- the secondary colours
- what is meant by the colour spectrum
- how the colour spectrum is used in the hair and beauty industries.

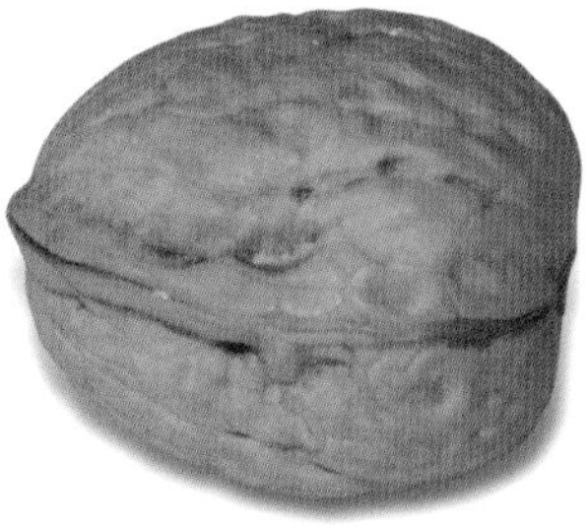

REVISION ACTIVITIES

SmartScreen 005 sample questions

Use the questions below to test your knowledge of Chapter 005 to see just how much information you've gained. This can help you to prepare for your assessments.

Turn to pages 491–492 for the answers.

WORDS TO FIND

Copy and complete the sentences below. Use these words to help you fill in the gaps.

primary	complementary	red	green
secondary	hair	yellow	image
colour	beauty	violet	create
spectrum	blue	orange	industry

1 Red, blue and yellow are known as ________ colours.

2 Orange, purple and green are known as ________ colours.

3 The colour green is made by mixing blue and ________ colours together.

4 When you mix red and blue together, the colour produced is ________ .

5 ________ colours are colours that are opposite the primary colours on the colour star.

6 The colour ________ is made up of the following colours: red, ________, yellow, ________, ________, indigo and violet.

7 Having a good understanding of ________ is important in the hair and beauty industries. It is taken into account when choosing hair, make-up and nail enamel products.

TEST YOUR KNOWLEDGE FURTHER

Now answer these questions:

1 Name the three primary colours.

2 Is it possible to mix colours together to get primary colours?

3 What are secondary colours?

4 Name the three secondary colours.

5 Copy and complete the table.

yellow	+		=	green
blue	+		=	violet
red	+	yellow	=	

6 What are complementary colours?

7 Copy and complete the table below to find the complementary colours for the three primary colours.

Primary colour	Which two primary colours are mixed together to get the complementary colour?	What complementary colour is produced from mixing them together?
Red		
Yellow		
Blue		

8 Which of the primary and secondary colours are classed as 'warm colours'?

9 Which of the primary and secondary colours are classed as 'cool colours'?

10 How is the colour spectrum used in the hairdressing and beauty therapy industries?

006 SKIN CARE

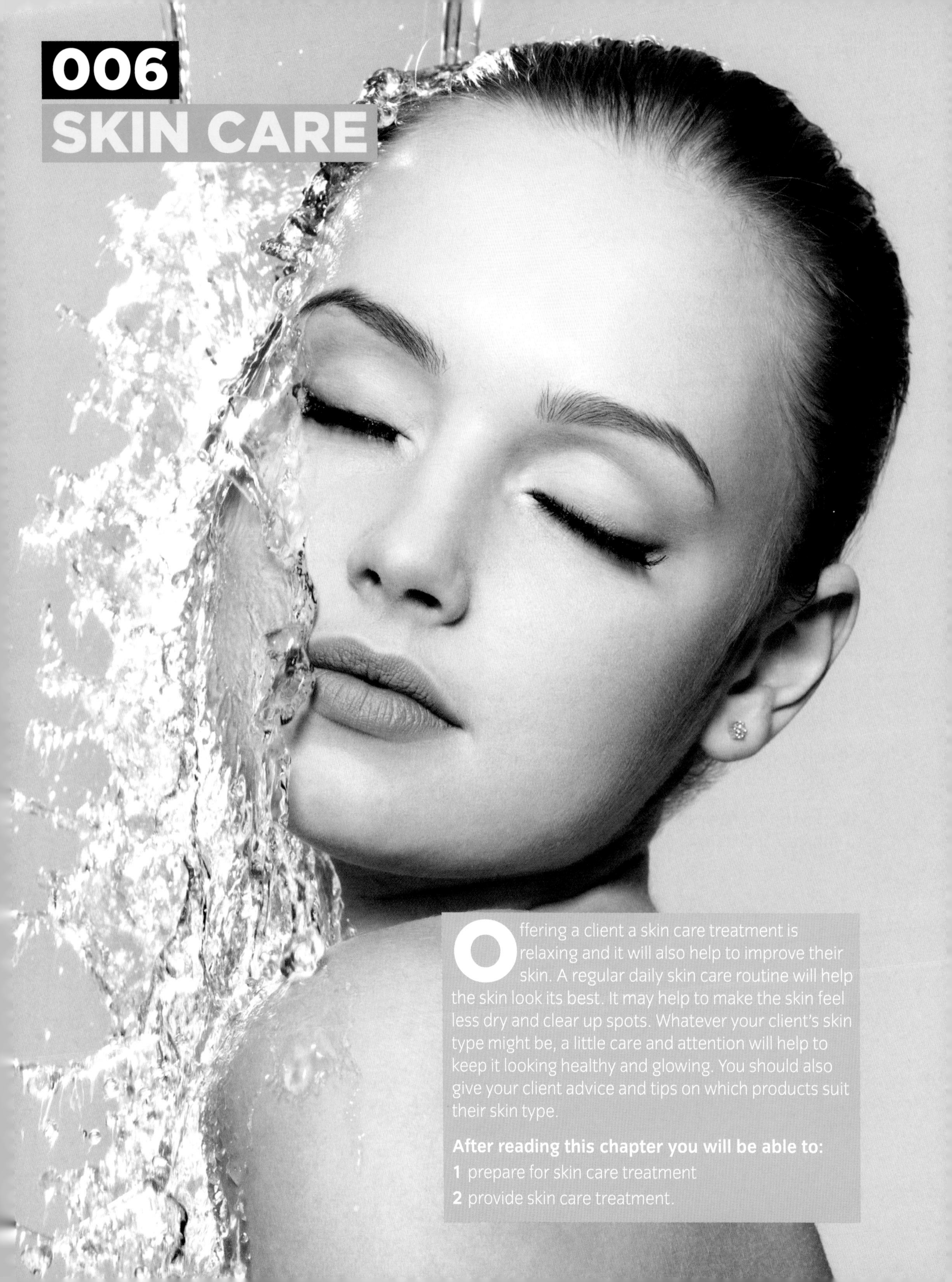

Offering a client a skin care treatment is relaxing and it will also help to improve their skin. A regular daily skin care routine will help the skin look its best. It may help to make the skin feel less dry and clear up spots. Whatever your client's skin type might be, a little care and attention will help to keep it looking healthy and glowing. You should also give your client advice and tips on which products suit their skin type.

After reading this chapter you will be able to:

1 prepare for skin care treatment

2 provide skin care treatment.

PREPARE FOR SKIN CARE TREATMENT

Requirement
Something that must be done

Before you begin the skin care service it's important to be prepared. Health and safety **requirements** should be carried out for every treatment, but knowing how to set up your treatment area, which products and tools you should use and how to carry out a proper consultation are also musts for skin care treatments.

SAFE AND HYGIENIC WORKING PRACTICES

It is important that you work in a safe and clean way. You should keep your treatment area tidy and only use tools and equipment that have been properly cleaned, which means they are **hygienic**. This will help to reduce the risk of harm to you and your clients and help to **prevent cross-infection**. This will make you look more **professional**.

Hygienic
Clean and germ free

Prevent
Stop something from taking place

Cross-infection
Passing of germs from one person to another

Professional
Someone who behaves in the correct way and has the right skills to do the job

ACTIVITY

Go to Chapter 113 Following health and safety in the salon and list all of the health and safety laws that you should follow when carrying out a skin care treatment.

TEAMWORK

You must always work in a professional way with your colleagues in the salon. Ways in which you can do this are:

- helping each other set up for a treatment and also tidy away
- following instructions from your supervisor/tutor when you are asked to do a job, such as helping to set up a treatment room
- working safely and hygienically in the salon
- keeping your voice level low so that it does not disturb the clients in the salon.

HANDY HINTS

Go to Chapter 113 Following health and safety in the salon and read up on more detailed information on health and safety, including PPE, COSHH, HASAWA and methods of sterilisation.

ACTIVITY

As a group, make a group **contract** of how you will behave and work together in the salon. You could include the following:

- how you should behave
- how you can help each other
- how to deal with problems between you
- how to motivate and encourage each other
- how to work professionally in the salon
- what steps to take if someone breaks the contract
- what your roles are in the salon
- what your tutor's roles are in the salon.

Once you and your tutor have agreed the contract, type it up and all sign to say that you agree to it.

HANDY HINTS

Do not use your fingers to remove products from the pots. This is not hygienic and may spread germs. Use a clean spatula instead. This is known as the 'cut out method'.

Contract
A formal agreement

THE SALON ENVIRONMENT

The treatment area should be prepared in a professional way:

- All products, tools and equipment should be clean and hygienic.
- They should be placed safely and tidily on the trolley.
- The couch should be covered for hygiene reasons with a couch cover and couch roll tissue.
- The room temperature should not be too hot or too cold. The ideal temperature for a treatment room is between 16–18 degrees Centigrade.
- The room should be well ventilated. This means that fresh air continually replaces stale air. It will also stop the atmosphere in the treatment room from becoming stuffy.
- The lighting should be suitable for a skin care treatment. The room needs to be well lit so that you can see clearly what you are doing.

HANDY HINTS

See Chapter 115 for further details on teamwork.

HANDY HINTS

If it is possible, dim the lights during the treatment; this will help the client to relax.

PREPARING FOR THE SKIN CARE TREATMENT

Before the client arrives, it is important that you get yourself and the treatment area prepared. All of the products, tools and equipment need to be ready. This will make sure that the treatment flows well and will also give the client a good first impression. It will help the client to relax and have confidence in you.

SmartScreen 006 handouts 1 and 2

You will need to have the following products, tools and materials on your trolley:

- Skin care products:
  - eye make-up remover
  - cleansers
  - toners
  - moisturisers.

You should have products suitable for oily, dry, combination and normal skin types.

- Skin care tools and equipment:
  - headband
  - spatula (placed in a jar containing Barbicide)
  - tissues
  - bowls
  - gowns
  - towels
  - cotton wool (needs to be dampened)
  - blanket (in case the client gets cold)
  - waste bin (with bin liner and lid)
  - treatment plan and pen.

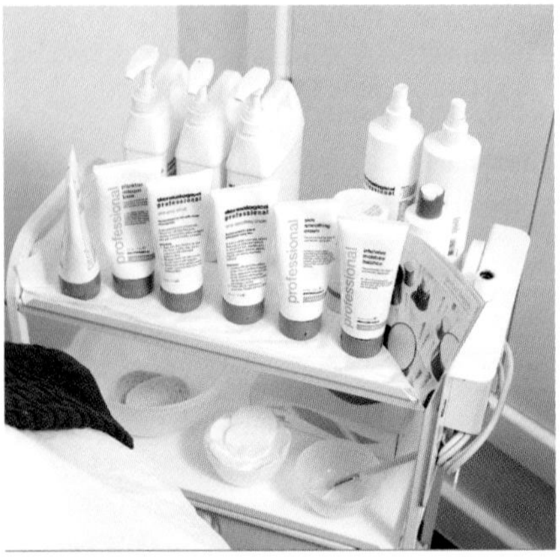

Professional beauty trolley set up

BASIC TOOLS AND EQUIPMENT

Some items, such as couch covers, are used in most beauty therapy treatments. The table lists them and their use in skin care.

Tools/equipment	What is it used for?	Hygiene steps to follow
Headband 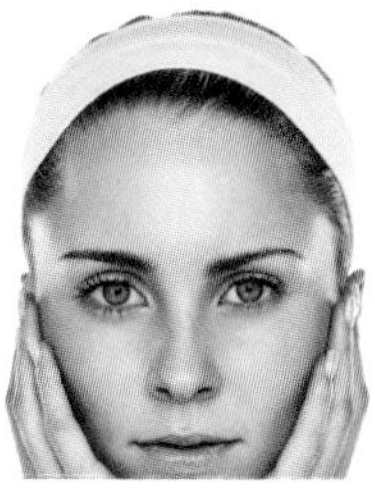	Will keep the client's hair off their face. It will also protect the hair from skin care products.	Machine wash on a high temperature to destroy harmful germs and get rid of dirt and grime.
Head cap 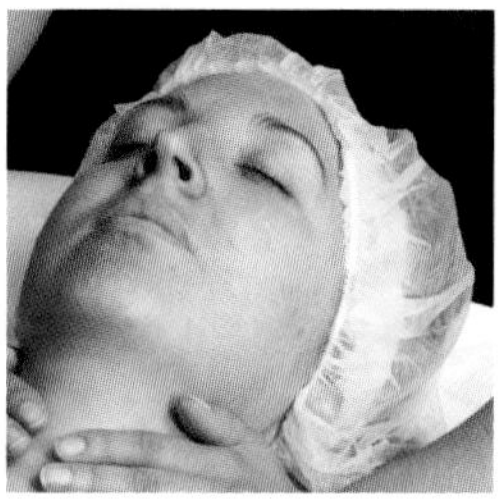	Can be either towelling or disposable; used to contain the hair, keeping it away from the face; ideal if your client has long hair. This is usually kept in place by a headband.	Machine wash the towelling ones on a high temperature to destroy harmful germs and get rid of dirt and grime. Throw away the disposable ones.
Tissues 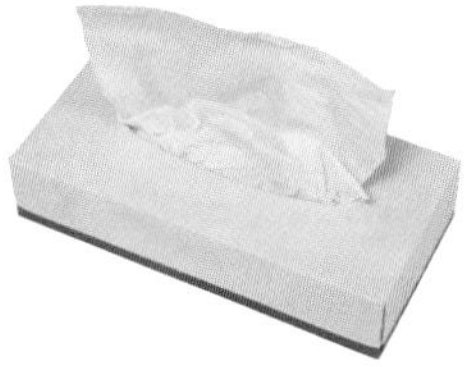	Can be used to blot the skin after the toner is applied.	Throw away after use.
Bowls 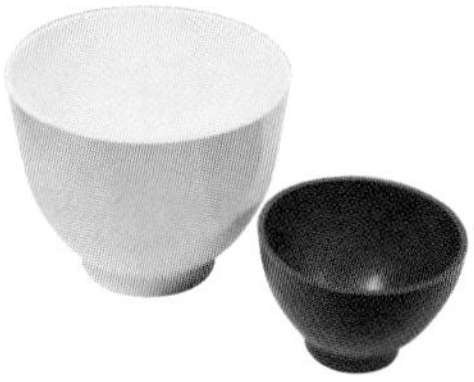	Used for warm water to dampen the cotton wool.	Wash in warm, soapy water and then disinfectant.
Gown 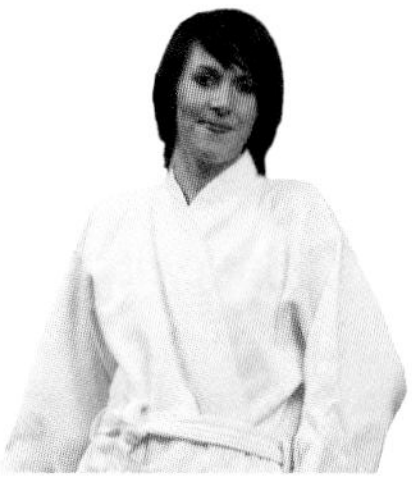	Will cover the client and help to protect their clothes from products. It will also help to keep them warm.	Machine wash on a high temperature to destroy harmful germs and get rid of dirt and grime.

Tools/equipment	What is it used for?	Hygiene steps to follow
Towels 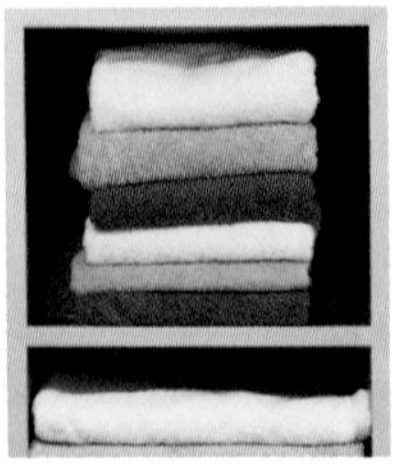	Used to cover the treatment couch and also the client. They can also help to keep the client warm during the treatment.	Machine wash on a high temperature to destroy harmful germs and get rid of dirt and grime.
Cotton wool 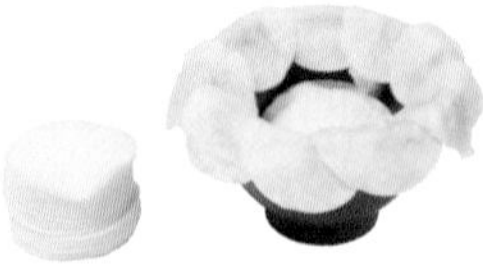	Used to remove the cleanser from the face. It is also used to apply the toner. It should be dampened with warm water before use.	Use clean, damp pads for each client. Throw away in the bin after use.
Cotton buds 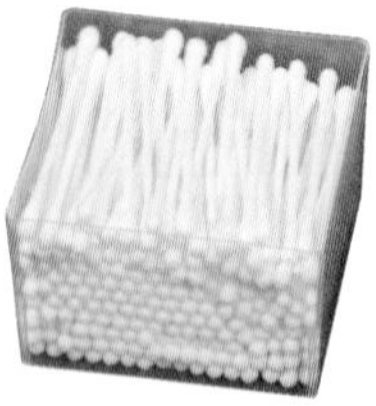	Used to remove stubborn traces of mascara and eye liner; they can be used dry or damp.	Use new cotton buds for each client. Throw away in the bin after use.
Treatment plan 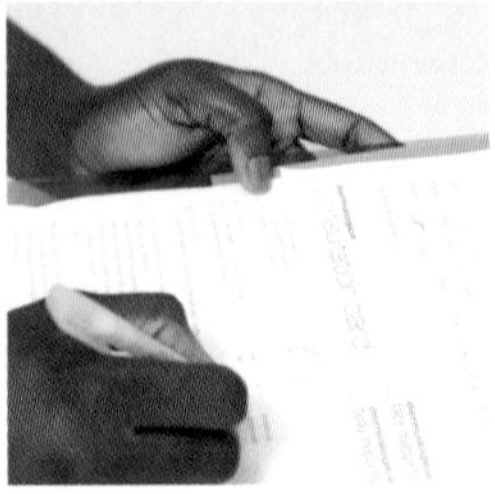	Records the treatment details, eg products used.	File away in a safe and secure place.
Blanket 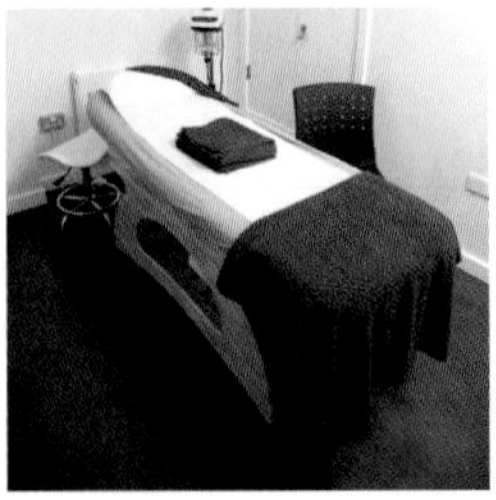	Can be used to keep the client warm during the treatment.	Machine wash on a high temperature to destroy harmful germs and get rid of dirt and grime.
Waste bin 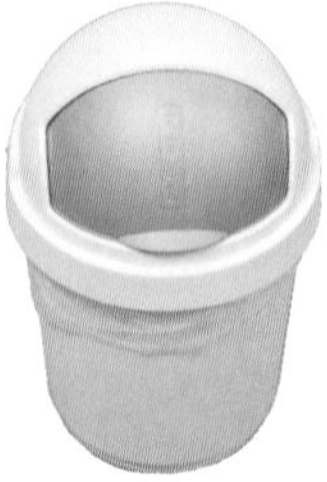	Should be lined with a bin liner and have a lid. Used for throwing away waste materials (such as cotton wool and tissues).	Empty the bin regularly. Place the contents into a large black bin bag and tie up.

Tools/equipment	What is it used for?	Hygiene steps to follow
Couch cover 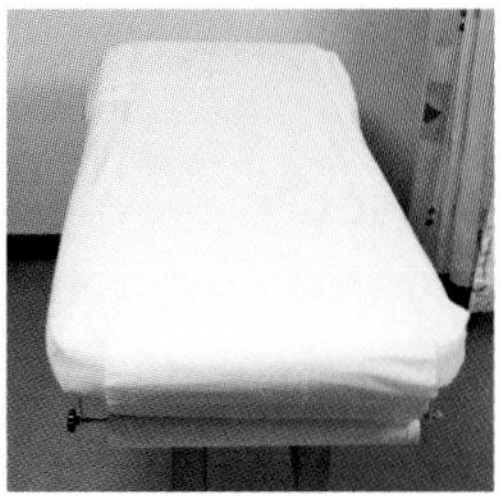	Placed over the couch for hygiene reasons.	Machine wash on a high temperature to destroy harmful germs and get rid of dirt and grime.
Spatulas 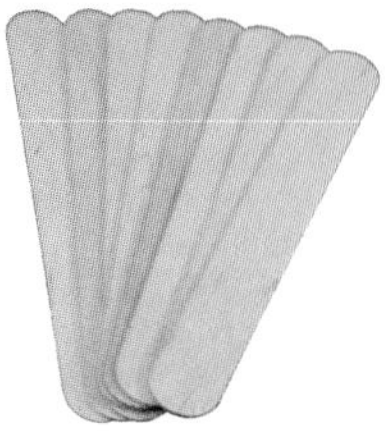	Used to scoop products out from pots. These can be plastic or wooden. The wooden ones are **disposable**.	Wash the plastic spatulas in warm, soapy water and then disinfectant. Place in an ultraviolet cabinet to store them hygienically. Throw away the wooden ones.
Barbicide and jar 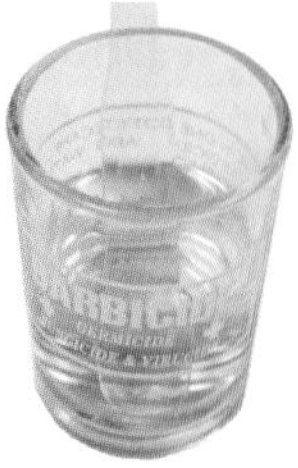	A disinfectant – the spatula can be placed in this during the treatment.	After use, pour the Barbicide down the sink. Rinse the jar with water and dry.

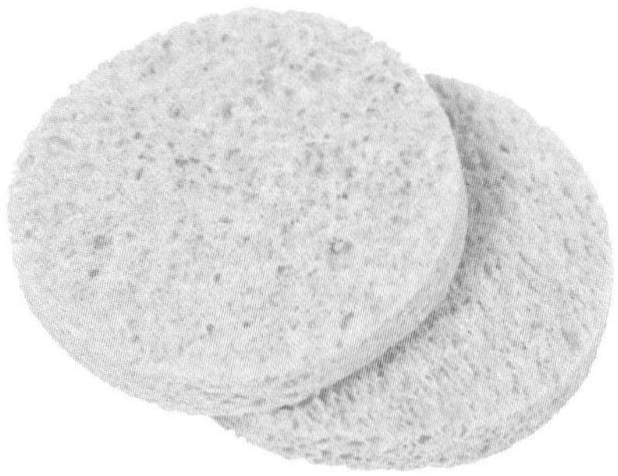

Sponges may also be used to remove facial products from the skin. They are often given to the client at the end of the treatment to use at home. This is for hygiene reasons

HANDY HINTS

Use warm water to dampen your cotton wool pads as this will feel nicer on the skin. It will also help to relax the client.

Disposable

Made to be thrown away after it has been used

SmartScreen 006 worksheet 1

PRODUCTS USED IN A SKIN CARE TREATMENT

It's important to know the products that are used in a skin care treatment, and which skin type they should be used for. This table provides a useful guide.

Skin care product	What is it used for?	Different types	Skin type they are used for	How is it used?
Eye make-up remover 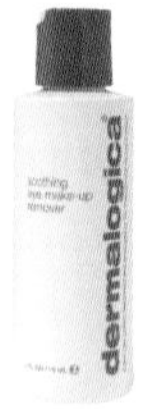	Removes eye make-up	Most of them come in a liquid or gel form. There are different ones that are designed to remove waterproof mascara.	All skin types	Apply either to a spatula, onto the back of the hand (cotton bud is dipped into the product) or to warm, damp cotton wool pads.
Cleansers 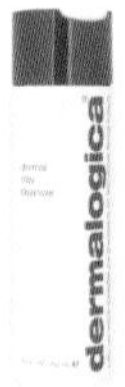	Remove make-up and surface dirt from the skin	Face washes (foaming cleanser)	Oily and **combination skin** types	Becomes a foaming cleanser when mixed with water. It is massaged onto the skin with clean hands. Wash off using warm water and damp cotton wool pads, a skin care cloth or a sponge.
		Lotions	Oily, combination and normal skin types	Usually applied to damp cotton wool, then wiped over the face.
		Milk	Oily, combination, normal and **sensitive skin** types	Usually applied to damp cotton wool, then wiped over the face.
		Creams	Normal, sensitive and dry skin types	Usually applied to the face with clean hands, then gently massaged in. Removed using warm, dampened cotton wool pads or sponges.

HANDY HINTS

There are lots of manufacturers and product houses. The products displayed here are not the only products used for facials.

Combination skin

A mixture of more than one skin type (usually dry and oily)

Sensitive skin

Skin type that is easily irritated. Gentle products should be used on this skin type

Skin care product	What is it used for?	Different types	Skin type they are used for	How is it used?
Toners 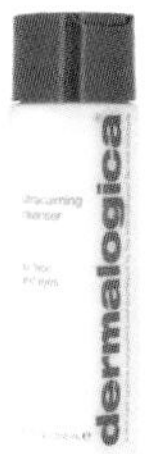	**Refreshes** the skin. Removes the last traces of the cleanser. Tightens the **pores**.	Fresheners (very mild)	Dry, sensitive and normal skin types	Applied to damp cotton wool pads – these are then gently wiped over the skin. Sometimes they can be sprayed over the skin; always make sure the client has their eyes and mouth closed.
		Toners (slightly stronger)	Normal skin type	
		Astringents (strong)	Oily and combination skin types	
Moisturisers	Helps to stop the skin from drying out. Makes the skin feel soft and supple.	Lotion (lighter product) 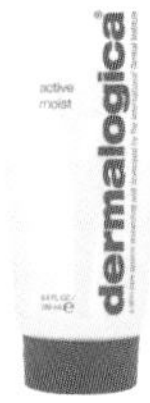	Oily and combination skin types	Use a clean spatula to remove the moisturiser from a jar container. If the moisturiser is in a pump bottle or a tube, it can be squeezed straight into clean hands. Apply to the fingertips and gently tap over the skin. It is then lightly massaged in until it has been **absorbed** into the skin.
		Mousse 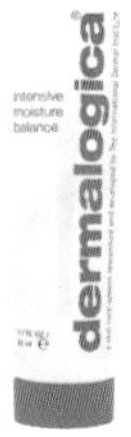	Normal skin type	
		Cream 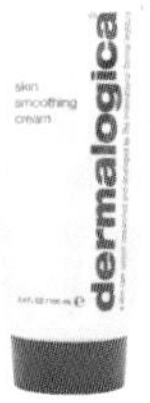	Normal and dry skin types	

ACTIVITY

Bring in the skin care products that you are using on your skin. Have a look at what other students in your group are using. Discuss the reasons why they are using them (such as the cost, the packaging, etc).

ACTIVITY

Take a look on the internet at the cleansing products that are available. See if you can find ones for all of the skin types that you have just read about.

Refreshes
Cools

Pores
Very tiny holes found on the surface of the skin. Sweat comes out of these

Absorbed
Taken in

SmartScreen 006 handouts 5, 6, 7

SmartScreen 006 worksheet 4

Consultation
Discussion and examination of the client before the treatment starts

Contra-indication
A condition that will prevent a treatment being carried out

Restrict
Limit; make it difficult for a treatment to be carried out

SmartScreen 006 handouts 10 and 11

CONSULTATION

Before you start the treatment you will need to carry out a **consultation** with the client. Remember to ask your tutor for help if you need it.
A consultation is carried out for the following reasons:

- to find out why the client is having the treatment
- to check what skin type the client has
- to discuss what products you are going to use
- to check for any **contra-indications** and skin conditions that may prevent or **restrict** the treatment.

HANDY HINTS

Go to Chapter 102 Presenting a professional image in the salon and read up on how to communicate and behave in a professional way.

SmartScreen 006 handout 8

COMMUNICATION AND BEHAVIOUR

Before you can carry out a consultation, you need to know how to communicate and behave well. When you first meet your client, make good eye contact and greet them with a smile. This will give them a positive first impression and also help to put them at ease. Remember to:

- speak clearly
- have a friendly approach (such as smiling)
- listen to the client and respond politely
- give the client your full attention and respect.

Routine
Something that you do regularly in the same order

Sebum
An oil produced by the skin; helps to keep the skin soft and supple

Skin texture
How rough or smooth the skin is

LOOKING AT THE SKIN

Once you feel confident in your communication skills, you can carry out the consultation. For skin care treatments it's important to ask the client about their skin, but you must also look closely at their skin before you start. You will then be able to choose the correct products for their skin type.

Skin types

During the consultation you will need to find out what skin type the client has. This will affect your choice of skin care products. Choose products that are suitable for their skin type.

Skin type	What causes it	How would you recognise it?
Normal 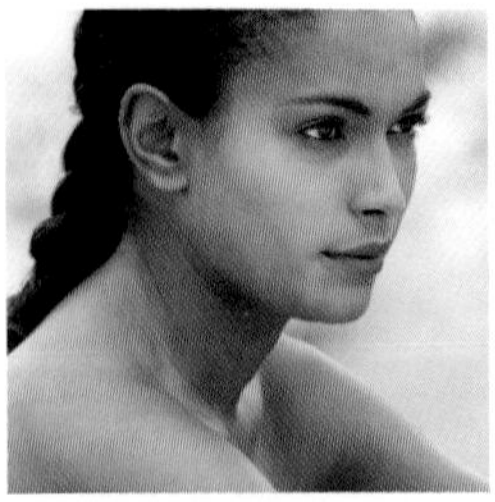	The ideal skin type. You will help to achieve this with a good skin care **routine**. This skin type has a good balance of oil (**sebum**) and water (sweat).	▪ Even **skin texture** ▪ Feels soft ▪ Skin colour is even ▪ Does not feel tight ▪ Feels firm to touch
Oily/greasy 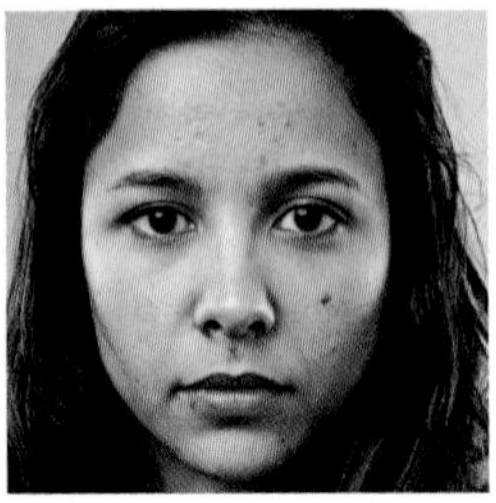	Too much of the skin's oil (sebum) is produced.	▪ Shiny ▪ Spots (pustules) ▪ Blackheads (comedones) ▪ Large pores ▪ Wet/sticky on surface

Skin type	What causes it	How would you recognise it?
Dry 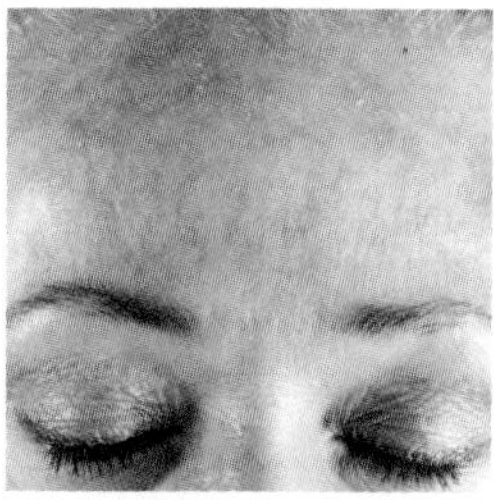	Not enough of the skin's oil is produced.	▪ Flaky patches ▪ Dull ▪ Feels tight ▪ Small pores ▪ Whiteheads (blocked oil under the skin) ▪ Fine lines
Combination 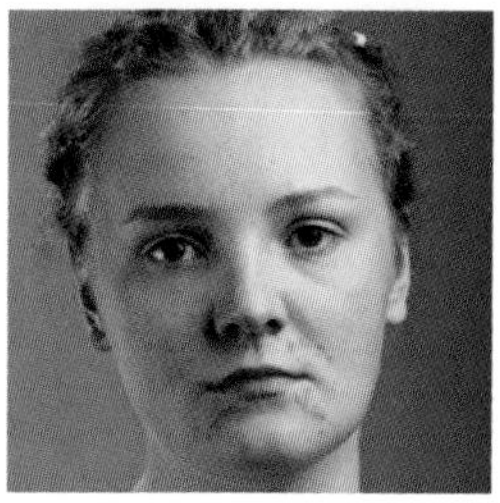	A combination of any of the above skin types.	▪ Usually dry cheeks ▪ Oily skin on the 'T' zone (forehead, nose and chin)

ACTIVITY

Look at the skin care products that you are currently using. Find out if they are the correct products for your skin type.

ACTIVITY

Skin care quiz

To help you work out what your skin type is, have a go at answering the following multichoice questions. Choose the best answer from **a** to **d**:

SmartScreen 006 worksheet 3

1 How does your skin feel after you wash it?
- **a** tight
- **b** smooth
- **c** cleaner
- **d** dry in some areas and smooth in others

2 How does your skin look?
- **a** flaky patches and dull
- **b** fresh and bright
- **c** shiny with some spots
- **d** spots on the forehead, nose or chin, but flaky patches on the cheeks

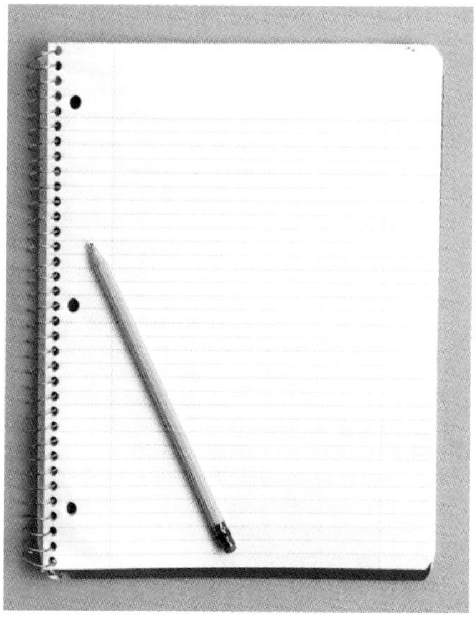

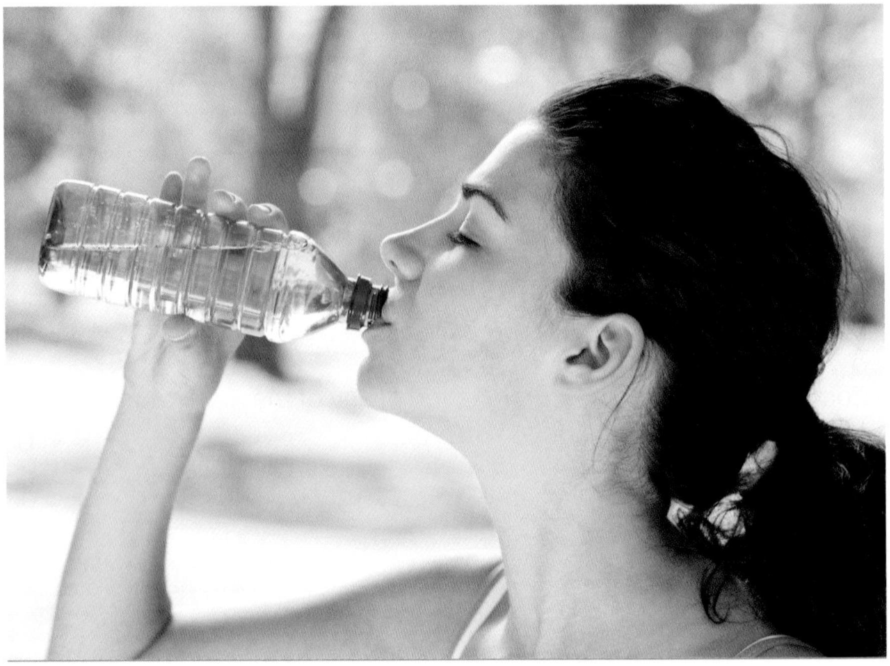

Drinking lots of water is good for your skin

HANDY HINTS

As well as following a good, regular skin care routine, eating healthily and drinking lots of water will also help to keep your skin looking great.

3 How often do you get spots?
- **a** hardly ever
- **b** never
- **c** often
- **d** sometimes on the forehead, nose or chin areas

4 How does your skin feel after using a toner?
- **a** stings
- **b** feels OK
- **c** feels fresher
- **d** feels fresh in some areas but stings in others

5 How does your skin feel if you put a thick moisturiser on it?
- **a** soaks into the skin
- **b** feels ok
- **c** makes it feel very greasy
- **d** makes it feel greasy on the forehead, nose and chin, but soaks in on the cheek area

Now add up how many **a**s, **b**s, **c**s or **d**s you scored. The one that is the highest will tell you which of the following skin types you have:

Mostly **a**s: Your skin type is dry.
Mostly **b**s: Your skin type is normal.
Mostly **c**s: Your skin type is oily.
Mostly **d**s: Your skin type is combination.

SmartScreen 006 handout 4

CONTRA-INDICATIONS TO A SKIN CARE TREATMENT

As part of the consultation you should also be able to spot any contra-indications that may prevent or restrict this treatment. If you see any signs of the contra-indications mentioned below, you need to speak to your tutor. They will help you explain to the client that the treatment cannot go ahead. Remember that you are not a doctor. You should not name the condition in case you are wrong. Your client will need to go to their doctor, who can treat them properly.

Conditions that prevent a skin care treatment

Certain skin and eye conditions prevent you from carrying out a skin care treatment. All the skin and eye conditions below are **contagious**. For this reason you must never treat a client with these conditions.

- **bacterial infections** such as impetigo, conjunctivitis, boils and styes
- viral infections such as a cold sore
- fungal infections such as ringworm
- **parasitic infections** such as scabies and head lice.

Contagious
Describing a condition that can be passed from one person to another

Bacterial infections
Infections caused by bacteria. Signs of a bacterial infection can include redness, heat, swelling and pain in one part of the body

Parasitic infections
Infections caused by tiny insects or worms that live either under or on the skin

Condition	What is it?	What does it look like?	How may it affect the treatment?
Impetigo 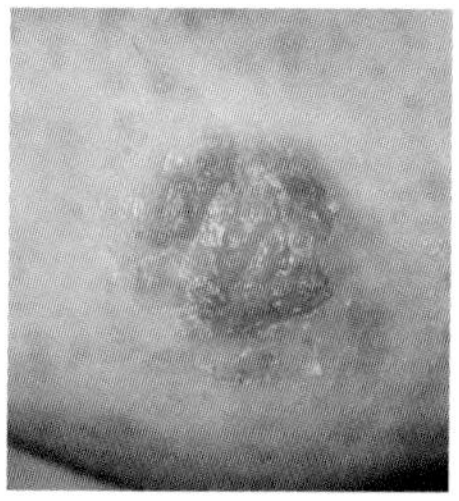	An **infectious** condition. It is caused by bacteria getting into the cracks of skin.	Yellow, clear-filled spots, which dry into yellow or honey-coloured crusts.	The client will need to go to their doctor for treatment. This condition can be spread from one person to another. You can catch it by either touching the infected area or from towels that have come in contact with the infected skin.
Conjunctivitis 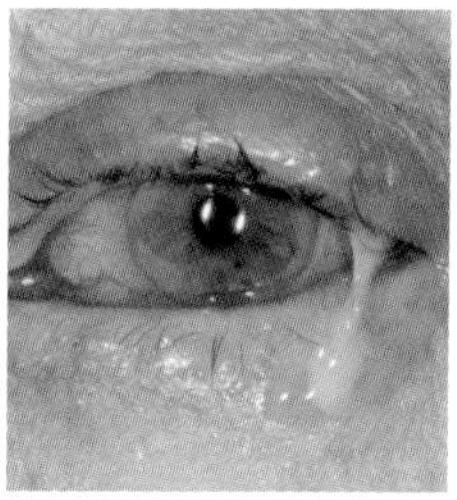	An infectious condition that affects the eye.	The eye becomes sore, red and itchy. Sometimes pus is present.	The client will need to go to their doctor for treatment. This condition can be spread from one person to another. You can catch it by touching the infected area.
Boil 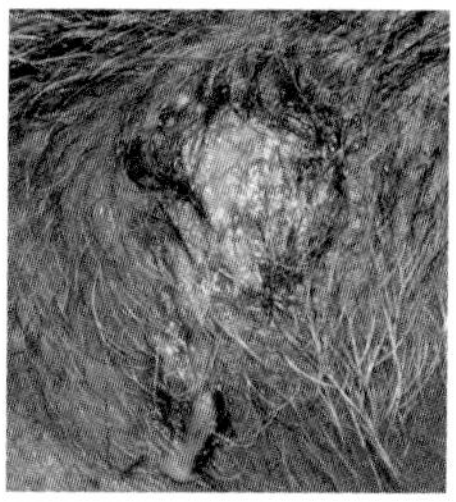	An infectious condition of the **hair follicle**.	Red, painful swelling with a hard centre that contains pus. It forms around a hair follicle. Usually found at the back of the neck.	The client will need to go to their doctor for treatment.

Infectious
Another word for contagious; catching

Hair follicle
A pocket in the skin that contains the hair

Condition	What is it?	What does it look like?	How may it affect the treatment?
Stye 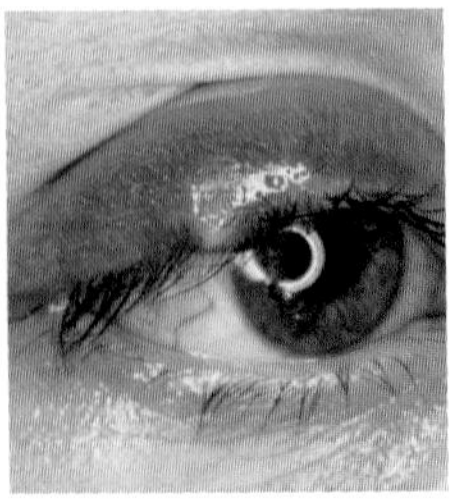	An infectious condition of the eye.	A small boil at the bottom of an eyelash follicle; a raised, sore, red swelling.	The client will need to go to their doctor for treatment. This condition can be spread from one person to another. It is also very painful.
Cold sore 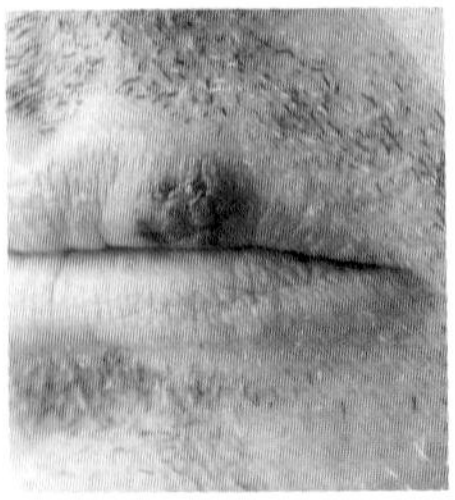	An infectious viral condition of the skin.	Red, itchy skin. Crusts form that can weep pus. Usually found around the mouth and nose.	The client will need to go to their doctor for treatment. This condition can be spread from one person to another.
Ringworm 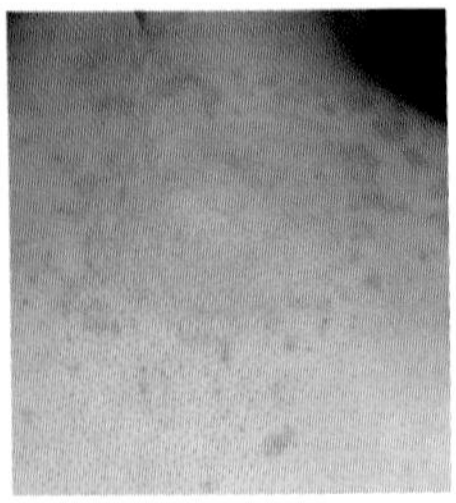	An infectious condition of the skin.	Red circular rash on the skin.	The client will need to go to their doctor for treatment. This condition can be spread from one person to another.
Head lice 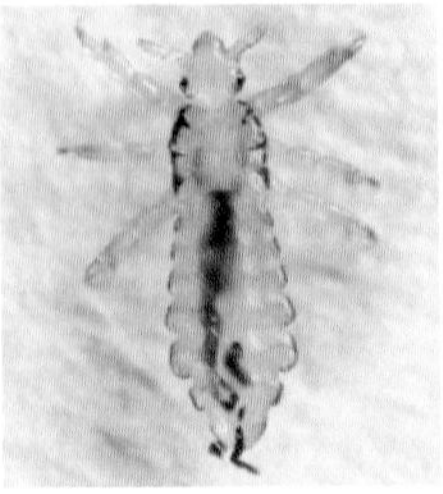	Small insects that live on the scalp and feed on blood.	They lay tiny eggs called nits, which stick onto the hair. The nits look like tiny white balls. When the lice move around it makes the scalp very itchy.	The client will need to go to their doctor for treatment. This condition can be spread from one person to another by close contact.

SmartScreen 006 handout 3

SmartScreen 006 worksheet 2

HANDY HINTS

If the client has an infectious condition, do not treat them. Speak to your tutor who will ask them to see their doctor.

Conditions that might restrict a skin care treatment

The following conditions may restrict the treatment in some way. They are not **contagious**, but you may have to change your treatment. Check with your tutor if you think your client may have any of these conditions.

Sensitive
Easily irritated

Condition	What is it?	What does it look like?	How may it affect the treatment?
Recent scars 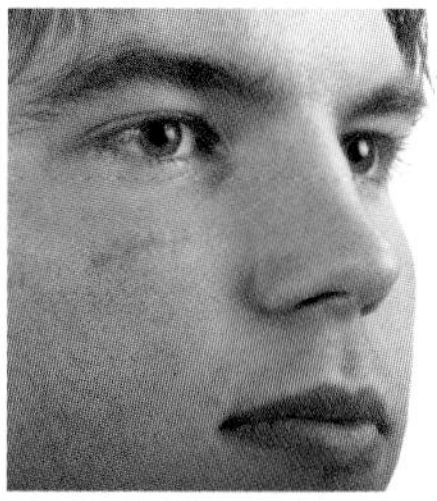	Damage to the skin.	It may be red in colour.	Do not work over this area if it is painful.
Eczema 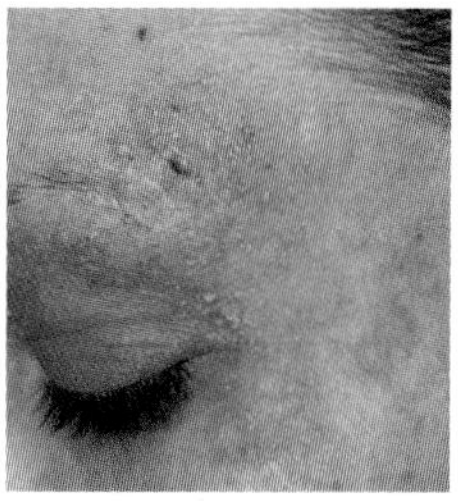	A skin condition that cannot be passed from one person to another.	Dry, flaky skin which may be cracked.	If the skin is broken or painful, do not work over the area. If the skin is not broken or painful, use cream products to help with the dryness.
Psoriasis 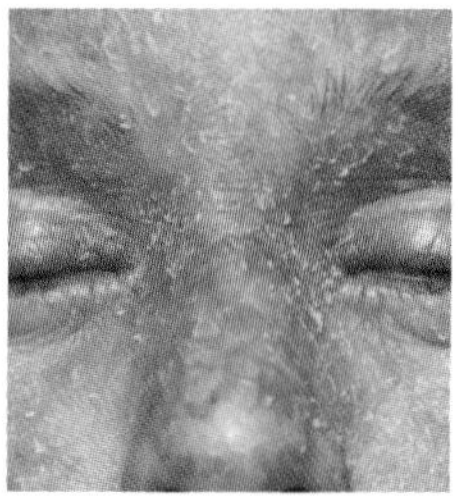	A skin condition that cannot be passed from one person to another.	Dry silvery scales on red skin.	If the skin is sensitive, do not work over the area. If the skin is not sensitive, use cream products to help with the dryness.
Bruising or cuts 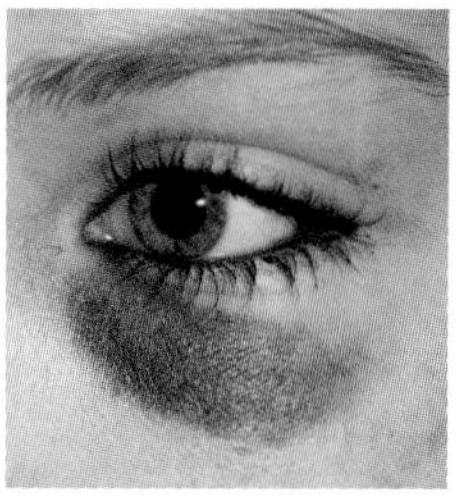	Damage to the skin.	It may look blue, red or yellow in colour.	Do not work over this area as it may be **sensitive**.
Allergies 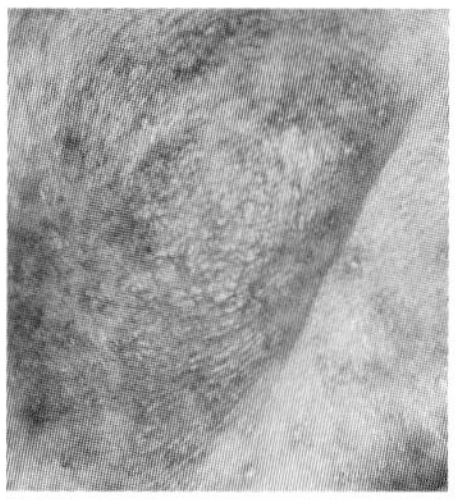	Something that causes a reaction.	Can cause redness, itching, swelling and burning of the skin.	If the client has an allergy to the products that you are using, do not use them. If an **allergic reaction** happens during the treatment, stop straight away and remove the product gently using cool water.

Allergic reaction
When the body over reacts to something (eg facial products); may cause a rash, itchiness and redness

Condition	What is it?	What does it look like?	How may it affect the treatment?
Mature skin 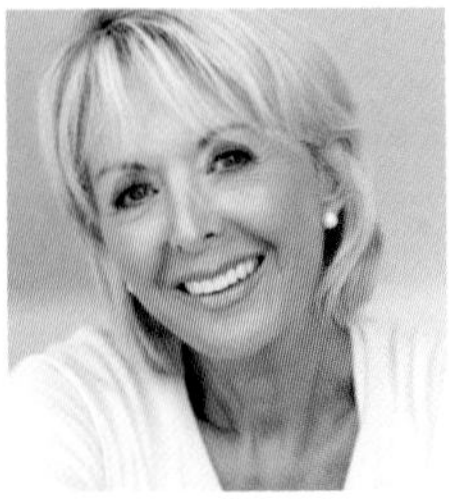	The skin is classed as mature after age 25 because the skin starts to age.	Wrinkles start to form and the skin starts to sag.	Use products that are suitable for a mature skin, such as products for dry skin. These contain more oil, so will help to moisturise the skin.
Sensitive skin 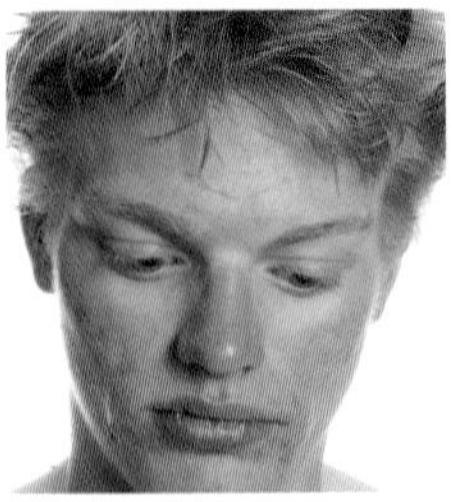	When the skin gets easily irritated by products.	The skin may look red, be itchy, hot to the touch and tend to burn easily in the sun.	Use products that are gentle on the skin. Work very gently.

HANDY HINTS

If your client has an allergic reaction and it does not get better soon after the treatment, they will need to see their doctor.

ACTIVITY

Carry out a role-play exercise with a partner. One of you can be the therapist and the other the client. Pretend the client has one of the conditions listed above. How would you explain to them in a professional way the effect it would have on the skin care treatment?

PROVIDE SKIN CARE TREATMENT

BASIC SKIN CARE TREATMENT ROUTINE

Before starting the skin care treatment, you must make sure that your client is prepared:

- Make sure the client is resting comfortably on the couch and is warm. Use a blanket if the client is cold.
- Place a headband around their head (to keep the hair off the face).
- Make sure that you have all the products ready that are suitable for your client's skin type.

SmartScreen 006 handout 8

HANDY HINTS

A simple skin care routine will only take a few minutes. Ideally it should be done twice a day – in the morning and at night.

HANDY HINTS

Remember to wash your hands before and after the treatment to prevent cross-infection.

HANDY HINTS

Keep your nails short. You don't want to scratch the client!

CLEANSING ROUTINE

A basic skin routine should include the regular and correct use of a cleanser, toner and moisturiser. Look back at the products chart on pages 166 and 167 if you need to remind yourself of the products to use for each skin type.

The following routines are to be used as a guide only – your tutor may teach these routines differently.

HANDY HINTS

Always work very gently over the eye area.

THE EYE CLEANSE

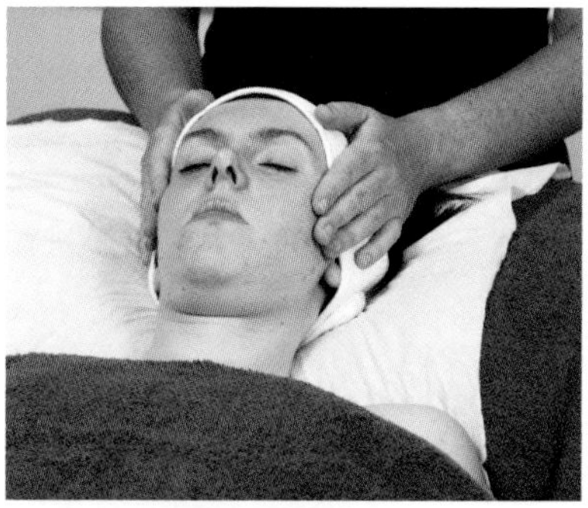

STEP 1 – Start by placing your hands on the sides of the client's head. This will help to prepare them for the treatment. It will also help them to relax.

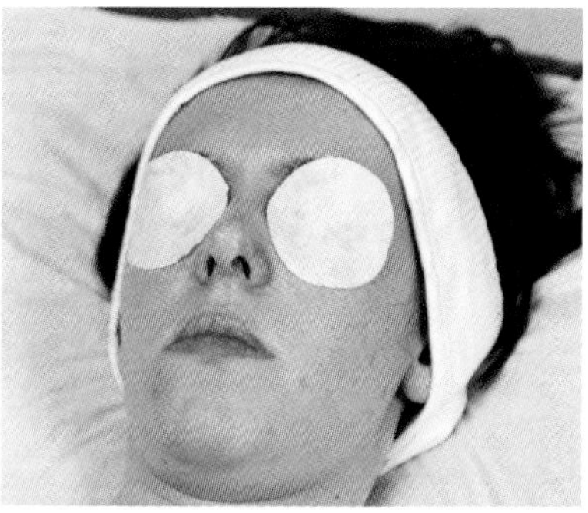

STEP 2 – Apply the eye make-up remover to damp cotton wool and place over both eyes. Gently circle the pads on both eyes to start to loosen the eye make-up, supporting the eye area as you work. Remove the pads.

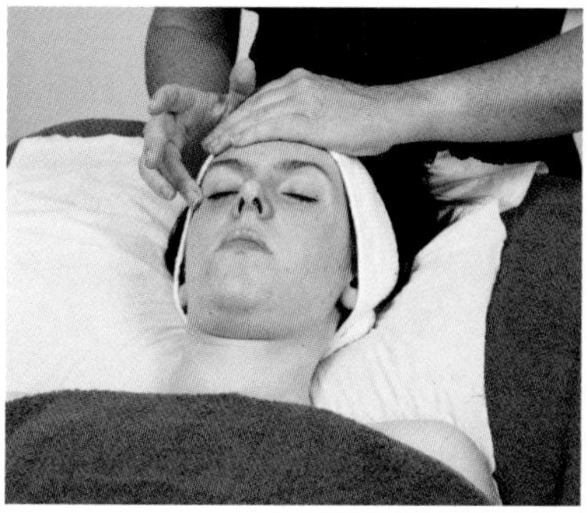

STEP 3 – Place a small amount of eye make-up remover on the back of one hand. Place this hand on the forehead for support and gently apply the eye make-up remover with the ring finger of the other hand. Use circular movements over the eye. Stroke down on the lashes to remove the mascara.

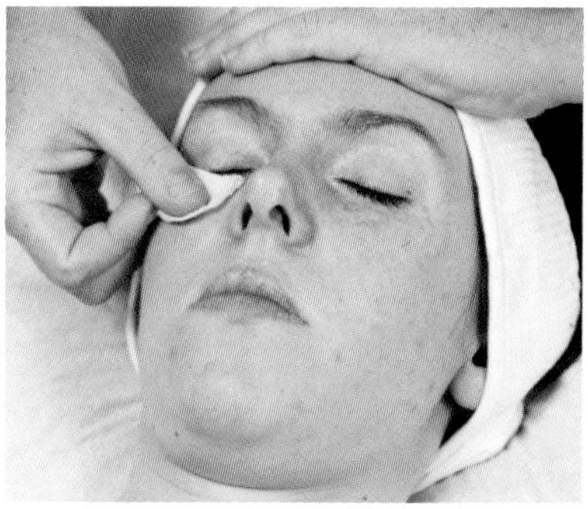

STEP 4 – Using dampened cotton wool pads, stroke down over the lids and lashes until all the make-up has been removed.

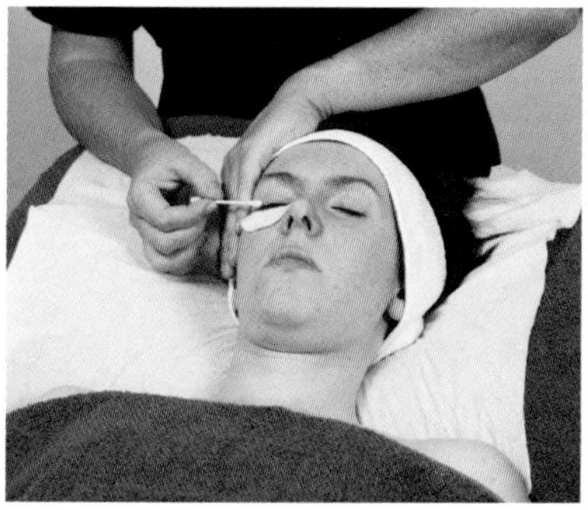

STEP 5 – If needed, use a cotton bud or tipped orange wood-stick to remove the last traces of mascara and eye liner.

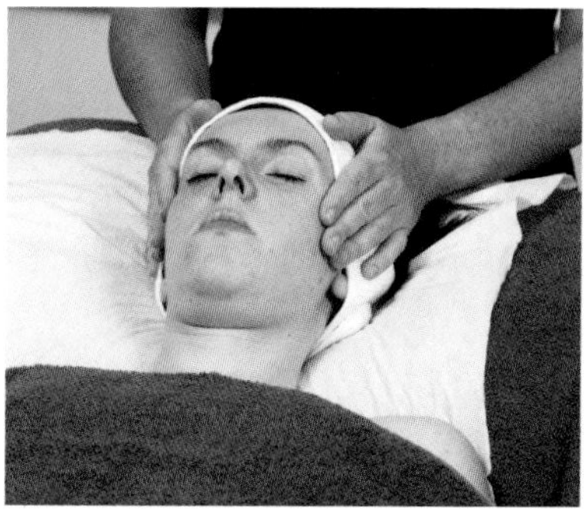

STEP 6 – Finish by placing your hands on the sides of the client's head. This will complete the eye cleanse.

HANDY HINTS

Eye make-up remover can often also be used for the lip cleanse.

THE LIP CLEANSE

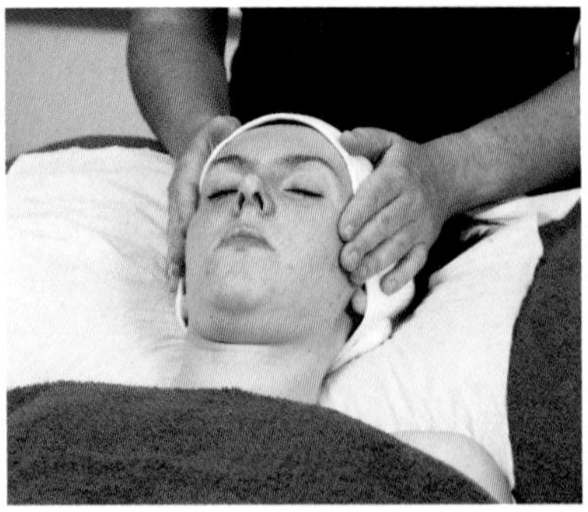

STEP 1 – Start by placing your hands on the sides of the client's head. This will help to prepare them for the lip cleanse.

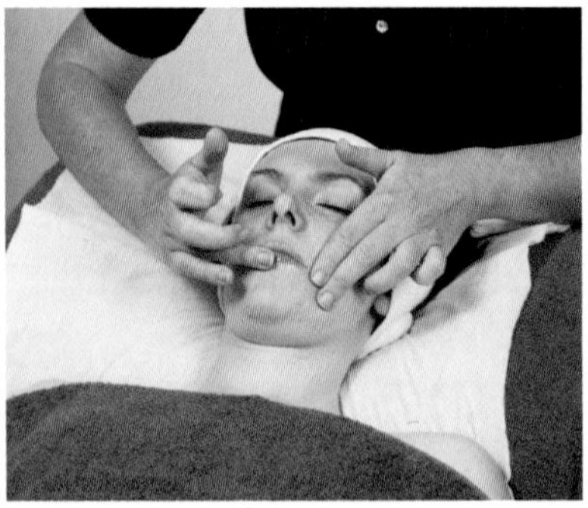

STEP 2 – Place a small amount of eye make-up remover on the back of one hand. Use this hand to support the side of the lip area. Gently apply the eye make-up remover with the ring finger of the other hand. Use circular movements over the lips. This will help to remove any lipstick.

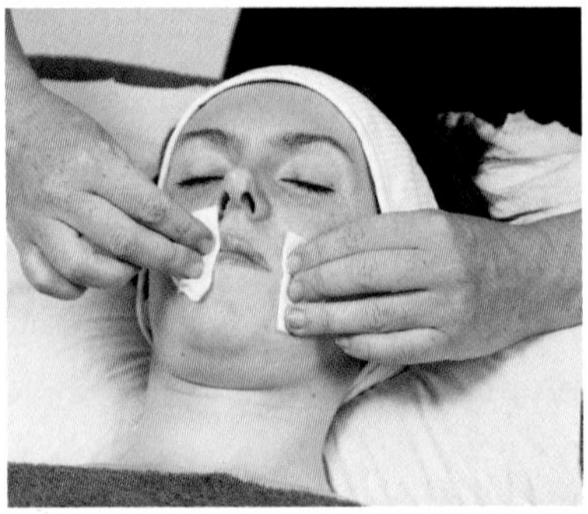

STEP 3 – Using dampened cotton wool pads, stroke across the lips until all the lipstick has been removed.

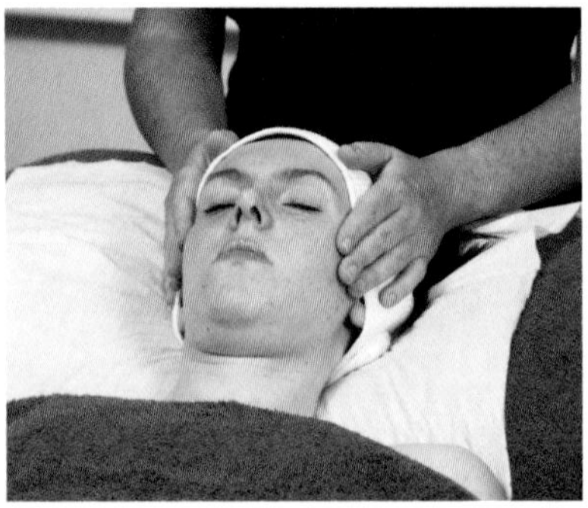

STEP 4 – Finish by placing your hands on the sides of the client's head. This will complete the lip cleanse.

HANDY HINTS

Do not ask the client any questions when you are doing the lip cleanse. They may end up eating the cleansing product by answering you!

THE FACE CLEANSE

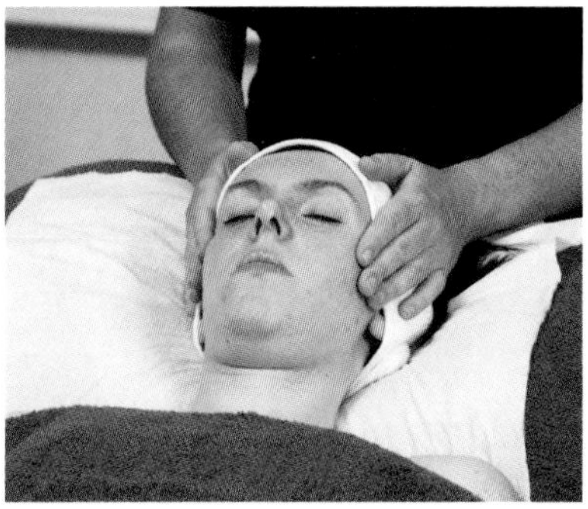

STEP 1 – Start by placing your hands on the sides of the client's head. This will help to prepare them for the face cleanse.

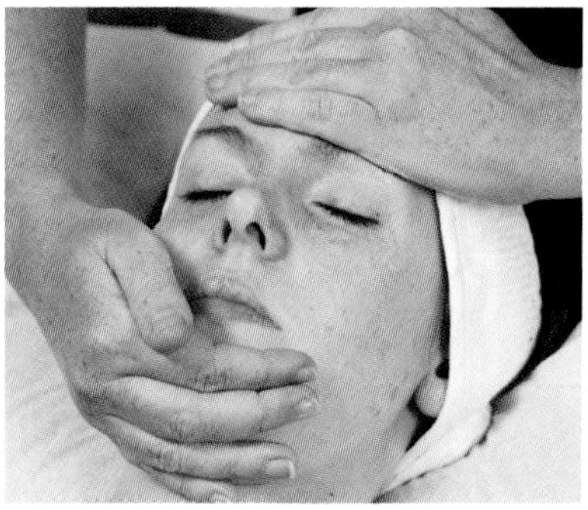

STEP 2 – Apply the most suitable cleanser for the client to the palms of your hands (to warm it up). Apply the cleanser in smooth strokes to the face and neck.

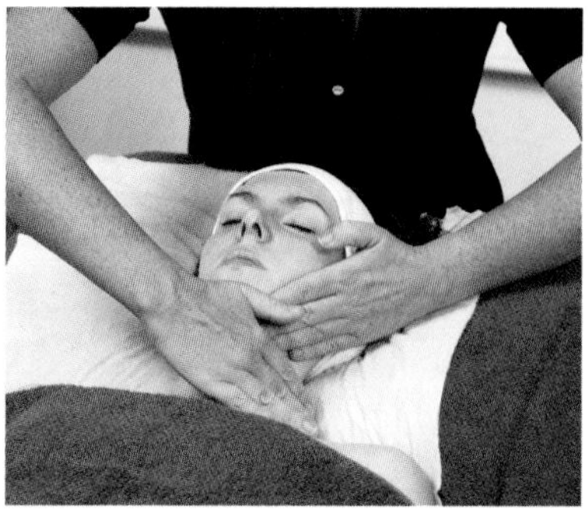

STEP 3 – Use alternate strokes up the neck.

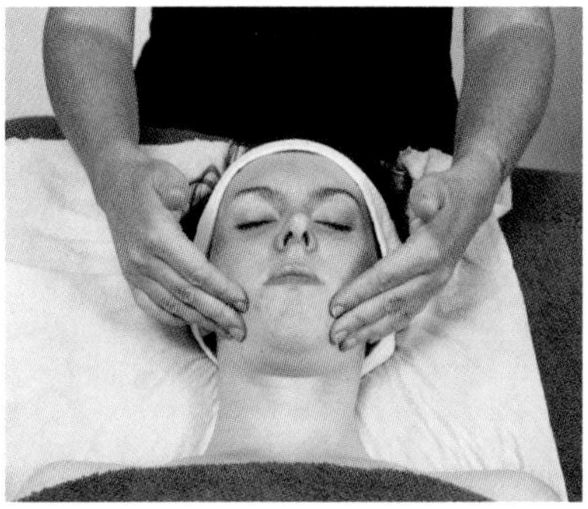

STEP 4 – Use finger circles along the outer jaw to the chin.

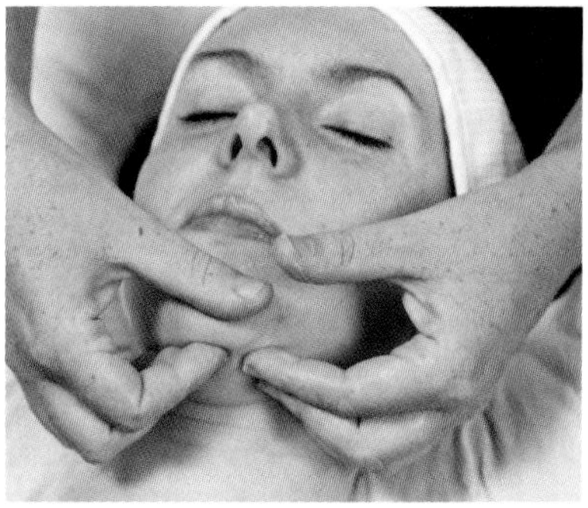

STEP 5 – Use thumb circles on the chin.

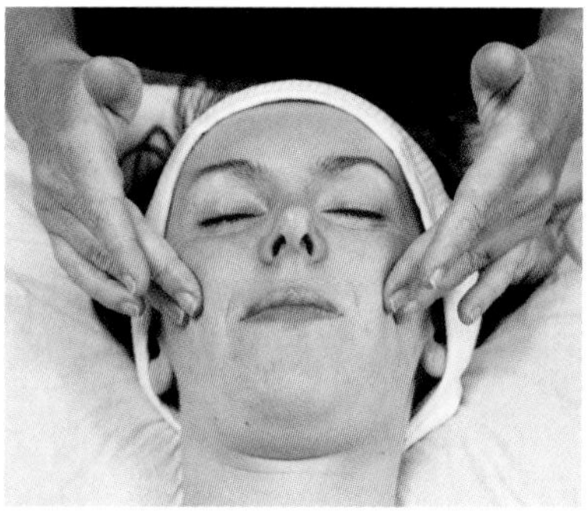

STEP 6 – Use finger circles along the cheeks.

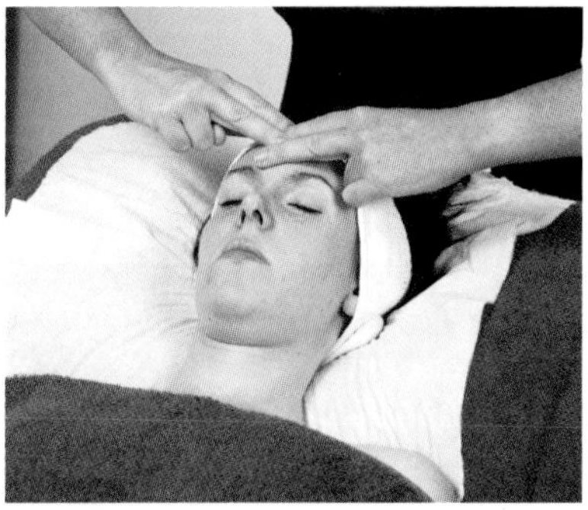

STEP 7 – Use alternate finger slides between the brows to the forehead.

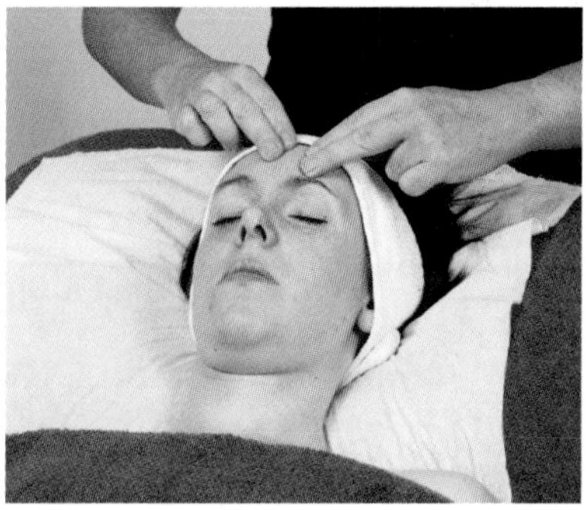

STEP 8 – Use finger circles along the forehead.

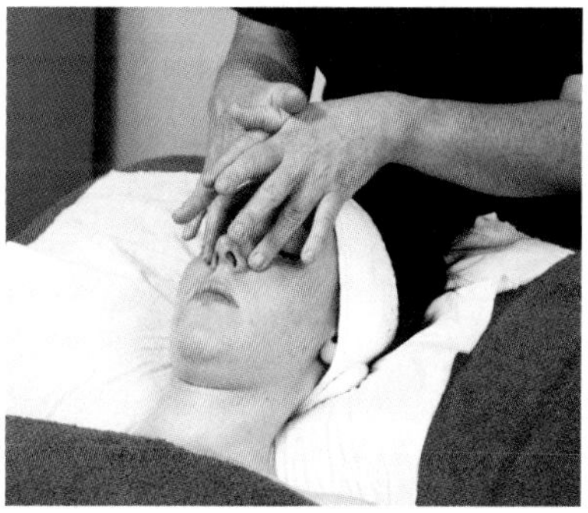

STEP 9 – Use alternate finger circles on the sides of the nose.

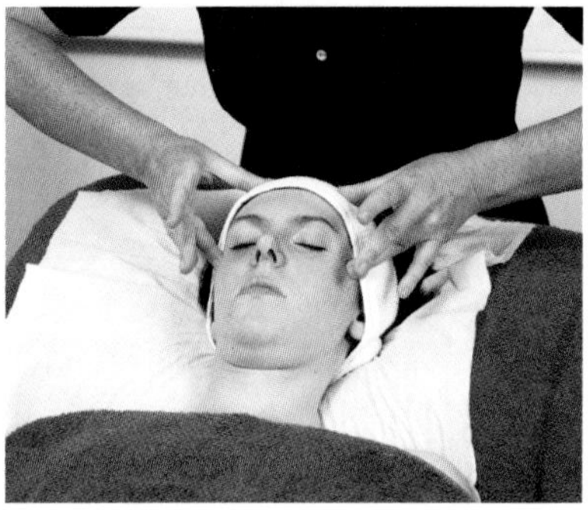

STEP 10 – Press and circle the fingertips on the **temples**.

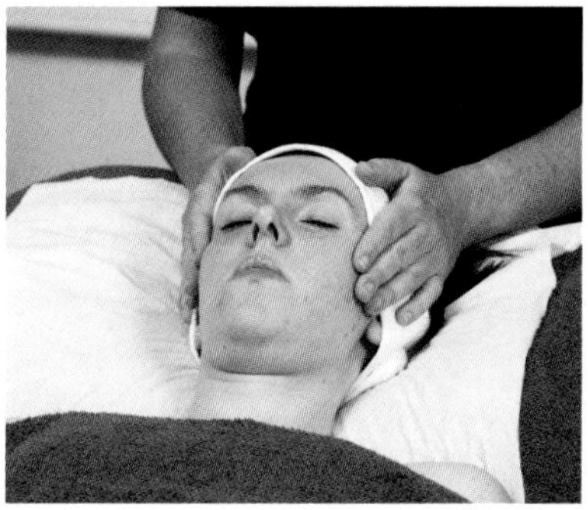

STEP 11 – Finish by placing your hands on the sides of the client's head. This will complete the face cleanse.

Temples

The areas at the sides of the head, by the side of the eyes

THE TONE

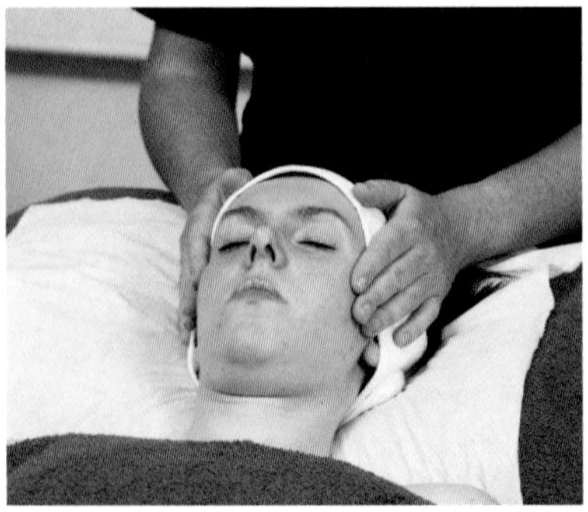

STEP 1 – Start by placing your hands on the sides of the client's head. This will help to prepare them for the toner.

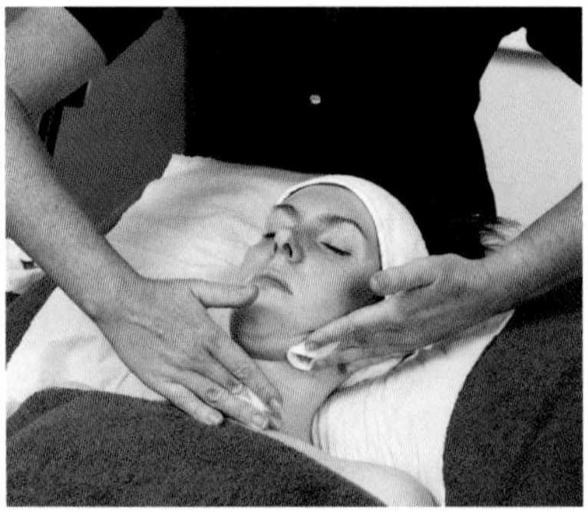

STEP 2 – Apply the most suitable toner for the client to two damp cotton wool pads. Start at the sides of the neck; wipe upwards on the neck. The toner can also be gently sprayed over the face. Make sure your client keeps their eyes and mouth closed.

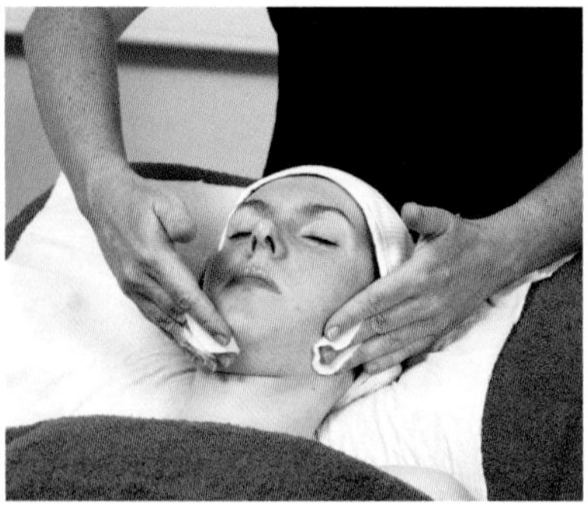

STEP 3 – Use alternate sweeping strokes across the jaw line.

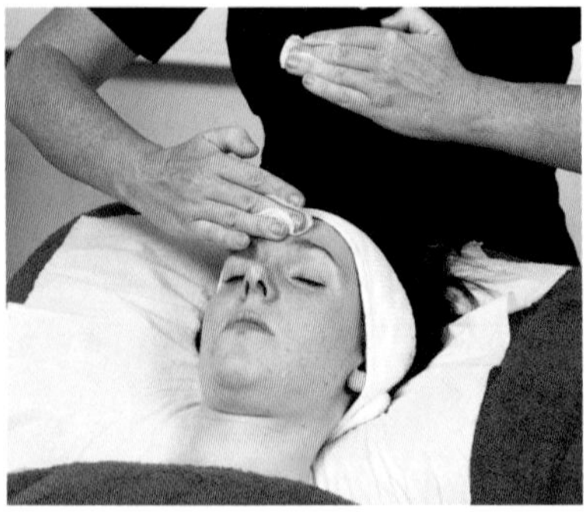

STEP 4 – Use alternate strokes up the cheeks, nose and forehead.

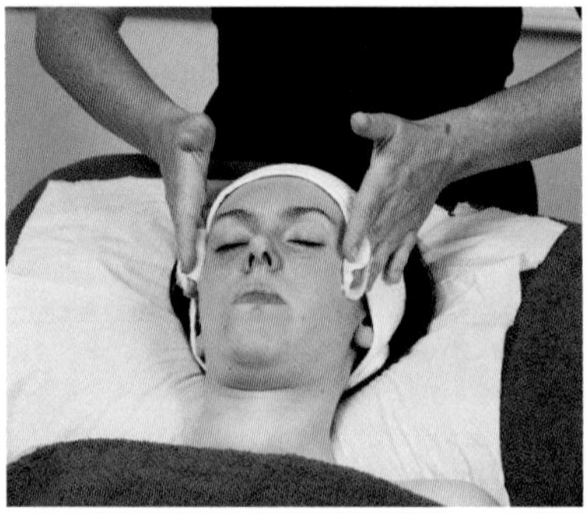

STEP 5 – Press and circle the cotton pads on the temples to finish.

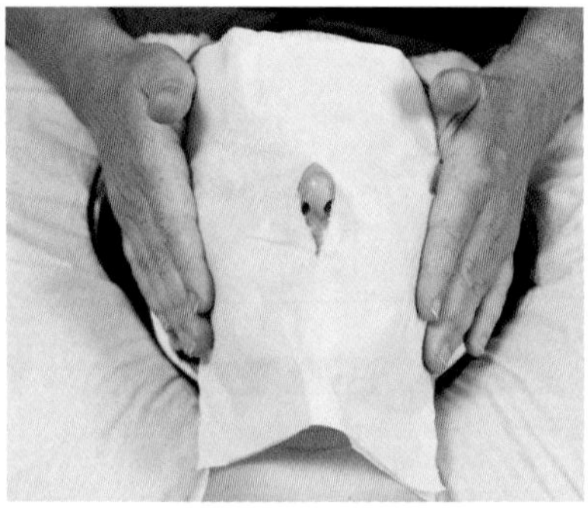

STEP 6 – Blot the skin dry. Place a tissue over the client's face (with a hole for the nose).

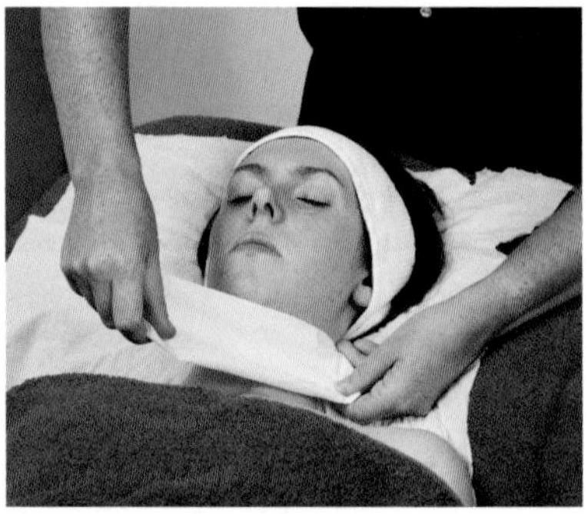

STEP 7 – Fold the tissue in half and blot the neck area.

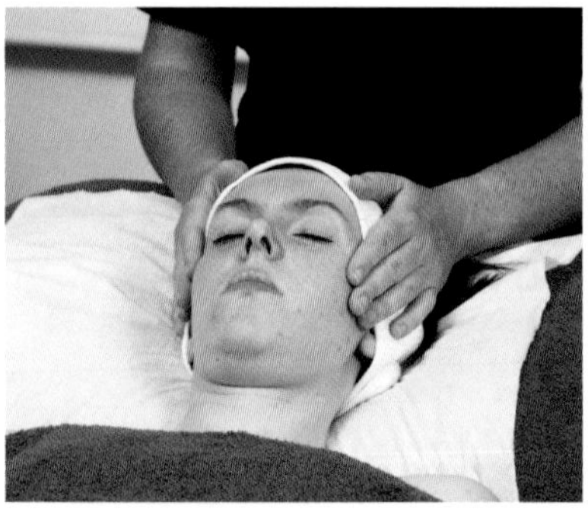

STEP 8 – Finish by placing your hands on the sides of the client's head. This will complete the face cleanse.

HANDY HINTS

Dampen the cotton wool pads with warm water. This will be more relaxing for the client. You can do this easily if you have a bowl of warm water on your trolley.

HANDY HINTS

Remember to tone and blot the skin before applying the moisturiser.

APPLYING THE MOISTURISER

The moisturiser you use will depend on the client's skin condition. Once you have chosen the correct product, you are ready to moisturise your client's skin.

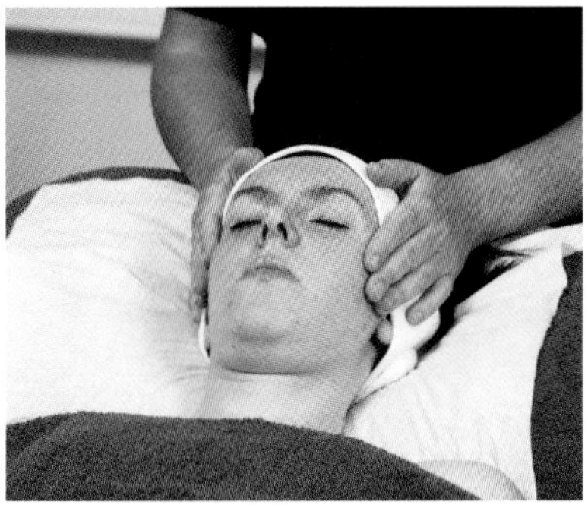

STEP 1 – Start by placing your hands on the sides of the client's head. This will help to prepare them for the moisturiser.

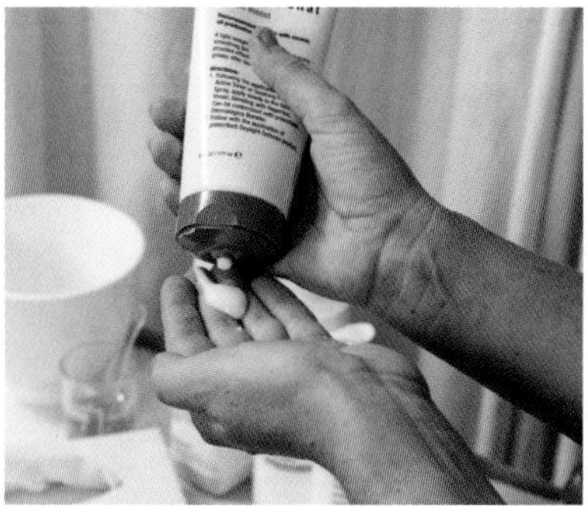

STEP 2 – Place a small amount of moisturiser in the palm of your hand.

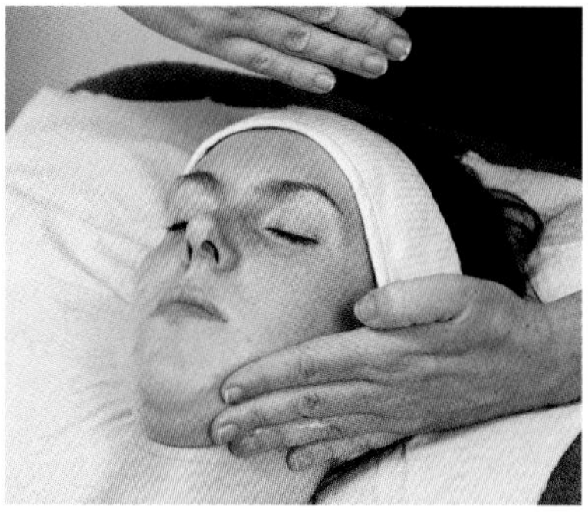

STEP 3 – Apply moisturiser in smooth strokes up the neck.

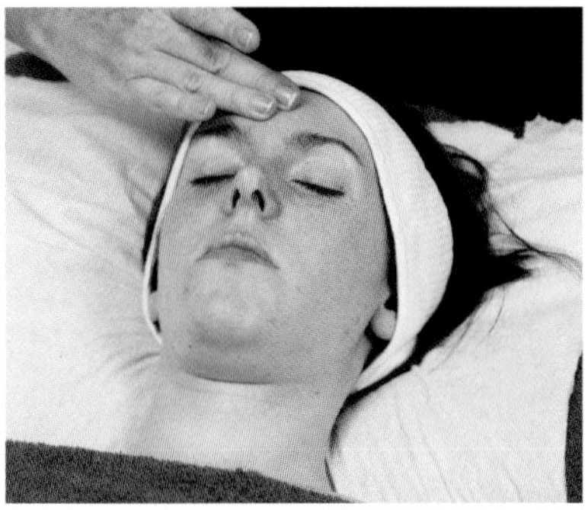

STEP 4 – Continue with sweeping strokes along the cheeks, nose and forehead.

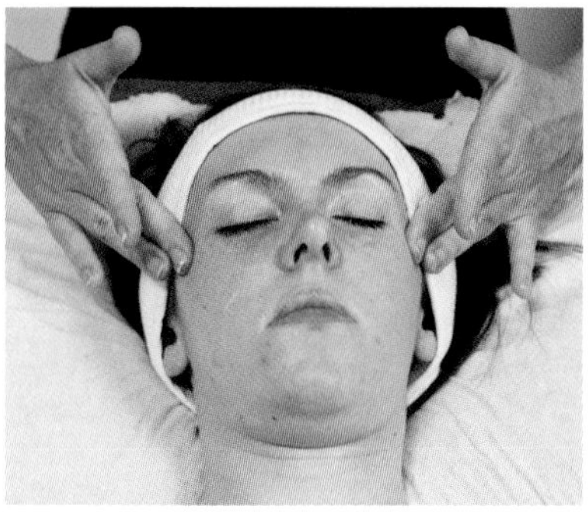

STEP 5 – Press and circle the temples to finish.

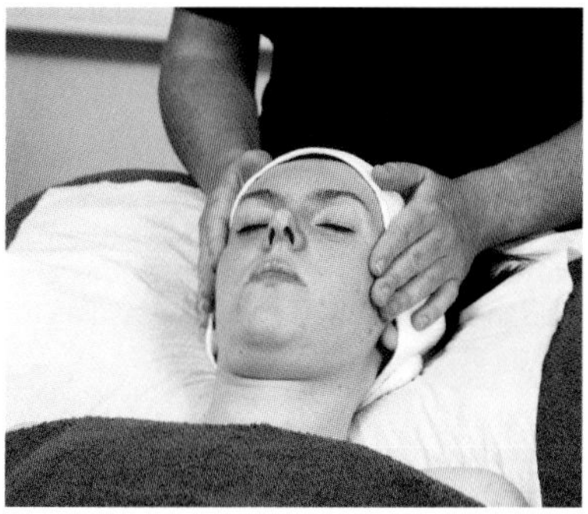

STEP 6 – Finish by placing your hands on the sides of the client's head. This will complete the moisturising part of the facial.

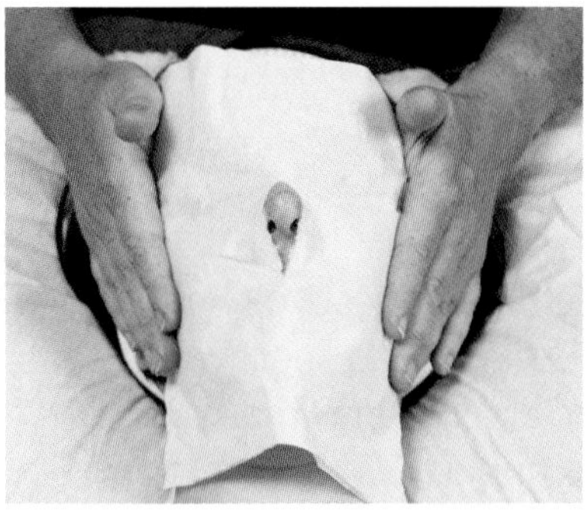

STEP 7 – If needed, blot the skin with tissue. This will remove any moisturiser that has not soaked into the skin.

AFTER THE TREATMENT

After you have finished the treatment, make sure that you record everything you have done on the client's treatment plan. You may also include any tips that you have given to the client such as the products that you would recommend for their skin type. It's also a good idea to suggest they follow a regular skin care routine at home.

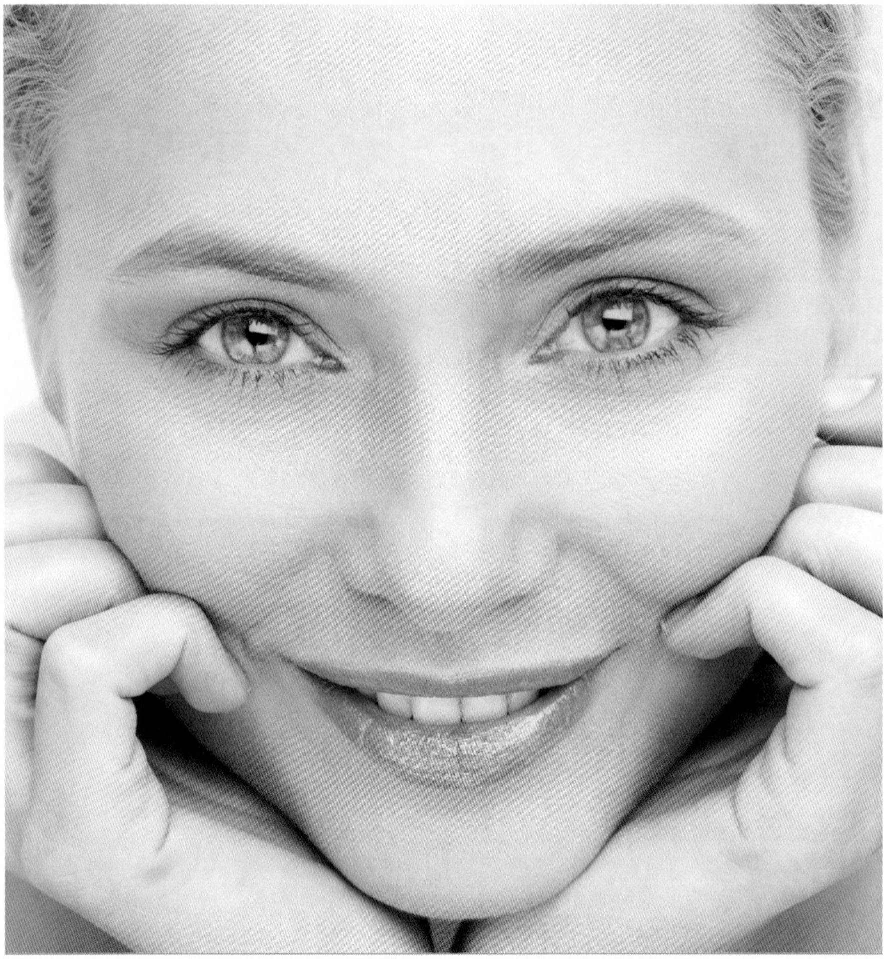

A healthy skin

HANDY HINTS

Remember to include the products that you have used on your treatment plan. This will help if the client comes in again or wants to buy any of the products.

HANDY HINTS

It is important to ask the client if they enjoyed the treatment. This will make sure that they leave happy and help you to improve your skills.

ACTIVITY

In a group or with a partner, make a list of ways in which you can work hygienically when carrying out a skin care treatment.

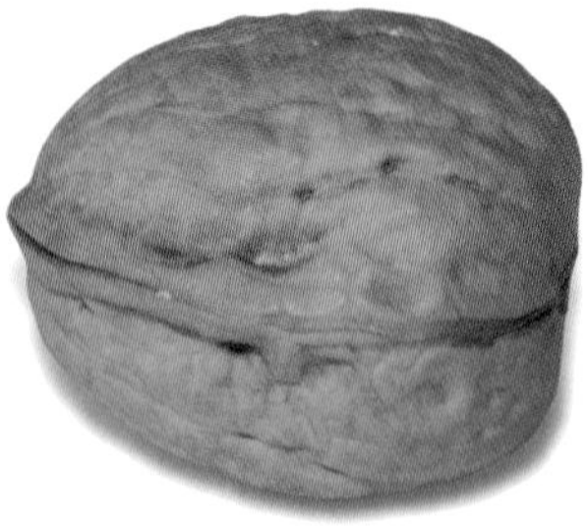

IN A NUTSHELL

You are now at the end of the chapter. Before you test your knowledge with the revision activities, check the following list to see if you feel confident in all the areas covered. If there are still any areas you're unsure of, go back over them in the book and ask your tutor for extra support:

- what preparation is needed for a basic skin care treatment
- what products, tools and equipment you will need
- how to use the products, tools and equipment safely and hygienically
- how to carry out a skin care treatment
- how to communicate and behave in a professional manner
- the main skin types.

REVISION ACTIVITIES

Use the questions below to test your knowledge of Chapter 006 to see just how much information you've gained. This can help you to prepare for your assessments. Turn to pages 493–494 for the answers.

SmartScreen 006 sample questions

WORDS TO FIND

Copy and complete the sentences below. Use these words to help you fill in the gaps.

cleanser	tissue	combination	bowl
toner	communication	hygiene	towels
moisturiser	oily	skin type	Barbicide
preparation	dry	spatula	safety

1 If you use tools and equipment that are clean, this is an example of good ______________________.

2 A product that is used to remove facial make-up is called a ______________________.

3 A ______________________ is used to hygienically remove products from jars or pots.

4 After you have applied the toner, a ______________________ is used to blot the skin dry.

5 Before your client arrives, ______________________ of all of your tools, equipment and products is important. This will make sure that you have everything ready for the treatment.

TEST YOUR KNOWLEDGE FURTHER

1 Copy and complete the table to show which skin type suits each of the skin care products. You can choose from the following skin types: oily, combination, dry, normal.

Skin care product	Type of skin care product	Which skin types it is suitable for
Cleansers	Face wash	
	Lotion	
	Milk	
	Cream	
Toners	Freshener	
	Toner	
	Astringent	
Moisturisers	Lotion	
	Mousse	
	Cream	

2 For what reason would you use a blanket in a treatment?

3 a What does a cleanser do?
b What does a toner do?
c What do–es a moisturiser do?

4 Copy and complete the table. You may use the following skin types: oily, combination, dry, normal.

Skin type description	Which skin type is this describing?
▪ Usually dry cheeks and oily skin on the 'T' zone (forehead, nose and chin)	
▪ Even skin texture ▪ Feels soft ▪ Skin colour is even ▪ Does not feel tight ▪ Feels firm to touch	
▪ Shiny ▪ Spots ▪ Blackheads ▪ Large pores	
▪ Flaky patches ▪ Dull ▪ Feels tight ▪ Small pores ▪ Whiteheads	

5 Name **two** positive ways in which you can communicate with your client.

6 Why is it important to smile at your client?

7 Why should you not ask the client questions during the lip cleanse?

8 During a skin care treatment, which do you apply first – the toner or the cleanser?

9 Give **two** reasons why a client may have a skin care treatment.

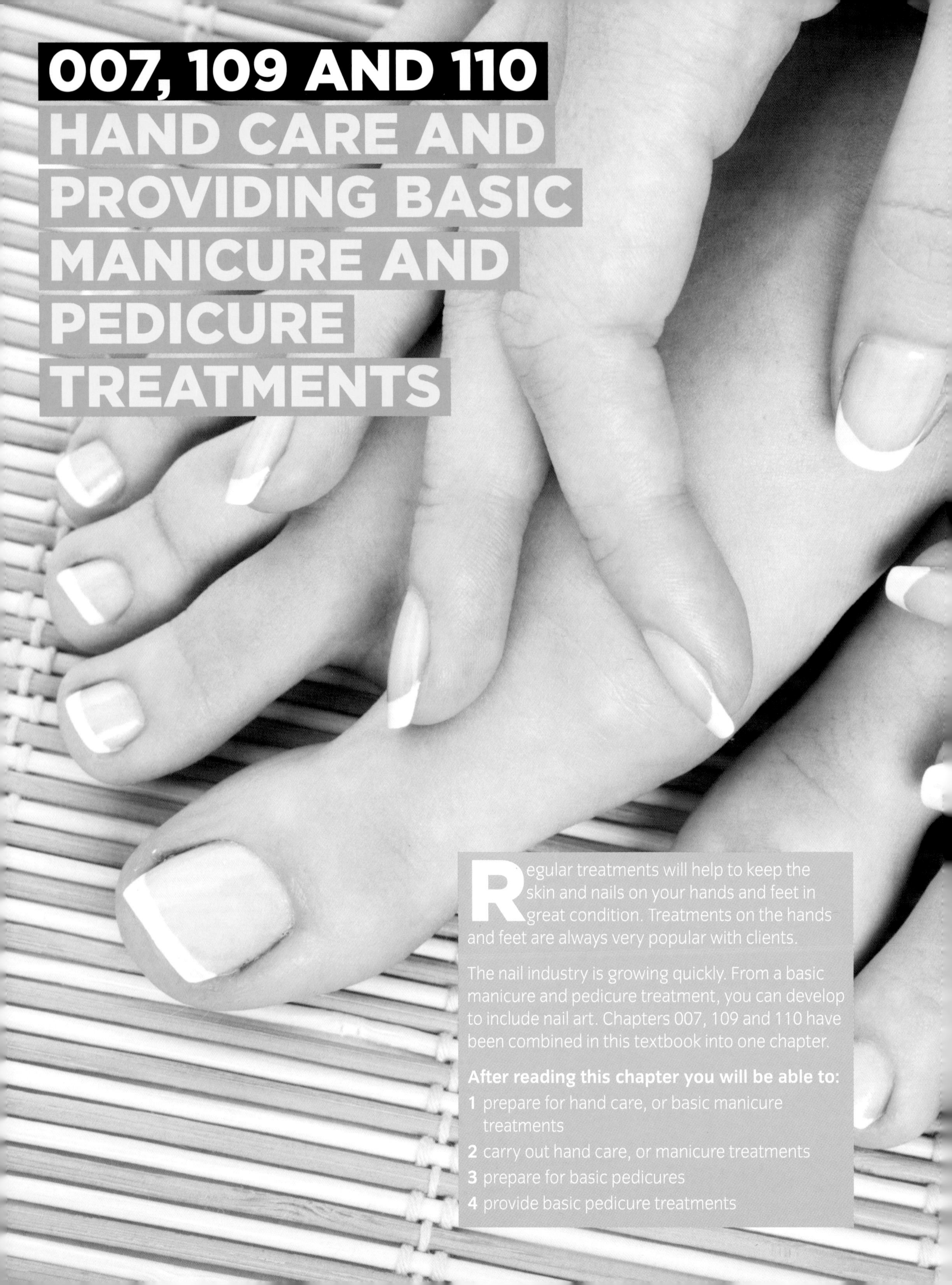

007, 109 AND 110
HAND CARE AND PROVIDING BASIC MANICURE AND PEDICURE TREATMENTS

Regular treatments will help to keep the skin and nails on your hands and feet in great condition. Treatments on the hands and feet are always very popular with clients.

The nail industry is growing quickly. From a basic manicure and pedicure treatment, you can develop to include nail art. Chapters 007, 109 and 110 have been combined in this textbook into one chapter.

After reading this chapter you will be able to:

1 prepare for hand care, or basic manicure treatments
2 carry out hand care, or manicure treatments
3 prepare for basic pedicures
4 provide basic pedicure treatments

PREPARE FOR A HAND CARE, BASIC MANICURE OR PEDICURE TREATMENT

Before you begin the nail treatment it's important to be prepared. Health and safety requirements should be carried out for every treatment, but knowing how to set up your treatment area and carrying out a proper consultation are also musts for nail services.

HANDY HINTS

The word 'manicure' comes from the Latin 'manus' – hand – and 'curo' – care.

HANDY HINTS

The word 'pedicure' comes from the Latin 'pedi' – foot – and 'curo' – care.

SAFE AND HYGIENIC WORKING PRACTICES

It is important that you work in a safe and clean way. You should keep your treatment area tidy and only use hygienic tools and equipment. This will help to reduce the risk of harm to you and your clients and prevent cross-infection. The client will also have more confidence in you and you will look more professional.

It is your responsibility to be aware of health and safety legislation to protect yourself, your clients and your colleagues.

The main safe and hygienic working practices that you need to know for a manicure and pedicure treatment are:

- PPE – 'Personal Protective Equipment', eg using towels and tissue roll to cover your client's clothes. The therapist may also wear **non-latex gloves** when looking at the client's feet at the start of the pedicure.
- COSHH – 'Control Of Substances Hazardous to Health', eg using nail-enamel remover safely in a **well-ventilated** area. This will help to remove the strong smell of this product from the room.
- HASAWA – 'Health And Safety At Work Act', eg ensuring that all equipment, tools and products are clean and safe to use for each client.
- Methods of sterilisation and disinfection: if tools and equipment are sterilised, all germs that may be present on them are killed and they are then safe to use on a client. Disinfection of tools and equipment will kill some germs but not all of them. Disinfectants will also help to prevent germs from growing. An example is placing the spatula in a container of disinfectant, such as Barbicide, during the treatment.
- Clean treatment area: wipe over your treatment area with a clean cloth and disinfectant after you have finished. This will help to prevent cross-infection.
- Clean your hands by washing them in warm water with an **antibacterial** soap at the start of the treatment and then again at the end. This will help to stop germs from passing from one person to another.

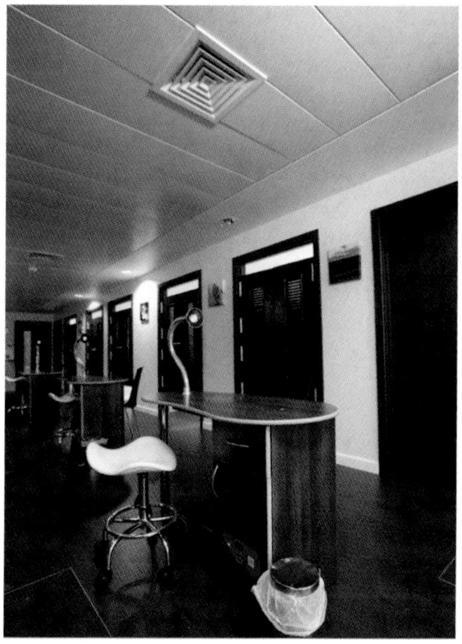

A professional working area for nail services

Non-latex gloves
Gloves that are unlikely to cause irritation to the skin

Well-ventilated
Where stale air is replaced by fresh air to help get rid of smells and odours

Antibacterial
Something that kills or slows down the growth of bacteria

HANDY HINTS

Go to Chapter 113 Following health and safety in the salon for detailed information on PPE, COSHH and HASAWA.

HANDY HINTS

Nail 'enamel' is another word for nail 'varnish'. Both are used in this chapter.

SmartScreen 007 handouts 4 and 9

THE SALON ENVIRONMENT

It is important that you have prepared your treatment area before your client arrives for their treatment. Think about the client's comfort and what you need to do your job well.

The treatment area should be prepared in a professional way:

- All products, tools and equipment should be clean and hygienic.
- Products, tools and equipment should be placed safely and tidily on the trolley.
- If a couch is to be used for the client, the couch should be covered for hygiene reasons with a couch cover and couch roll tissue.
- If a workstation is being used, it should be cleaned with a suitable product, such as disinfectant, and covered for hygiene reasons with couch roll tissue.
- If chairs are to be used, then both chairs should be placed facing each other (there will be a workstation between the chairs for a hand care or manicure treatment). The therapist's chair should be slightly lower to help stop you getting back and shoulder ache.

HANDY HINTS

Remember to wash your hands before and after the treatment. This will help to stop cross-infection (spreading of germs).

HANDY HINTS

Go to Chapter 113 Following health and safety in the salon and read up on health and safety legislation.

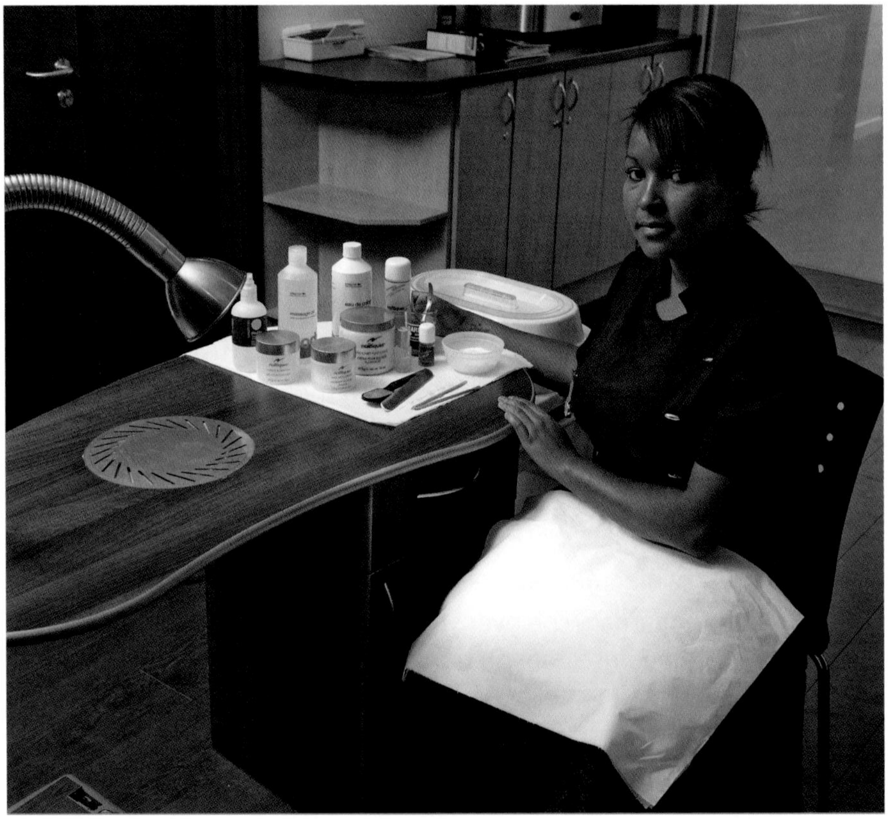

A professional set-up for a manicure treatment

SmartScreen 007 handout 1

The following should also be thought about:

- The room temperature should not be too hot or too cold. The ideal temperature for a treatment room is between 16–18 degrees Centigrade.
- The air in the room should be well ventilated. This means that fresh air continually replaces stale air. It will stop the air in the treatment room from becoming stuffy, and will also prevent strong smells from building up, eg from the nail-enamel remover.
- The lighting should be suitable for a manicure and pedicure treatment. The treatment area needs to be well lit so that you can see clearly what you are doing.

PREPARING FOR THE HAND, FOOT OR NAIL SERVICE

Before the client arrives, it is important that you get yourself and the treatment area prepared. All of the products, tools and equipment need to be ready. This will make sure that the treatment flows well and will also give the client a positive first impression. It will help the client to relax and have confidence in you.

BASIC TOOLS AND EQUIPMENT

Some items, such as couch covers, are needed for most beauty therapy/ nail services. The table lists them and describes their use in hand and nail care.

Tools/equipment	What does it do?	How is it used?
Cotton wool 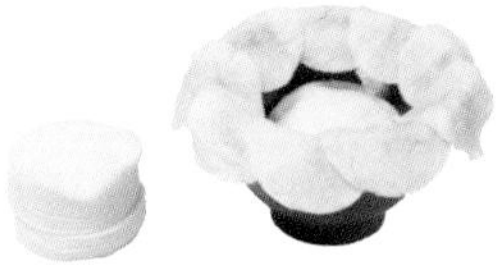	Used with the nail-varnish remover. Also used to wipe over the arms and hands with the disinfectant gel/spray.	▪ Apply the disinfectant spray or nail-varnish remover to the cotton wool pad. ▪ Throw away after use.
Treatment plan 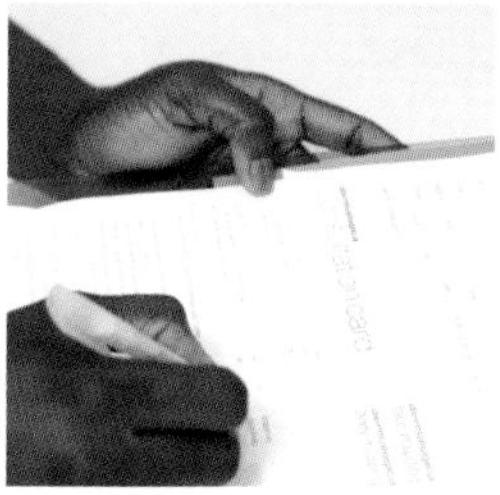	Records the treatment details, eg products used.	▪ Write down details of the treatment on the plan. ▪ Make sure that you write neatly and clearly, being careful to record the correct information.

Tools/equipment	What does it do?	How is it used?
Waste bin 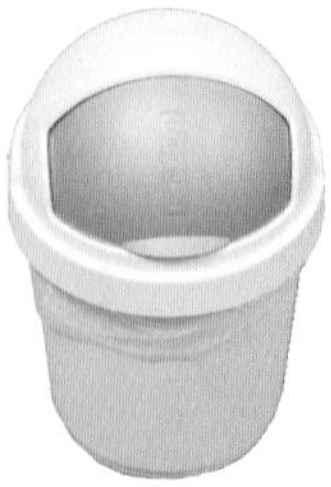	Used for throwing waste materials in, such as cotton wool and tissues.	▪ Waste bins should be lined with a bin liner and have a lid. ▪ Empty them into the main bin when they are full.
Couch cover 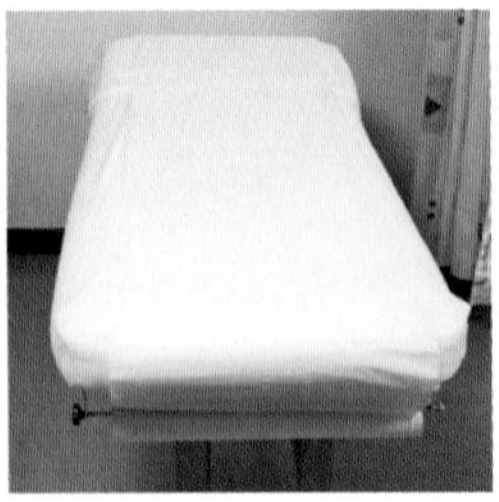	Placed over the couch for hygiene reasons. (Only if a couch is used for the treatment – normally a workstation or table is used for nail services.)	▪ Place a clean one over the couch. ▪ Cover with couch roll tissue. ▪ Machine wash on a high temperature after use to destroy harmful germs.
Couch tissue roll 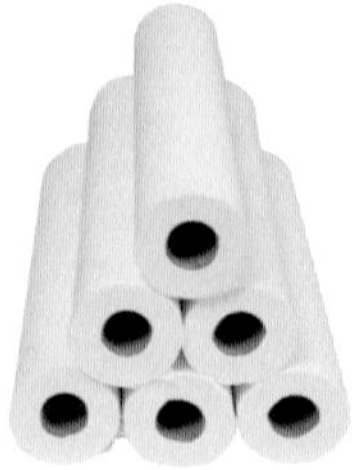	Placed over the workstation and on top of the couch cover for hygiene reasons.	▪ Dispose of after use. ▪ Use a fresh one for each new client.
Towels 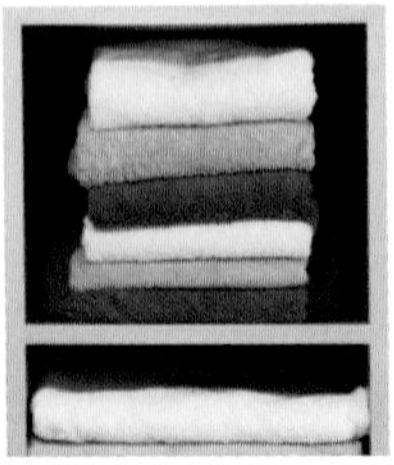	Used to cover the treatment area. Also used to dry the client's hands or feet after they have been soaked, and to rest the client's hands or feet on during the treatment.	▪ Place over the treatment area, then cover with couch roll tissue. ▪ Machine wash on a high temperature after use to destroy harmful germs.
Tissues 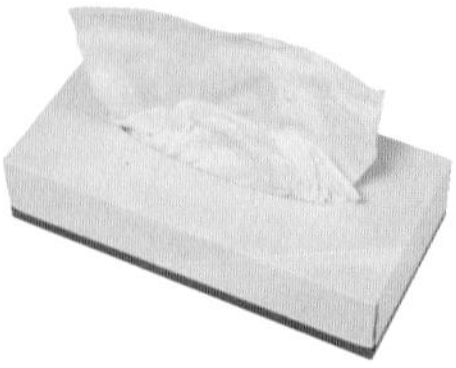	Used to place the client's hands on before varnishing. This will help to protect the treatment area.	▪ Place the client's hands on here before you **enamel** the nails. ▪ Throw away after use.

Enamel

To apply nail varnish

Tools/equipment	What does it do?	How is it used?
Nail file 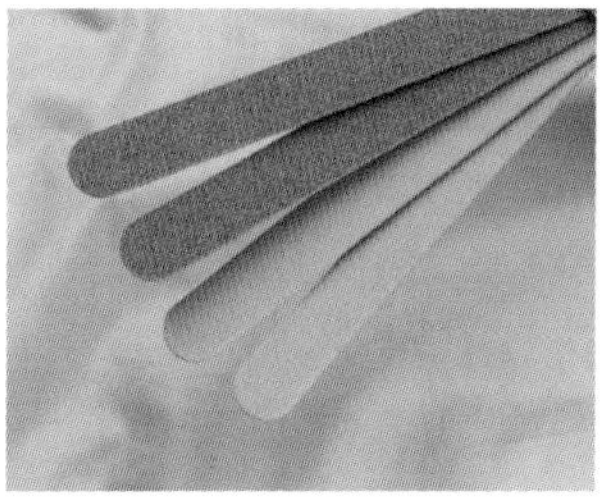	Helps to shape the **free edge** of the nail, remove rough edges and make it feel smooth.	▪ Use the rough side for reducing the nail length. ▪ Use the fine side for finishing off and smoothing. ▪ File the nails from side to centre only. If you use the file from side to side (in a 'seesaw' action) this may split the nail. ▪ Throw away after each client or use an antibacterial/ disinfecting spray after each client.
Barbicide and jar 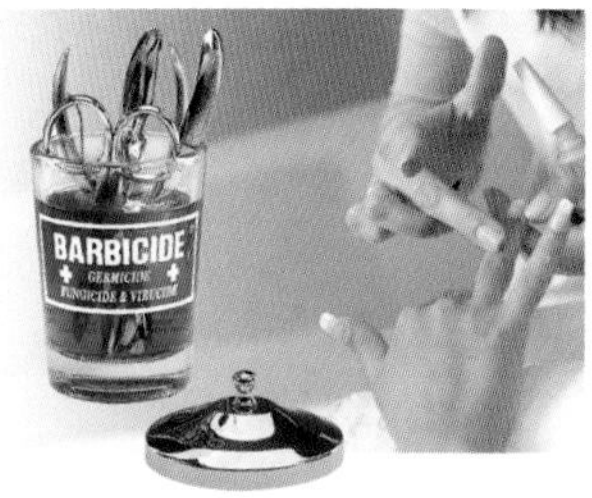	A disinfectant – spatulas and orange-wood sticks can be placed in this during the treatment.	▪ **Dilute** the Barbicide according to the **manufacturer**'s instructions. ▪ Rinse down the sink after use.
Spatulas 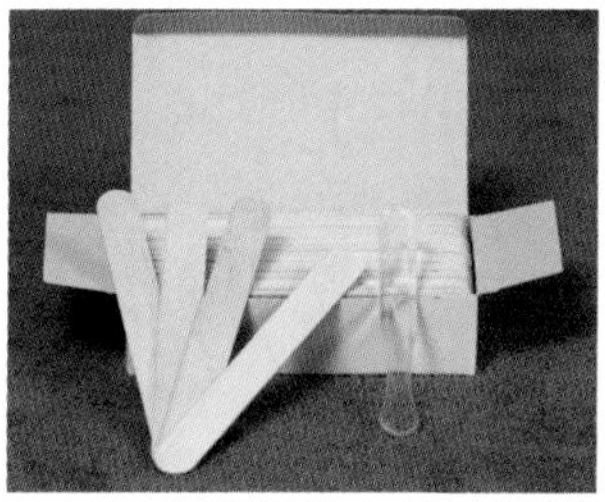	Used to scoop the cuticle cream from the pot. Can be plastic or wooden – the wooden ones are disposable.	▪ Keep in the Barbicide jar during the treatment for hygiene reasons. ▪ After the treatment, wash plastic spatulas in warm, soapy water and then disinfectant. Place in an ultraviolet cabinet to store them hygienically. ▪ Throw away wooden ones after each client.

Free edge
The white part of the nail found at the tip of the finger (the part that gets bitten if you bite your nails!)

Dilute
Mix with water to make less strong

Manufacturer
A company that makes a product

Tools/equipment	What does it do?	How is it used?
Manicure/finger bowl 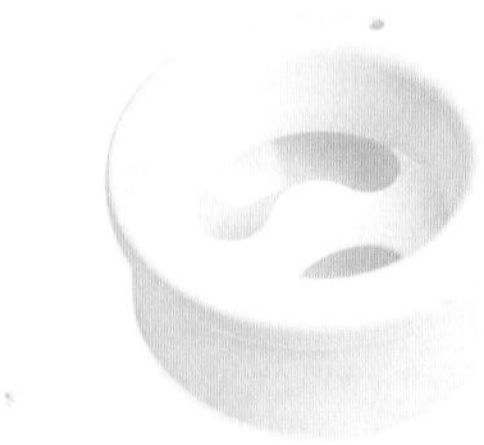 Pedicure bowl 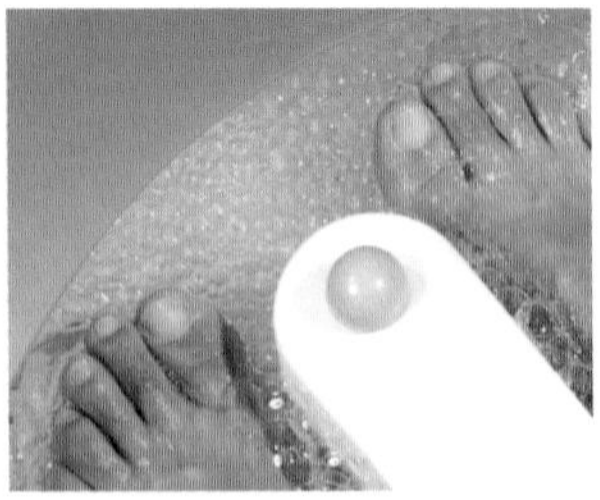	Used to soak the hands or feet. Add hand or foot soak before adding warm water. The warm, soapy water helps to clean and soften the skin and cuticles.	▪ Fill with warm, soapy water. ▪ Once cuticle cream has been massaged into the cuticles, place the client's fingertips or feet in the bowl to soften the cuticles. ▪ After use, clean using warm, soapy water and then disinfectant. Dry thoroughly.
Orange stick 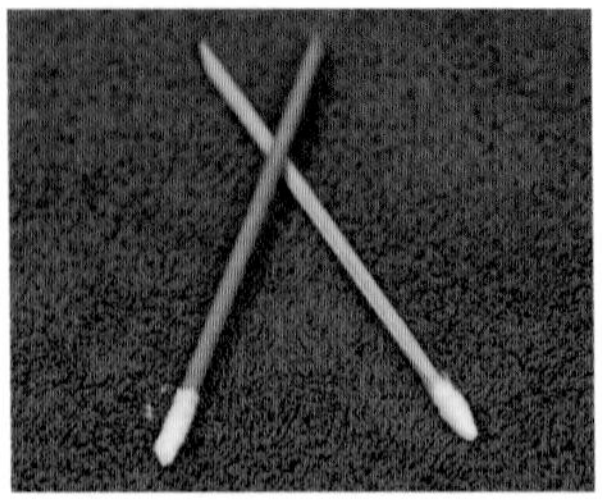	Can be tipped with cotton wool and used to gently ease back the cuticles, or remove nail varnish from the edges of the nail.	▪ Apply cotton wool to the end of the orange stick. This makes it less sharp so that it can be used safely to gently push back the cuticles. ▪ Place in the Barbicide jar during the treatment when not in use. ▪ Throw away after use.

HANDY HINTS

Why not give the client the nail file after the treatment? Take the cost of it into account and include this in your treatment price.

HANDY HINTS

Nail files are sometimes called 'emery boards'.

HANDY HINTS

Do not use your fingers to remove products from the pots. This is not hygienic and may spread germs. Always use a clean spatula.

HANDY HINTS

A foot spa can also be used to soak the client's feet in. These are very relaxing as the water bubbles around the feet.

ACTIVITY

Look back at the tables of the tools and equipment used in a hand care, manicure or pedicure treatment. Copy the table below and for each item listed, tick the column that applies to what you do with it after the treatment. This means that you will be working with them in a hygienic way.

Tools/equipment used in a hand care, manicure or pedicure treatment	**Disposable – throw away after use/ between clients**	**Wash in warm, soapy water, then wipe over with disinfectant**	**Machine wash on a high temperature**
Cotton wool			
Towels			
Tissues			
Nail file			
Plastic spatula			
Manicure/finger bowl			
Pedicure bowl			
Orange stick			

Now discuss your answers and mark them with your tutor.

PRODUCTS USED IN A HAND OR FOOT TREATMENT

There are many products you need to know about that are used in a hand or nail treatment. This table will help you.

HANDY HINTS

Place the products, tools and equipment on your trolley (or nail station) in the order that you will use them. This will also help you to remember the routine.

Manicure/ pedicure product	**What does it do?**	**How is it used?**
Disinfectant or anti-bacterial gel 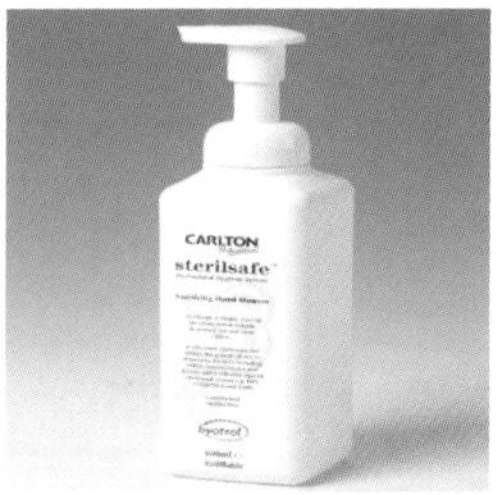	Used to clean the client's hands or feet before you start the treatment. Helps to remove dirt and germs and prevent cross-infection. Usually in gel or liquid form.	▪ Apply to cotton wool pads. ▪ Gently wipe down the arms, hands and fingers. ▪ Use a fresh piece of cotton wool for each hand.
Hand and foot soak 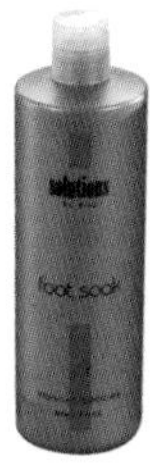	Helps to clean the hands or feet.	▪ Add a small amount to the manicure or pedicure bowl. ▪ Add warm water. Check with the client that the water is a comfortable temperature.

Manicure/ pedicure product	What does it do?	How is it used?
Nail-varnish remover 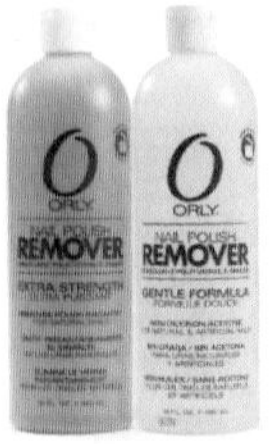	Removes nail varnish, dirt and grease from the nail. Can dry the **nail plate** if it is used a lot.	▪ Apply to cotton wool pads. ▪ Gently press onto the nail and hold for a few seconds, then wipe off. Use a clean surface for each wipe. ▪ Continue until all the nail enamel has been removed.
Cuticle cream 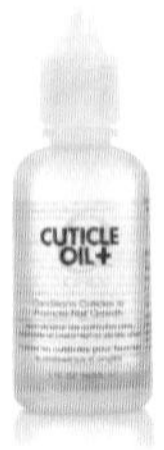	Softens the cuticles. Helps to prepare the cuticles for the cuticle work.	▪ Remove from the pot using a clean spatula. ▪ Apply a small amount to the cuticles on each finger or toe. ▪ Massage in using circular thumb movements.
Hand and arm/foot and leg lotion or cream 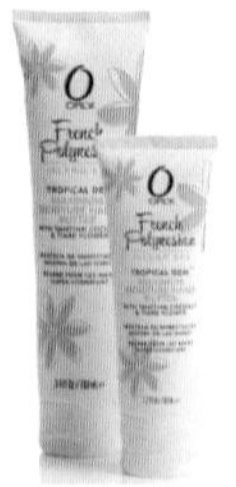	Used for massaging the arms, hands and fingers or lower leg, feet and toes. Helps to replace moisture in the skin. Makes the skin feel soft and smooth.	▪ Remove using a clean spatula (if in a pot). ▪ Warm in your hands first. ▪ Apply using smooth strokes. ▪ Carry out the massage routine (see later in the chapter).
Base coat 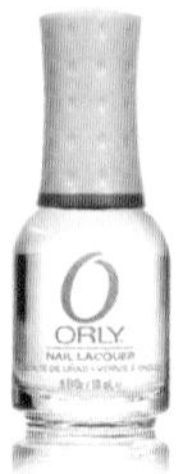	Provides a smooth base for the nail varnish. Helps to prevent the nails from becoming stained by the nail varnish.	▪ Apply one coat to clean nails.
Nail enamel 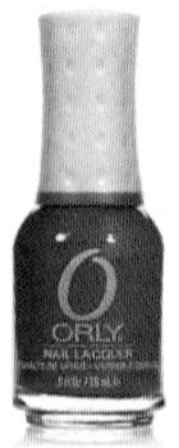	Available in lots of different colours. These give colour to the nail plate. Available in **matt**/cream or **pearlised** effects; choice of enamel depends on the finished effect needed.	▪ Apply on top of the base coat when it's dry. ▪ Always check the manufacturer's instructions before using. ▪ Apply two coats if using matt/cream enamel. ▪ Apply three coats if using pearlised enamel. This is because you do not normally put a top coat over this type of enamel because it already has a shiny look to it, so a top coat is not needed.

Manicure/ pedicure product	What does it do?	How is it used?
Top coat 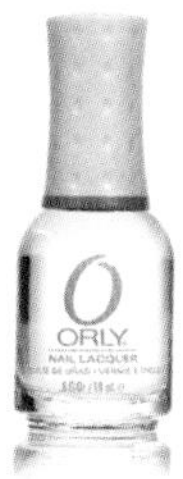	Provides an extra glossy finish to the nails. Helps to protect the nail varnish from chipping.	▪ Apply one coat once the nail varnish is dry ▪ Usually not applied over pearlised varnish as there is a shine already.

ACTIVITY

Paint some artificial nails with different coloured nail enamels. Stick these nails onto some card to make a display board (you can use a CD case for this). You can then use these to show your client what nail enamel colours you have. This will help them to choose the colour for their own nails.

Use this table to help you set up for the treatment:

Hand care (Chapter 007) and Manicure (Chapter 109)	Pedicure (Chapter 110)
✓ disinfectant or anti-bacterial hand gel	✓ disinfectant or anti-bacterial foot gel
✓ nail soak	✓ foot soak
✓ manicure/finger bowl	✓ pedicure bowl
✓ nail-varnish remover	✓ nail-varnish remover
✓ cuticle cream	✓ cuticle cream
✓ hand and arm lotion or cream	✓ foot and leg lotion or cream
✓ base coat	✓ base coat
✓ nail enamels (different colours)	✓ nail enamels (different colours)
✓ top coat	✓ top coat
✓ nail file	✓ nail file
✓ Barbicide and jar	✓ Barbicide and jar
✓ spatulas	✓ spatulas
✓ tissues	✓ tissues
✓ cotton wool	✓ cotton wool
✓ treatment plan	✓ treatment plan
✓ couch tissue	✓ couch tissue
✓ towels	✓ towels
✓ couch cover	✓ couch cover
✓ orange stick (Chapter 109 only)	✓ orange stick
✓ waste bin with a lid (containing a bin liner)	✓ waste bin with a lid (containing a bin liner)

Disinfectant or anti-bacterial gel
A product that helps to kill some germs; disinfectant does not work as well as sterilising

Nail plate
The main part of the nail

Matt
Dull, with no shine

Pearlised
Shiny appearance

HANDY HINTS
Nail enamel is also called nail varnish.

HANDY HINTS
Dark-coloured nail enamels are more likely to stain the nail plate. Remember to use a base coat before you apply the enamel to stop this from happening.

SmartScreen 007 handout 11

SmartScreen 007 worksheet 3

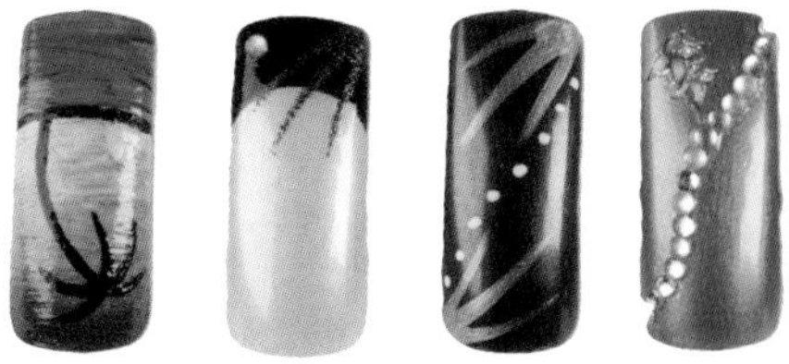

HANDY HINTS
Always follow the manufacturer's instructions as products vary. This will also make sure you are using the products safely.

> **HANDY HINTS**
> Make sure that the chairs that you use are the right height for you and the client. This will make sure that you are both comfortable. It will also stop you and the client from getting back- and neckache.

You will also need the following in your treatment area:

- suitable chairs for you and the client
- treatment couch or nail workstation.

BASIC STRUCTURE OF THE NAIL

Before you can carry out a consultation for hand and nail services, you need to have an understanding of the nail structure.

Nail part	Description
Nail plate	Forms the main part of the nail. It is hard and protects the nail bed from damage.
Nail bed	Lies underneath the nail plate. It contains a blood supply which helps the new nail cells to grow. It is this part that gives the nail its colour.
Nail wall	The skin that is found at the sides of the nail. It helps to protect the nail from damage and infection as it grows.
Cuticle	The skin that is found around the base of the nail. It helps to stop dirt and bacteria getting under the skin around the nail. It should be soft and loose. If it is dry and sticks to the nail plate it will be stretched as the nail grows. Eventually it will tear, causing rough and sometimes painful skin known as a **hangnail**.
Free edge	This is the part of the nail that grows past the fingertip. It is usually white. It is the part of the nail that is filed and shaped (or bitten!). It helps to protect the fingertip.

Hangnail
Loose bit of cuticle around the side of the nail; can be sharp and sore

The structure of the nail

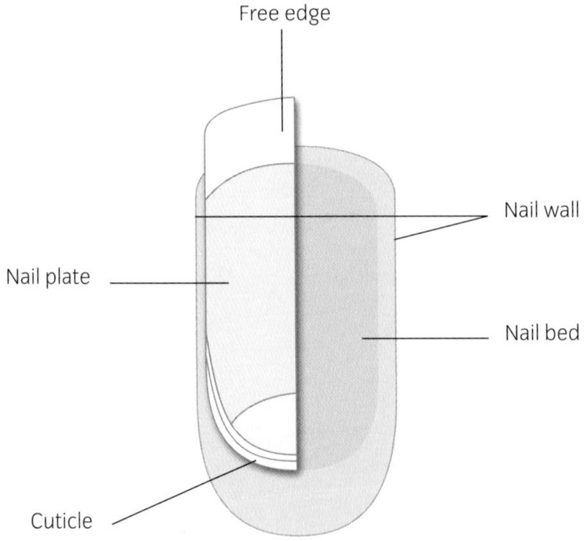

> **HANDY HINTS**
> If the blood supply to our nails is good, then the nails will look pink. If the blood supply to our nails is poor, then the nails may look white or pale.

SmartScreen 007 handout 8

SmartScreen 007 worksheet 2

CONSULTATION

Before you start the treatment you will need to carry out a consultation with the client to determine the treatment **objectives**. This is carried out for the following reasons:

- to find out why they are having the treatment. Reasons for treatment may include:
  - to improve their skin, nail or cuticle condition
  - make their skin feel softer
  - to improve the appearance of their hands or feet
- to have their nails painted for a special occasion, such as a party or wedding
- to make themselves feel better by having a relaxing treatment
- to discuss what products you are going to use, such as the colour of nail varnish
- to complete a treatment plan with your client. This includes all details of the treatment, such as client's details and nail enamel colour used.

Objectives
Aims; what the client would like to gain from the treatment

During the consultation you will need to find out about the condition of the client's nails, skin and cuticles. This will help you to choose the right products for them.

SmartScreen 007 handout 7

SmartScreen 007 worksheet 1

COMMUNICATION AND BEHAVIOUR

You must use your communication and behavioural skills at all times, but they are very important in a consultation. Remember that first impressions are important. Your client will need to get a positive first impression of you, so take the following into account when meeting your client:

- Smile.
- Greet them by their name.
- Shake their hand and introduce yourself to them.
- Ask them to walk with you to the treatment area.
- Help them to sit down on the chair.
- Make sure your body language is open, eg your arms are open and not crossed.

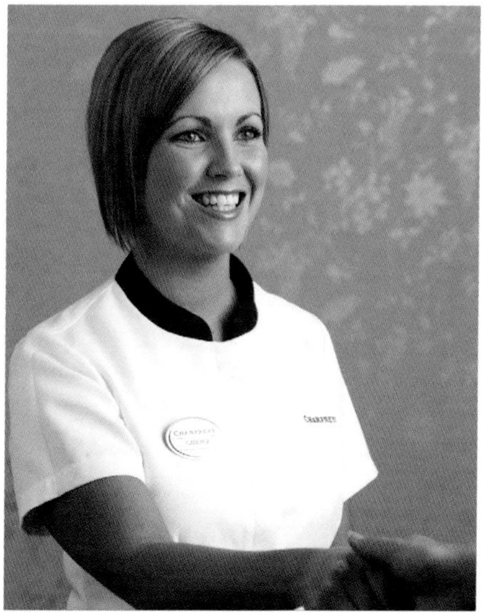

Always try your best to give the client a good impression of the salon

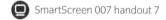

All of these tips will help to give a positive first impression. This will make the client feel relaxed and at ease.

Remember also to:

- speak clearly
- have a friendly approach (remembering to smile, for instance)
- listen to the client and respond politely
- give the client your full attention and respect
- try to use words that the client will understand. If you use any technical words used in manicure or pedicure (such as cuticle or free edge) make sure that you explain to the client what they mean. This will help them to understand what you are saying to them.

SmartScreen 007 handout 6

HANDY HINTS

Go to Chapter 102 Presenting a professional image in the salon and read up on how to communicate and behave in a professional way.

You will also need to work in a professional way with your colleagues in the salon. Ways in which you can do this are:

- helping each other set up for a treatment and also tidy away
- following instructions from your supervisor/tutor when you are asked to do a job, such as sweeping the floor
- working safely and hygienically in the salon
- keeping your voice levels low so that it does not disturb the clients in the salon.

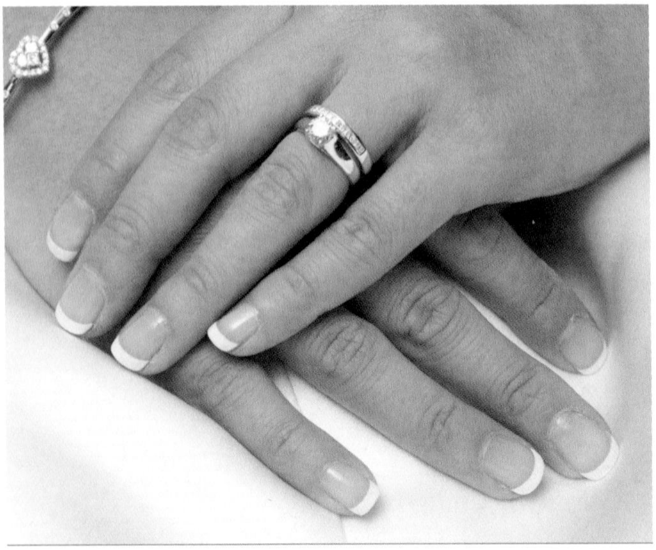
Well manicured fingernails

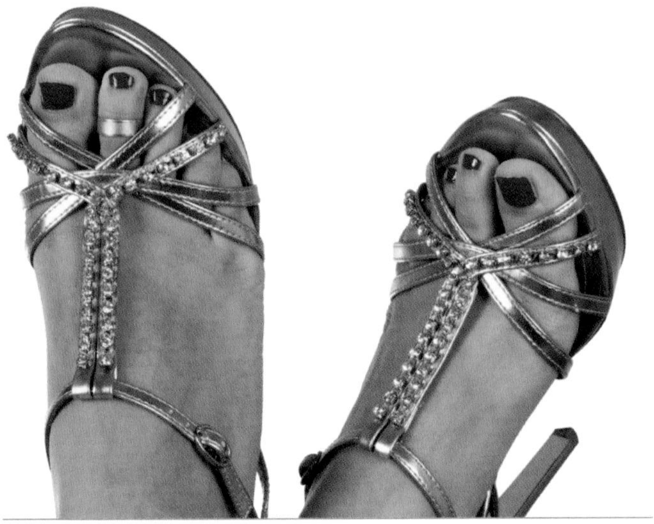
Nicely painted toenails

FACTORS THAT WILL INFLUENCE THE TREATMENT

In order to make sure that you are providing a safe treatment for your client, you will need to be aware of the following **factors**. You will need to look at the client's hands or feet at the start of the treatment. Ask your tutor if you need help to identify any factors.

Factors
Things you have to think about. A factor such as nail length may need you to change the service slightly

HANDY HINTS
Remember to ask your tutor for help when you are checking for these factors with your client.

Factor	Description	How may it affect the treatment?
Allergy 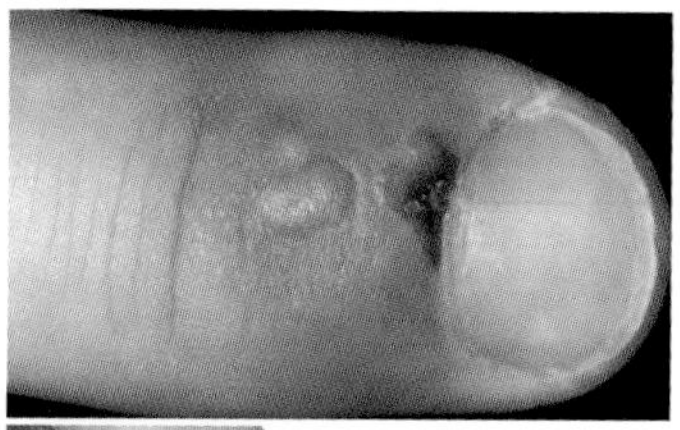 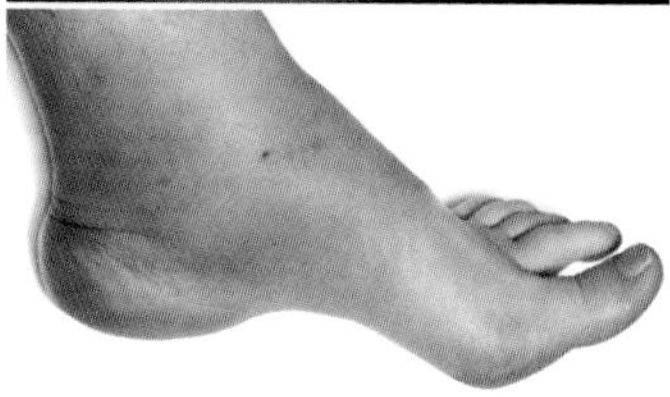	When the body overreacts to products. The skin may become red, itchy, swollen and feel hot.	Ask the client before you start the treatment if they are allergic to any of the products that you are using. If they are, you must not use them. If your client has an allergic reaction to the products during the treatment, remove the product straight away with cool water. Speak to your tutor who may refer the client to see their doctor.
Nail length 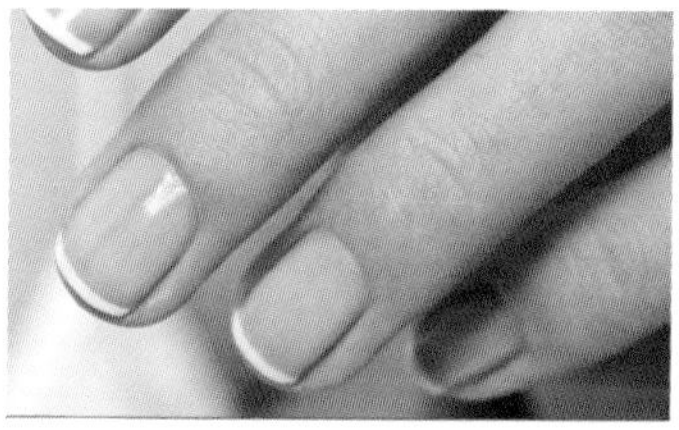 Short fingernails 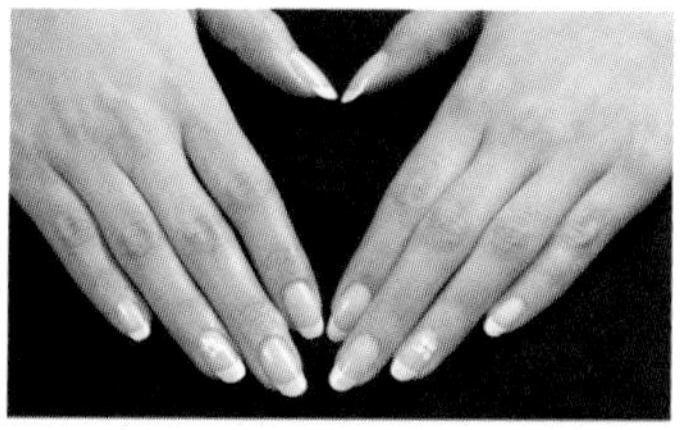 Long fingernails 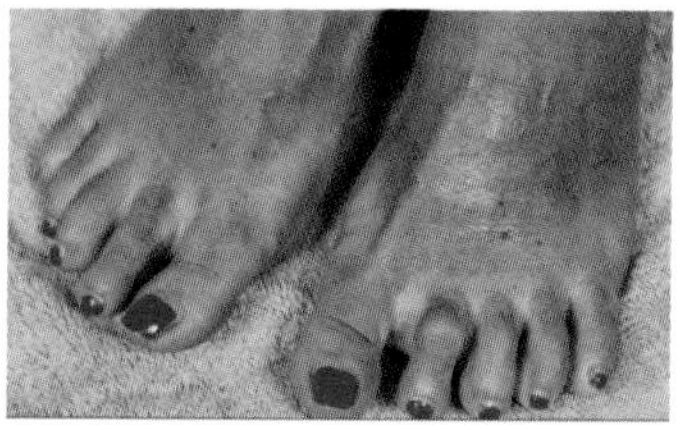 Short toenails 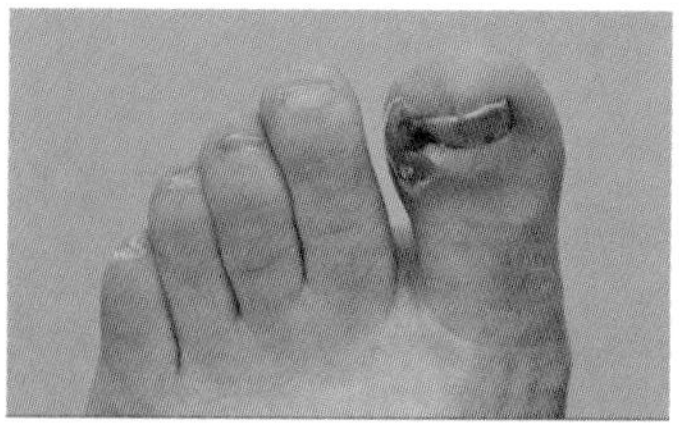 An ingrowing toenail	Hands: some clients will want a short length; others will prefer a longer length. Feet: most clients will want their toenails short, so that they do not rub on their shoes. Ideally, toenails should be filed straight across.	Ask the client what length they would like their nails to be. You will then know how short to file them. Toenails are cut straight across to stop them from growing into the skin at the sides of the nail. This is called an **ingrowing toenail**. Some clients may want the corners just slightly curved or the nails left slightly longer in the summer when sandals are worn.

Factor	Description	How may it affect the treatment?
Skin condition 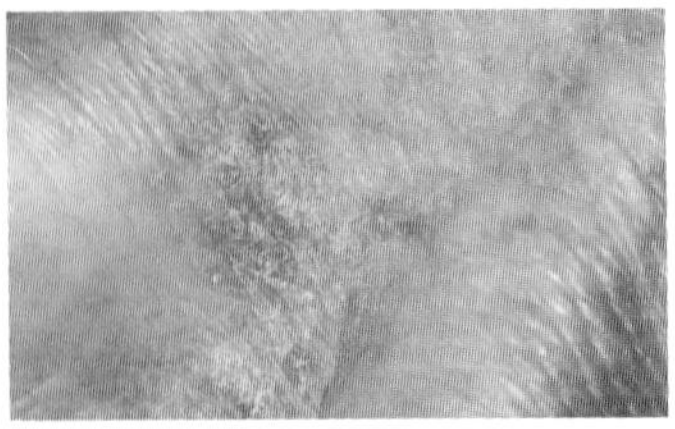 Dry skin on a thumb 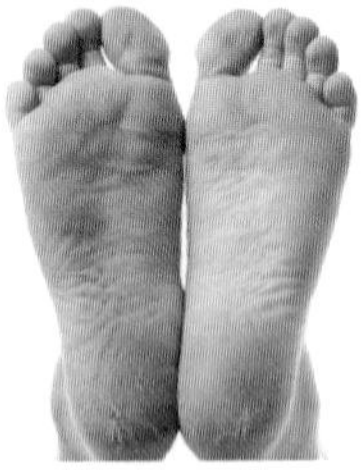 Well moisturised feet	The client's hands or feet may be dry. The manicure/pedicure will help to make the hands/feet feel soft and moisturised.	The client's skin condition will affect which products you choose. If the skin is dry, then more hand and arm or foot and leg lotion may be needed. You can also spend a little bit longer on this part of the treatment if the skin is dry.
Nail condition 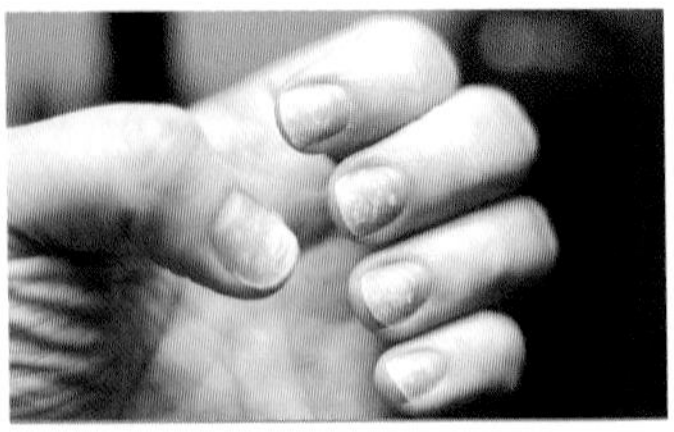 Broken fingernails 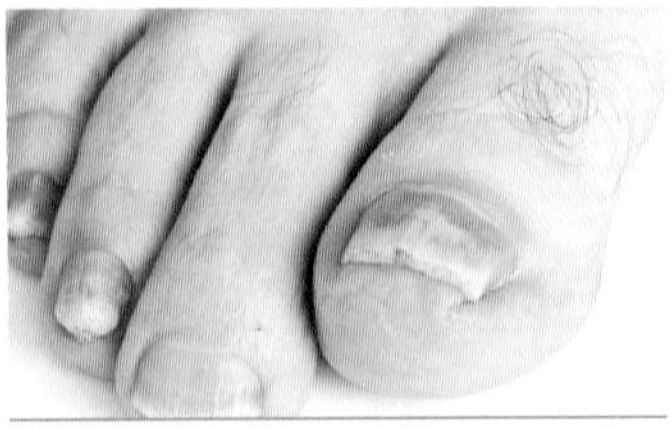 Broken toenails 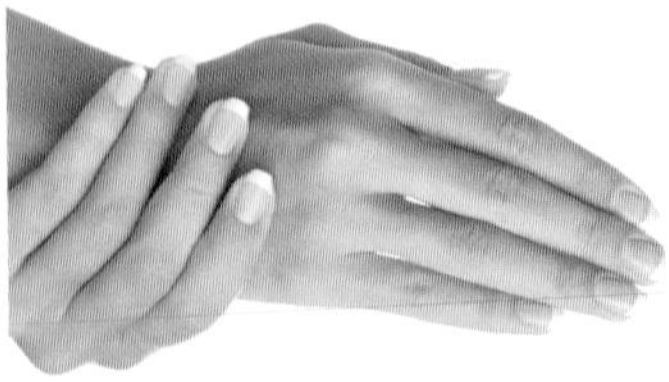 Fingernails in good condition	Nails that are in poor condition may feel rough and break easily. Nails that are in good condition will feel smooth and will not break easily.	If the client's nails are in poor condition, you may have to spend more time on helping to improve it. This may mean filing rough, broken nails or massaging cream into the skin around the nails.

Ingrowing toenail
Where the nail grows into the skin at the side of the toenail

Skin condition
How the skin looks and feels

Nail condition
How the nails look and feel

Factor	Description	How may it affect the treatment?
Surrounding cuts and abrasions 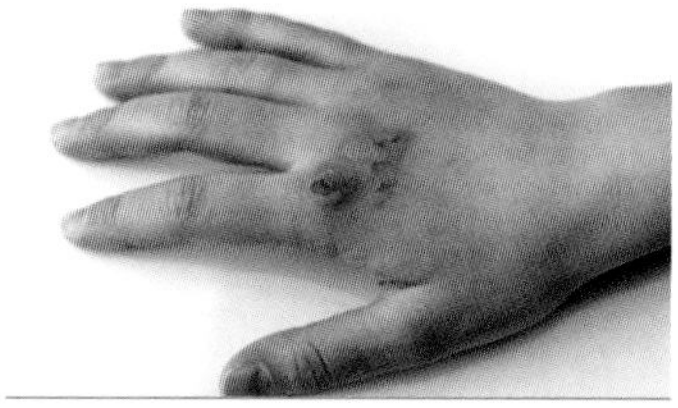 Abrasion on a hand 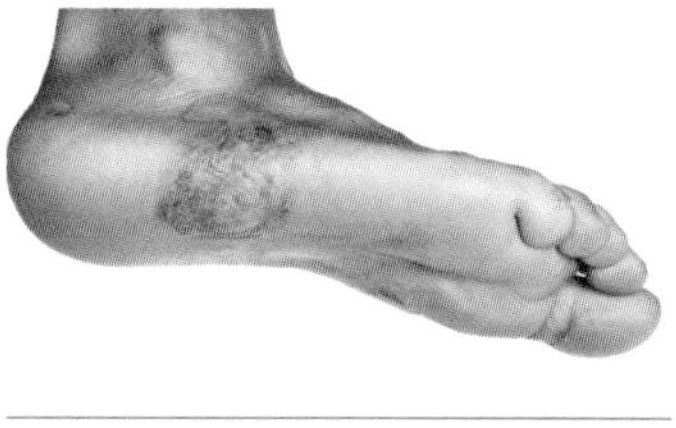 Abrasion on a foot	Cuts or scratches on the skin or around the nail area on the hands or feet.	If the client has these around the nail or on their skin, you will need to avoid the area. This is because it may be sensitive and could make the condition worse.
Bruising and swelling 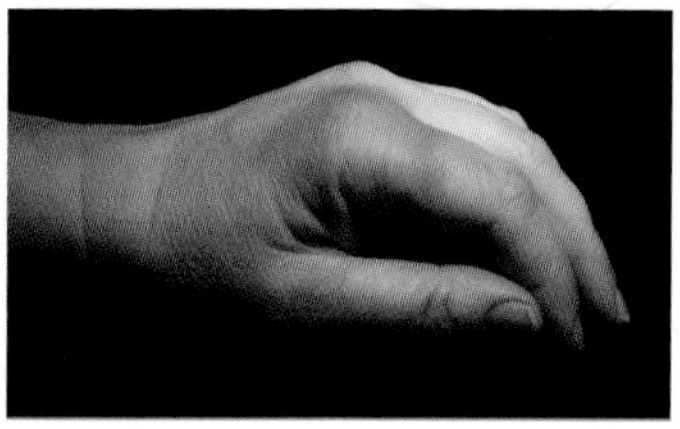 Bruising on a hand 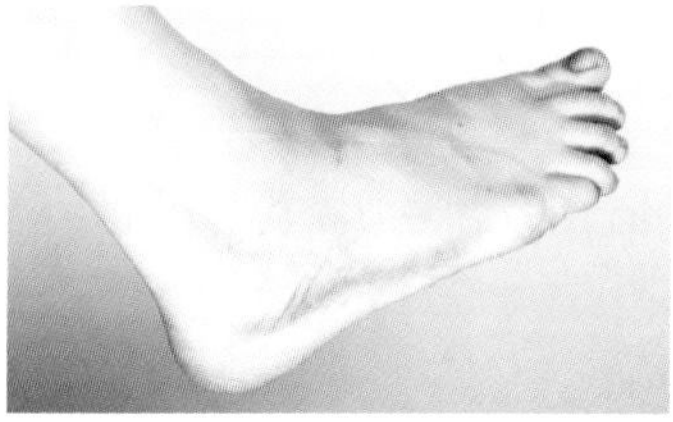 Bruising on a foot	Bruises are caused through injury to the skin (such as bumping into a table). They can appear blue, purple and sometimes yellow in colour. They can be sensitive and painful to touch.	If the client has these on their hand, fingers or around the nails, you will need to avoid the area. This is because it may be sensitive and could make the condition worse.
Severe nail damage 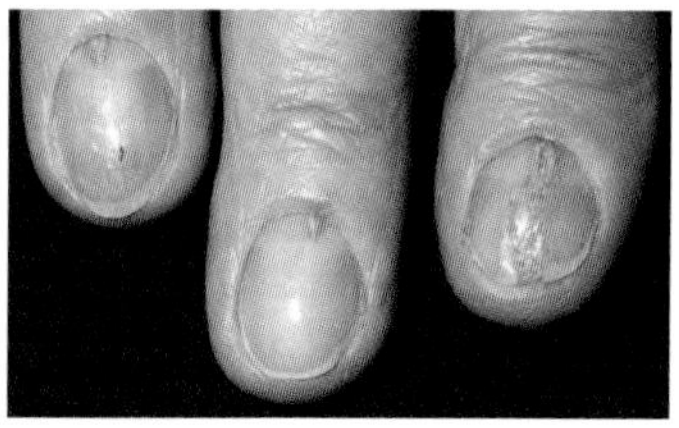 Fingernails with severe damage	When the nail has been damaged through some sort of injury. The nail and skin may be bruised or the nail have scratches around it.	If the client has **severe** nail damage you will not be able to work on this area. This is because it may be sensitive and could make the condition worse.

Severe
Very serious

SmartScreen 007 handout 5

HANDY HINTS

Your client may come to you with short nails but would like to grow them. You can offer advice on how they can look after their nails to help them grow. This will include regular application of hand cream and filing off any rough nail edges.

HANDY HINTS

Any cuts in the area will need to be covered with a waterproof plaster to prevent cross-infection.

HANDY HINTS

Ask your tutor to help you with giving the client advice.

ACTIVITY

Work in pairs. Draw around your partner's hands on a piece of paper. Take a look at their hands and mark on the hand drawing if they have any of the above conditions.

When you have finished, compare your findings with others in your group.

LOOK AT THE HANDS AND NAILS

You will need to assess the client's hand and nail condition before you start the manicure or pedicure treatment. You will then be able to work out which products to choose for your client. Things that you are looking for include:

- nail condition
- cuticle condition
- condition of skin on the hands/feet and around the nails
- nail shape.

ACTIVITY

Research on the internet the different types of base coat and top coat that are available with different product companies. Print off your findings and discuss them in small groups.

- How many different base and top coat products have you found?
- What are they used for?

Nail condition	Description	Advice
Ridged nails 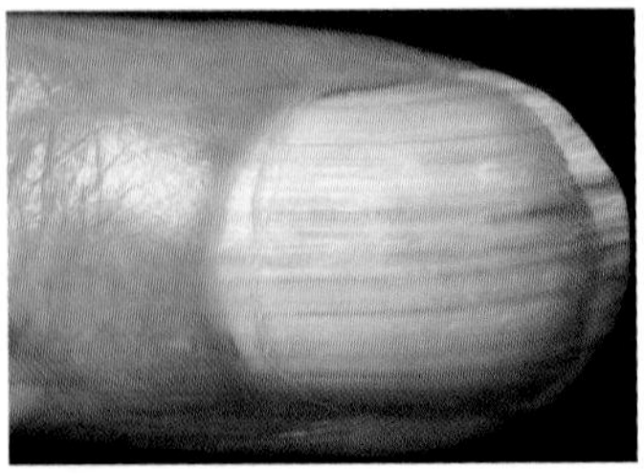	Lines on the nail plate.	Recommend a good base coat. This will help to make the nail plate feel smooth.
Brittle nails 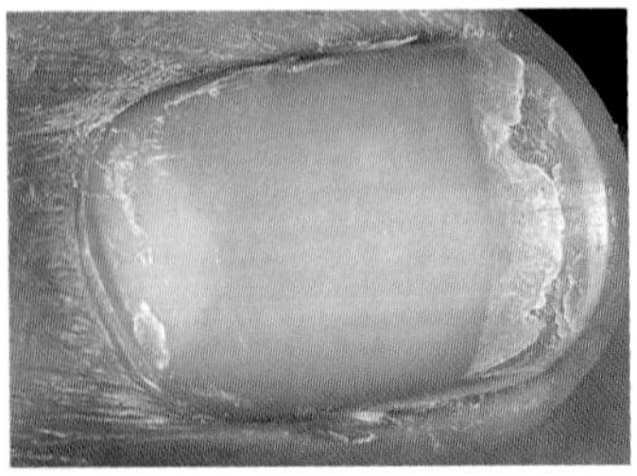	Nails that peel off and break easily.	Moisturise the nail and massage the cuticle area using cuticle cream.

Ridged
Having lines that run down the nail

Brittle
Breaks easily

Nail condition	Description	Advice
Weak nails 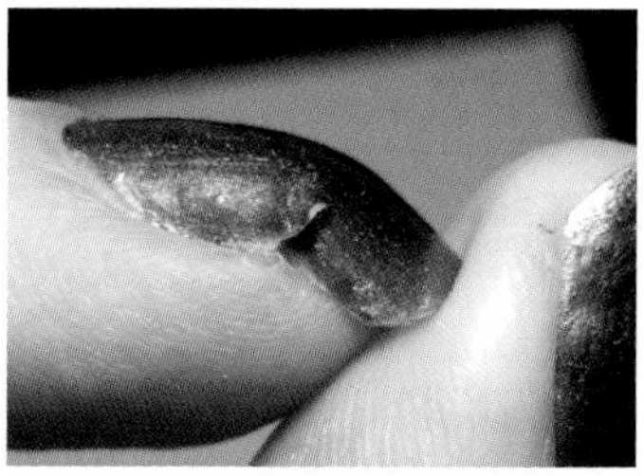	These nails break and split easily.	Keep nails short. Moisturise the nail and massage the cuticle area.
Slight nail **separation** 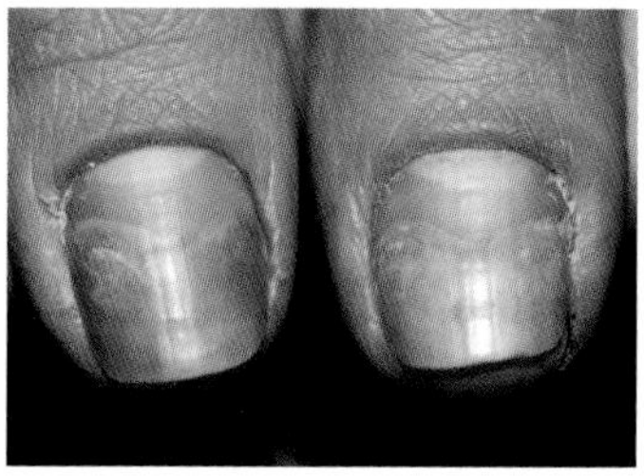	The nail lifts up from the nail bed. It may be caused by injury to the nail, such as trapping it in a door.	This may be sensitive so do not treat this nail.

Separation
Coming apart

Cuticle condition	Description	Advice
Healthy 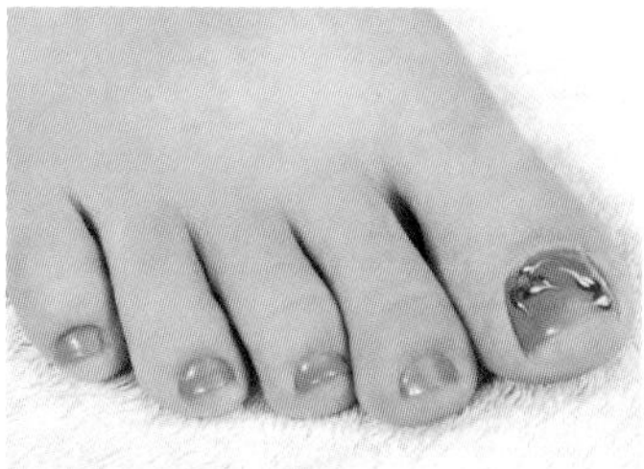	The cuticles are in good condition. They are soft and not too thick.	Maintain the cuticle area by moisturising regularly with cuticle cream.
Splitting 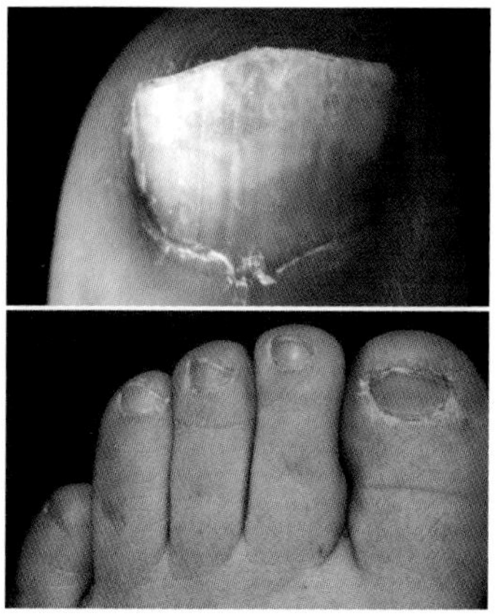	When the cuticles become dry they can split and become rough.	Massage in cuticle cream every night. Use hand cream after washing to help keep the cuticles moisturised.
Overgrown 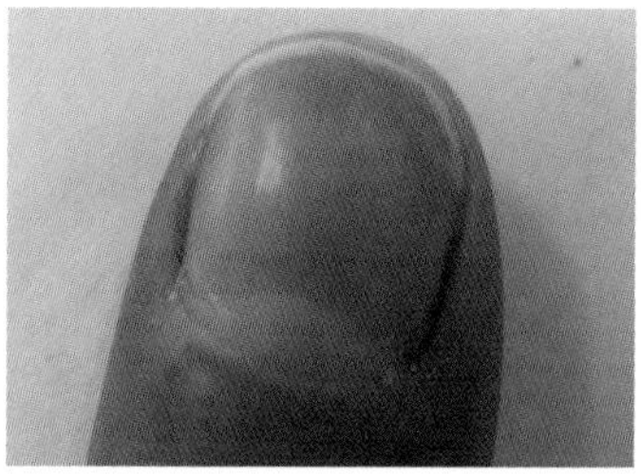	If the cuticles are not kept soft and looked after they can become thick and stick to the nail plate.	Have regular manicures to gently push back the overgrown cuticle. Massage in cuticle cream every night to keep the cuticle moisturised.

Cuticle condition	Description	Advice
Dry 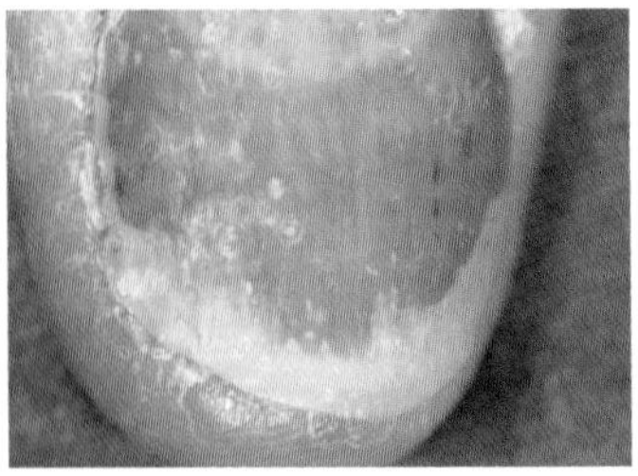	If the cuticles are not regularly moisturised they will become dry and may feel rough.	Massage in cuticle cream every night. Use hand cream after washing.

Skin on the hands and around the nails	Description	Advice
Smooth and soft 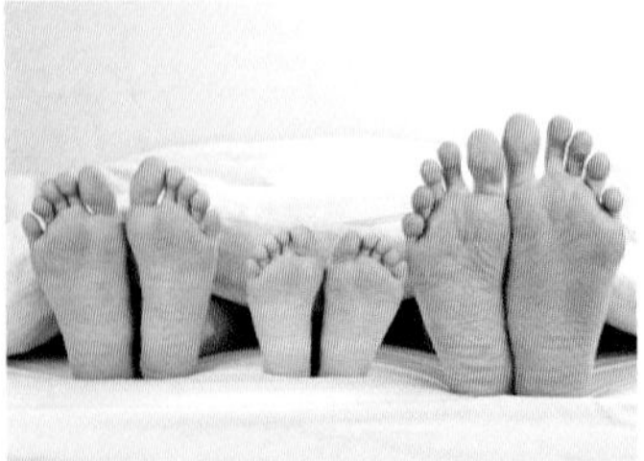	If the skin is well moisturised it will feel soft and smooth to the touch.	Maintain the skin condition by moisturising regularly.
Dry and rough 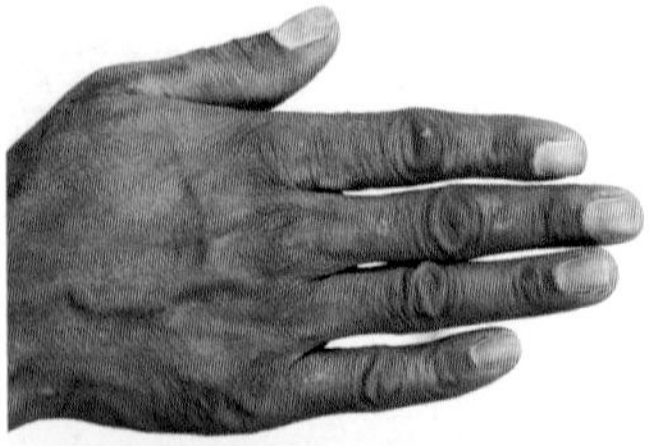 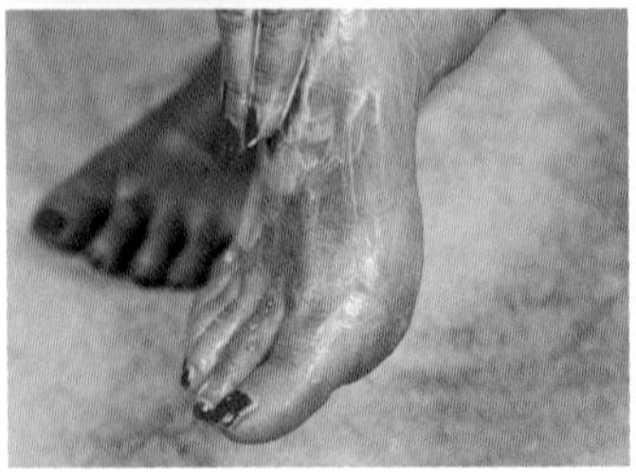	If the skin is dry it will look and feel rough.	Have regular manicures and pedicures. Massage in hand/foot cream every night. Use hand cream after washing.
Warm 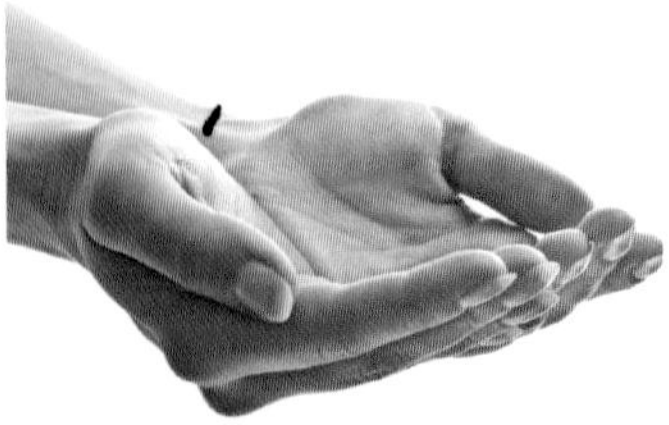 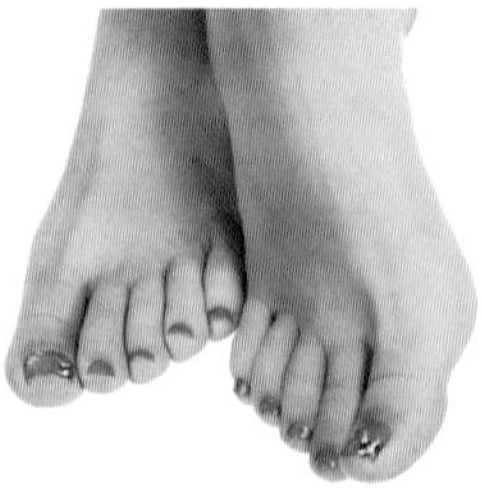	If the feet and hands are warm, this means that the blood supply to the area is good. This will help to keep the skin, cuticles and nails in good condition. They should look pink; not too red or pale.	Maintain the skin condition by moisturising regularly.

Skin on the hands and around the nails	Description	Advice
Cold 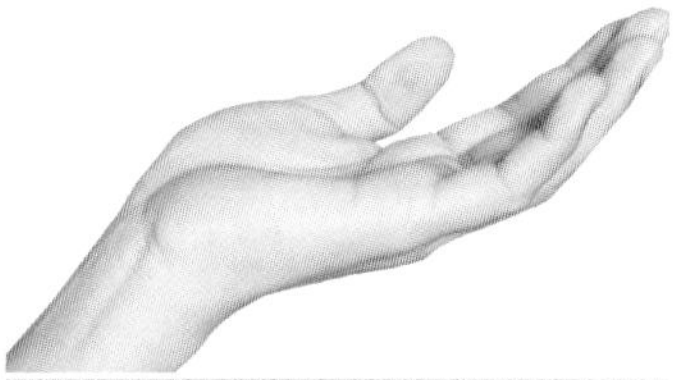 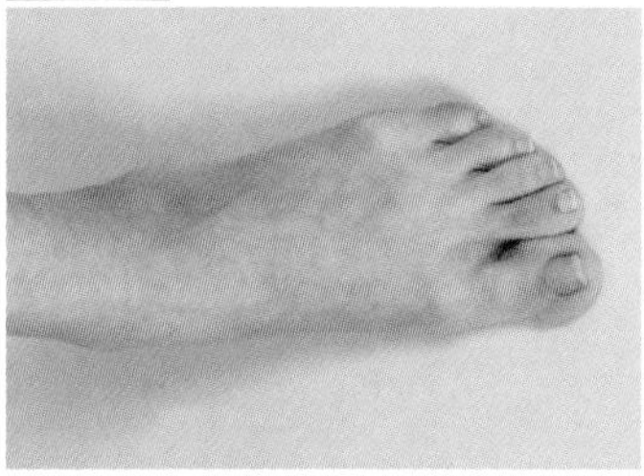	If the feet and hands are cold, this means that the blood supply to the area is poor. The skin will look pale in colour and feels cold to the touch. Massage will help to improve the **blood circulation**.	Massage in hand/foot cream every night to increase the circulation and warm the hands/feet up.

ACTIVITY

Have a look at your own hands and feet. When was the last time you did the following?

- filed your nails
- massaged cream into your hands or feet
- applied nail varnish.

Do you care for your hands and feet?

Blood circulation
The movement of blood to all parts of the body

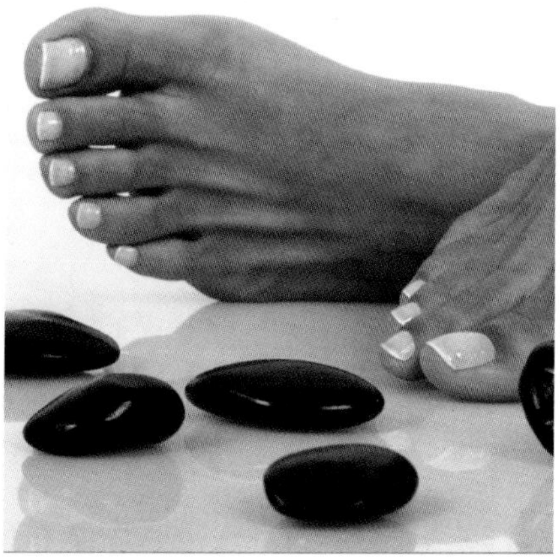
Healthy-looking feet and toenails

NAIL SHAPES

During the consultation, discuss with the client what nail shape they would like. It is important to do this at the start of the treatment and before you start to file the nails. This will make sure that the client will be pleased with the final shape. The toenails are usually filed straight across (or slightly curved at the edges).

ACTIVITY

Working in pairs, with one of you being the therapist and the other the client, take it in turns to pretend that the client has one of the conditions mentioned above. Practise what advice you would give to a client with this condition.

Unlike toenails, there are many possible fingernail shapes, as shown in the following table:

Nail shape	Description
Oval 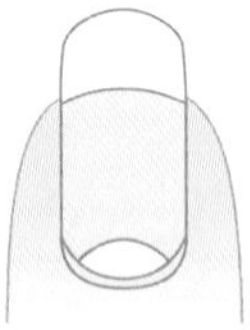	Can make the fingers look longer. It is therefore good for short fingers.
Rounded 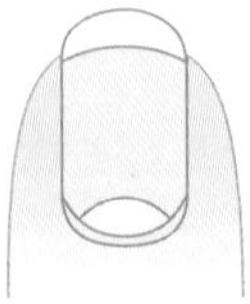	**Popular** for shorter nails. The free edge is shaped following the curve of the end of the finger.
Square 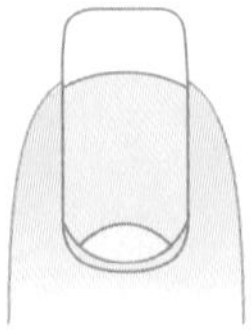	A popular shape for longer nails. The free edge is shaped straight across. This shape looks really nice on someone who has long fingers.
Squoval 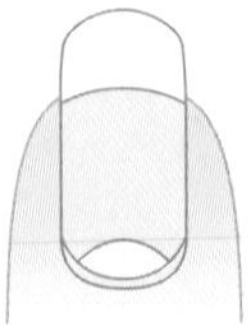	A combination of square and oval nail shapes. The nail is filed to a square finish and then gently rounded at the edges. This shape is ideal for longer nails.
Pointed 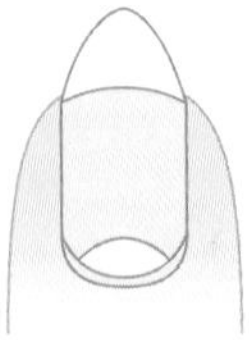	A very sharp nail shape. It is not often recommended as a nail shape because it can make the nail very weak at the sides. The nail can break easily if knocked and often splits at the sides of the nail.

SmartScreen 007 handout 13

Popular
Liked by a lot of people.

HANDY HINTS

It is important to confirm with the client what nail shape they would like. Discuss this during the consultation part of the treatment. You don't want the client to leave unhappy because you filed all of their long nails too short!

HANDY HINTS

At the start of the treatment allow time for the client to choose the colour of nail enamel that they would like.

ACTIVITY

Why not paint some artificial nails with the different coloured nail varnishes that you have? You can then make a display of them to show your client. This will help them choose their favourite colour.

CARRY OUT A HAND CARE, BASIC MANICURE OR PEDICURE TREATMENT

You are now ready to carry out the treatment. Before you start, do a final check to make sure your client is comfortable and that you have all your tools and products ready.

HAND CARE AND BASIC MANICURE TREATMENT ROUTINE

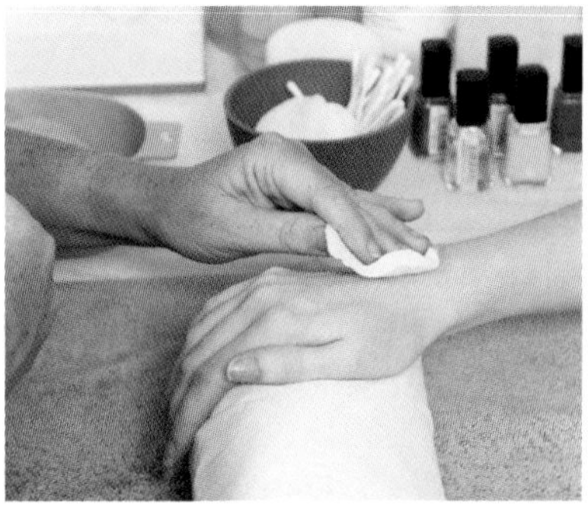

STEP 1 – Start by wiping over the client's arms and hands with disinfecting spray or gel. Use a clean piece of cotton wool for each hand. This will remove germs from the skin.

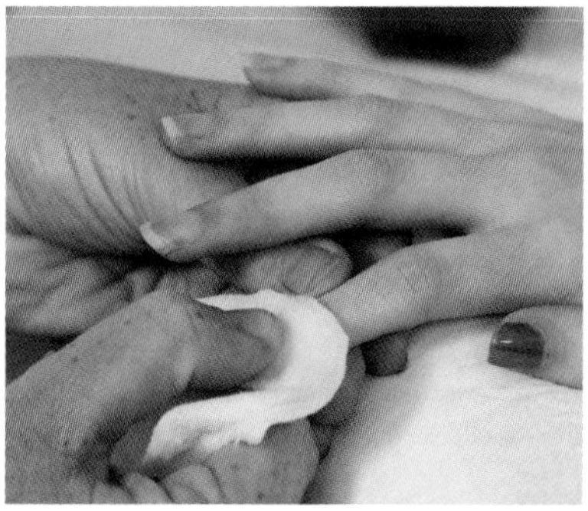

STEP 2 – Remove any nail enamel from the nails using cotton wool pads with nail-enamel remover on them.

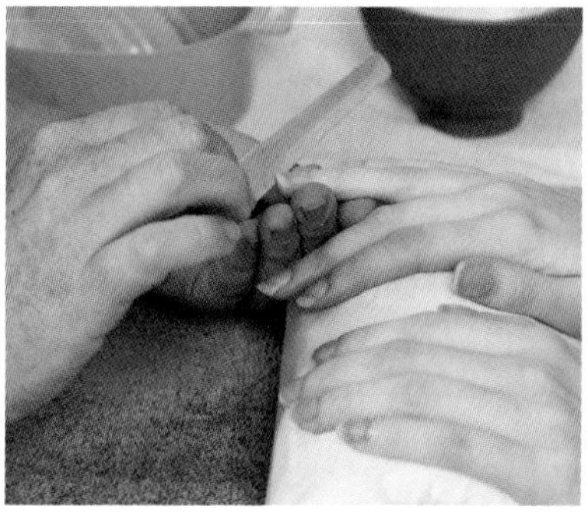

STEP 3 – File the nails. Work from side to centre. Finish with a bevel action (working downwards on the tip of the nail). This will help to stop the nail from splitting.

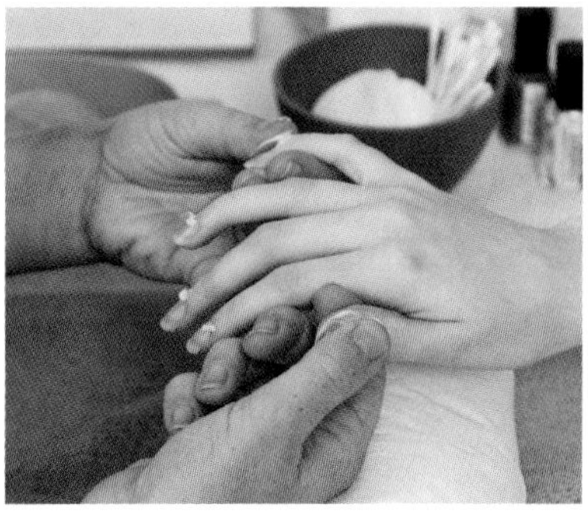

STEP 4 – Apply cuticle cream to the cuticle area. Massage it in to help soften the cuticles.

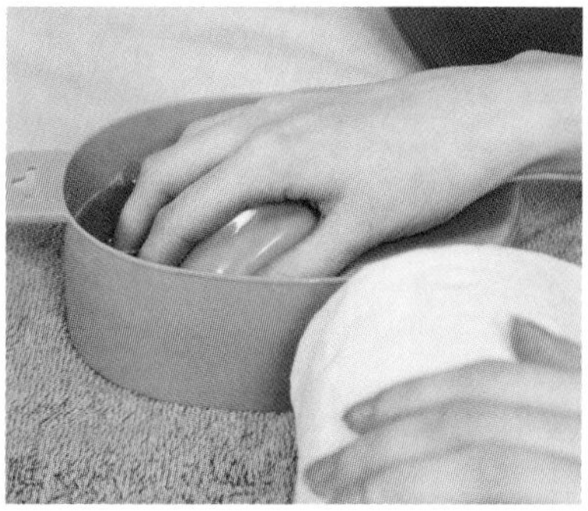

STEP 5 – Place the fingertips in the manicure bowl. This should contain warm, soapy water. Repeat steps **1** to **5** on the other hand.

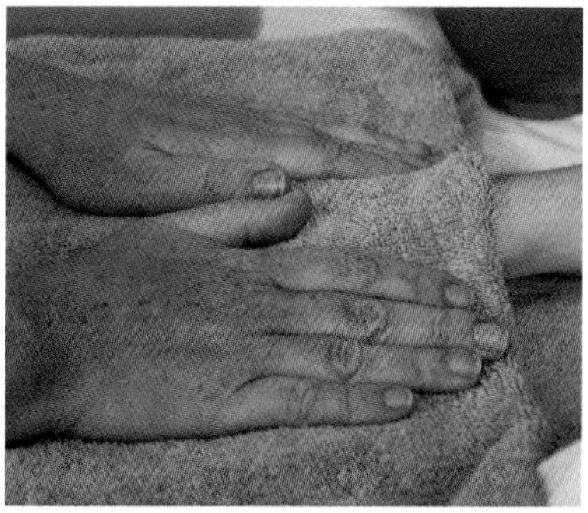

STEP 6 – Remove the first hand from the manicure bowl. Dry it off using a small hand towel.

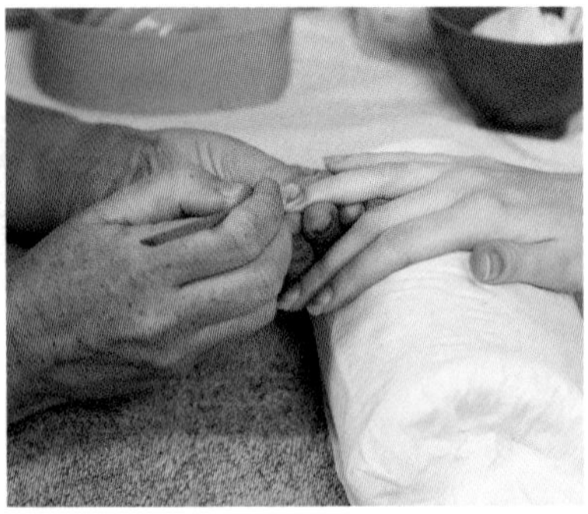

STEP 7 – Gently ease back the cuticles. Use an orange stick tipped with cotton wool. Repeat steps **6** and **7** on the other hand. (**NB**: step **7** should only be carried out for Chapter 109 Manicure)

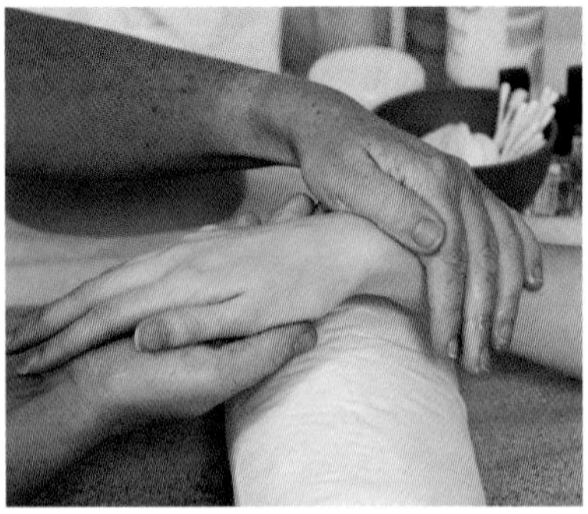

STEP 8 – Taking one hand, apply massage lotion/cream to the arm and hand.

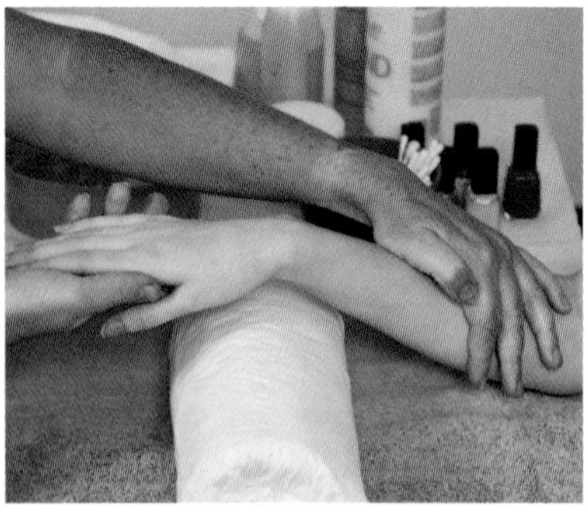

STEP 9 – Massage up the arm using **alternate** sweeping strokes.

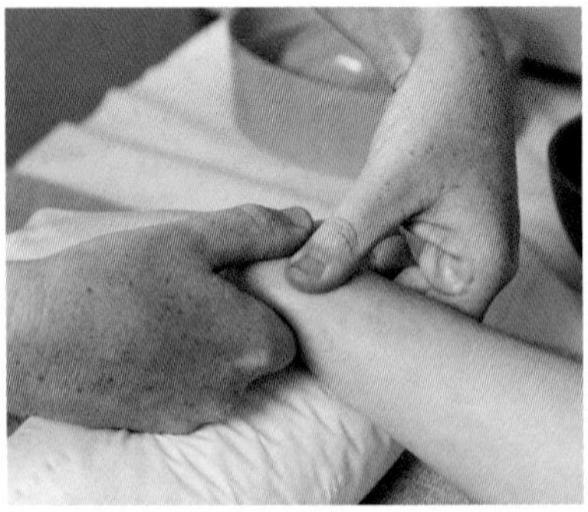

STEP 10 – Massage using thumb circles, working from the wrist to the elbow.

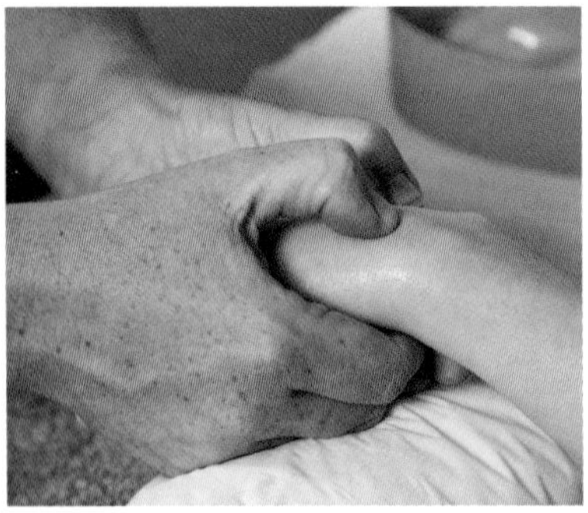

STEP 11 – Massage around the wrist using thumb circles.

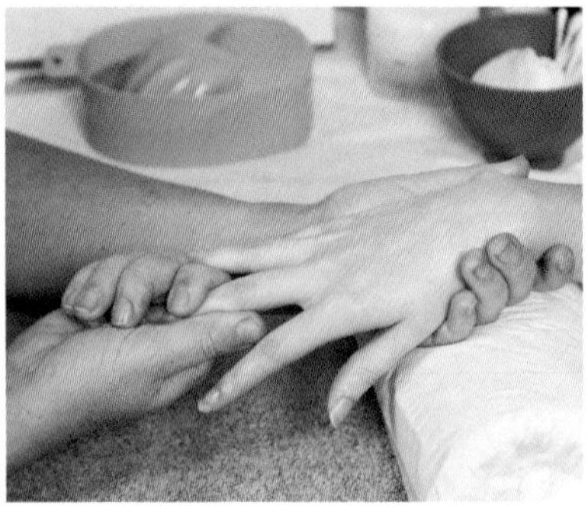

STEP 12 – Massage around and down the fingers.

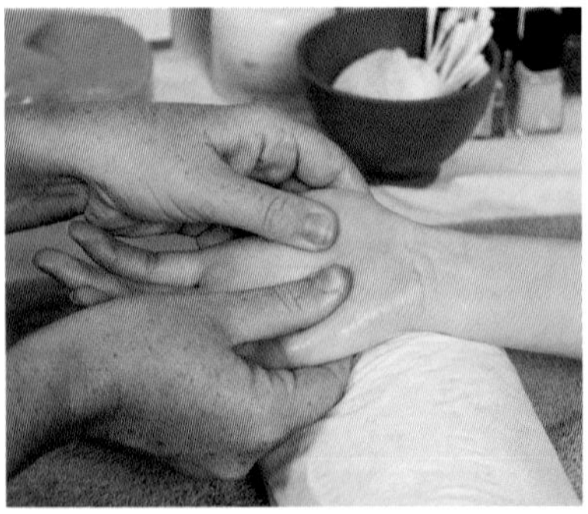

STEP 13 – Massage the palm.

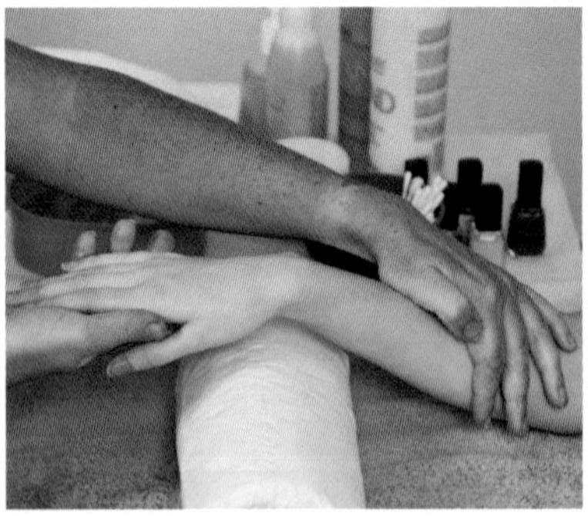

STEP 14 – Massage up the arm using alternate sweeping strokes. Repeat steps **8** to **14** on the other arm and hand.

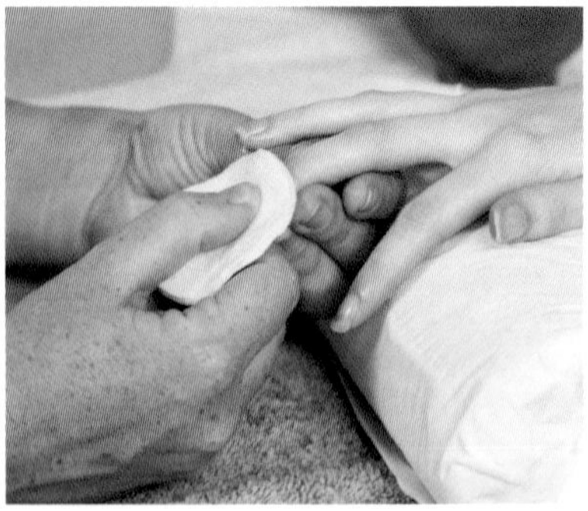

STEP 15 – Remove cream from the nails using nail-varnish remover.

Alternate
One after the other

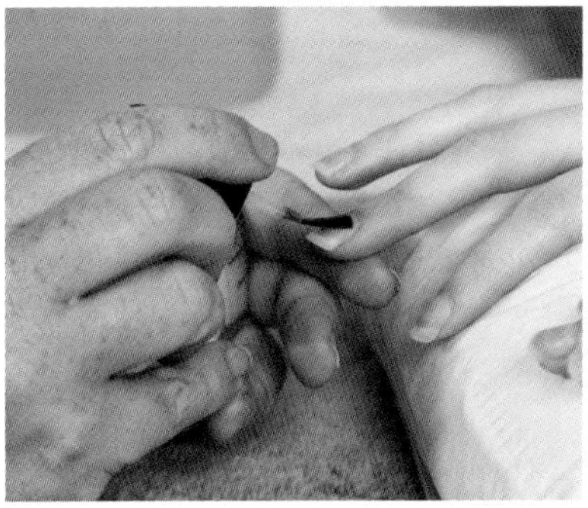

STEP 16 – Apply the base coat.

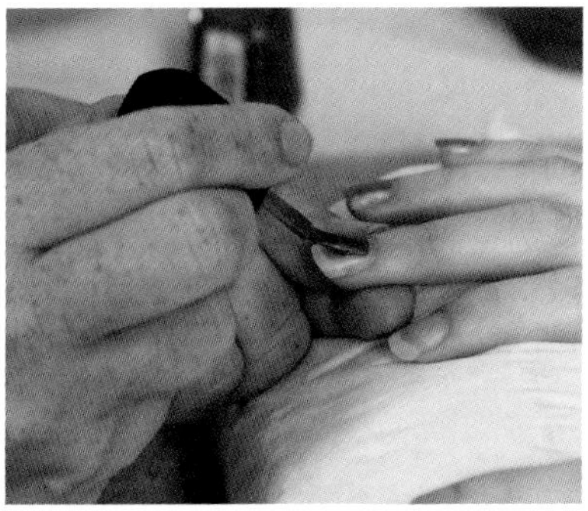

STEP 17 – Apply the coloured nail varnish.

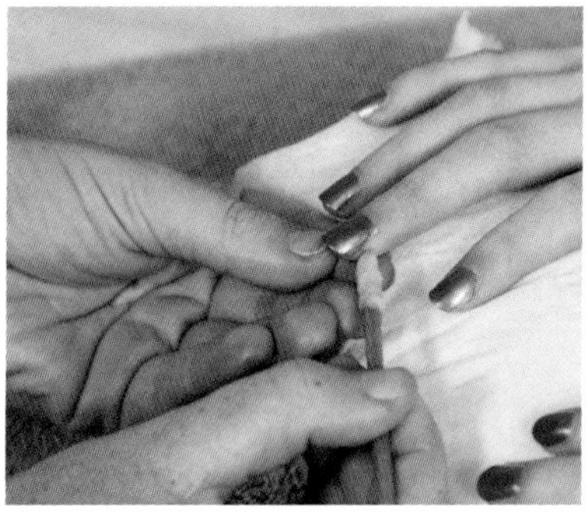

STEP 18 – Remove any smudged varnish with an orange stick tipped with cotton wool that has been dipped into nail-varnish remover.

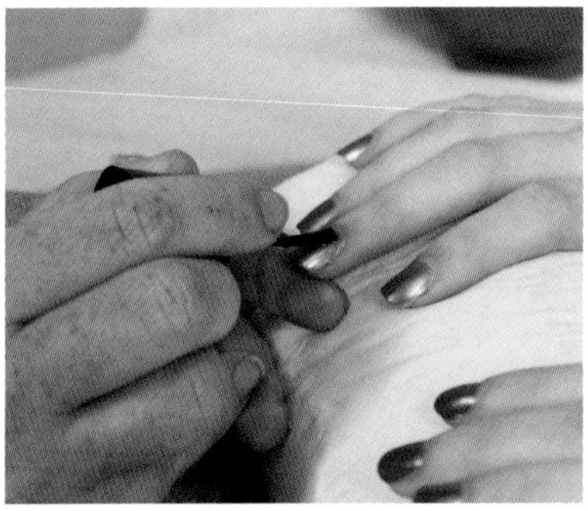

STEP 19 – Apply the top coat.

HANDY HINTS

Make sure that the water in the manicure bowl is not too hot! Check with your client that the temperature is OK for them.

HANDY HINTS

Suggest to the client that they put on their coat before you apply the base coat and enamel. This will help to stop them smudging their nails afterwards.

HANDY HINTS

Keep your own nails short. You don't want to scratch the client!

SmartScreen 007 handouts 3 and 10

BASIC PEDICURE TREATMENT ROUTINE

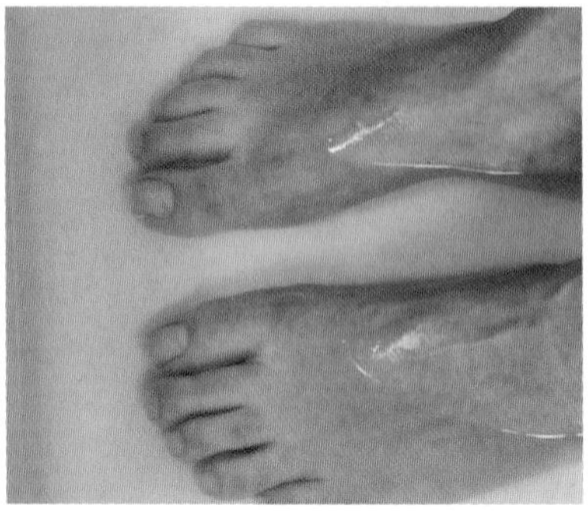

STEP 1 – Start by placing the client's feet into the pedicure bowl. This should be filled with warm, soapy water.

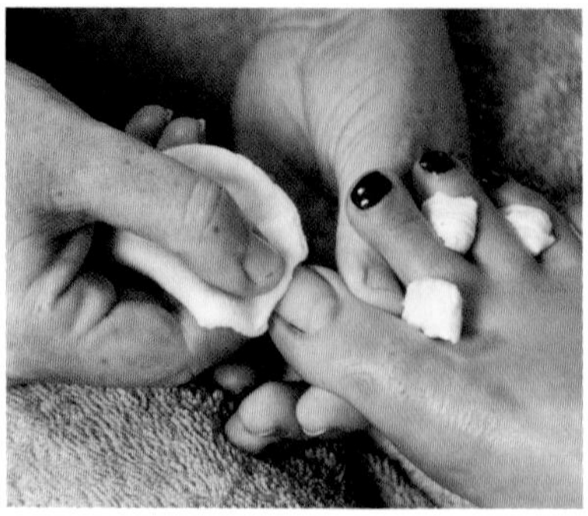

STEP 2 – Remove one foot and dry on a towel. Remove any nail enamel from the nails using cotton wool pads with nail-enamel remover on them.

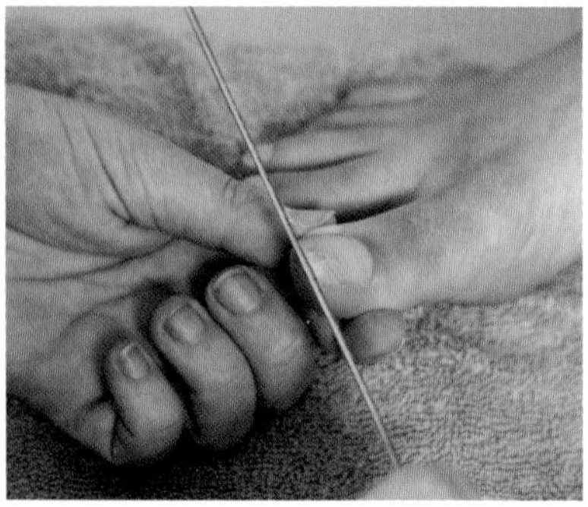

STEP 3 – File the nails straight across. Work from side to centre. Finish with a bevel action (working downwards on the tip of the nail). This will help to stop the nail from splitting.

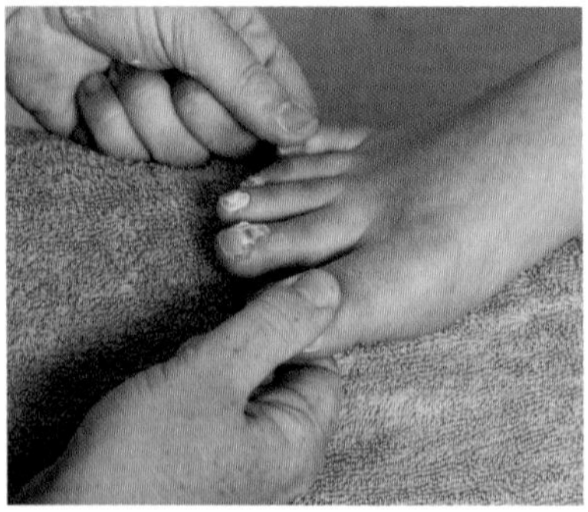

STEP 4 – Apply cuticle cream to the cuticle area. Massage it in to help soften the cuticles. Place the foot back into the pedicure bowl. Repeat steps **1** to **4** on the other foot.

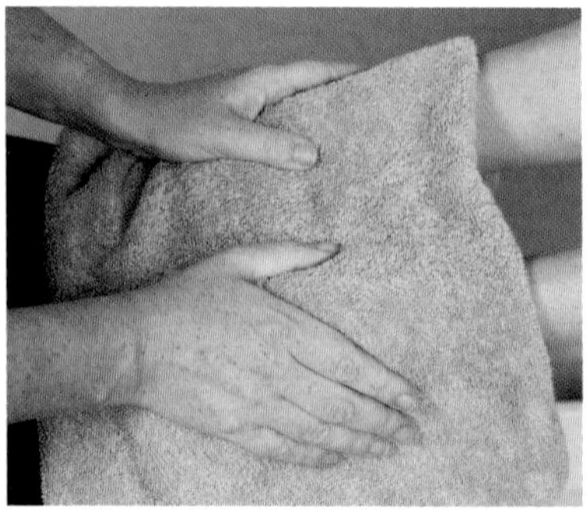

STEP 5 – Remove the first foot you worked on from the pedicure bowl. Dry it off using a towel.

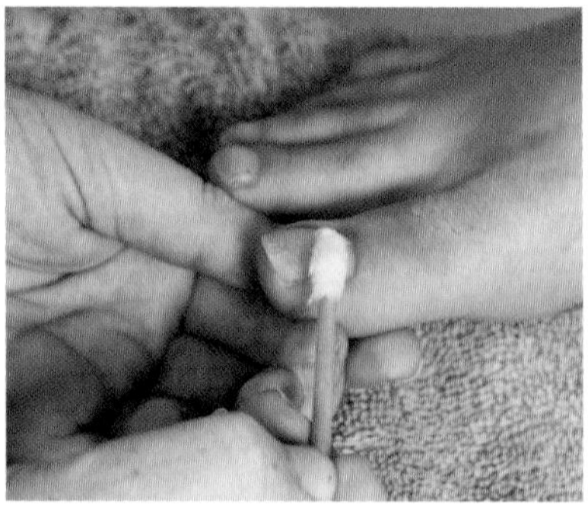

STEP 6 – Gently ease back the cuticles. Use an orange stick tipped with cotton wool. Wrap the foot in a towel. Place by the side of the pedicure bowl.

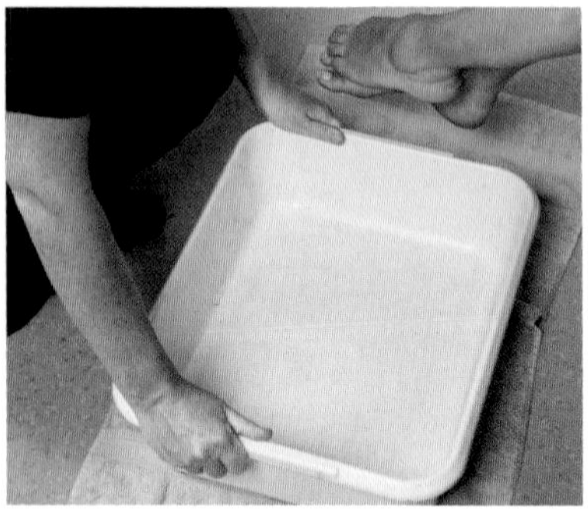

STEP 7 – Repeat steps **5** to **6** on the other foot. Then move the pedicure bowl safely out of the way.

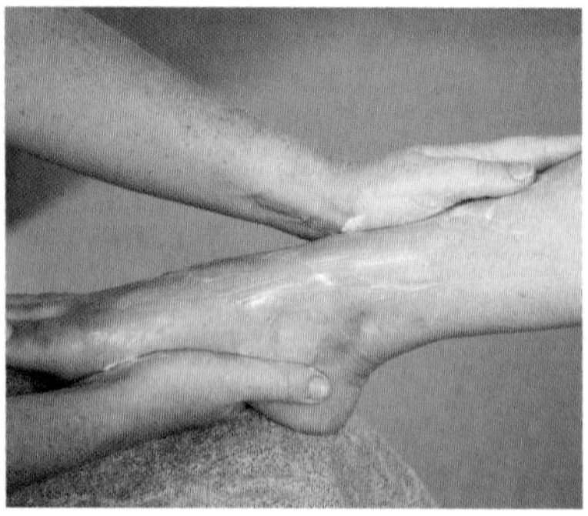

STEP 8 – Taking one foot, apply massage lotion to the lower leg and foot.

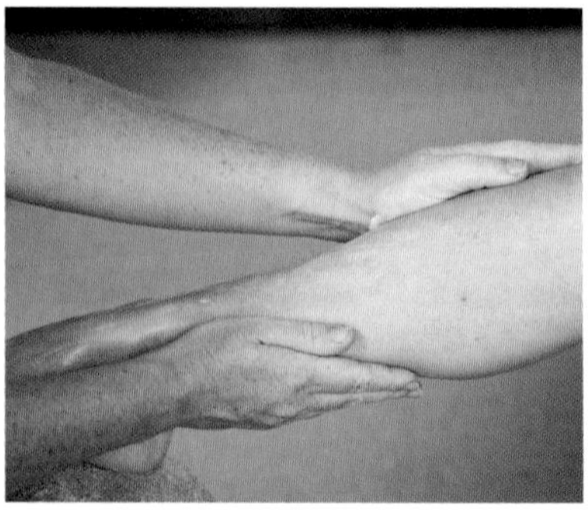

STEP 9 – Massage up the lower leg using alternate sweeping strokes.

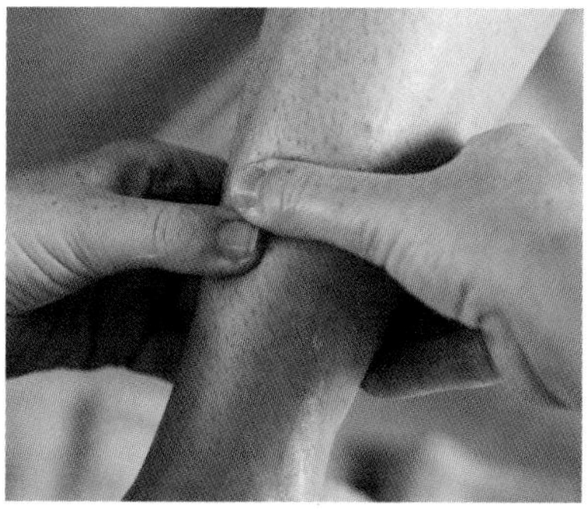

STEP 10 – Massage using thumb circles, working from the ankle to the knee.

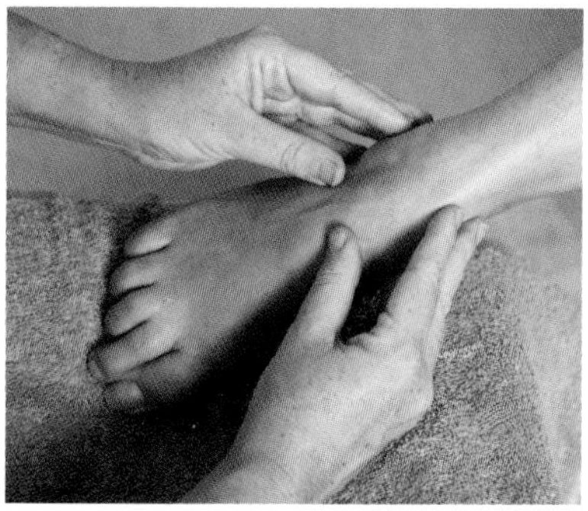

STEP 11 – Massage around the ankle using circular movements of the fingertips.

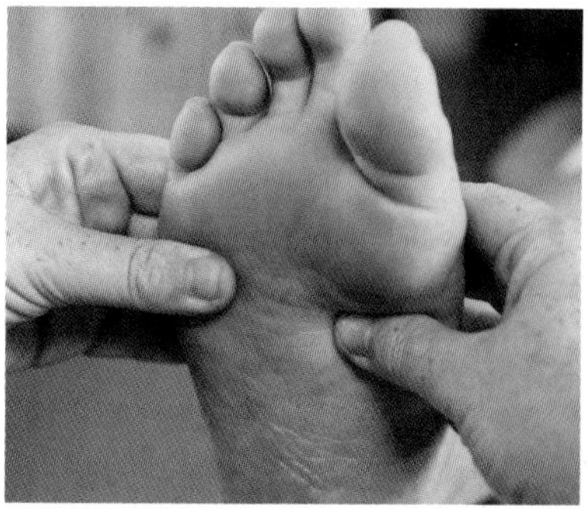

STEP 12 – Make 'scissor' movements using the thumbs up and down the sole of the foot.

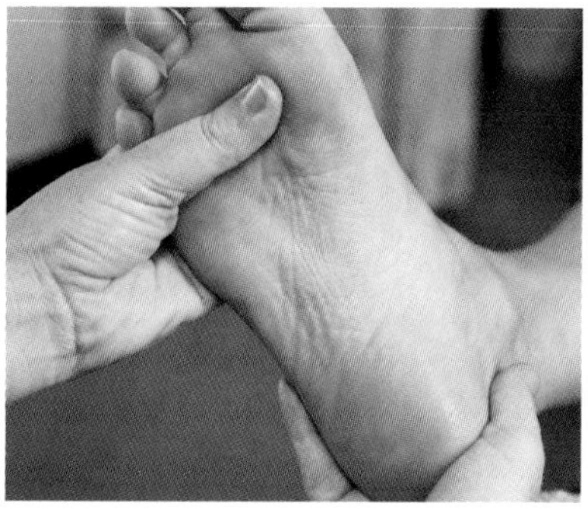

STEP 13 – Circle and rotate the toes.

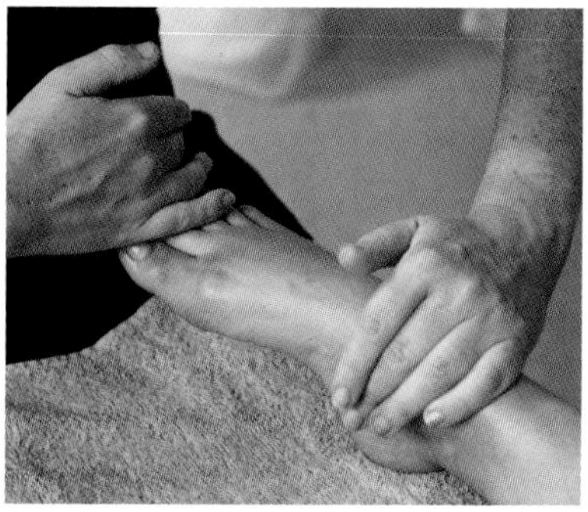

STEP 14 – Make alternate finger strokes on the top of the foot.

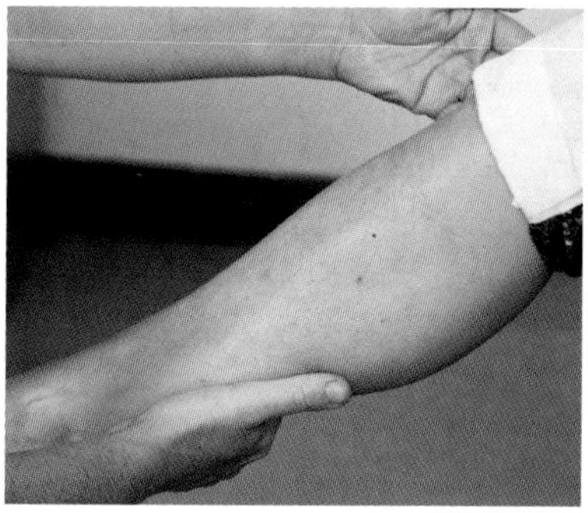

STEP 15 – Massage up the back of the lower leg using alternate sweeping strokes.

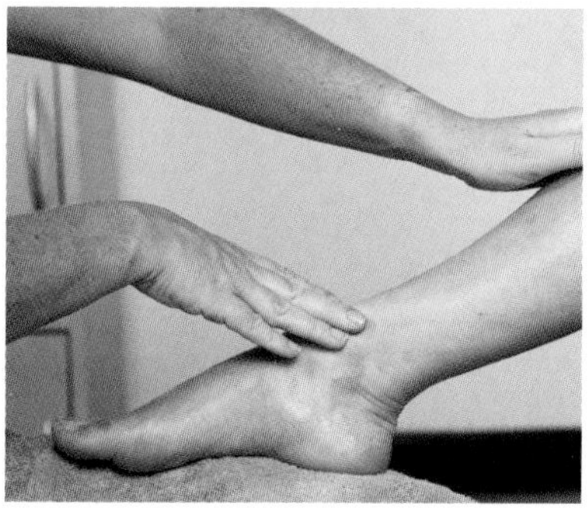

STEP 16 – Finish with alternate strokes down the lower leg. Repeat steps **8** to **16** on the other leg and foot.

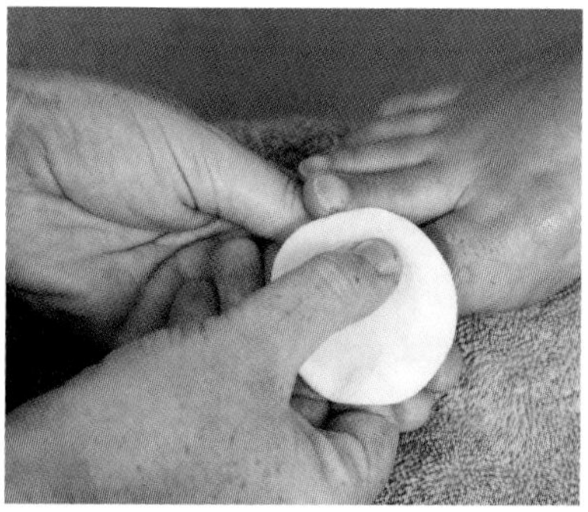

STEP 17 – Apply nail-varnish remover to cotton wool. Wipe over each nail on both feet to remove any massage lotion.

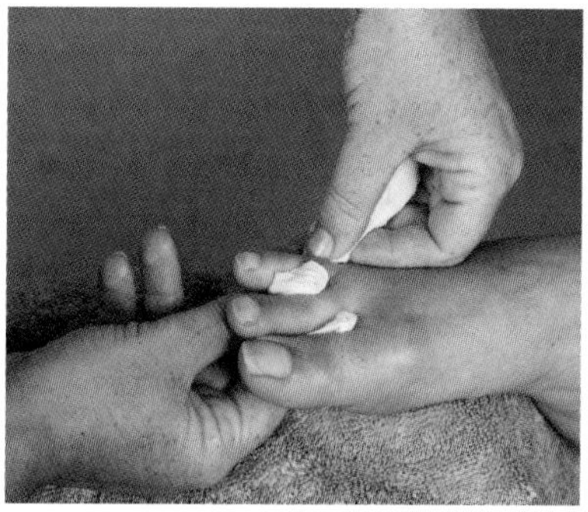

STEP 18 – Place tissue between the toes on both feet. This will help to separate the toes and stop the nail enamel from getting smudged.

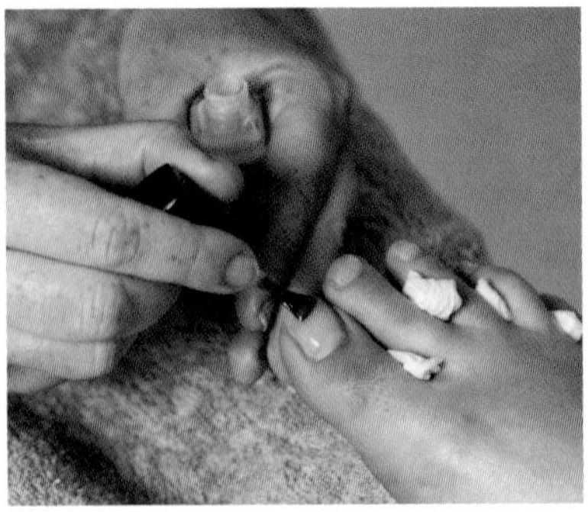

STEP 19 – Apply the base coat to each nail.

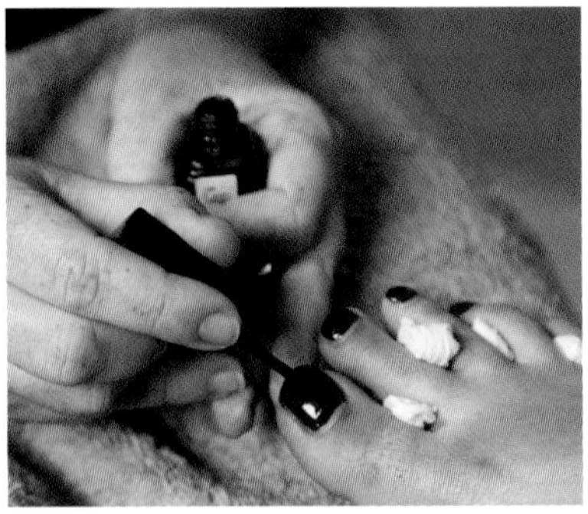

STEP 20 – Apply the coloured nail enamel to each nail.

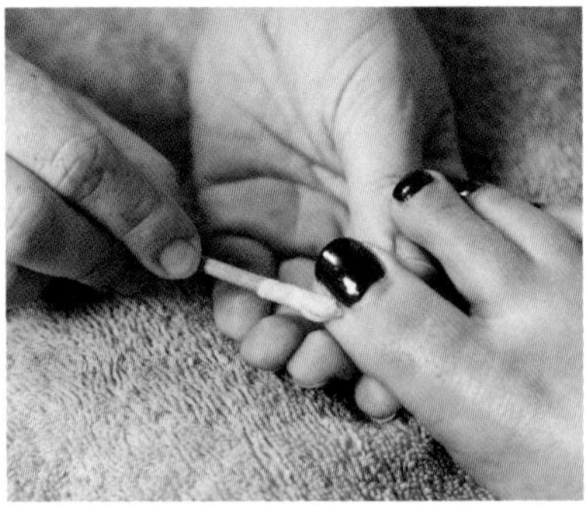

STEP 21 – Remove any smudged varnish from around the sides of the nail. Use an orange stick tipped with cotton wool that has been dipped into nail-varnish remover.

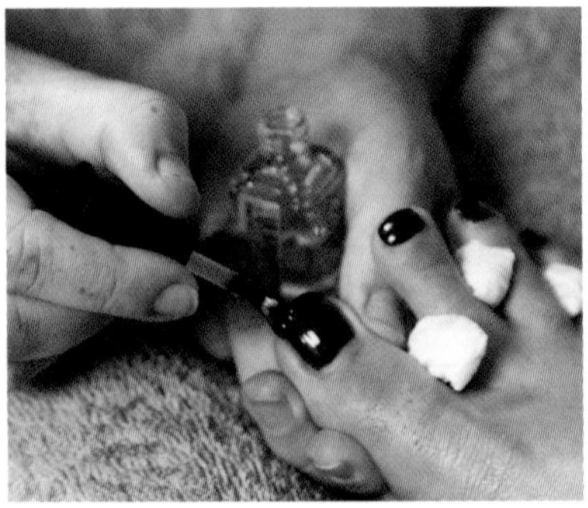

STEP 22 – Apply the top coat.

HANDY HINTS

Make sure that the water in the foot bowl is not too hot!

HANDY HINTS

Remember to cut the toenails straight across and not to shape them at the sides. This will help to stop ingrowing toenails.

CONTRA-ACTIONS

This is something that may happen during or after the treatment.

Possible contra-action	Description
Erythema 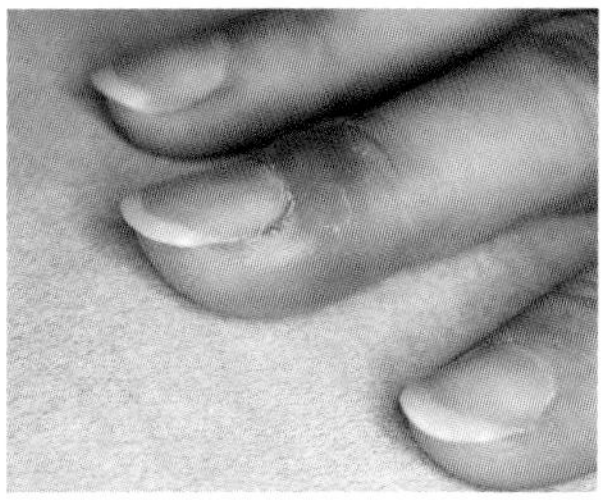	Skin may become red and feel hot.
Irritation 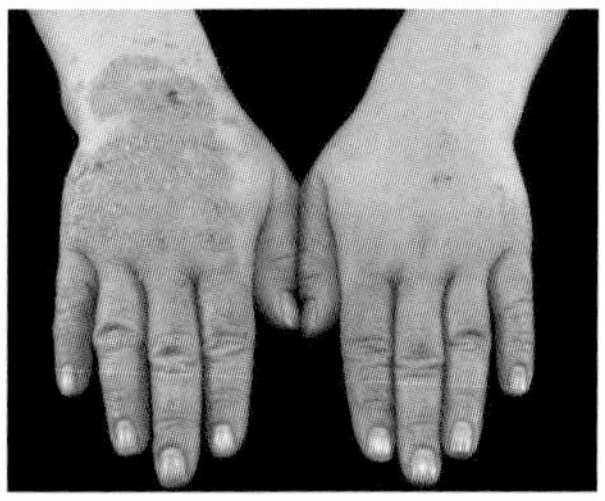	This may occur as a rash and may be itchy.
Swelling 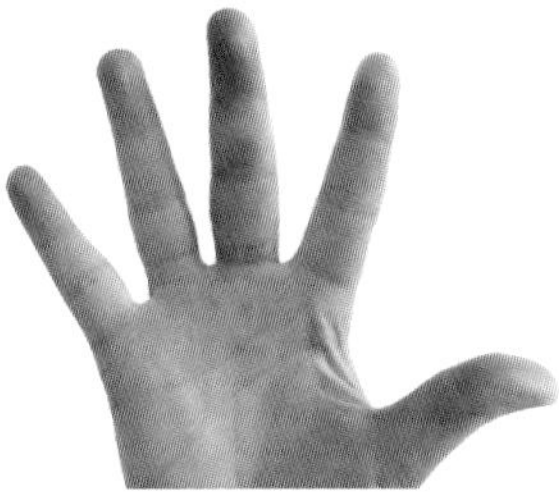 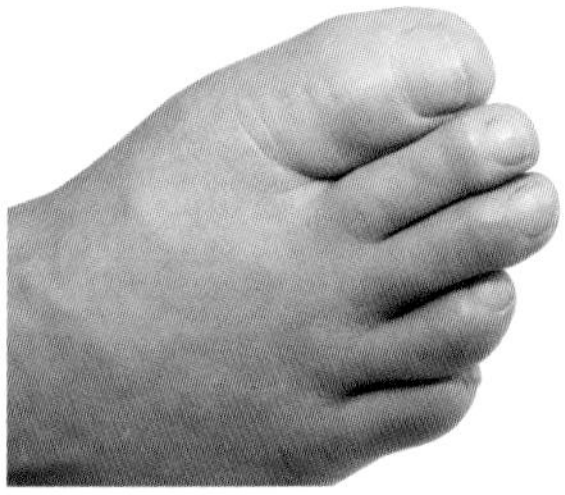	The fingers or toes may become enlarged, and look and feel puffy.

If the client has any of the above reactions either during the treatment or afterwards:

- stop the treatment straight away
- report this to your tutor or supervisor
- remove the product with cool water and apply soothing lotion.

If the condition does not improve, check with your tutor. They may tell the client to see their doctor.

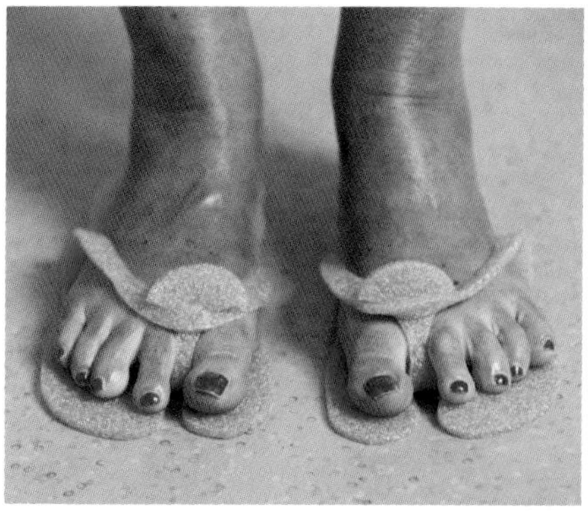

HANDY HINTS

When clients book in for a pedicure treatment, ask them to either wear or bring some open-toed sandals with them. This will help to prevent smudging of their nail enamel. Disposable footwear can also be given to the client to wear after the treatment to help stop smudging.

Erythema
Reddening of the skin

HANDY HINTS

It takes longer for toenails to grow than fingernails. Toenails grow about 0.3–1 mm per week. It can take about eight months for a new toenail to grow back completely.

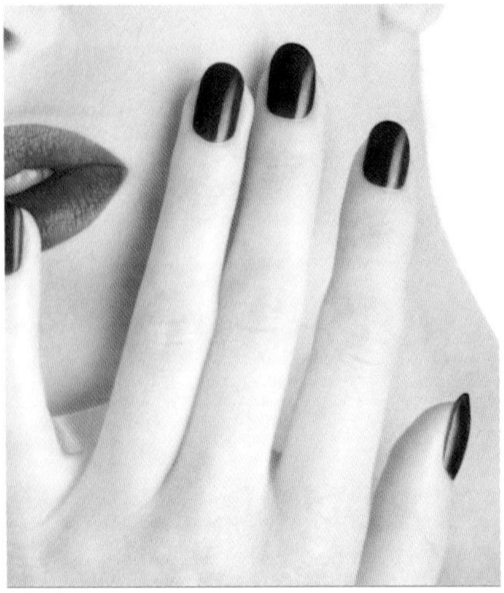

Well manicured hands and nails

AFTER THE TREATMENT

After you have finished the treatment, make sure that you write down everything that you have done on the client's treatment plan. You may also include the following aftercare advice tips for the client:

- Use a hand or foot cream regularly to keep the hands and feet soft and moisturised.
- File the nails regularly to help to stop them from breaking.
- Have regular manicure and pedicure treatments.

You will also need to make sure that your treatment area and equipment are cleaned with disinfectant. Also, all of your products should be put away tidily and in their correct storage place. This will make sure that the treatment area is ready for the next therapist to use.

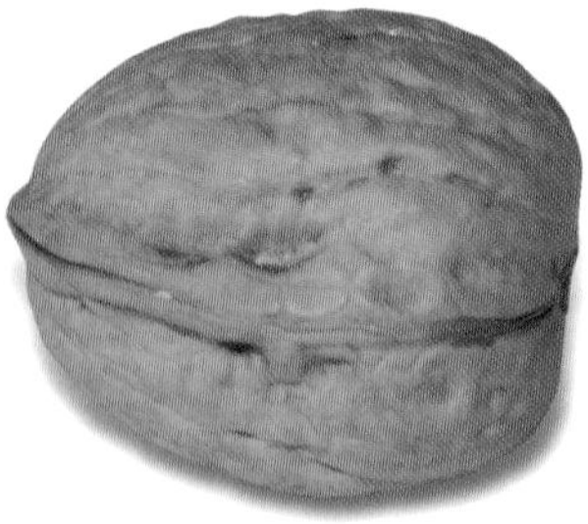

SmartScreen 007 handout 12

HANDY HINTS

Remember, having beautiful hands and feet does not just include the nails. Advise your client to moisturise their hands and feet daily with a good hand or foot cream.

IN A NUTSHELL

You are now at the end of the chapter. Before you test your knowledge with the revision activities, check the following list to see if you feel confident in all the areas covered. If there are still any areas you're unsure of, go back over them in the book and ask your tutor for extra support:

- what preparation is needed for a basic manicure and pedicure treatment
- looking at hands, feet and nails to see what condition they are in
- identifying factors that influence the treatment
- what products, tools and equipment you will need
- how to use the products, tools and equipment safely and hygienically
- how to carry out a hand care, basic manicure and pedicure treatment
- how to communicate and behave in a professional manner
- the main nail shapes
- how to identify the basic structure of the nail
- state possible contra-actions and how to respond to them.

REVISION ACTIVITIES

Use the questions below to test your knowledge of Chapters 007, 109 and 110 to see just how much information you've gained. This can help you to prepare for your assessments.

Turn to pages 495–496 for the answers.

CROSSWORD

See if you can answer the questions and write in the answers.

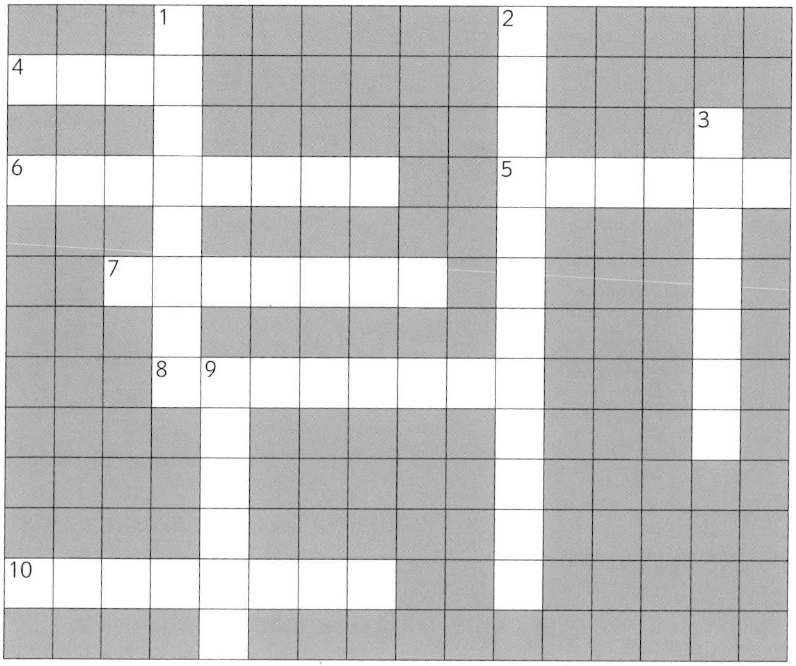

Across

4 This is used to shorten and shape the nail

5 A nail shape

6 A treatment that cares for the hands

7 The skin around the base of the nail

8 When the skin becomes red

10 Germs that can cause an infection

Down

1 A treatment that cares for the feet

2 A discussion with the client before the treatment starts

3 Describing nails that peel off and break easily

9 Lines on the nail plate

WORDS TO FIND

Copy and complete the sentences below. Use these words to help you fill in the gaps.

allergies	file	pedicure	ridges
enamel	massage	square	base coat
cuticle	oval	round	top coat
manicure	erythema	nail	feet

1 A ____________________ is a treatment that cares for the hands.

2 During the consultation, it is important to check whether your client has any ____________________ to the products that you are using. This will help to stop any adverse reactions from happening.

3 Nail ____________________ is applied to the ____________________ plate to give it colour.

4 If you apply a ____________________ coat before the nail enamel, it will help to stop the nail enamel from staining the nail plate.

5 A ____________________ is a treatment that cares for the feet.

6 A ____________________ is applied after the nail enamel and will help to protect the enamel and prevent it from chipping.

7 The skin around the base of the nail is called the ____________________ .

8 A nail ____________________ is used to shorten and shape the nails.

9 Oval, rounded, pointed, squoval and ____________________ are all types of nail shape.

TEST YOUR KNOWLEDGE FURTHER

Read the sentences below and state whether they are true or false.

1 The spatula and orange stick can be placed in Barbicide during the treatment. True or false?

2 Towels should be machine washed at a high temperature. True or false?

3 Nail-varnish remover is applied to the nails with a tissue. True or false?

4 A treatment plan should include details of the treatment, such as the colour of varnish used. True or false?

5 Cuticle cream helps to remove nail varnish. True or false?

6 Massage will make the skin feel dry. True or false?

7 Good communication will help to relax the client. True or false?

8 A top coat is applied before the nail varnish. True or false?

9 An oval shape is good for short nails. True or false?

10 Erythema is an example of a contra-action. True or false?

11 After soaking the fingertips, the cuticles can be gently eased back using a spatula. True or false?

12 A good therapist will ensure that the treatment area is prepared before the client arrives. True or false?

13 Dry cuticles would benefit from a manicure treatment. True or false?

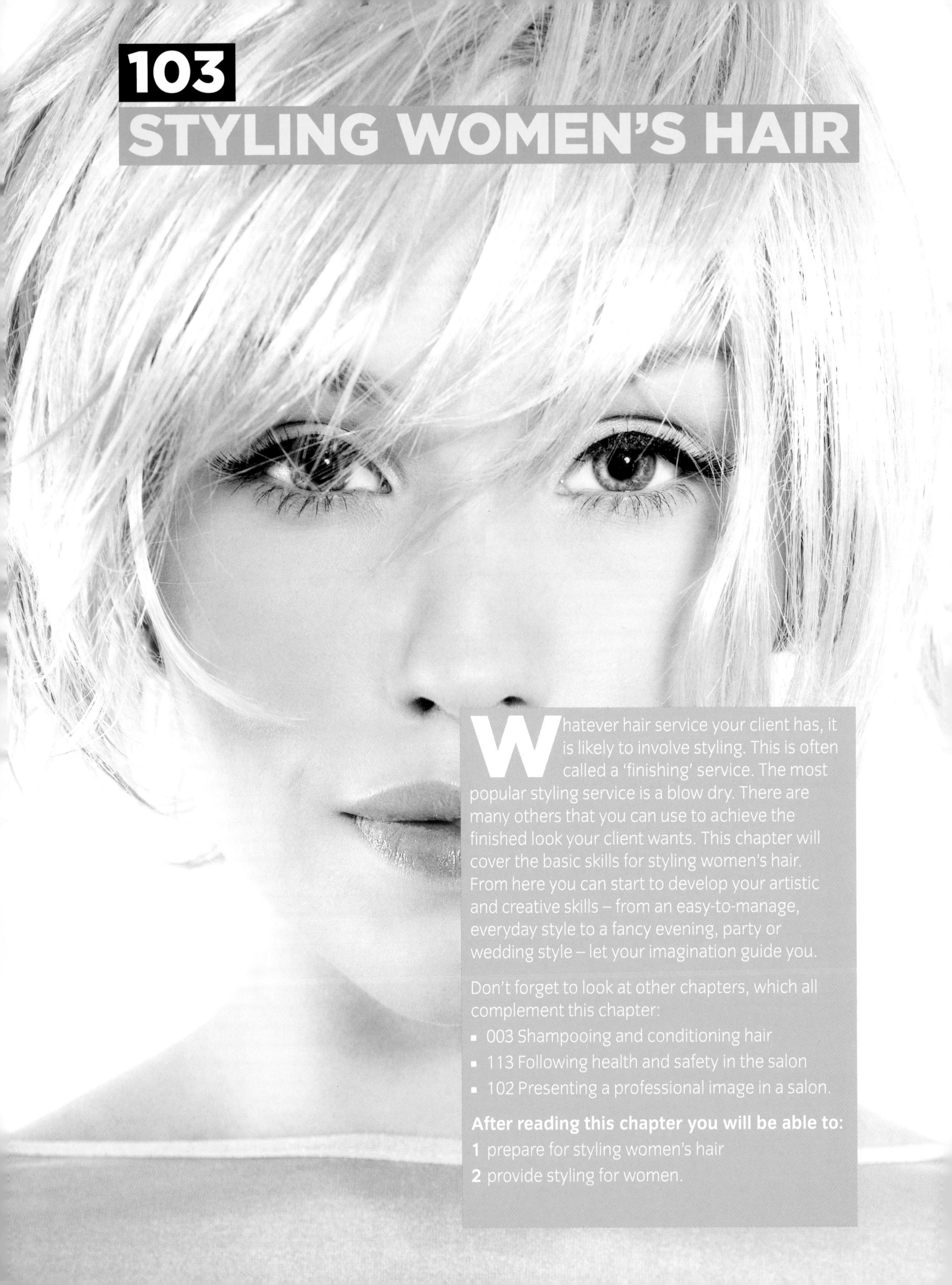

103 STYLING WOMEN'S HAIR

Whatever hair service your client has, it is likely to involve styling. This is often called a 'finishing' service. The most popular styling service is a blow dry. There are many others that you can use to achieve the finished look your client wants. This chapter will cover the basic skills for styling women's hair. From here you can start to develop your artistic and creative skills – from an easy-to-manage, everyday style to a fancy evening, party or wedding style – let your imagination guide you.

Don't forget to look at other chapters, which all complement this chapter:

- 003 Shampooing and conditioning hair
- 113 Following health and safety in the salon
- 102 Presenting a professional image in a salon.

After reading this chapter you will be able to:

1 prepare for styling women's hair

2 provide styling for women.

PREPARE FOR STYLING WOMEN'S HAIR

This part of the chapter looks at factors that influence the choice of hair-styling techniques for women, and the importance of the preparation procedures for styling women's hair.

THE BASIC TECHNIQUES FOR STYLING WOMEN'S HAIR

There are several basic techniques that can be used for styling women's hair.

BLOW DRYING

Blow drying is the most popular of all the styling **techniques**. The style is usually affected by the cut, which puts the shape into the hair. Blow drying puts the finish to that shape. It can be carried out on all lengths of hair. Hair that is very fine and **sparse** may not be suited to blow drying. It is carried out on wet hair.

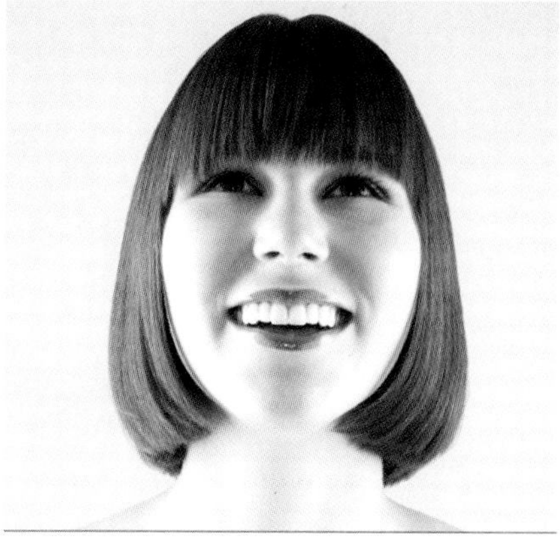

A classic 'bob' blow dry

Techniques

The way things are done

Sparse

Thin; less than the average number of hairs on the scalp

SmartScreen 103 handout 3

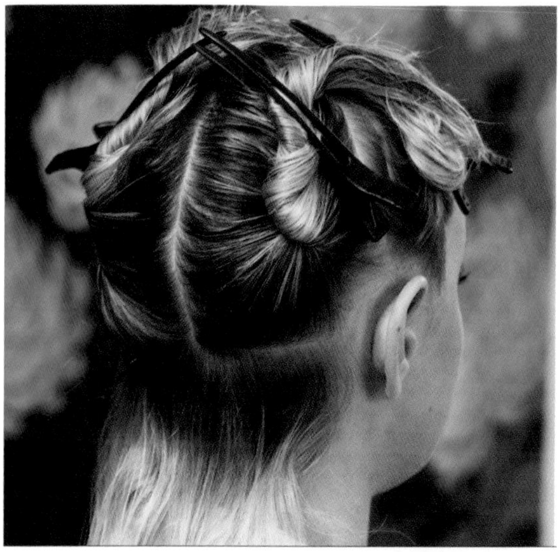

The hair is divided into sections. These are held in place with sectioning clips. Smaller sections are taken from these

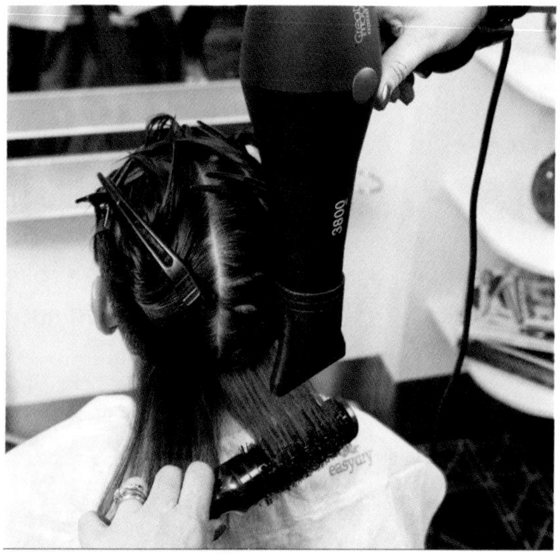

The stylist uses a hand-held dryer to provide the hot air needed to dry the hair

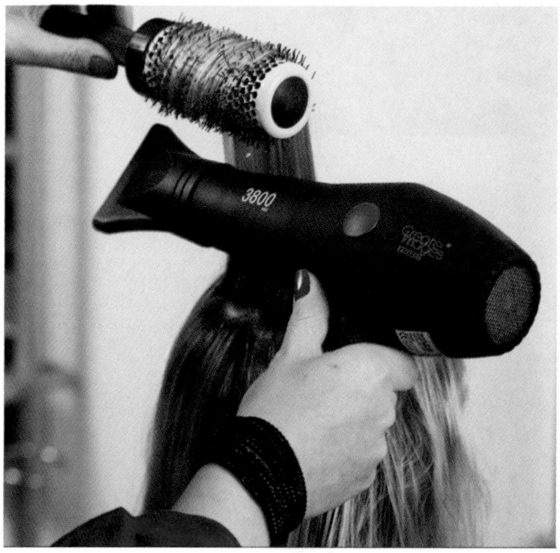

The hair is placed on a brush and held in the direction needed. The hot air from the dryer is directed on to the hair to dry it in that direction

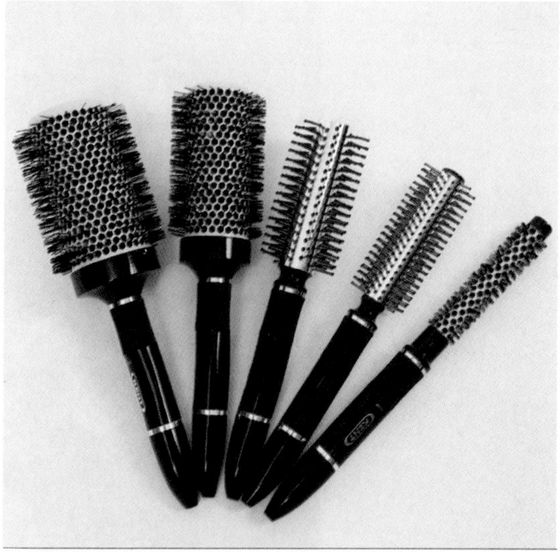

Different types of brush are used to give root lift and smoothness to the style

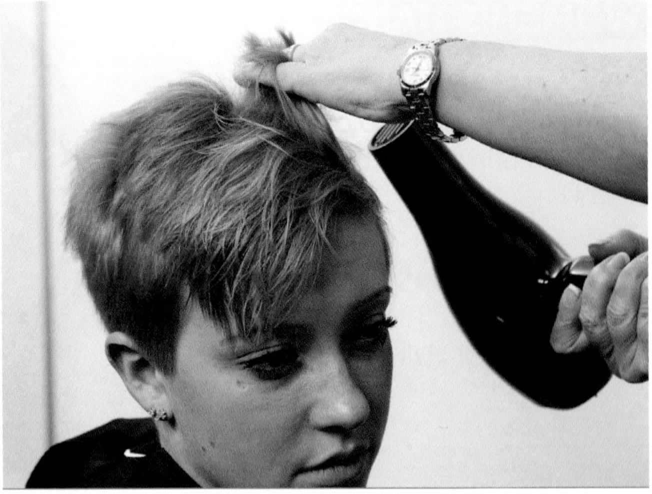

Finger drying

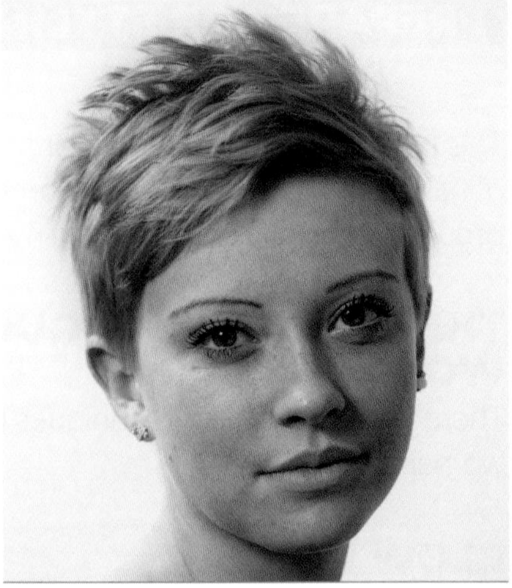

The finished look

FINGER DRYING

Finger drying is a technique similar to blow drying. The hair is dried using the fingers instead of a brush. It is carried out on wet hair. It will give soft, natural-looking styles.

The fingers are used to lift the hair and mould it into shape.

ROLLER SETTING

Roller setting is a widely used styling technique. It is carried out on wet hair. The hair is wound on rollers and dried under a hood dryer. The rollers are removed and the hair is brushed and combed into the desired shape. Different size rollers are used for different effects. When the hair is dried it is brushed and combed into position.

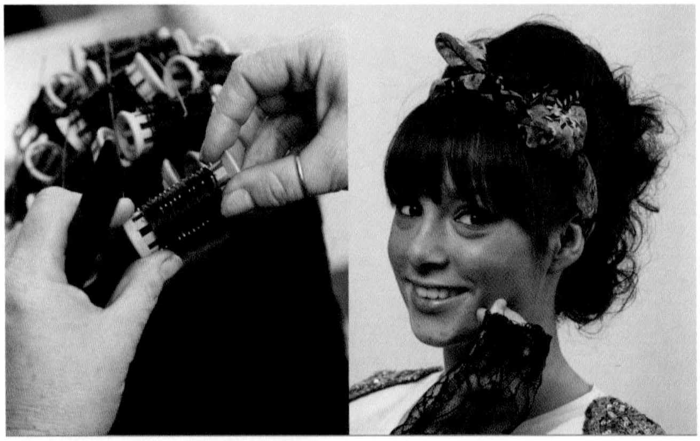

Small rollers are used to give tighter curls

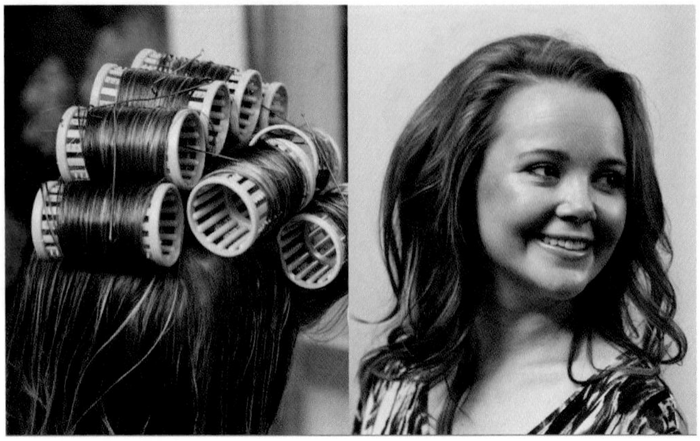

Larger rollers give softer curls

SmartScreen 001 handout 4

HAIR UP

Roller setting is very useful for styling longer hair. It is often used for a 'hair up'. This is a style on long hair where the hair is secured with pins and grips. It is used to create styles for special occasions such as weddings, evenings out and parties.

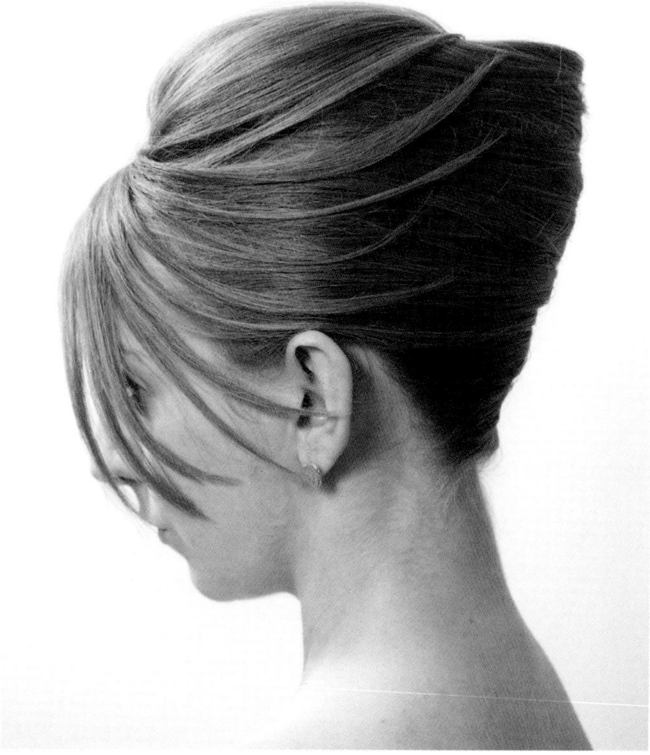

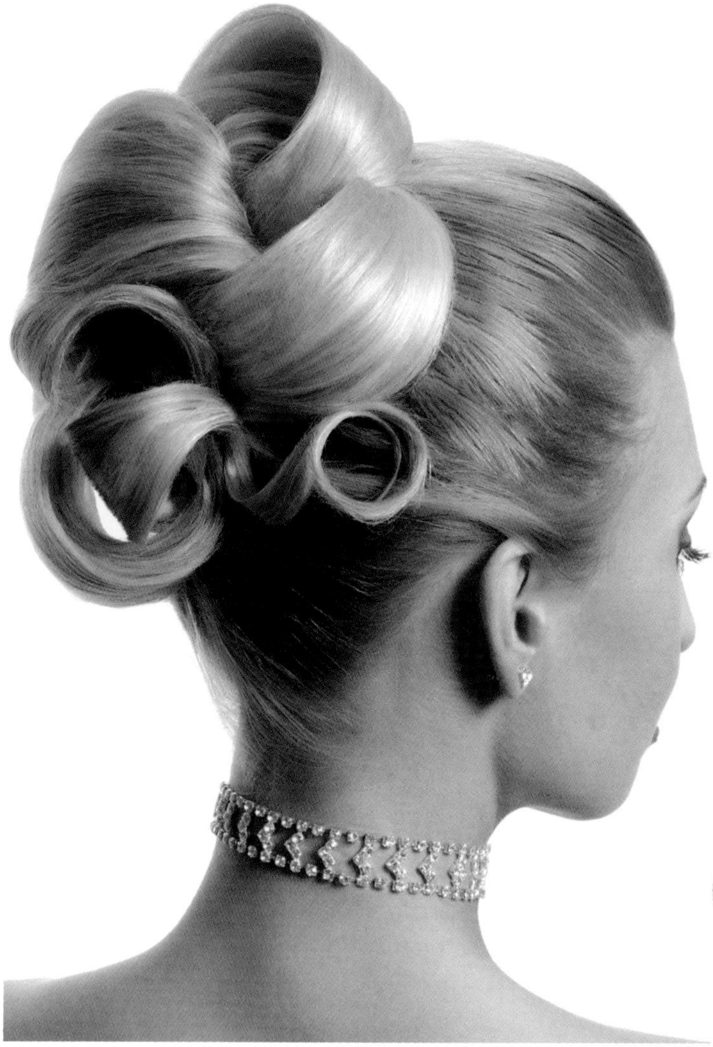

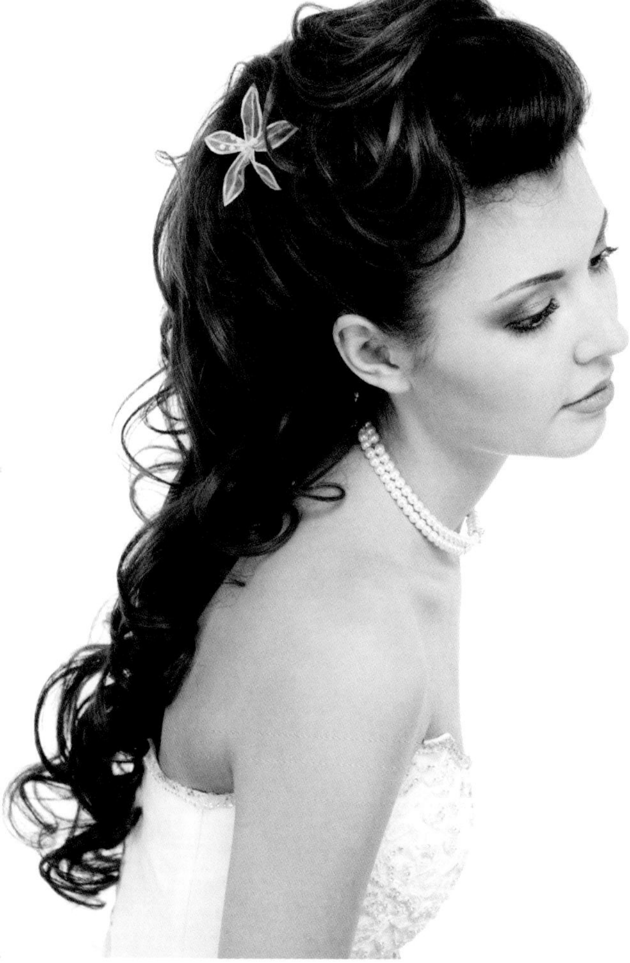

PIN CURLING

Pin curling is a method of styling where the hair is formed into a curl and then fixed in place with a clip. This technique is used to achieve wave movements in the hair. It can also be used with a roller set to give some movement in the short hair in the nape area. Pin curling is carried out on wet hair. The hair is dried and then brushed and combed into shape.

There are three types of pin curl:

Pin curl type	How it is made	Effect
Barrel-spring curls	A section of hair 2.5 cm square is taken and the points are formed into a circle the same size as the square. The circle is wound to the roots, keeping the hair flat to the head. The curl is secured flat by placing a clip diagonally across the square.	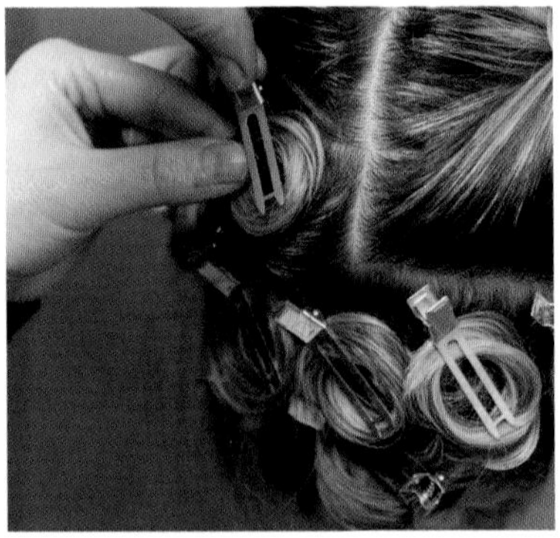 Gives a flat wave effect
Clock-spring curls	These are similar to barrel-spring curls but they are closed at the centre. Instead of forming a circle the same size as the square, you make the first circle as small as you can. Then wind and secure as before.	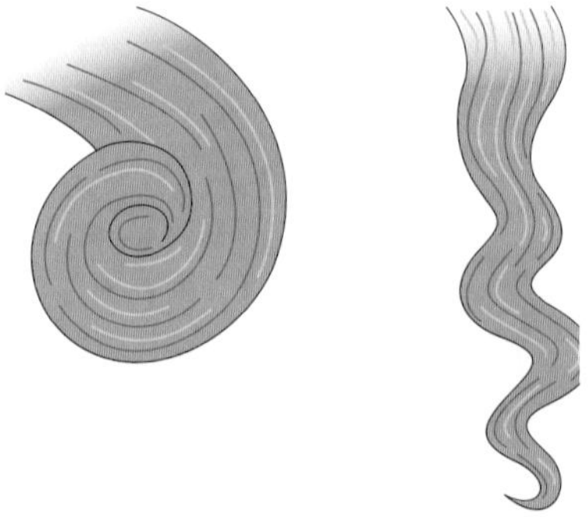 Used to give ringlets around the hairline
Barrel curls	Barrel curls look like curls that have been made with rollers. A 2.5 cm section is wound down from the point to the root. It is secured through the base with a clip.	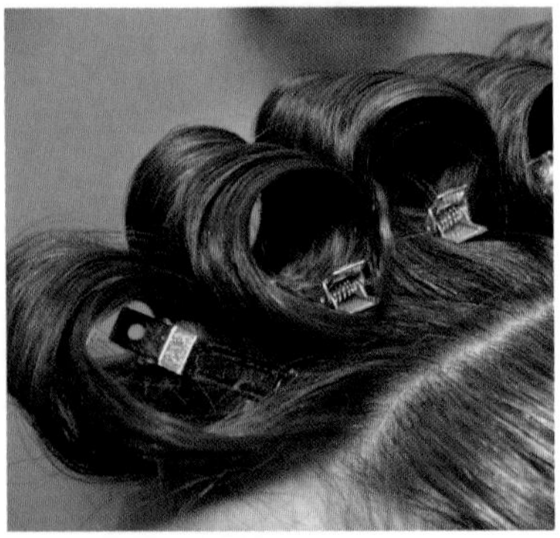 Can be used in place of rollers to give root lift and curl

The next group of styling methods are carried out on dry hair. They can be used on their own to style the hair or as part of other methods. The appliances used are heated and the heat produces the finish. Care must be taken to prevent damage to the hair by using too much heat.

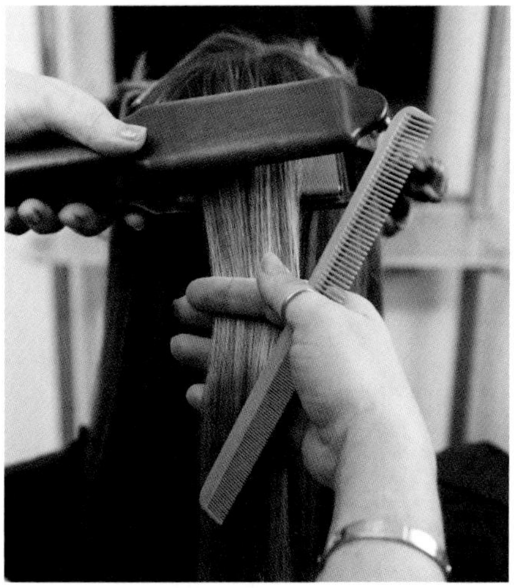

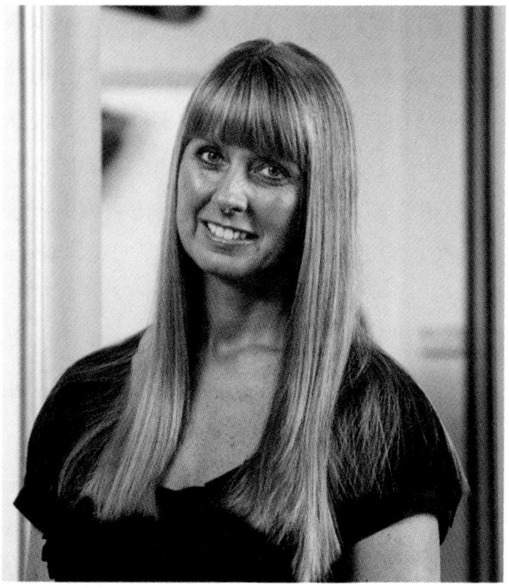

STRAIGHTENING AND SMOOTHING

This method is used to produce straight hair with a smooth finish. It is usually carried out on longer length hair. It can be used on hair with some natural curl to give a straight finish. It can also be used after blow drying to get a smooth finish to the style.

This technique uses straighteners. The hair is sectioned into small sections. The straighteners are closed around the section. They are then slid gently down the section from the root of the hair to the point.

CURLING

This is a styling technique often used to add lift and curl to a blow dry. It can also be used to 'freshen up' a blow dry or set after a few days. It is very useful on fine hair to give body. Care should be taken not to use too much heat.

This technique uses tongs. The hair is sectioned into small sections. The points of the hair are placed in the tongs and the tongs are wound down to the root. Take care not to burn the scalp. After a few seconds the tongs are unwound. The hair should look like it does when you take the rollers out when setting. The hair is then brushed or combed into shape when it has cooled.

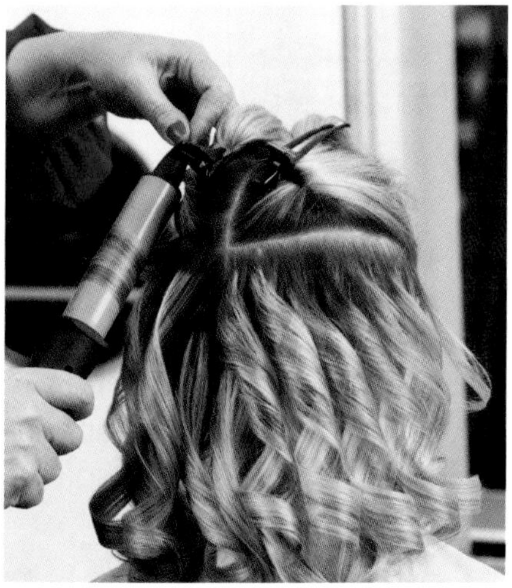

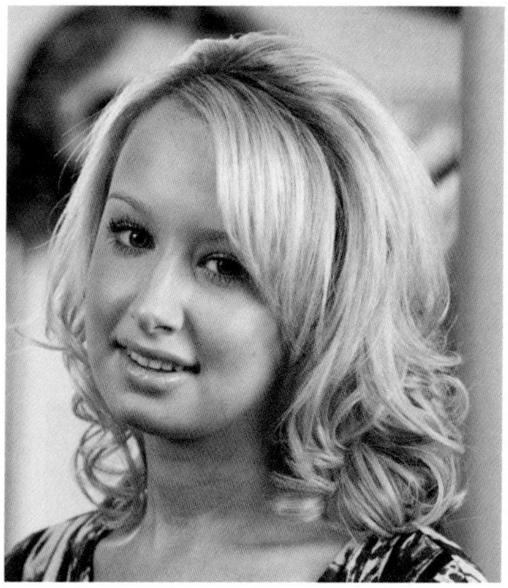

ACTIVITY

Find some pictures of styles that are achieved by these styling techniques. Make some notes of how they were done. Keep your pictures for your assignment.

FACTORS THAT CAN INFLUENCE YOUR CHOICE OF STYLING TECHNIQUES

Factors
Things to consider about the subject

There are many **factors** that you will need to take into account when you are deciding which technique you are going to use to achieve the style the client wants. They will also help you decide how to use the selected technique.

FACE SHAPE

People have different-shaped faces. Here are five of the more common ones.

Face shape	Ideal styles for this face shape
Oval 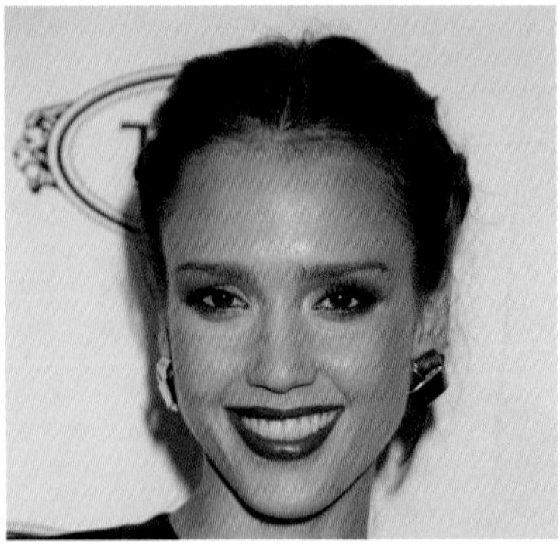 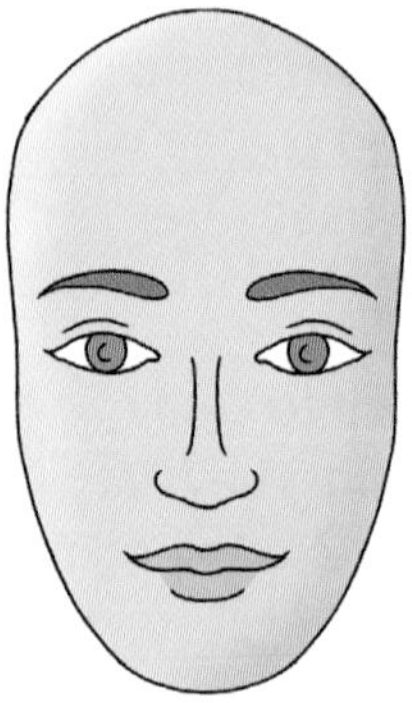	This face shape does not need any correcting. It is the ideal face shape. You can add height or width as you wish; soft curls or straight smooth finishes.
Square 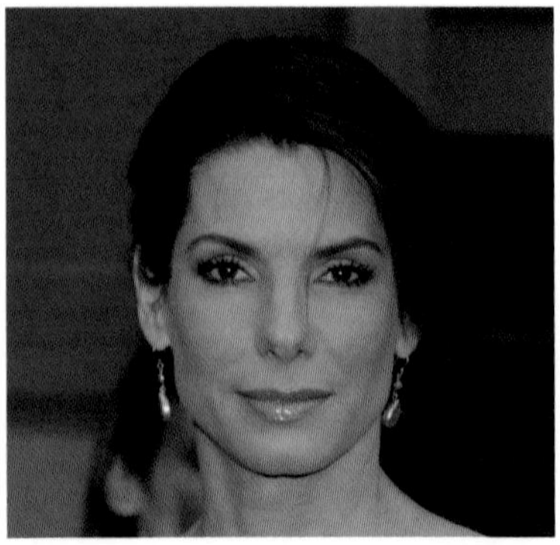 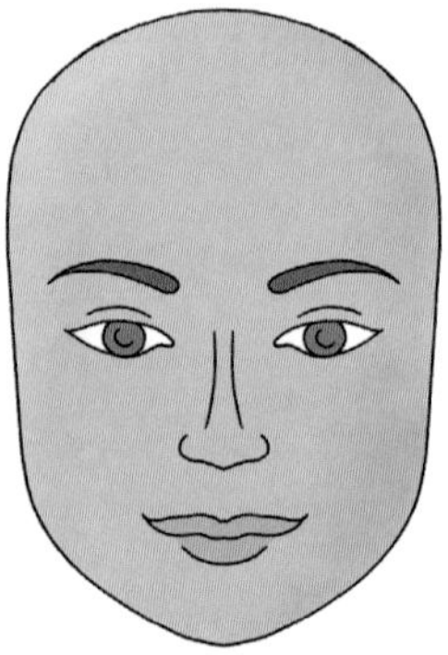	Square faces need to have some height and not too much width. Go for a softer, curlier look rather than straight, hard lines.
Oblong 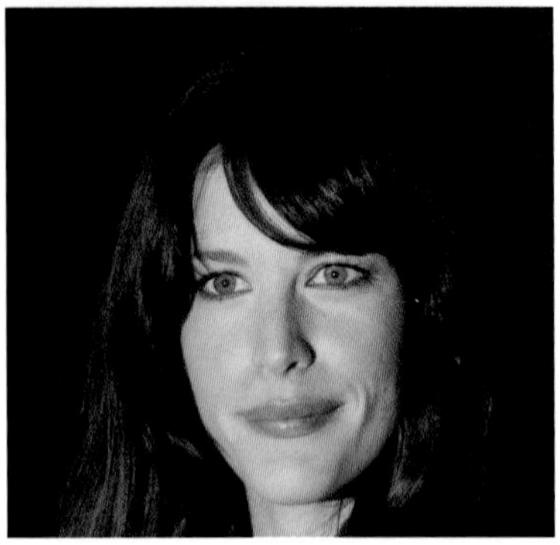 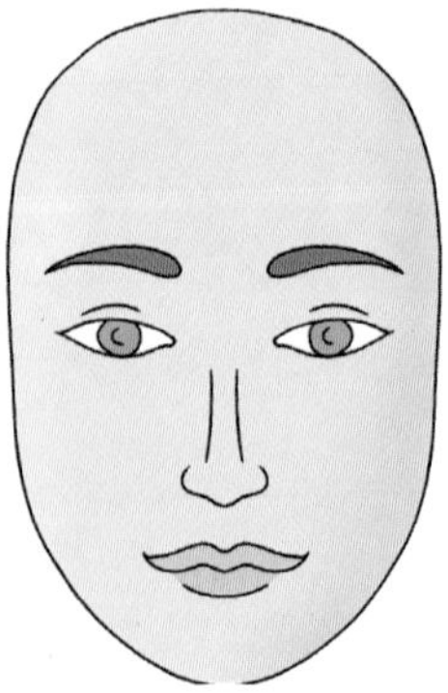	Oblong faces are similar to square faces. They tend to be angular. Avoid height in the style and straight, hard lines. Soft waves will soften this face shape.

Face shape	Ideal styles for this face shape
Heart 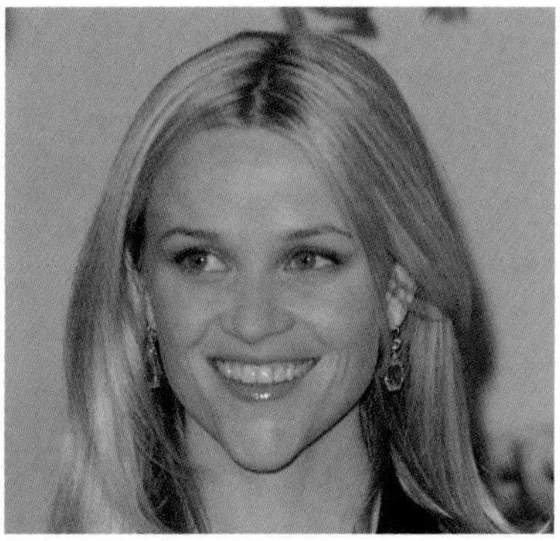 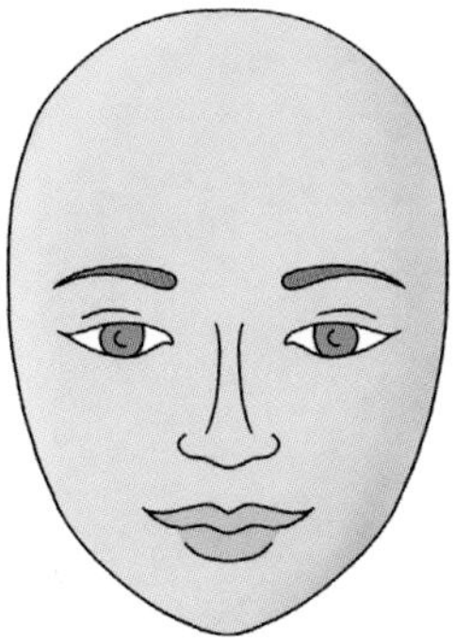	Heart-shaped faces are wider at the top and narrower at the bottom, so try to avoid width at the top and add width at the bottom.
Round 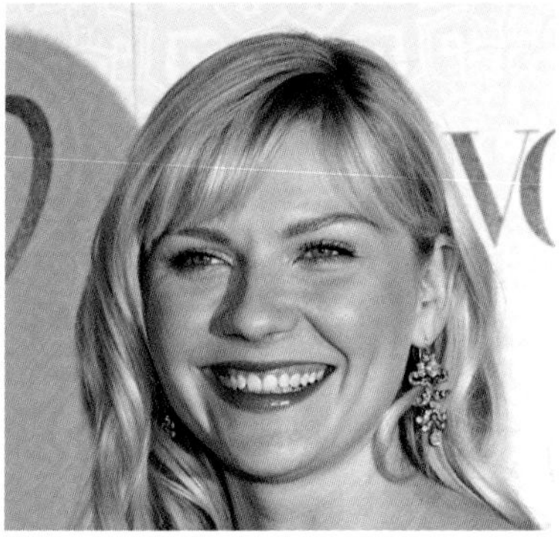 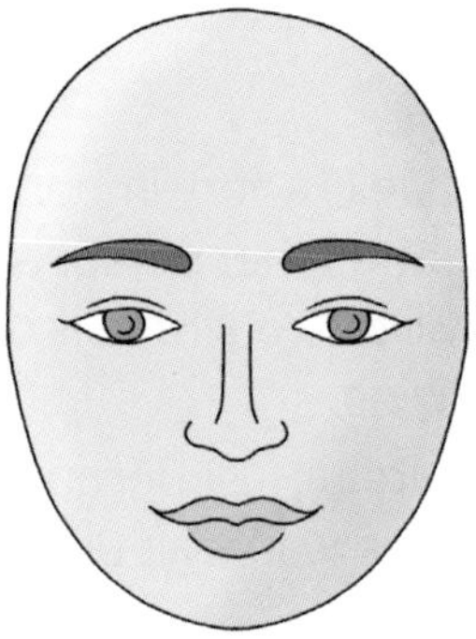	A round face needs to have added height and flatter sides to reduce the width of the face.

ACTIVITY

With other members of your group, decide each other's face shape. Make notes on the styles that would suit each member. Compare your decisions with the others.

HEAD SHAPE

Head shapes will also be different. Look at the head from the front and from the side. Your style should balance the shape of the head. Add volume or height if the head is small. Keep the style flat if the head is large or wide.

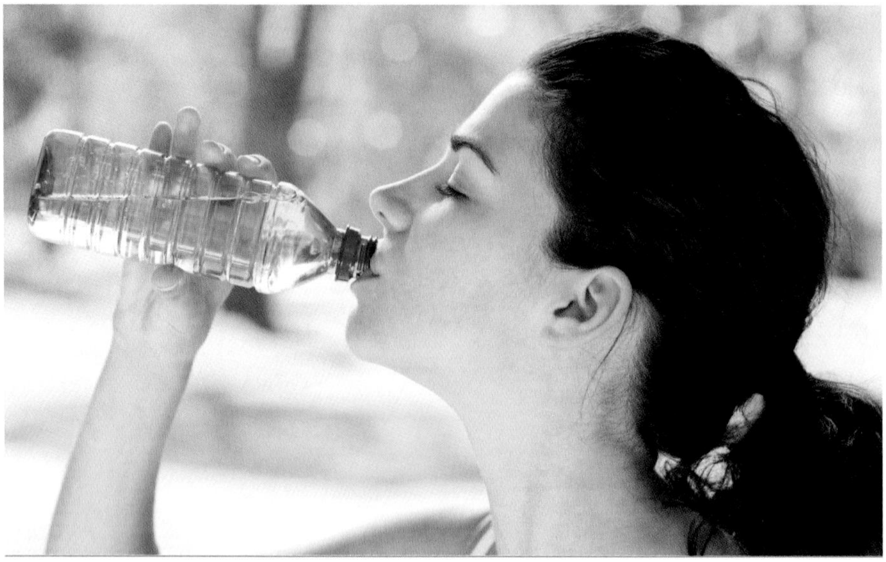

Ask your client if they play any sports before you decide on a hairstyle

LIFESTYLE

The client's lifestyle is a very important factor in the styling process. It will tell you a lot about her personality and give you clues as to her likes and dislikes. It will tell you if she is outgoing or quiet. You should take note of the following:

- Her age – be careful; just because she may be of the older generation doesn't mean she wants an old-fashioned style.
- Her job – this is most important. The client's style has to fit into her job role. She may want a short, easy-to-manage style.
- How much make-up she wears or the style of make-up.
- Is the client sporty? If so, an easy-to-manage style is important.

The next group of factors are about the client's hair.

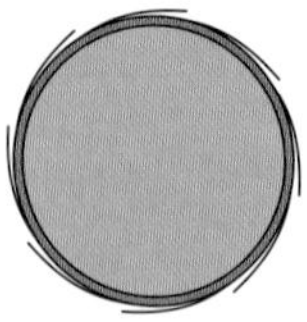

Very fine hair

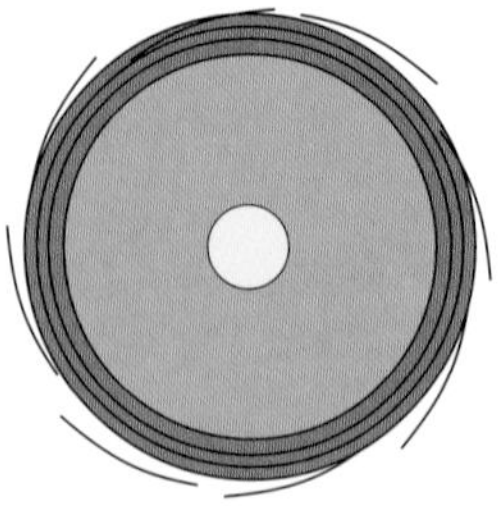

Average hair

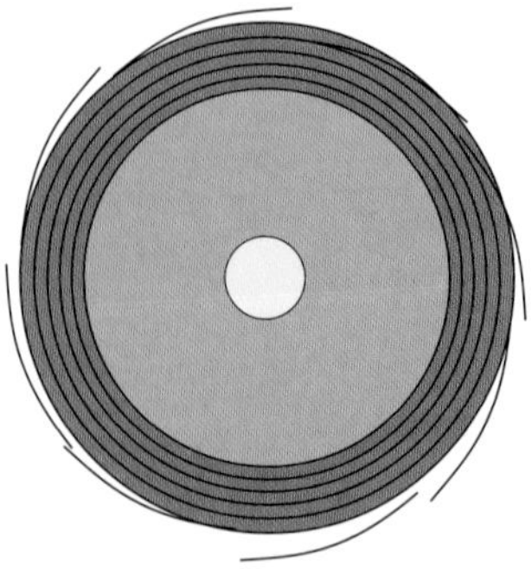

Very coarse hair

HAIR TEXTURE

Hair texture is about the thickness of each individual hair. It is not about the number of hairs on the head.

- Fine: this texture is more suited to shorter styles. The hair may look thinner if it is longer and will need root lift. This texture of hair may be weaker than other textures – take care when using heated appliances; do not use too much tension.
- Medium: this texture is ideal, and is suited to long and short styles.
- Coarse: this texture can have a rough look, and can sometimes be harder to curl because the hair will be strong and resistant. Be careful when selecting a style as there may be too much hair for you to achieve the look you want.

Deciding the texture of the client's hair is done by looking at a few hairs and feeling them.

ACTIVITY

With other members of your group, look and feel each other's hair and decide what texture the hair is. Compare your **analysis** with the rest of the group.

Analysis
The result of looking at something carefully

HAIR DENSITY

Density describes the number of hairs on the head. There are around 120,000 hairs on the average scalp.

- Sparse: this means that there are less than the average number of hairs on the scalp. Like fine hair, it is more suited to shorter styles.
- Abundant: this means that there are more hairs than average on the scalp. Like coarse hair, it may take longer to dry and could be strong and difficult to curl.

The density can be decided by looking at the scalp. The more skin you can see the less hair the client has.

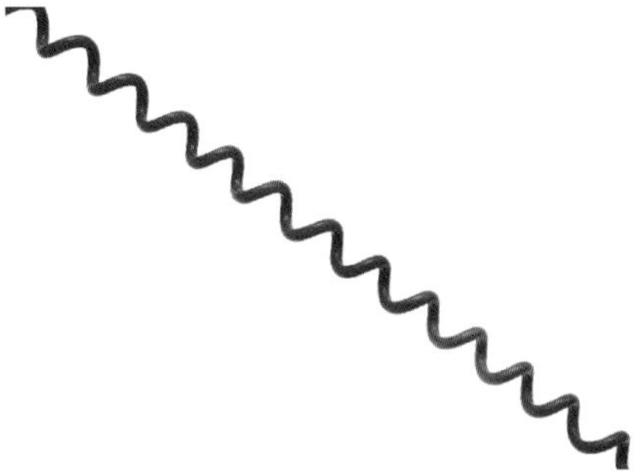

Hair in bad condition; does not return once stretched

HAIR ELASTICITY

Hair is naturally elastic; it can stretch and go back to its original shape. If the hair is fine it may not have as much elasticity as coarse hair. This weakness may cause the hair to break if too much tension is put on it. Hair that has been damaged by chemical treatments such as colour or perm will be weaker than normal hair. Using excessive heat can cause the same damage.

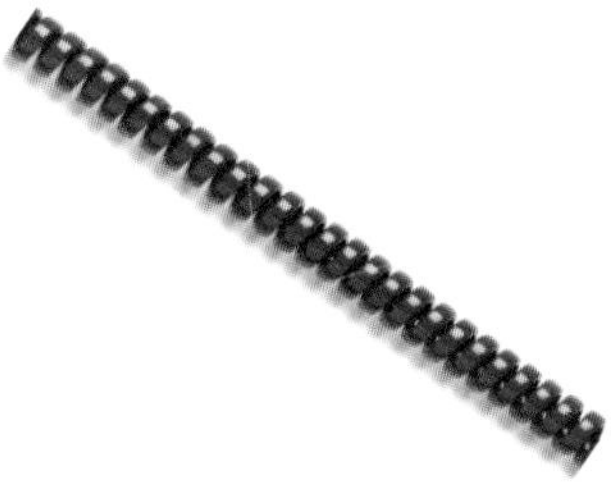

Hair in good condition; returns to original state once stretched

HAIR CONDITION

Hair type	How you recognise it	Effect on the styling service
Normal 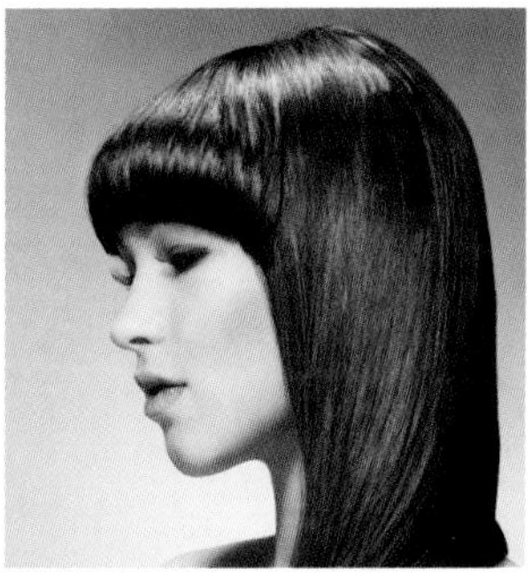	Will shine and look good. Feels smooth to the touch.	This hair type will not present any major problems when styling.
Oily/greasy 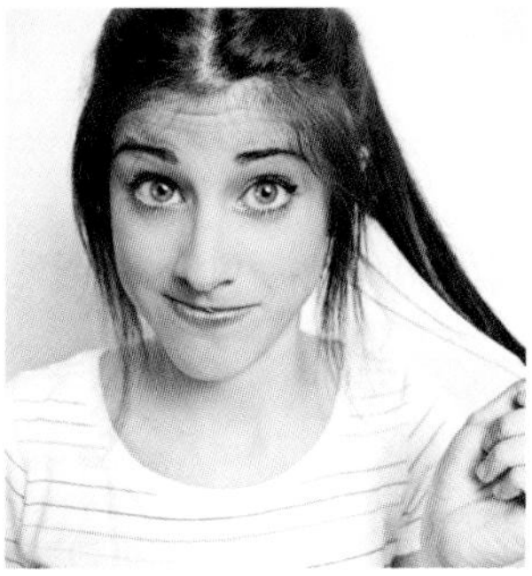	Will look dull and greasy. Feels sticky to the touch.	The hair will need frequent washing, so easy-to-manage styles will be more practical.

Hair type	How you recognise it	Effect on the styling service
Dry 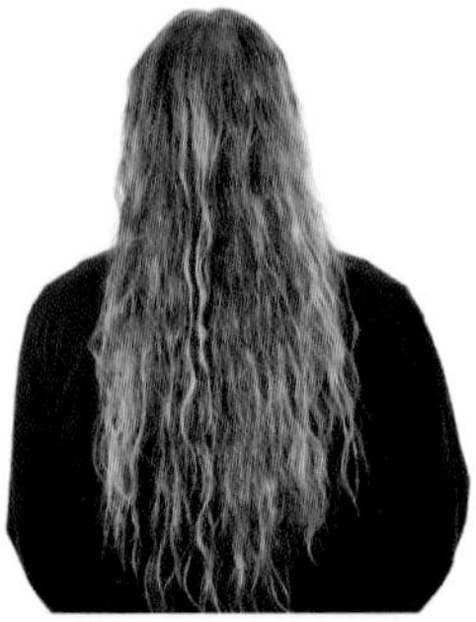	Will look dull and straw-like. Feels rough to the touch.	The hair will need regular conditioning to help achieve a smooth finish. Don't use too much heat.
Dandruff 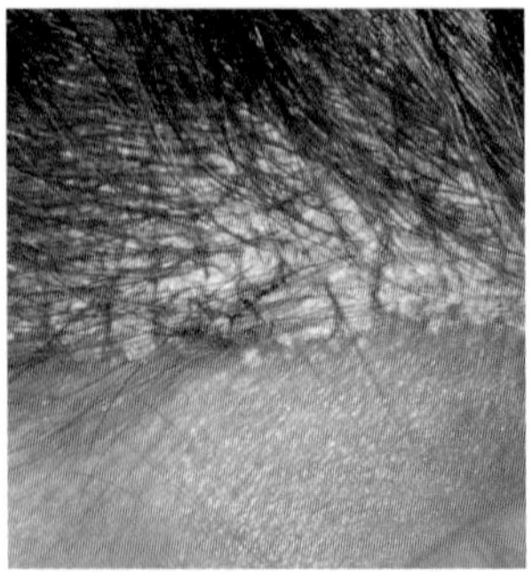	Appears and feels the same as dry hair. There will be white flakes in the hair and on the shoulders.	The hair will need regular conditioning to help achieve a smooth finish. Don't use too much heat. The condition should be treated.
Damaged 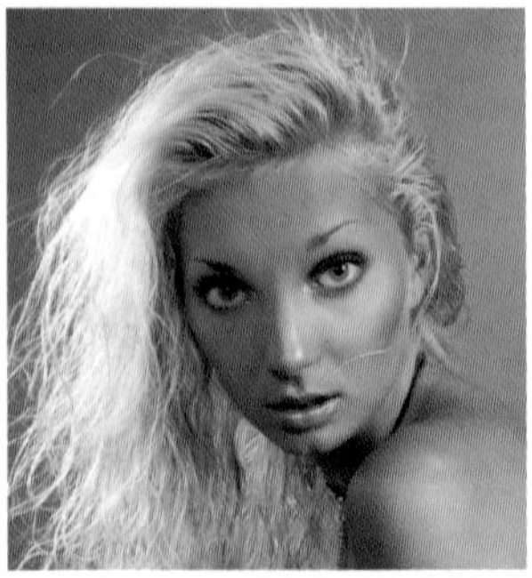	May look dull and straw-like. Feels rough to the touch. Points of the hair may look spiky.	If the hair is damaged as a result of other services, like perming or colouring, the hair may be weak. Treat the hair carefully. Don't use too much heat or too much tension.

Deciding hair condition is done by looking at and feeling the hair. You may also need to ask some questions.

ACTIVITY

Working in a group, determine what hair condition each member of the group has. Check your answers with the others.

HAIR TYPE

The client's hair will be straight, curly or wavy. If the client has straight hair you may need to add root lift and body to your style. Straight hair tends to lie flat to the head.

With curly hair, if you want a straight, smooth style you may need to use straighteners. If your client has very wavy hair this may present some styling problems. Hair with a strong natural wave will be difficult to change. You will have to go with the natural shape when you style the hair.

HAIR LENGTH

The length of the hair will affect your choice of style and styling technique. The longer the hair the more work it will need to keep it looking nice. It will also take longer to dry so extra time may be needed. Very short hair will limit your choice of style. There may not be enough hair to do what the client would like. Long hair is heavier so the weight may cause the curl to drop sooner than it would with short hair.

HAIR GROWTH CYCLE

Each hair does not grow **continuously**. A single hair has a life of between 18 months and seven years. At the end of its life it will fall out and after a short while another hair will grow in its place. About 100 hairs a day will reach the end of their life and fall out. This is why you get hairs in the brush or comb when you use them.

Continuously
Happening all the time without a break

There are three stages in the hair growth cycle:

- Active or growing period – lasts for 18 months to seven years. This is the anagen stage of the hair growth.
- Breaking down stage – lasts about two weeks. This is the catagen stage of hair growth.
- Resting – lasts about a month. This is the telogen stage of hair growth.

HANDY HINTS

Look at the images of the anagen, catagen and telogen stages on page 127.

Hair grows on average 1.25 cm a month. Some people's hair grows more each month than the average; some people's hair grows less than the average. Some people can grow their hair very long. Others will not be able to and will say that their hair gets to a certain length and then stops growing. How long the hair grows is decided by how much it grows every month and by its life cycle.

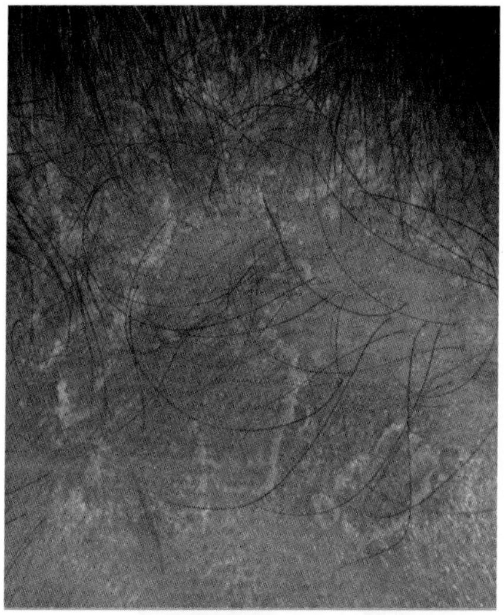

Scaly patches or rough areas on the scalp

ACTIVITY

In a small group, measure and record the length of each other's hair. Make a note of whether the hair is fine, medium or coarse. After a month, measure the hair again and calculate how much it has grown. Did the fine hair grow more or less than the coarse hair?

ADVERSE SKIN, SCALP AND HAIR CONDITIONS

Any disease or condition of the hair and scalp can affect your choice of styling technique and the style you decide to do. Some diseases and conditions may be contagious. This could stop you from carrying out any service on the client.

You should look at the hair and scalp when you are consulting with your client. Look for the following conditions:

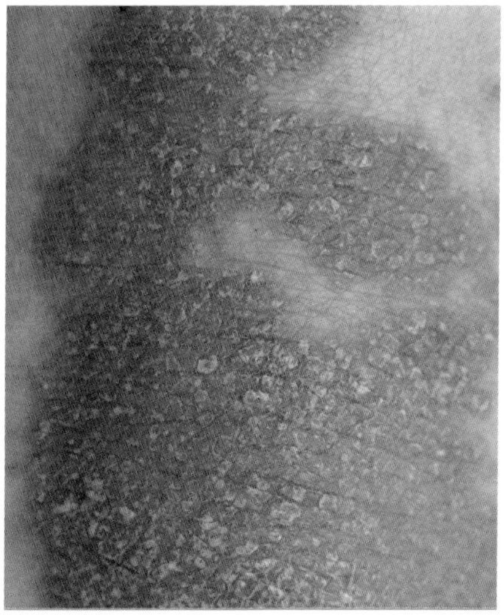

Red, inflamed patches

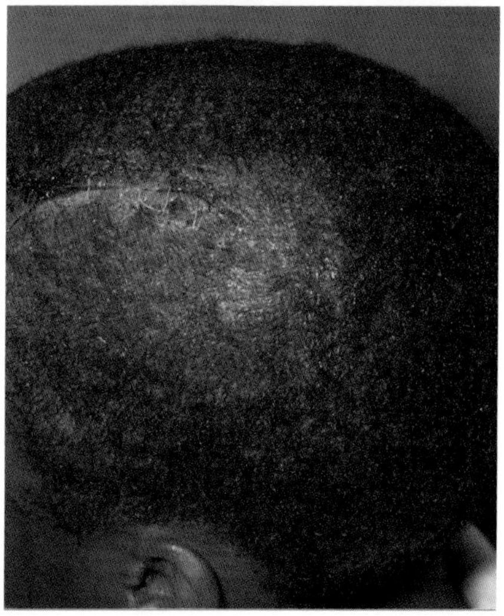

Cuts and abrasions on the skin

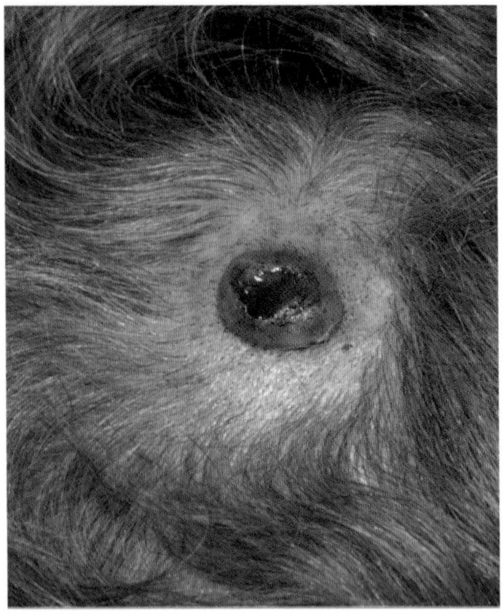
Lumps and bumps or raised areas

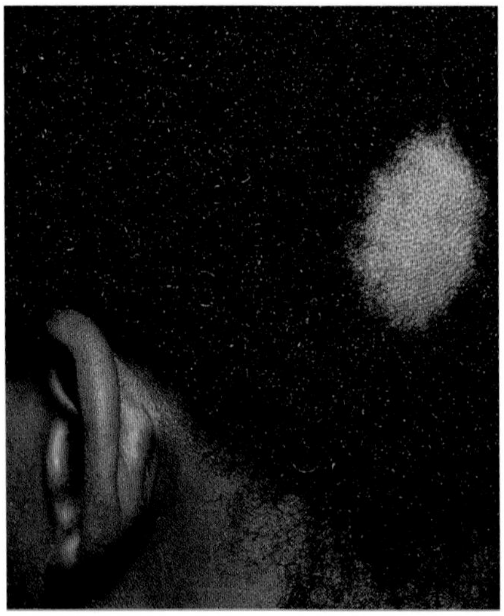
Bald patches

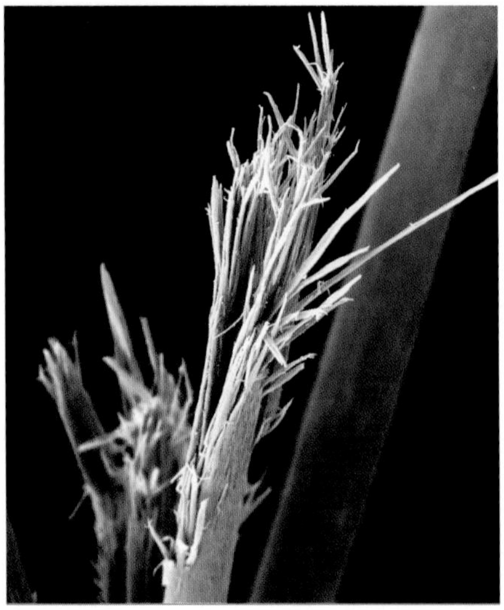
Hair breakage seen under the microscope

Colleague
Someone that you work with

HANDY HINTS
Remember to look for head lice when you are checking the scalp.

If there is anything unusual then you should ask a senior **colleague** to look and advise you. If you are unable to give the service then you may need to explain to the client that the treatment cannot go ahead. Remember that you are not medically trained. You should not name the condition in case you are wrong. Sometimes it may be necessary to advise the client to go to her doctor.

HAIR GROWTH PATTERNS

Hair growth patterns are places where the hair grows in a particular direction or directions. This may affect how the hair is styled. It can also affect how long or short the hair can be.

Look for the following when you do your consultation:

Growth pattern	How you recognise it	Effect on the styling service
Cowlick 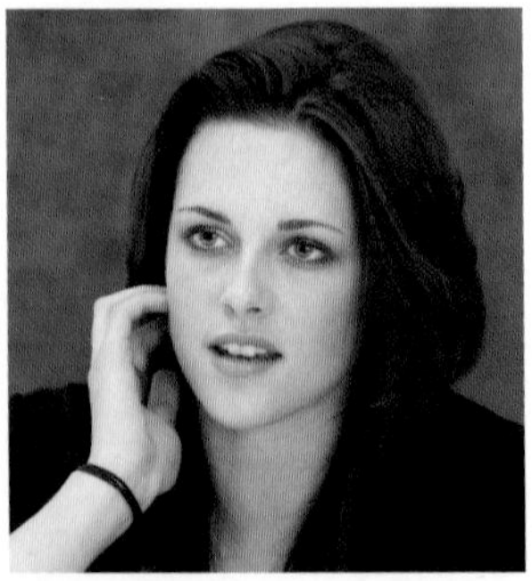	The hair falls to one side or the other at the front; sometimes forms a natural parting.	Full fringes will be difficult to achieve as the hair will part. Work with the direction of the hair.
Nape whorl 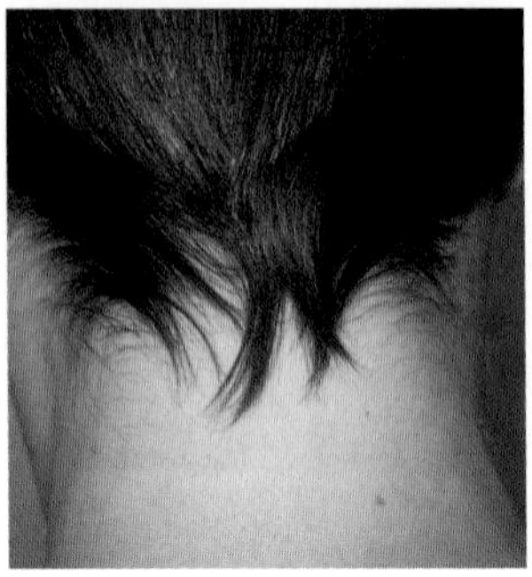	Nape whorls are found in the nape area. The hair grows upwards and inwards towards the middle. It can be on one side or both sides.	Longer styles will not be affected by nape whorls. On shorter styles, dry the hair flat with no root lift.

Growth pattern	How you recognise it	Effect on the styling service
Double crown 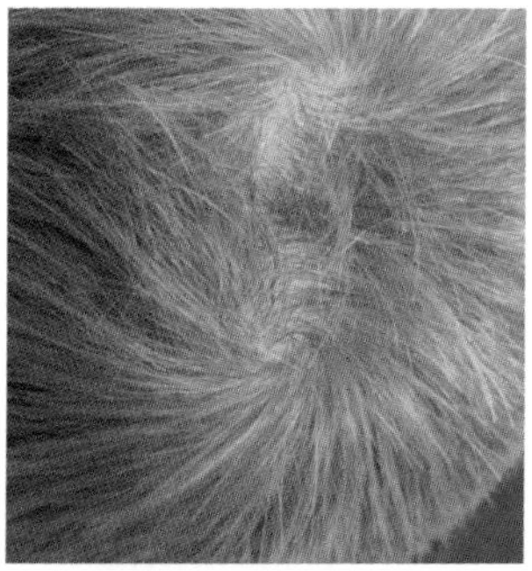	The hair forms two circles in the middle of the scalp.	If the hair is too short it may stick up. The hair should be left longer with good root lift.
Widow's peak 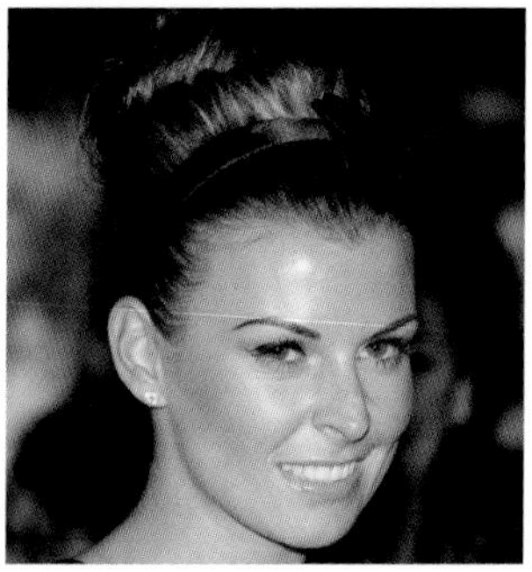	The hair grows to a defined point in the middle of the front hairline.	Fringes will difficult to achieve unless they are heavy. Styles where the hair is dressed back towards the crown are best.

FASHION TRENDS

Your client may want a hairstyle worn by their favourite pop star or celebrity. Sometimes this can be easy and sometimes it is difficult. The client may not have the right type of hair. It may be too short or too long. She may not have the same shape of face as the celebrity or the style might not be flattering to her body shape.

You may need to explain to the client that you may need to change the style because of her hair type or face shape.

ACTIVITY

Keep your eye on what styles and colours are popular at the moment. Keep up to date for your clients. There are many images of the latest styles in magazines or on the television. Cut out some pictures and make your own style book.

HANDY HINTS

Remember, you must be very tactful and polite when you discuss your client's face shape and lifestyle with her.

ACTIVITY

Select some pictures of your favourite pop stars or celebrities. Within your group, decide which of your colleagues could have the styles you have selected and which could not. Give reasons for your decisions and how you will tell the colleague they cannot have the style.

PREPARE THE WORK AREA

There are three reasons why you should prepare your work area ready to work:

1 It helps you to work safely and hygienically.

2 It looks good and gives the client the right impression.

3 It helps you to work efficiently.

Sterilised
Made free from germs and viruses

HANDY HINTS
Remember to make sure your appearance and your personal hygiene are up to standard. Read Chapter 102 to refresh your knowledge.

- Make sure you keep work surfaces clean by wiping regularly with a suitable cleaner.
- Mirrors should be cleaned to remove smears and smudges.
- Tools and equipment should be in their proper places and always cleaned and **sterilised** ready for use to help prevent passing on infection from one client to another.
- Sweep and clean the floor when necessary.
- Make sure the chair is clean.

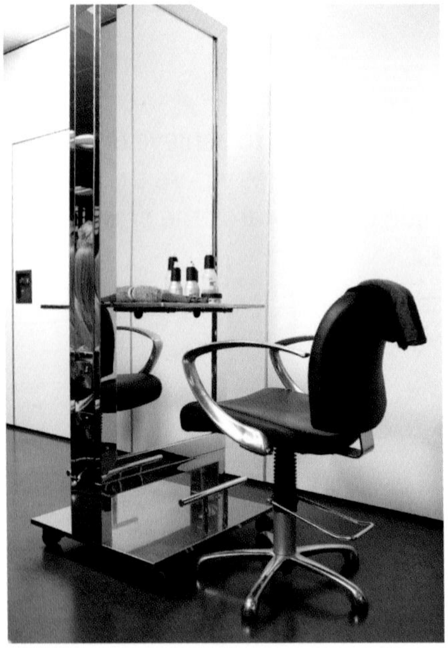

You may not be able to get all the things you need ready before the client arrives. When you have completed your consultation with the client, get the rest of the products and tools you need.

HANDY HINTS
Read Chapter 113 Following health and safety in the salon to learn about the employer's responsibilities and your responsibilities to provide a safe and healthy working environment.

SAFE AND HYGIENIC WORKING PRACTICES

Working safely and hygienically is very important. It is part of every practical skill you learn; it is part of every service you give to a client; it is part of the whole of your working day.

You should keep your work area tidy and only use **hygienic** tools and equipment. This will help to reduce the risk of harm to you and your clients and help to prevent **cross-infection**.

Hygienic
Clean and germ free

Cross-infection
When germs are passed from one person to another

The client will also have more confidence in you and you will look more professional.

When styling hair, the main safe and hygienic working practices that you need to know are:

- PPE – personal protective equipment. You may need an apron or non-latex gloves for any products you use if the manufacturer's instructions state this.
- COSHH – Control Of Substances Hazardous to Health. These regulations explain how to safely use any products that may be part of the service. They will also include using a **disinfectant** safely when cleaning tools and equipment.
- Electricity at Work Regulations. Checking all the electrical equipment you will use in the styling process is essential.
- HASAWA – Health and Safety at Work Act. You must make sure you check the work area for any hazards before you start work on the client. Make sure all the equipment, tools and products are clean and safe to use on the client.
- Methods of sterilisation. An example in a styling service is using a disinfectant such as **Barbicide** for combs.

Disinfectant
A cleaning fluid that kills germs and helps to prevent them growing

Barbicide
A liquid disinfectant

ACTIVITY

Go to Chapter 113 Following health and safety in the salon and list all of the health and safety laws that you should follow when carrying out a styling service.

HANDY HINTS

Go to Chapter 113 and read more about methods of sterilisation.

HYGIENE WHEN STYLING WOMEN'S HAIR

The following is a guide for keeping your styling tools and equipment ready for use.

Towels and gowns	Machine wash on a high temperature to destroy harmful germs.
Combs and brushes	Wash in warm, soapy water. Place in the sterilising jar.
Clips	Wash in warm soapy water and dry. Then place in the sterilising jar or the UV cabinet.
Rollers and pins	Wash in warm soapy water and dry.
Disposable gloves	Throw away after use. Use a new pair for each client.

PREPARE THE CLIENT

Preparing the client for styling services will involve the following:

1. gowning the client to protect their clothes
2. carrying out a consultation with the client
3. selecting the tools, equipment and products to be used
4. shampooing and, if necessary, conditioning the client's hair.

HANDY HINTS

Read more about preparing your client in Chapter 003 Shampooing and conditioning hair.

HANDY HINTS

Check regularly that the gown is still in place and the towels are not too wet. Change the towels if you need to.

GOWNING THE CLIENT

The first part of any service will be to protect the client and her belongings. For styling services, place a gown around the client to protect her clothes and a clean towel around her shoulders.

ACTIVITY

Practise preparing yourself, your work area and your client for a styling service. Work with a partner, taking it in turns to be stylist and client.

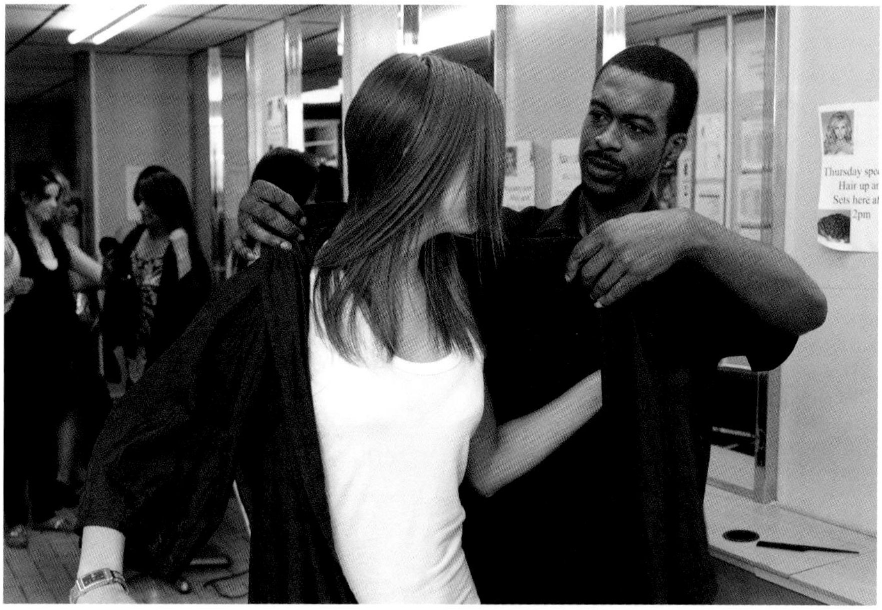

CONSULTATION

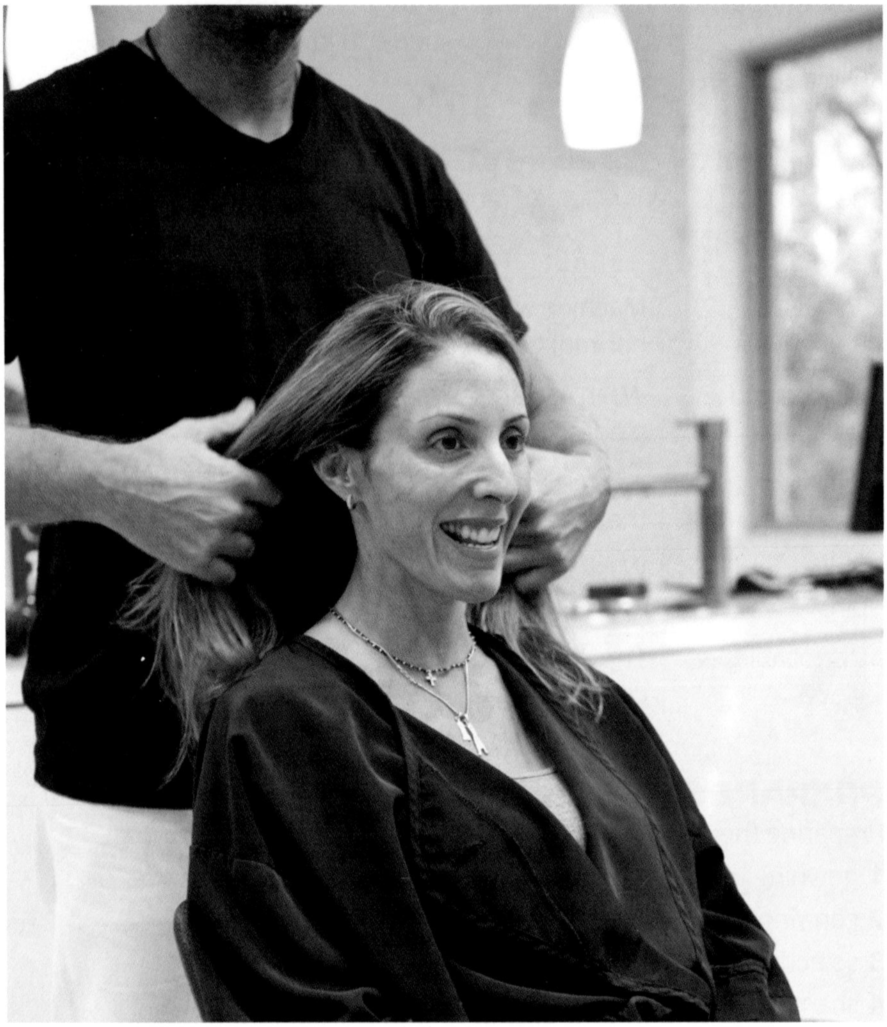

Consulting with the client allows you to find out what the client wants. It is how you decide what you are going to do.

Chapter 003 Shampooing and conditioning hair describes how to consult with your client to find out what shampoo and conditioner you will use and how you will carry out the service. If you are going to style the client's hair then you need to find out more information from the client.

- What does the client want the finished look to be? For example, a practical, easy-to-manage style, something for a wedding or an evening out, or something trendy and fashionable. This will help you decide which styling technique you need to consider using.
- Look at all the factors that can influence your choice of technique.
- Decide if you can achieve what the client has asked for. If you cannot then you will need to suggest something different.
- Select any products to use, such as mousse or setting lotion or heat protectors, etc.
- Decide how you will carry out the technique and the tools and equipment you need to use.

HANDY HINTS

Make sure you check the hair and scalp for diseases and conditions. If the client has a contagious disease you will not be able to carry out the service.

COMMUNICATION AND BEHAVIOUR

Consulting with your client will be a mixture of talking to her and looking and feeling her hair. You may be great at styling, but it won't really mean anything unless you're also very good at communicating with the client. You'll need to be confident about what you're doing, and think carefully about the types of question you're asking. Refer to Chapter 102 for more details about communication and behaviour.

HANDY HINTS

Don't forget to talk to the client while you are carrying out the service. For many clients a friendly chat is one of the reasons they visit the salon.

ACTIVITY

Make a list of all the things you need to find out from the client so you can decide what you are going to do:

- Include all the factors that may influence your decisions.
- Write down how you will find out the information, eg questioning the client, looking at or feeling the hair and scalp.
- Make a list of the questions you could ask the client.
- Working in pairs, try out your questions and observations to see if you get the information you need.

HANDY HINTS

Don't forget your posture when working. Good posture will influence the client's impression and be healthier for you.

SHAMPOO AND CONDITION THE CLIENT'S HAIR

When you have finished your consultation, the next step is to shampoo the hair ready for the styling service. Chapter 003 Shampooing and conditioning hair describes the method of shampooing and conditioning the hair ready for other services.

HANDY HINTS

Read Chapter 003 Shampooing and conditioning hair, to refresh your knowledge of the procedure.

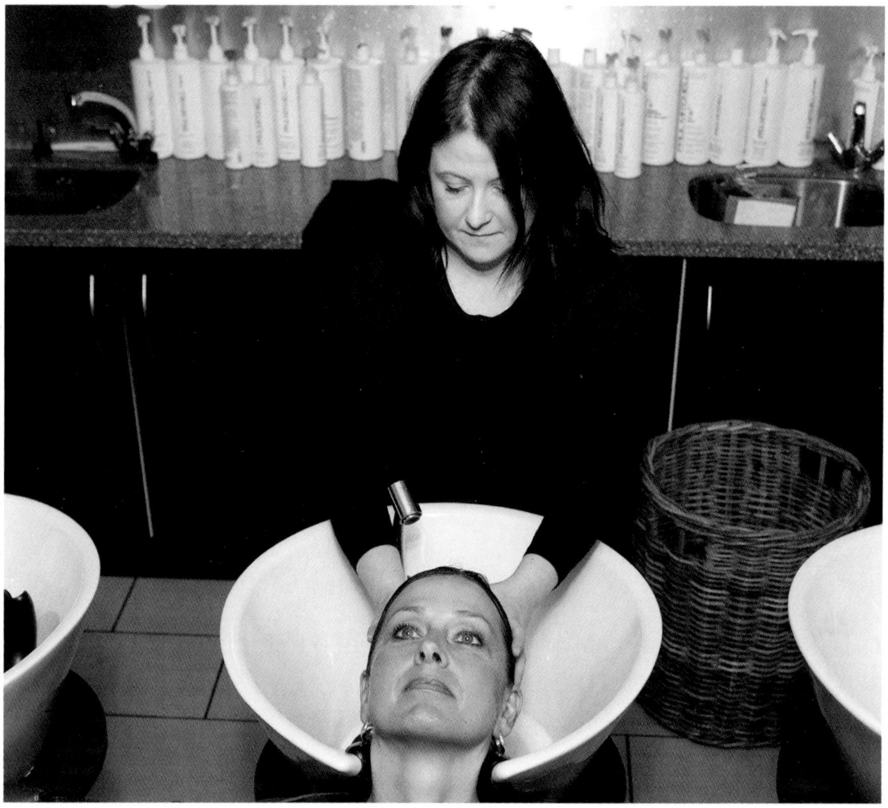

HANDY HINTS

When you towel dry after shampooing do not over dry the hair. For the styling process to work properly the hair should be moist but not dripping water. If the hair is too dry it will be difficult to get the shape you need.

Don't forget to use conditioner if the hair needs it. Make sure the client agrees to have it.

PROVIDE STYLING FOR WOMEN

This part of the chapter looks at appropriate products, tools and equipment for styling women's hair and the basic techniques for styling women's hair safely and professionally.

TOOLS AND EQUIPMENT USED IN BASIC STYLING TECHNIQUES

Tools and equipment	Use
Wide-toothed comb 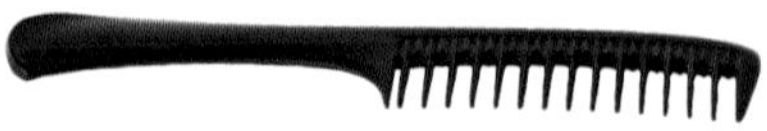	Used to detangle hair before styling.
Cutting comb 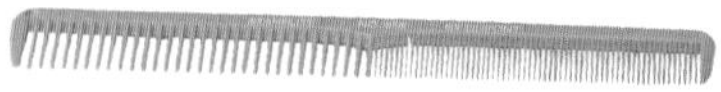	Used to split the hair into sections to keep it under control while you work.
Tail/pintail comb 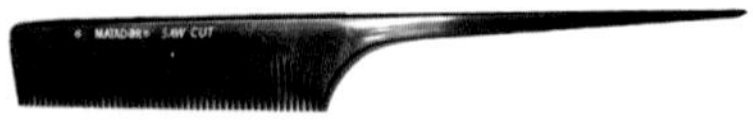	Used when setting and pin curling to make the sections to be wound on the roller or made into a pin curl.
Dressing out comb 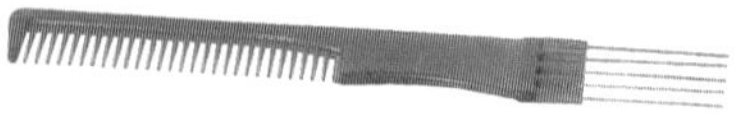	Used when the hair has been dried, to backcomb and dress the hair into shape and finish the style.
Sectioning clips 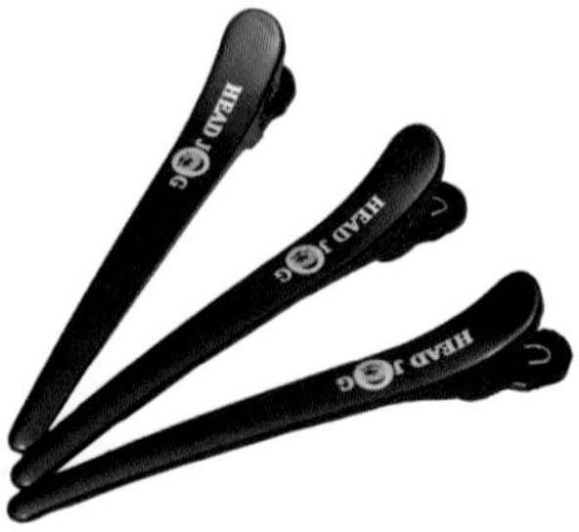	Used to secure the hair as you work.
Bristle brush 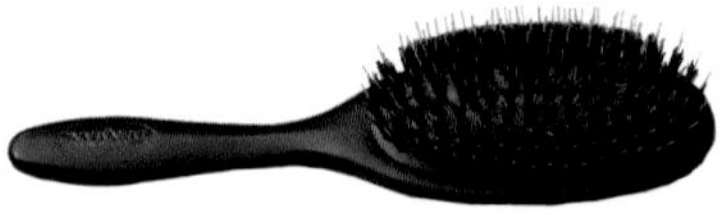	This is a soft brush used for general brushing and to remove roller marks when you are setting and dressing the hair.

Tools and equipment	Use
Denman brush 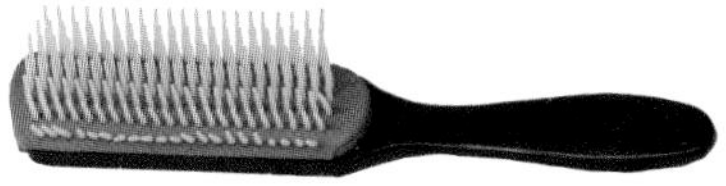	Used in blow drying to create a smooth, straight finish such as for a 'bob' style.
Vent brush 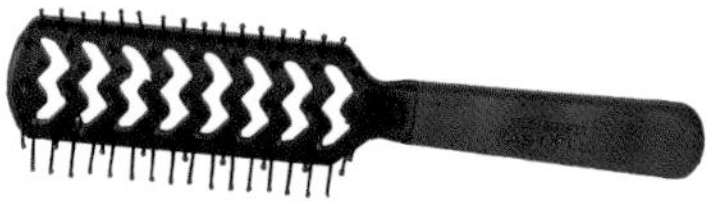	Used to create a textured straight finish when blow drying.
Radial brush 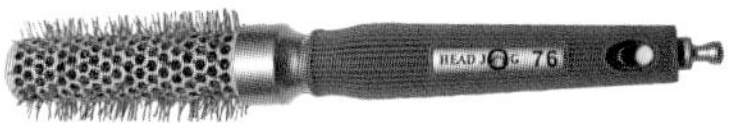	Radial brushes come in different sizes and are used to create root lift, curls and waves in hair of different lengths.
Rollers 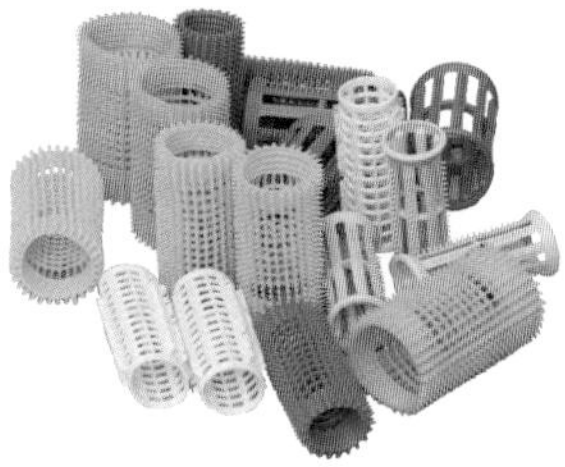	Rollers come in a range of sizes from small to large. They are used to set the hair. They produce lift, waves and curls.
Pins 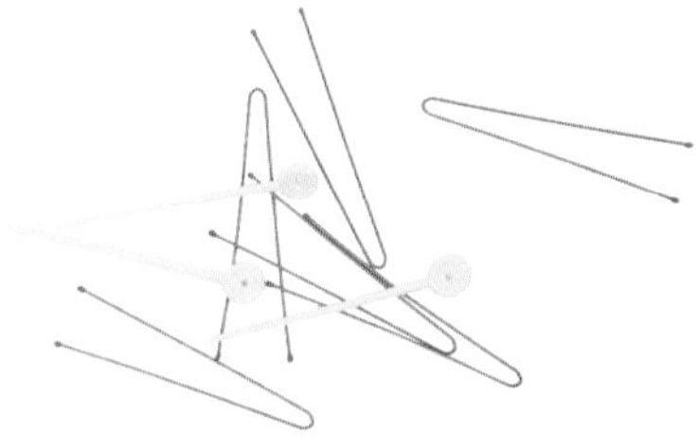	These are used to secure the rollers when setting the hair.
Pin curl clips 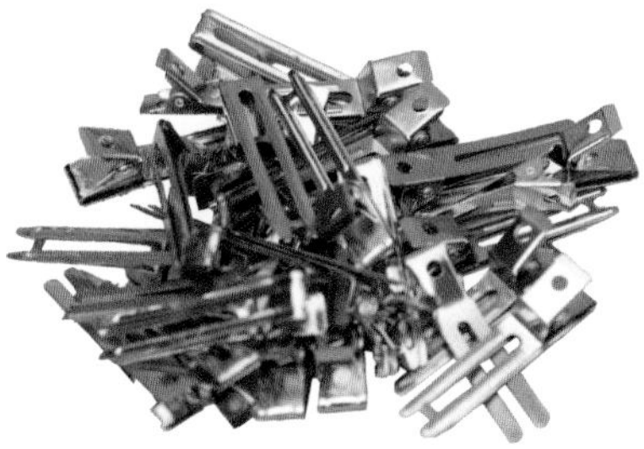	These are spring-loaded clips that are used to hold the hair in place when pin curling.

Tools and equipment	Use
Grips 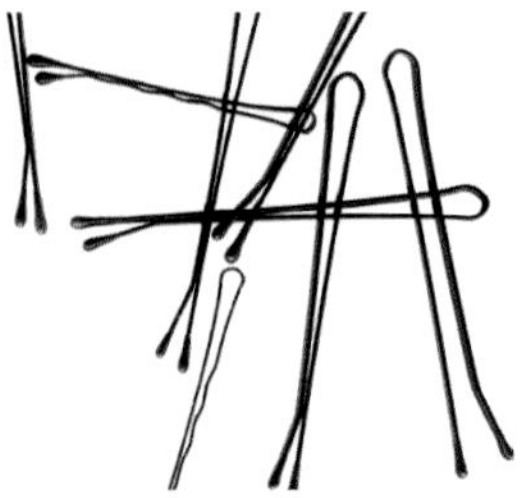	Sometimes called 'kirby' grips. They are used to hold hair in position when dressing out long hair in a hair-up style.
Hand-held dryer 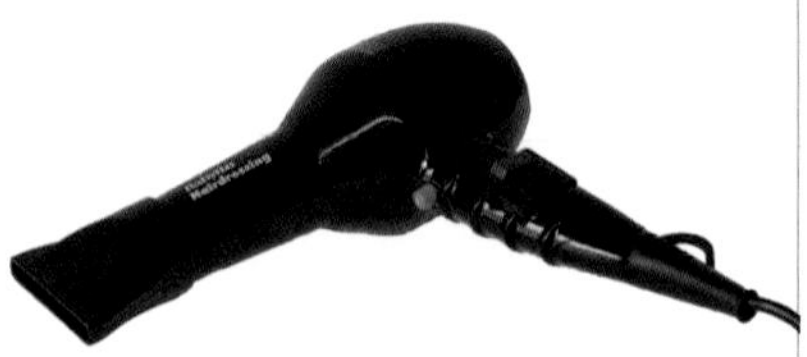	Used to dry the hair during blow drying. Has different heat settings and speeds.
Diffuser 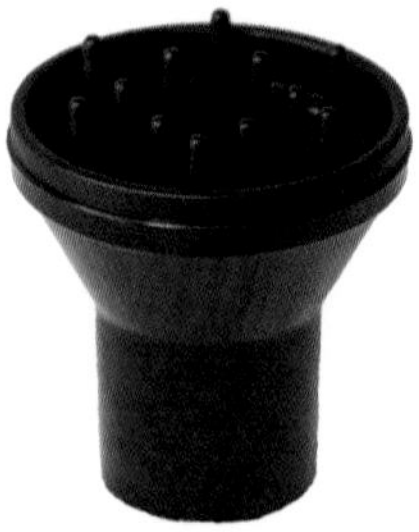	An attachment for a hand dryer used when finger drying. It spreads the air and decreases its force.
Nozzle 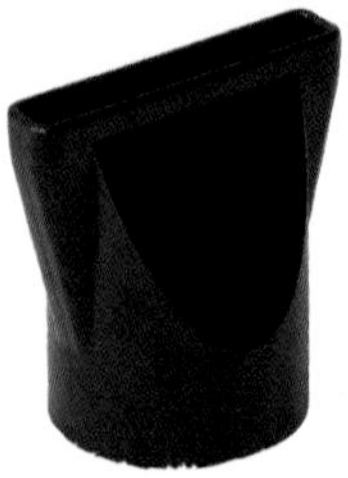	Another attachment for a hand dryer that allows you to direct the airflow and heat more accurately when blow drying.
Straightening irons 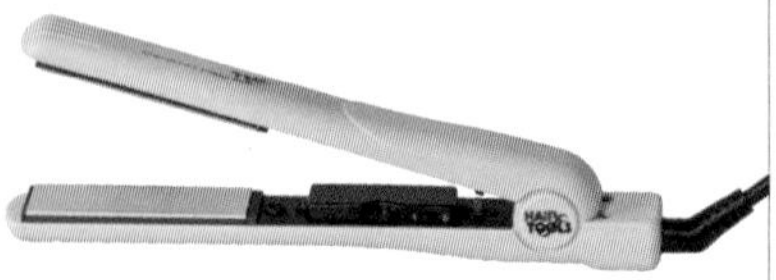	These have flat, heated surfaces that are used on dry hair to straighten and smoothe it.
Tongs 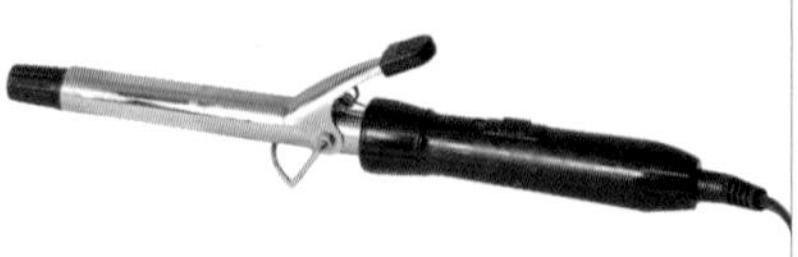	These have a round barrel shape that is heated. Used on dry hair to create curl and body.

Tools and equipment	Use
Hood dryer 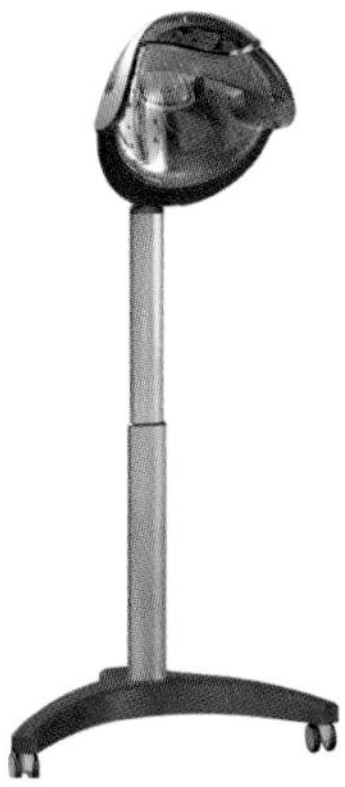	Used to dry hair that has been set.
Heated rollers 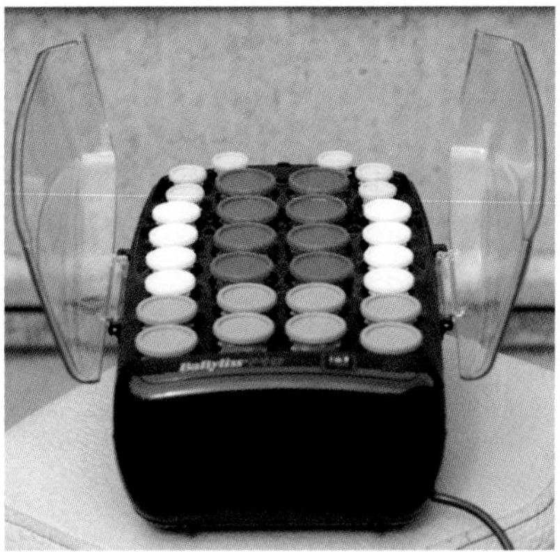	These are electrically heated rollers that are used on dry hair to refresh the style and shape.
Gown 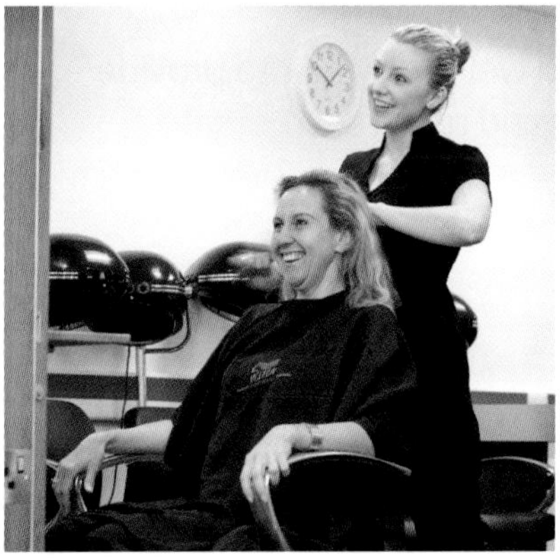	This will cover the client and help to prevent anything getting onto her clothes.
Towels 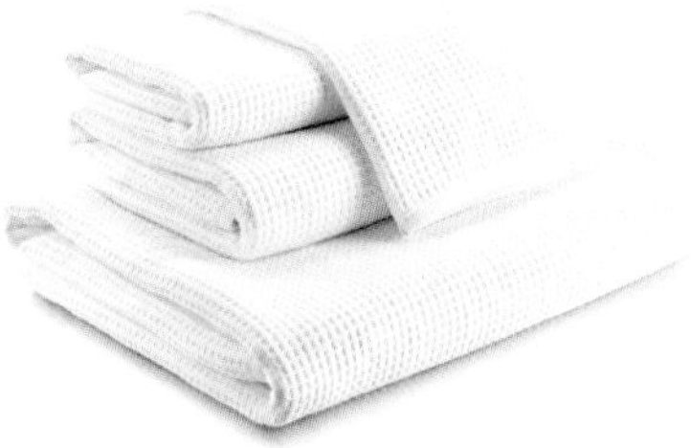	Used when shampooing and styling to prevent the client's clothing from getting wet.

Tools and equipment	Use
Hand mirror 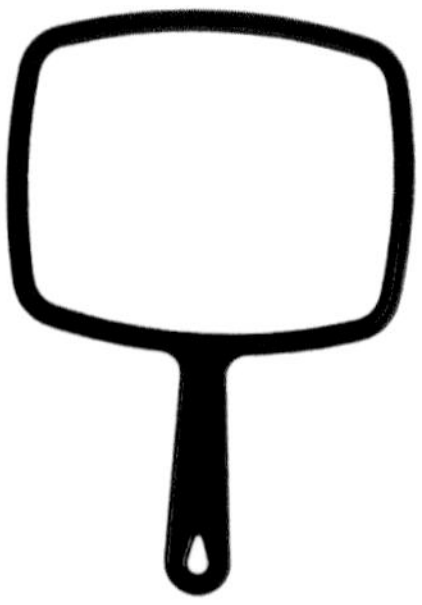	Used to show the client the back of her head so she can see the finished result.

PRODUCTS USED IN BASIC STYLING TECHNIQUES

Product	Use
Mousse 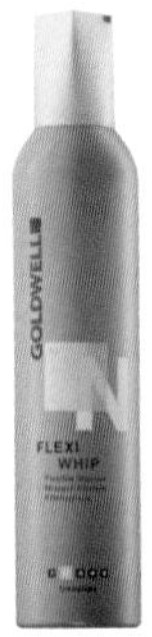	Used on wet hair before blow drying or setting. It gives support and hold to the style, making it last longer.
Gel 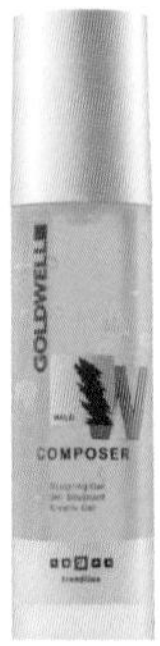	Used on wet or dry hair to provide volume and texture.
Blow dry/setting lotion 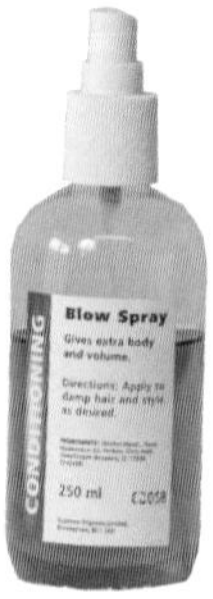	Similar to mousse but in liquid form; used on wet hair before blow drying or setting. Gives volume, lift and support for fine hair.

Product	Use
Hairspray 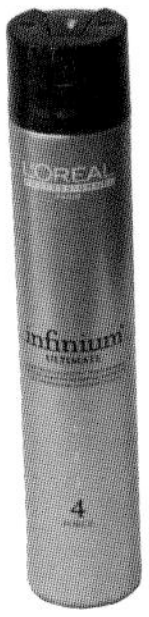	Sprayed lightly onto dry hair when dressing or drying is finished. It holds the hair in place and gives it shine.
Moisturiser 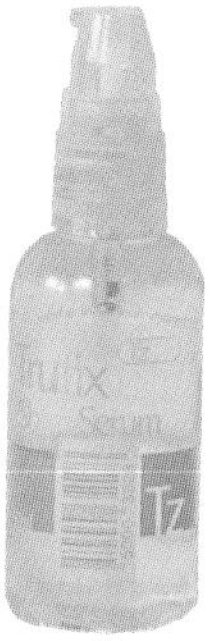	Used on wet hair when blow drying to help smoothe frizzy, curly hair to get a straighter look.
Wax 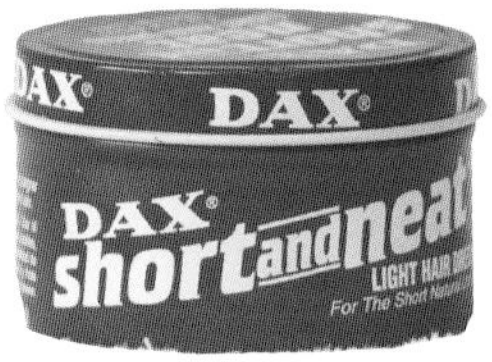	Applied to dry hair to achieve a 'spiky', 'messy' look. Can also be used to smoothe flyaway hair when doing a hair up.
Heat protector 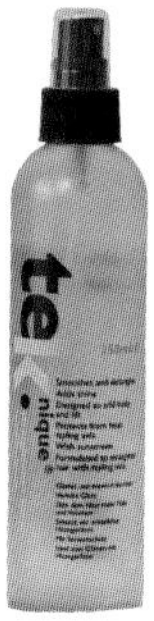	Sprayed onto dry hair before using heated appliances such as tongs, straighteners, etc. Protects the hair from the effects of the heat.

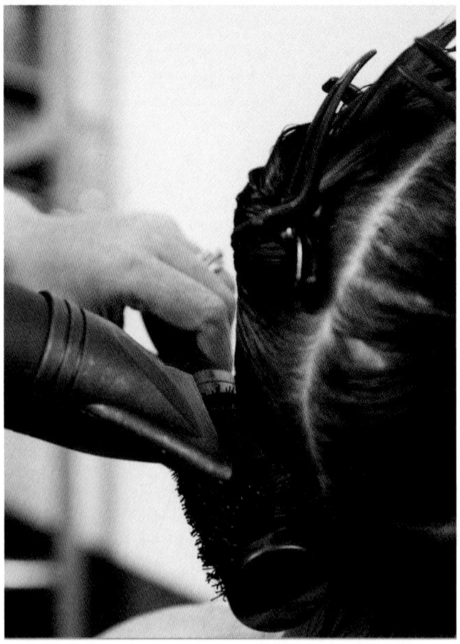

Holding the dryer still in one place or getting the dryer too close to the hair may burn the client's scalp

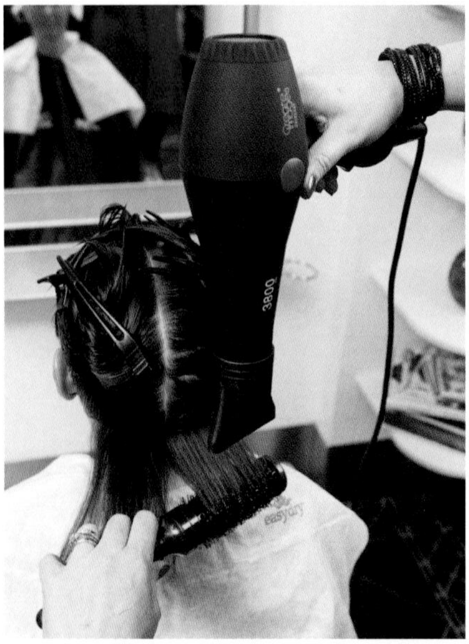

HANDY HINTS

Keep the hair tight so when you put the clip in it is not loose and floppy. You will have better control and it looks more professional to the client.

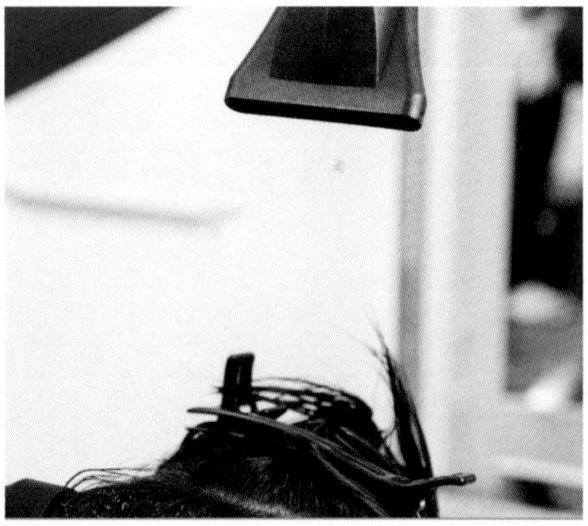

Stylist holding the dryer 15 cm from the scalp

BLOW DRYING THE HAIR

The most important thing to remember when you are blow drying is to have the hair under control. If the hair is not under control you will not get the shape and finish you want. Remember to work safely. You will be using heat to dry the hair. Concentrate on what you are doing all the time.

APPLYING PRODUCT

When you are ready to start your blow dry, apply any styling product that you wish to use. Be careful to follow the manufacturer's instructions.

Do not apply too much – use only as much as you need. Always avoid waste. This costs the salon money. It can also affect the result of your blow dry, making the hair sticky and dull.

SECTIONING THE HAIR

When you are blow drying medium to long hair divide it into sections. Use a sectioning clip to secure them. This will keep the hair out of the way as you dry each section.

A simple sectioning procedure would be:

Divide the hair into four sections. Part from the centre of the forehead to the centre of the nape; then from the crown to the back of the ear on each side. Secure each section with a clip.

Take one of the back sections and make a parting from the centre to the outside about 2 cm thick. (The size of the section will depend on the density of the client's hair.)

Re-secure the main section. Do the same on the other side.

You are now ready to blow the hair dry.

USING THE DRYER

The airflow from the dryer must always be away from the client's scalp. You need to direct the airflow in the direction of the style. Hold the dryer at least 10–15 cm away from the hair as you dry it. If the dryer is too close it can damage the hair.

BRUSHES

Your brush choice will depend on the look you want to achieve and the hair you are working with. For a straight style such as a classic bob, a Denman brush would be used. A radial brush will give lift and volume.

The airflow should be directed onto the brush. Do not direct the airflow to the hair between the brush and the scalp. This will spoil the shape you are looking to get.

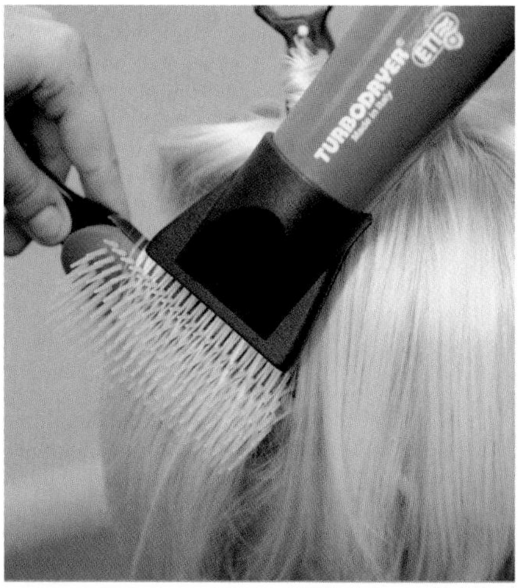

Using a Denman brush

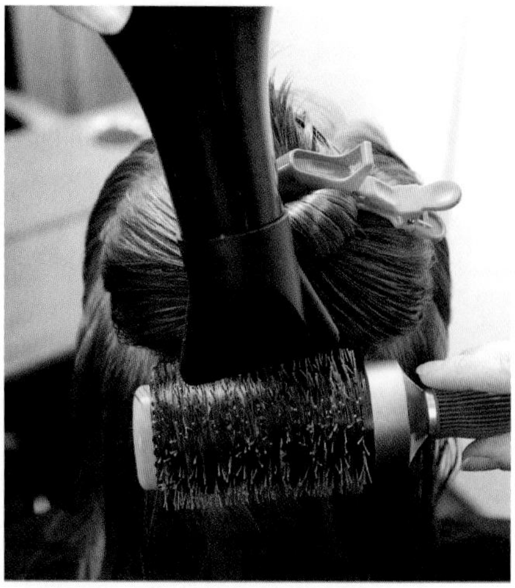

Using a radial brush

TENSION

Keep your tension even as you blow dry the hair. This will give you a smoother finish. Do not use too much tension as this may cause discomfort to the client.

ANGLES

Changing the angle of the brush and the dryer will help you get the shape you want. You need to practise holding the dryer and brush in both hands. Holding the dryer and brush in different positions is a must so you can move around the client and get the best result.

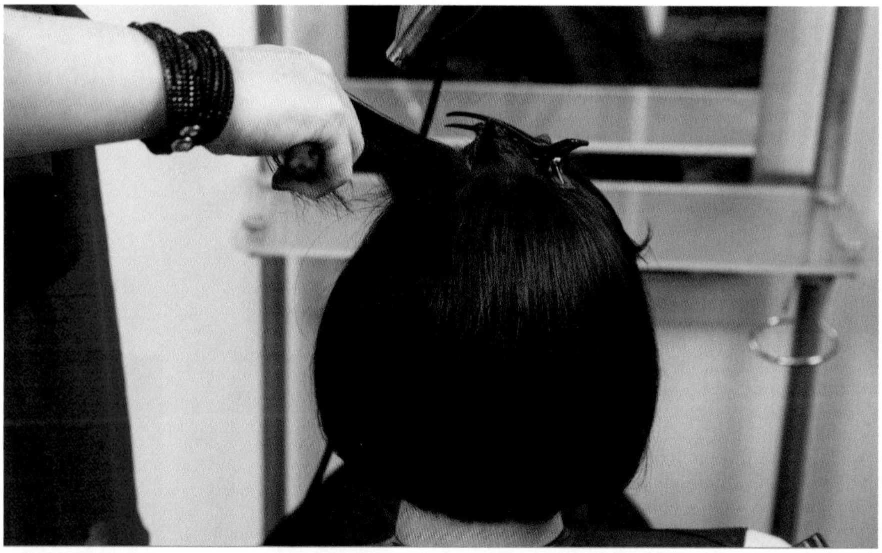

A 90 degree angle

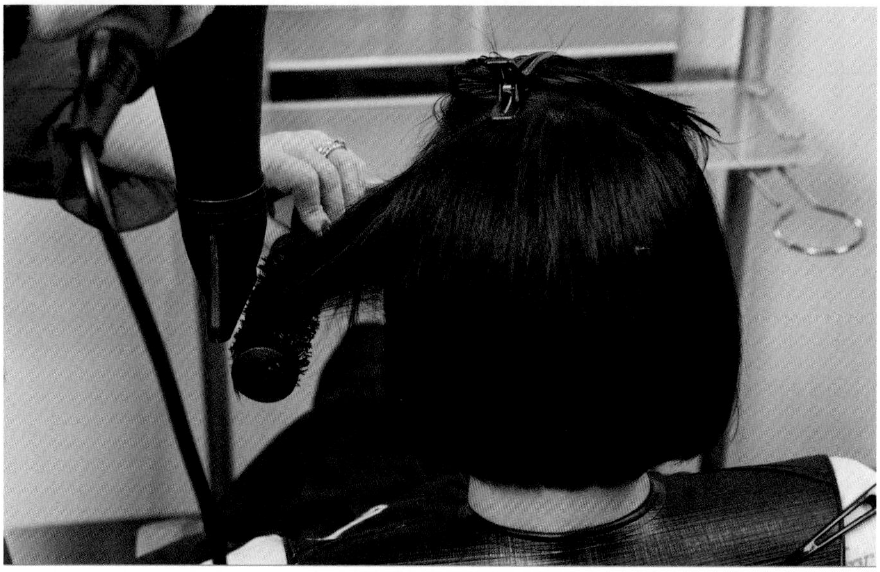

A 45 degree angle

STEP-BY-STEP BLOW DRYING A CLASSIC 'BOB' STYLE

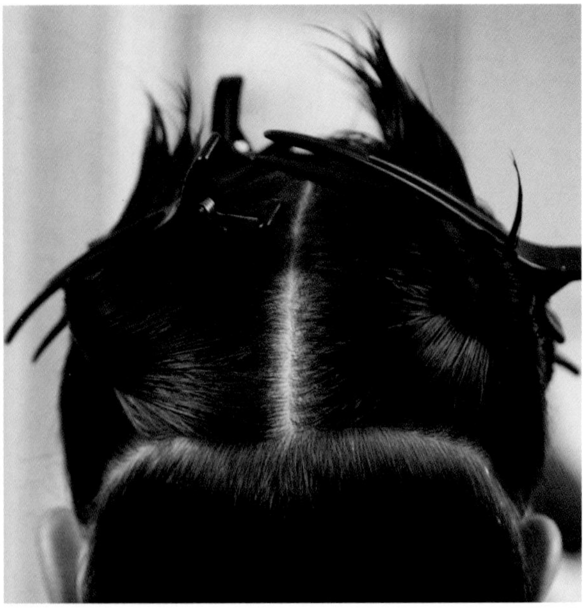

STEP 1 – Gown and prepare the client. Section the hair ready to start work.

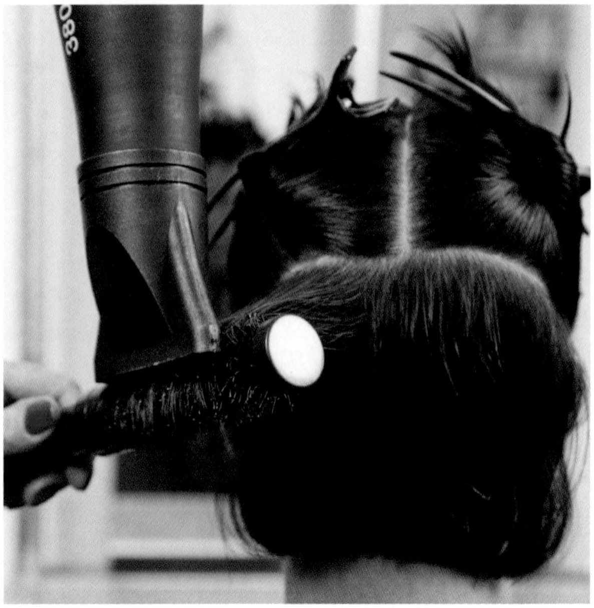

STEP 2 – Take a small section and roll the hair on the brush. Dry the hair from root to point. Direct the hot air in the direction you want it to go.

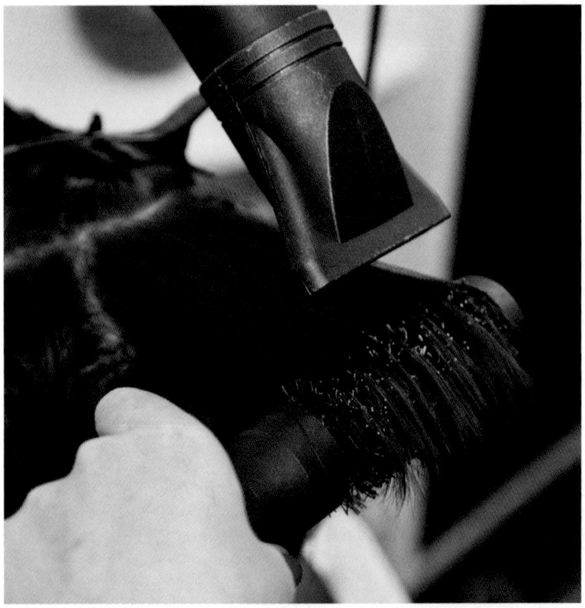

STEP 3 – Make sure the points of the hair are straight. Do not get the dryer too close to the hair or scalp.

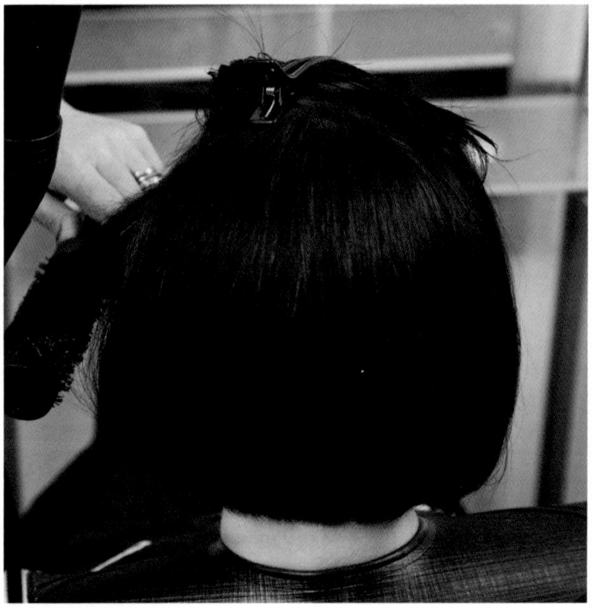

STEP 4 – Dry the hair in sections up to the crown. Then dry the sides and lastly the front.

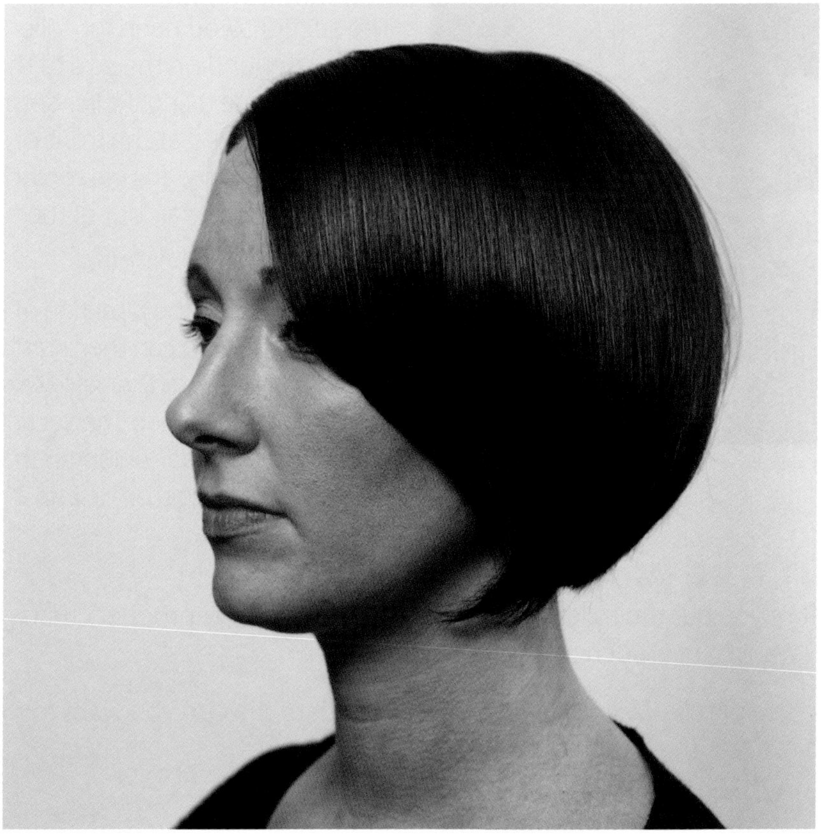

STEP 5 – Check the balance and make sure the client is happy with the finished style.

ROLLER SETTING AND DRESSING HAIR

In this technique the hair is wound on curlers of various sizes. This will give lift and curl to the hair. When the hair is dry the rollers are removed and the hair is brushed and combed into shape. This is called dressing the hair.

TENSION AND CONTROL

As with blow drying, keeping the hair under control is important. Using even tension when you are putting in the rollers will give you the direction and finish you want. Don't use too much tension as this can be uncomfortable for the client and can damage the hair.

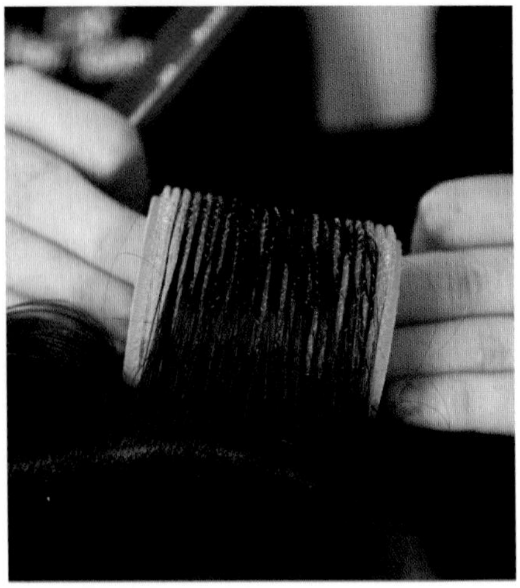
This section is the correct size

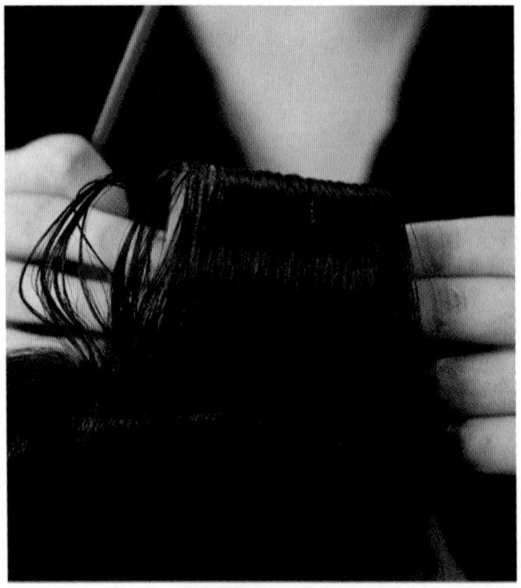
This section is too big

SECTIONING

The sections you need for roller setting depend on the size of the rollers you are using. Roller setting is usually started at the front of the head. This means you do not need to clip the hair out of the way as you do in blow drying.

Comb the hair in the direction of the finished style. You can then start to put your rollers into the hair. Make a section for each roller. The section should not be wider or longer than the size of roller you are using.

HANDY HINTS

If you are using metal pins they will get hot during drying and could burn the client's scalp.

PUTTING IN A ROLLER

Before you put the rollers in, don't forget to apply any products that you want to use, such as setting lotion.

The size of roller will depend on the strength of the curl you want to achieve and the length of the hair.

- Large rollers will give softer waves and curls.
- Smaller rollers will give tighter waves and curls.
- The longer the hair the larger the roller should be.
- The shorter the hair the smaller the roller should be.

The pattern you use when you put the rollers in is determined by the finished style you want to get. For example:

- If you want a fringe in your style then the rollers will be placed going to one side at the front.
- If you want the hair to cover the ears then the rollers will be wound downwards.

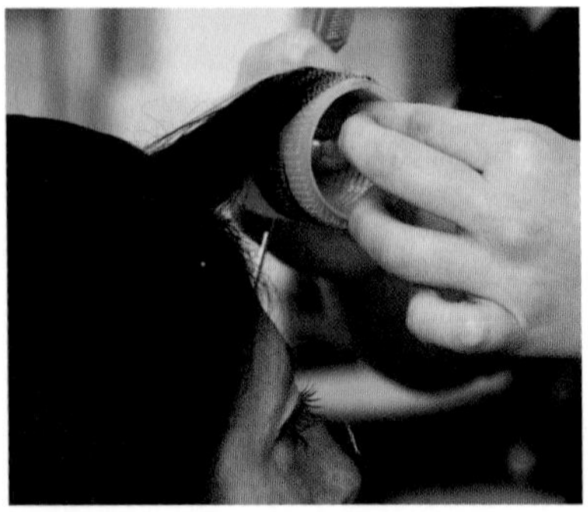
STEP 1 – For a full fringe wind the roller forwards.

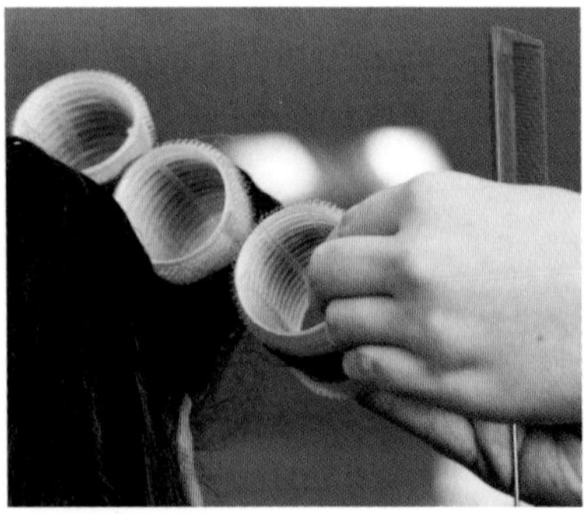
STEP 2 – Winding the rollers like this will let the hair cover the ear when you dress out your style.

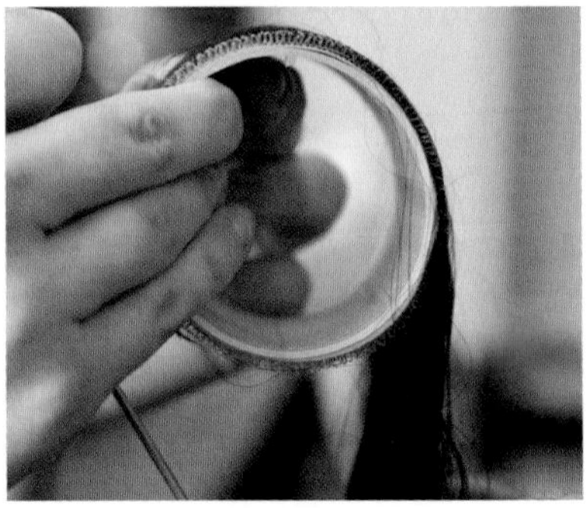
STEP 3 – To get height in the style make sure the roller sits on its own base.

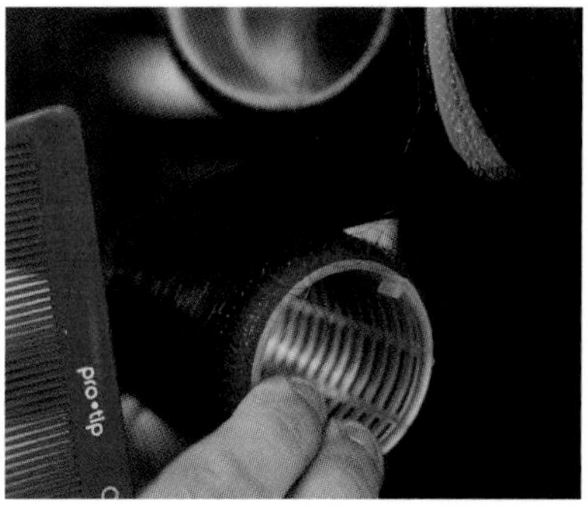

STEP 4 – To keep the style flat wind the roller so it sits off the base.

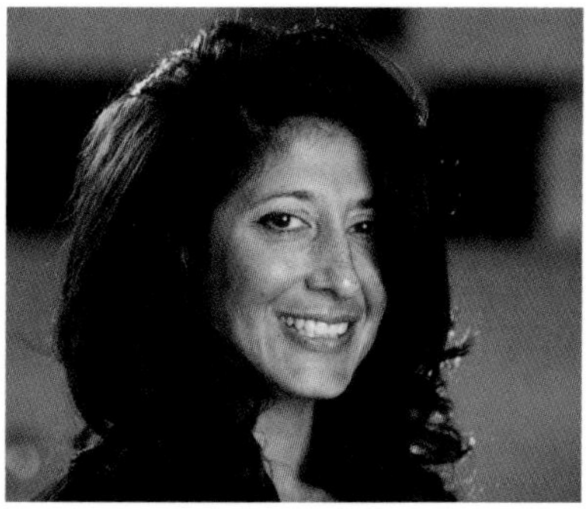

STEP 5 – The finished look.

To get lift when you set you must make sure the roller is sitting on its base. When you make the section, comb the hair up and away from you. Hold the hair at more than 90 degrees from the scalp and wind the roller back towards you.

If you do not want root lift, then when you comb the section hold it at less than 90 degrees from the scalp. When you wind the roller down it will not sit on its base. You will see a flat area from the root to the start of the roller. This will decrease the amount of root lift you get.

STEP-BY-STEP ROLLER SETTING AND DRESSING OUT

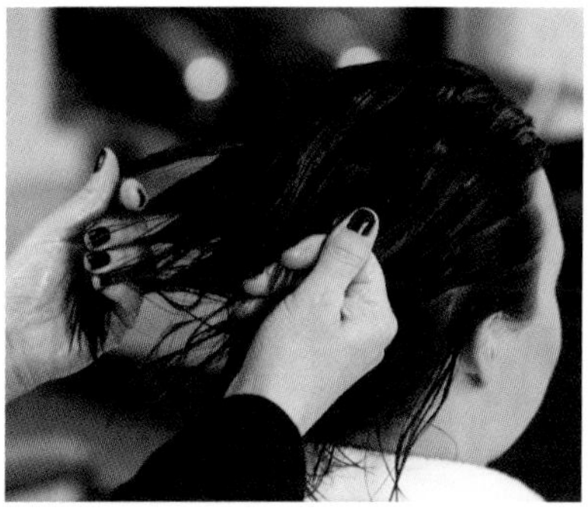

STEP 1 – Comb the hair into the direction you want it to finish.

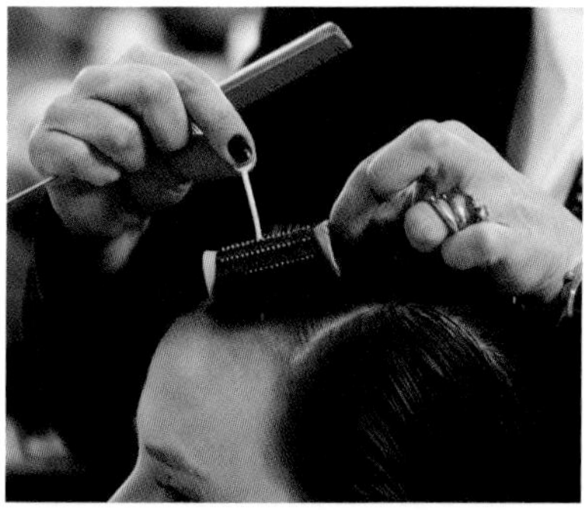

STEP 2 – Start at the front. Make a section and wind the roller in the direction you want it to go. Secure with a pin.

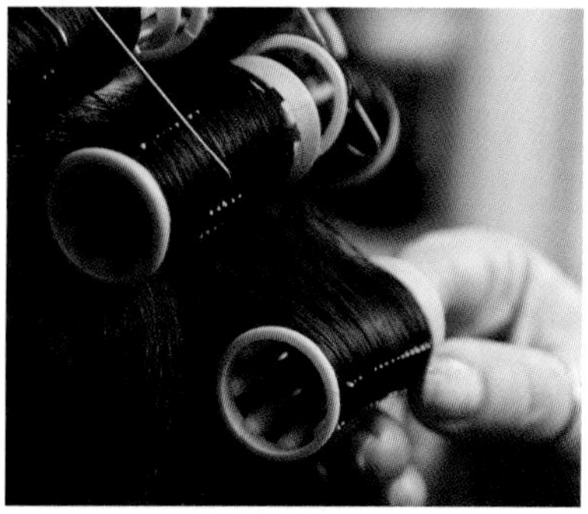

STEP 3 – Follow the pattern you decided during consultation. If you do not want root lift then 'drag' the roller down.

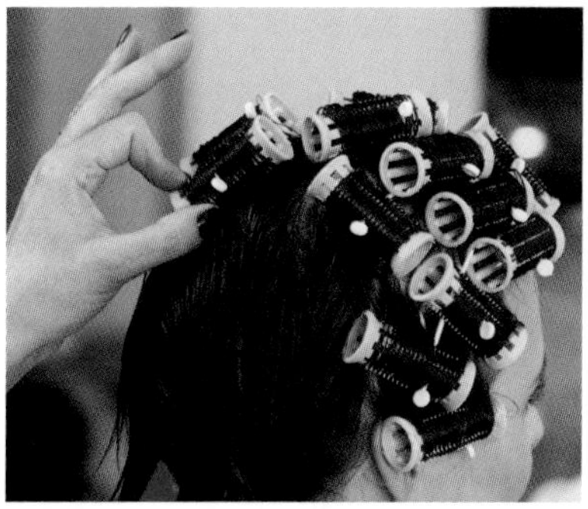

STEP 4 – Continue to take clean sections and use the size of roller to give you the right amount of curl for the style you have chosen.

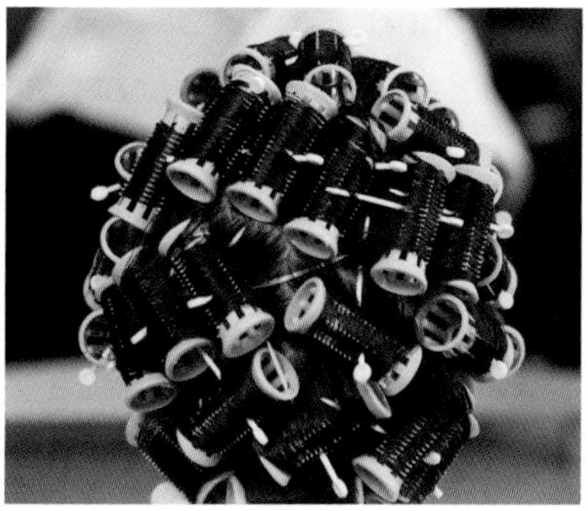

STEP 5 – When you have put all the rollers in check that they are in the right place and that they are secure but not too tight which may be uncomfortable for the client and damage the hair.

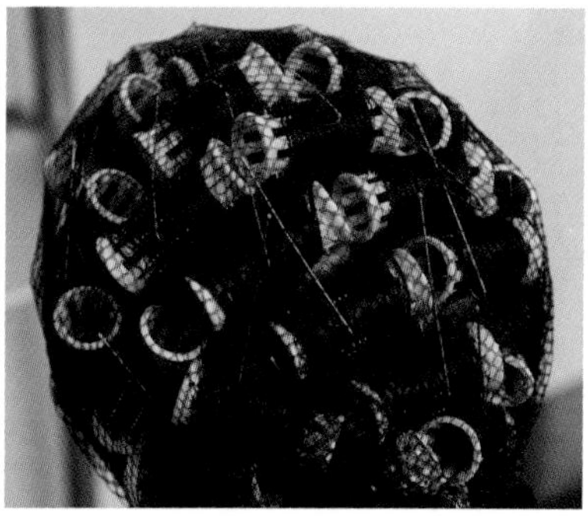

STEP 6 – Cover the rollers with a net and don't forget to use ear protectors.

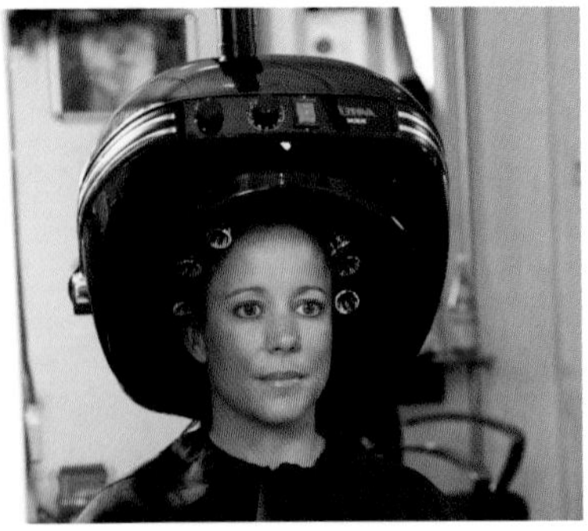

STEP 7 – Put the client under a hood dryer to dry. Make sure the temperature is comfortable.

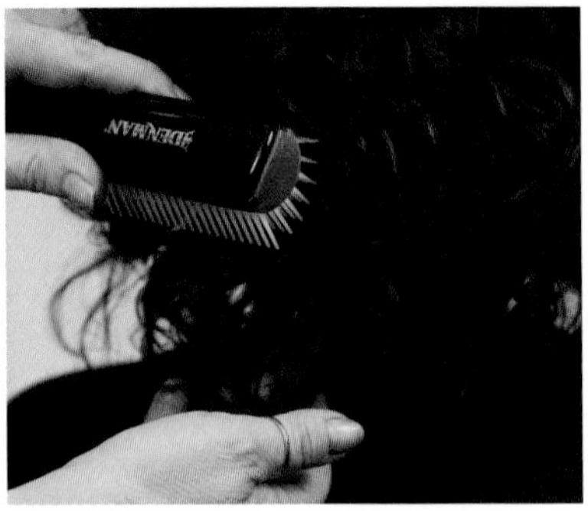

STEP 8 – Let the hair cool and then remove the rollers. Brush the hair in the direction of the style to remove the roller marks.

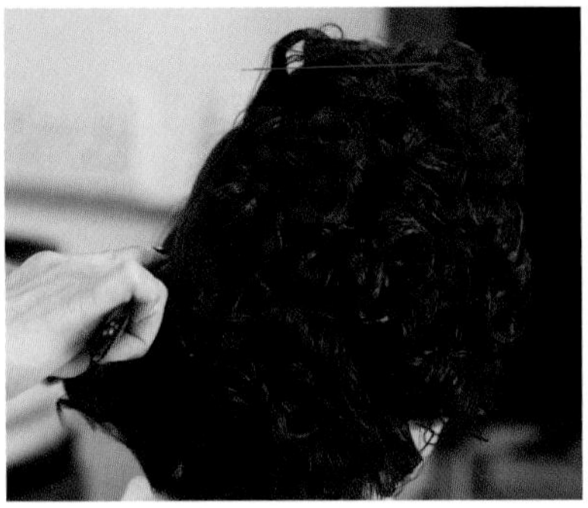

STEP 9 – Finish dressing your style by combing the hair into place. Use hairspray to hold the hair if required and make sure the client is happy with the finished result.

DRYING THE HAIR

When all the rollers have been put in, a hair net is tied over them. This keeps the rollers in place during drying. A hood dryer is used and takes between 15 and 30 minutes depending on the length and thickness of the hair. Ear pads are used to protect the client's ears from the heat of the dryer.

Make sure the hair is properly dry before you dress it out. Leave the hair to cool for a few minutes. This will make the set last longer. Remove the rollers carefully – being rough may cause the client discomfort.

DRESSING OUT

Using a bristle brush, brush the hair into the shape you want. This loosens and spreads the hair and removes any roller marks. Next, using the dressing out comb, comb and tease the hair into its final shape. This will also give a smooth finish to your style. Apply any finishing products such as hairspray.

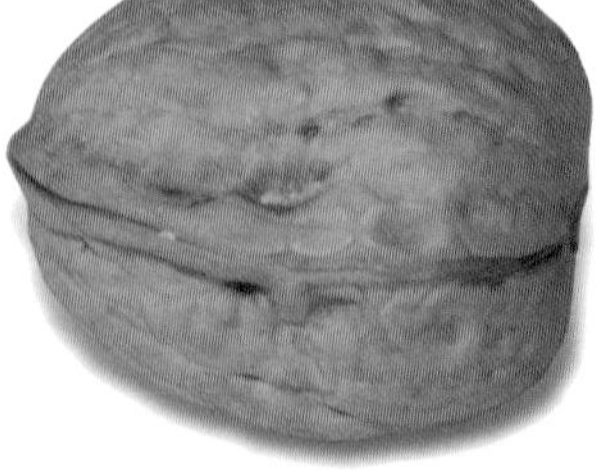

IN A NUTSHELL

You are now at the end of the chapter. Before you test your knowledge with the revision activities, check the following list to see if you feel confident in all the areas covered. If there are still any areas you're unsure of, go back over them in the book and ask your tutor for extra support:

- the basic techniques for styling women's hair
- the factors that can influence your choice of techniques
- how to prepare for styling women's hair
- the tools, equipment and products that are used in styling women's hair and selecting them
- following safe and hygienic working practices
- the importance of good communication, behaviour and attitude when styling women's hair
- styling women's hair using basic techniques.

REVISION ACTIVITIES

Use the questions below to test your knowledge of Chapter 103 to see just how much information you've gained. This can help you to prepare for your assessments. Turn to pages 496–498 for the answers.

WORDS TO FIND

Copy and complete the sentences below. Use these words to help you fill in the gaps.

contra-indication	tension	catagen	widow's peak
medium	towels	open	telogen
Barbicide	double crown	fine	anagen
ultraviolet cabinet	cowlick	gown	sectioned
coarse			

1 A ____________ and a ____________ are both types of growth pattern.

2 Tools used in styling hair can be sterilised using ____________ or an ____________.

3 ____________, ____________ and ____________ are the three stages of the growth cycle of hair.

4 If the hair grows to a point in the middle of the forehead this is called a ____________.

5 When you are blow drying the hair should be ____________ to keep it under control as you work.

6 The client's clothes should be protected by using a ____________ and ____________.

7 ____________, ____________ and ____________ are all types of hair texture.

8 Something that would prevent you from carrying out the service is called a ____________.

9 Questions that start with 'why', 'what', 'where' and 'how' are ____________ questions.

10 Using even ____________ when you are putting in the rollers will give you the direction and finish you want.

TEST YOUR KNOWLEDGE FURTHER

1 Name **four** basic styling techniques that can be used to style women's hair.

2 Name **four** factors that can influence your choice of technique.

3 Why is it important to prepare your work area before you start work on the client?

4 Name **three** styling products that can be used during styling and state what they are used for.

5 Name **four** tools or pieces of equipment that can be used for blow drying.

6 Why is it important to listen when you are consulting with the client?

7 What PPE would you use to protect your client when blow drying?

8 Why should the hair be sectioned when blow drying?

9 What size section should you use when putting in a roller?

10 Name **two** things that will promote a good atmosphere and image in the salon.

104 STYLING MEN'S HAIR

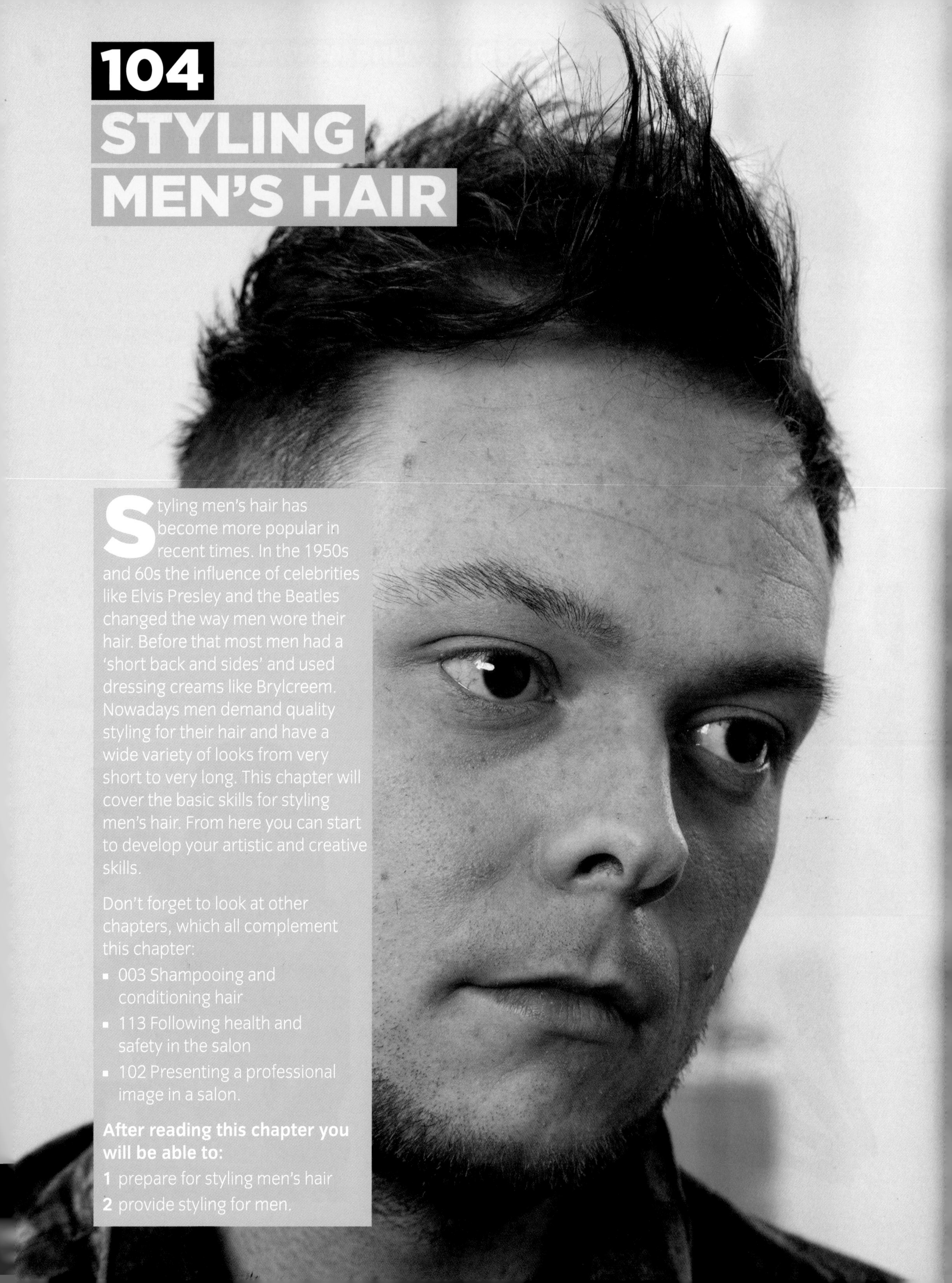

Styling men's hair has become more popular in recent times. In the 1950s and 60s the influence of celebrities like Elvis Presley and the Beatles changed the way men wore their hair. Before that most men had a 'short back and sides' and used dressing creams like Brylcreem. Nowadays men demand quality styling for their hair and have a wide variety of looks from very short to very long. This chapter will cover the basic skills for styling men's hair. From here you can start to develop your artistic and creative skills.

Don't forget to look at other chapters, which all complement this chapter:

- 003 Shampooing and conditioning hair
- 113 Following health and safety in the salon
- 102 Presenting a professional image in a salon.

After reading this chapter you will be able to:

1 prepare for styling men's hair
2 provide styling for men.

PREPARE FOR STYLING MEN'S HAIR

In this part of the chapter you will learn the basic techniques for styling men's hair, including factors that influence the choice of hair styling techniques for men and the importance of the preparation procedures for styling men's hair.

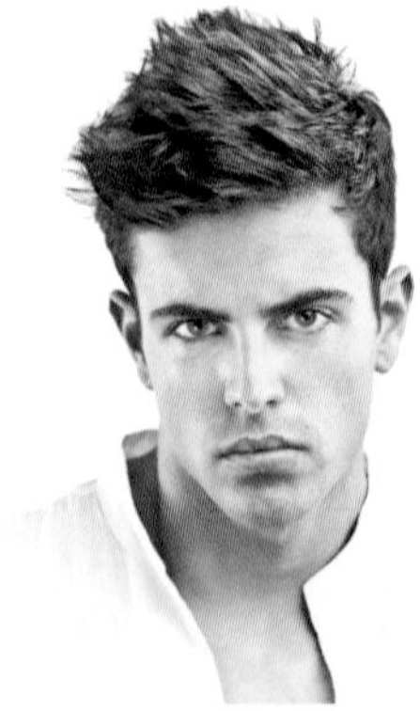

THE BASIC TECHNIQUES FOR STYLING MEN'S HAIR

BLOW DRYING

Blow drying is a widely used styling **technique**. The style is usually affected by the cut, which puts shape and direction into the hair. Blow drying puts the finish to that shape. It can be carried out on all lengths of wet hair. Modern fashion combines blow drying with the use of texturising and defining products (see products further on in the chapter).

- The barber/stylist will use a hand-held dryer to provide the hot air needed to dry the hair.
- The brush is used to direct the hair into the desired shape.
- The hot air from the dryer is directed on to the hair to dry it in that direction.
- On longer hair the brush can be used to add lift to the hair.
- Different types of brush are used to give root lift and smoothness to the style.

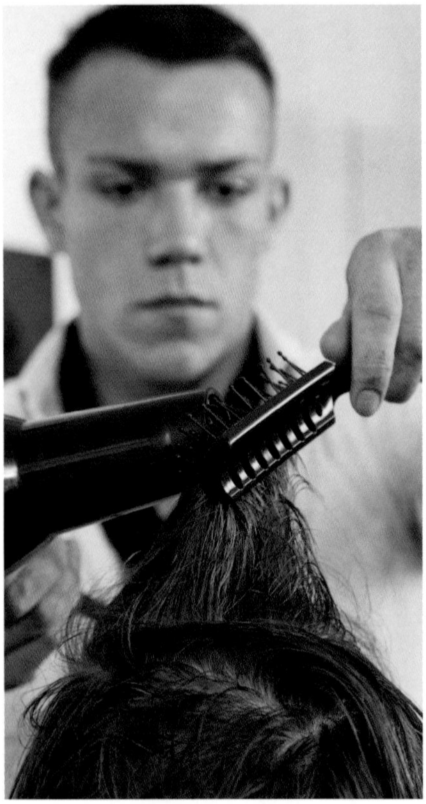

Technique
Procedure; the way things are done

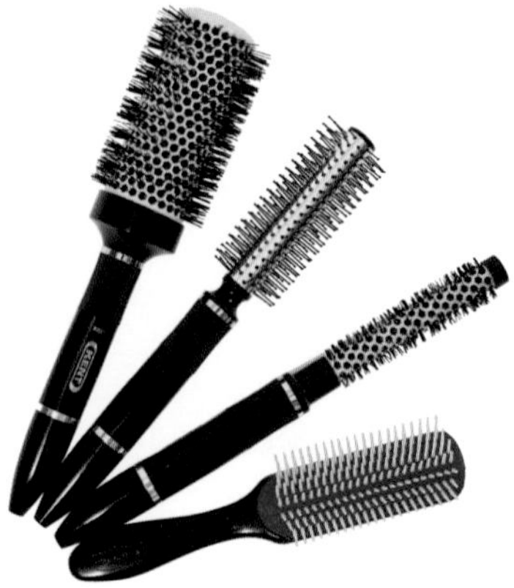

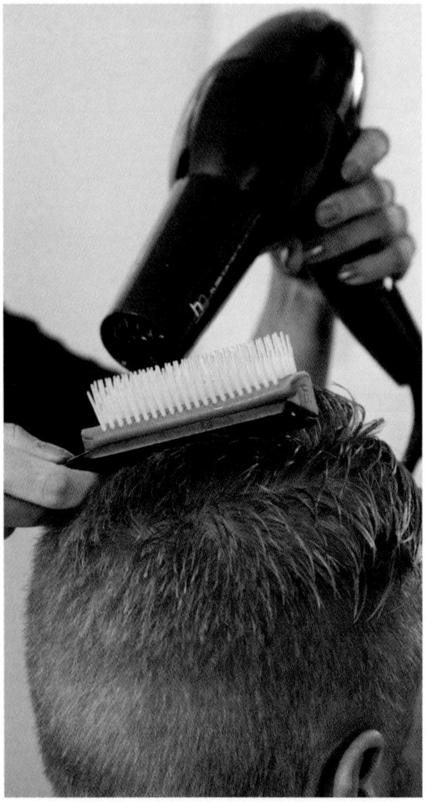

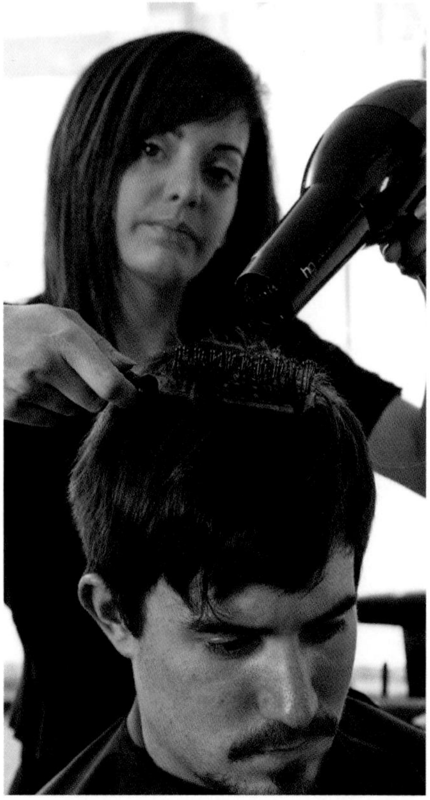

FINGER DRYING

Finger drying is a technique similar to blow drying. The hair is dried using the fingers instead of a brush. It will give soft, natural-looking styles and can be used on medium to long hair.

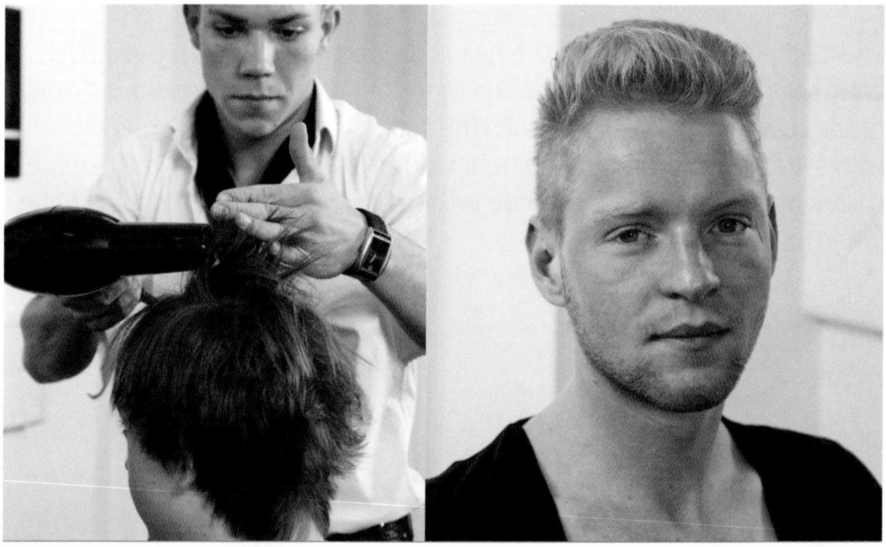

The fingers are used to lift the hair and mould it into shape. A diffuser is used with a hand-held dryer to gently dry the hair into the shape required

The next group of styling methods are carried out on dry hair. They can be used on their own to style the hair or as part of other methods. The **appliances** used are heated and the heat produces the finish. Care must be taken to prevent damage to the hair by using too much heat.

Appliances
Equipment used. In styling this might include a hairdryer and straighteners

STRAIGHTENING AND SMOOTHING

This method is used to produce straight hair with a smooth finish. It is usually carried out on longer hair. It can be used on hair with some natural curl to give a straight finish and can also be used after blow drying to get a smooth finish to the style.

This technique uses straighteners. The hair is divided into small sections. The straighteners are closed around the section and then slid gently down the section from the root of the hair to the point.

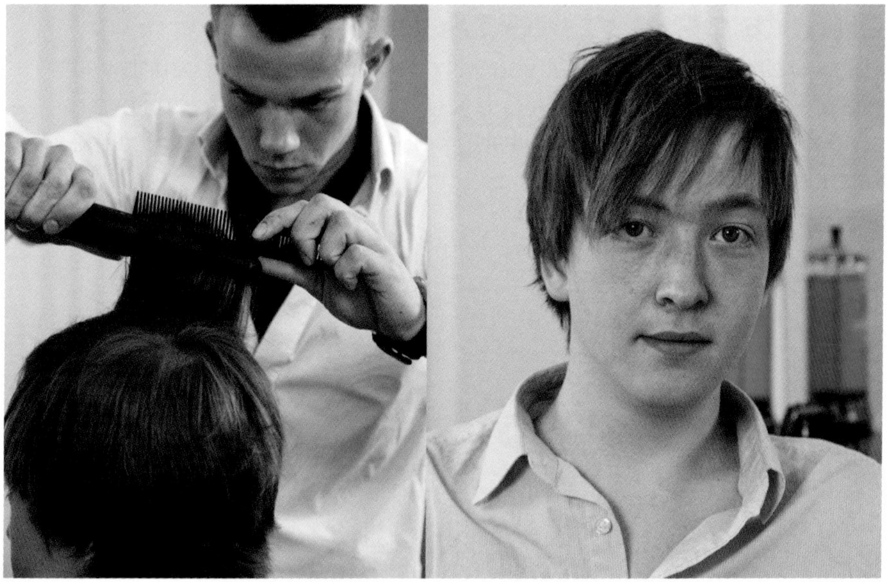

CURLING

This is a styling technique often used to add lift and curl to a blow dry. It can also be used to 'freshen up' a blow dry after a few days. It is very useful on fine hair to give body. Care should be taken not to use too much heat.

This technique uses tongs. The hair is divided into small sections. The points of the hair are placed in the tongs and the tongs are wound down to the root. Take care not to burn the scalp. After a few seconds the tongs are unwound. The hair should look like it does when you take the rollers out when setting. The hair is then brushed or combed into shape when it has cooled.

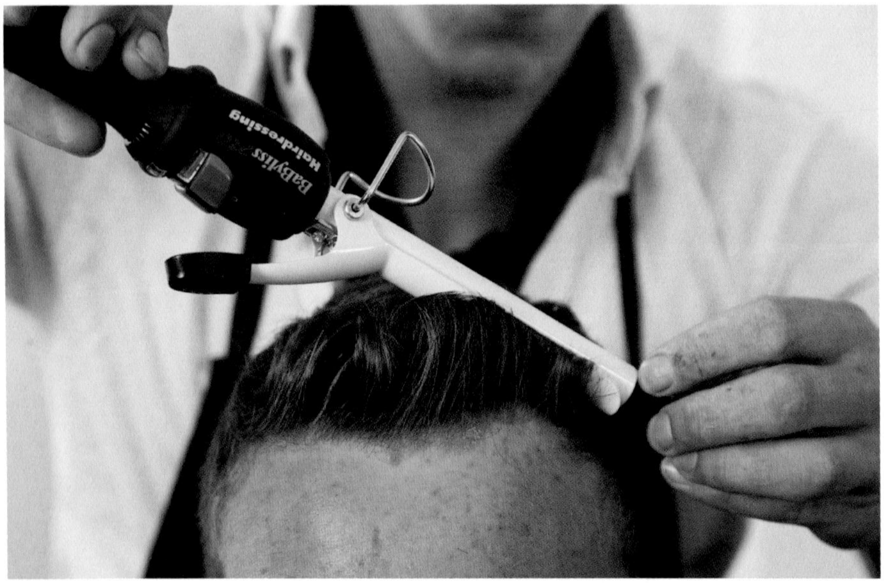

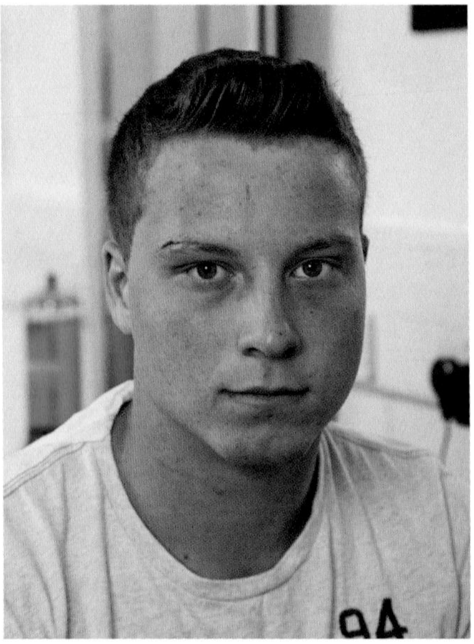

ACTIVITY

Find some pictures of styles that are achieved by these styling techniques. Make some notes of how they were done. Keep your pictures for your assignment.

FACTORS THAT CAN INFLUENCE YOUR CHOICE OF STYLING TECHNIQUES

There are many **factors** that you will need to take into account when you are deciding which technique you are going to use to achieve the style the client wants. They will also help you decide how to use the selected technique.

Factors
Things to consider about the subject

FACE SHAPE

People have different shaped faces. Here are four of the more common ones.

Face shape	Ideal styles for this face shape
Oval 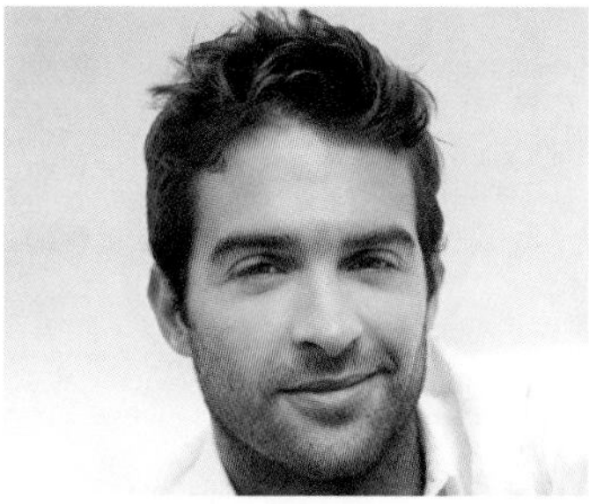	This face shape does not need any correcting. It is the ideal face shape. You can add height or width as you wish.
Square 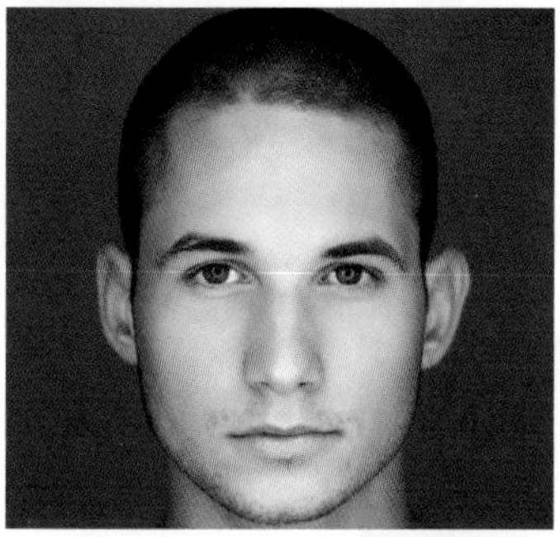	Square faces need to have some height and not too much width.
Oblong 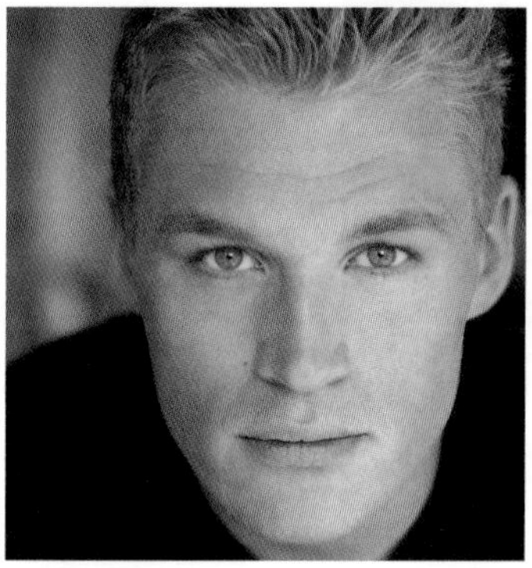	Oblong faces are similar to square faces. They tend to be angular. Avoid height in the style and straight hard lines.
Round 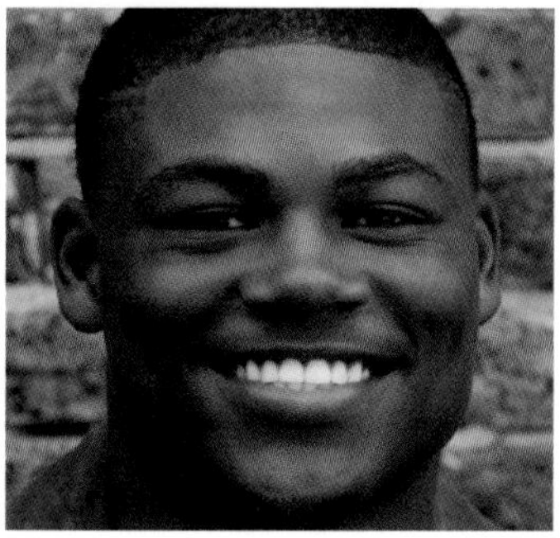	A round face needs to have added height and flatter sides to reduce the width of the face.

ACTIVITY

Look at these photographs of famous people. Try to work out what face shape they have. Collect examples of each of the face shapes mentioned above.

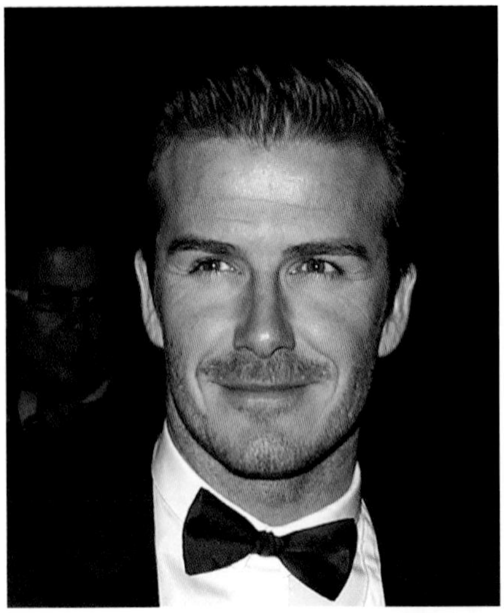

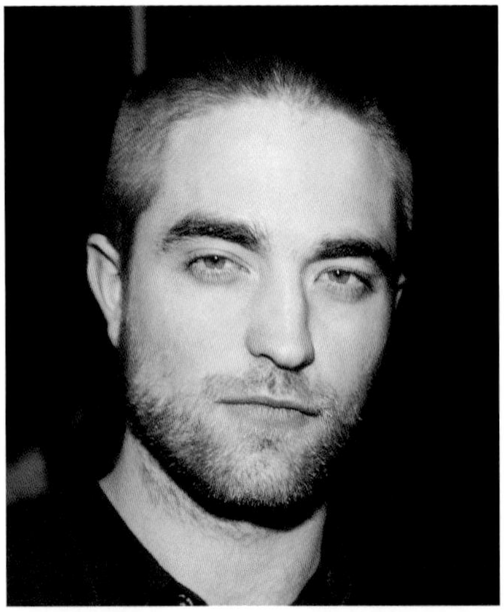

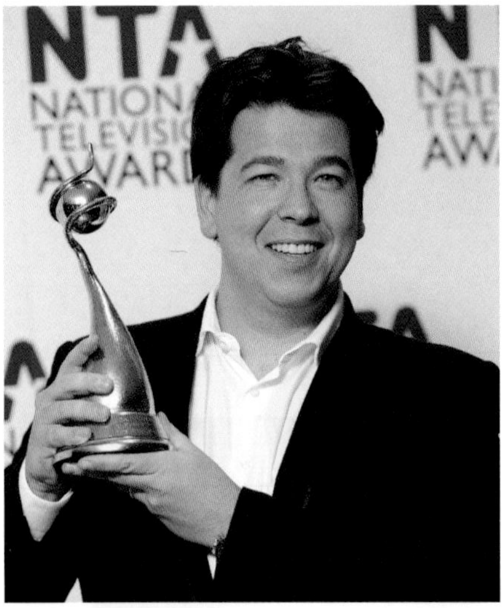

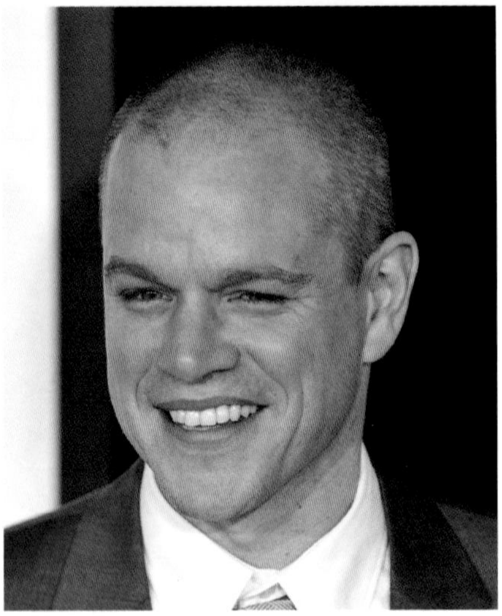

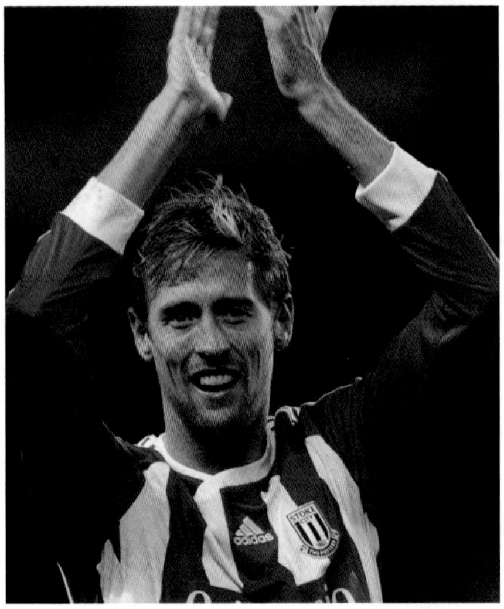

HEAD SHAPE

Head shapes will also be different. Look at the head from the front and from the side. Your style should balance the shape of the head. Add body or height if the head is small. Keep the style flat if the head is large or wide.

BODY SHAPE

The client's body shape can also affect the shape of the style you recommend for him.

- If the client is very thin, try and avoid styles with lots of volume or 'big' styles. It will make his head look bigger and out of proportion to the body.
- If the client is big bodied, don't go for close, short styles that will make the head look small.

You should look for 'balance' between the head and the body with your finished look.

LIFESTYLE

The client's lifestyle is a very important factor in the styling process. It will tell you a lot about his personality and give you clues as to his likes and dislikes. It will tell you if he is outgoing or quiet. You should take note of the following:

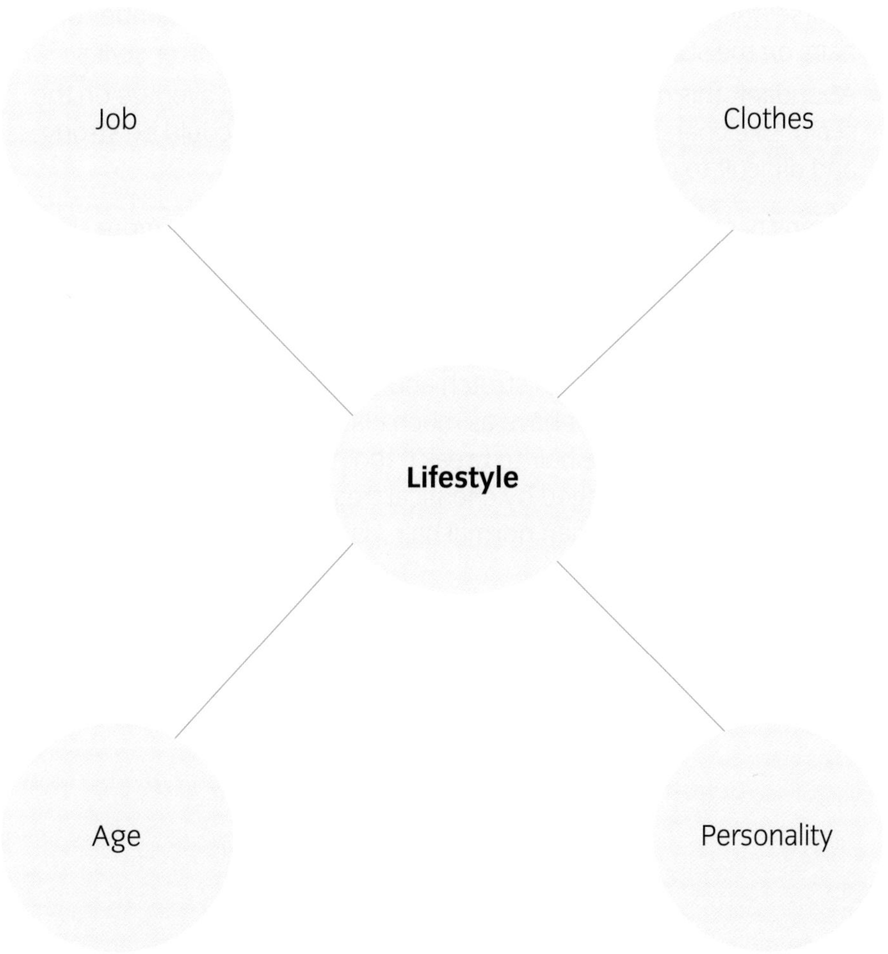

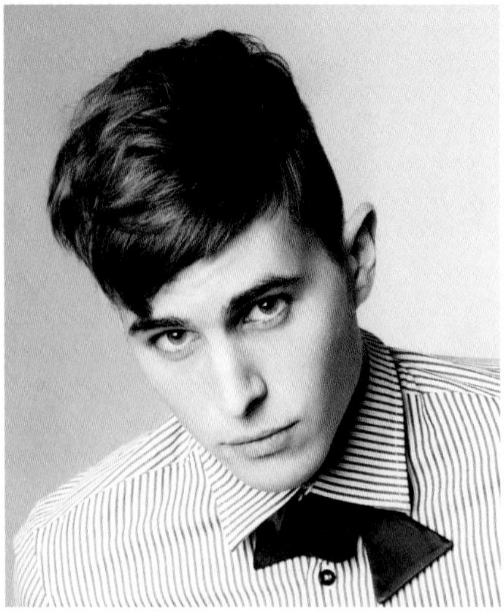

HAIR TEXTURE

Hair texture is about the thickness of each individual hair. It is not about the number of hairs on the head.

- Fine: this texture is more suited to shorter styles. The hair may look thinner if it is longer. This texture of hair may be weaker than other textures. Take care when using heated appliances. Do not use too much tension.
- Medium: this texture is ideal. Is suited to long and short styles.
- Coarse: this texture can have a rough look. It can sometimes be harder to curl because the hair is strong and resistant. Be careful when selecting a style as there may be too much hair for you to achieve the look you want.

Determining the texture of the client's hair is done by looking at a few hairs and feeling them.

ACTIVITY

With other members of your group, look and feel each other's hair and decide what texture the hair is. Compare your **analysis** with the rest of the group.

Analysis
The result of looking at something carefully

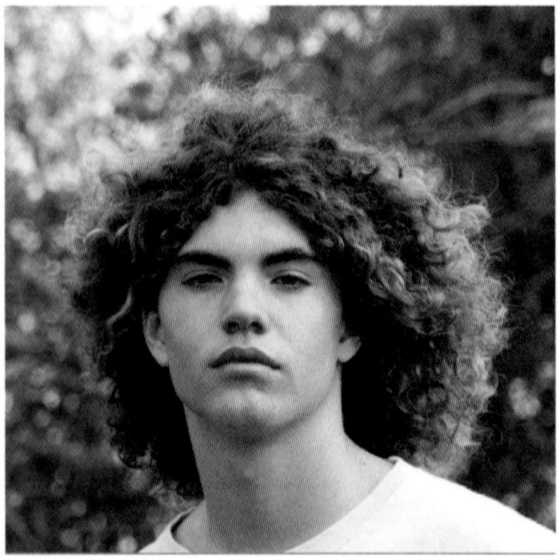

Abundant hair

HAIR DENSITY

Density describes the number of hairs on the head. There are around 120,000 hairs on the average scalp.

- Sparse: this means that there are less than the average number of hairs on the scalp. Like fine hair it is more suited to shorter styles.
- Abundant: this means that there are more hairs than average on the scalp. Like coarse hair it may take longer to dry and could be strong and difficult to curl.

The density can be determined by looking at the scalp. The more skin you can see the less hair the client has.

HAIR ELASTICITY

Hair is naturally elastic; it can stretch and go back to its original shape. If the hair is fine it may not have as much elasticity as coarse hair. This weakness may cause the hair to break if too much tension is put on it. Hair that has been damaged by chemical treatments such as colour or perming will be weaker than normal hair. Using excessive heat can cause the same damage.

HAIR CONDITION

Hair type	How you recognise it	Effect on the styling service
Normal 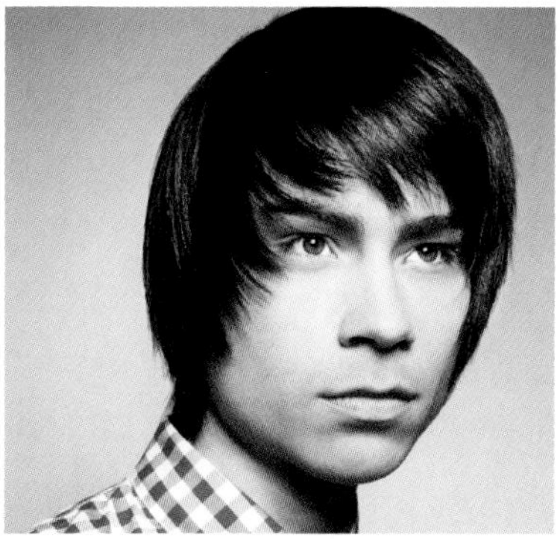	▪ Will shine and look good. ▪ Feels smooth to the touch.	This hair type will not present any major problems when styling.
Oily/greasy 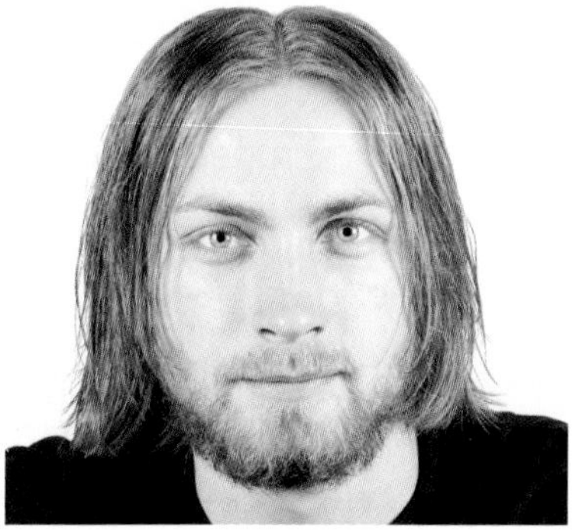	▪ Will look dull and greasy. ▪ Feels sticky to the touch.	The hair will need frequent washing, so easy-to-manage styles will be more practical.
Dry 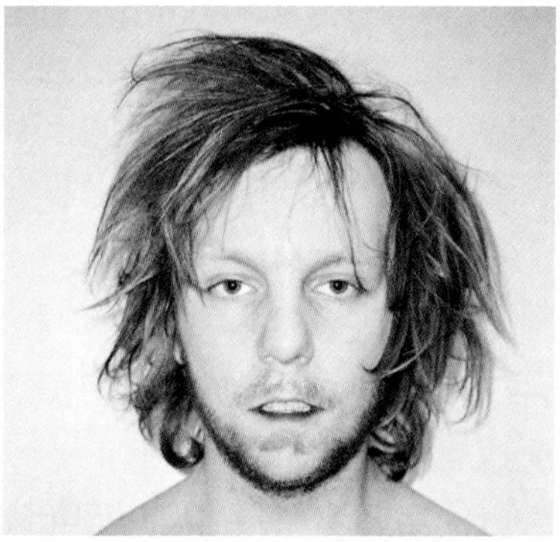	▪ Will look dull and straw-like. ▪ Feels rough to the touch.	The hair will need regular conditioning to help achieve a smooth finish. Don't use too much heat.
Dandruff 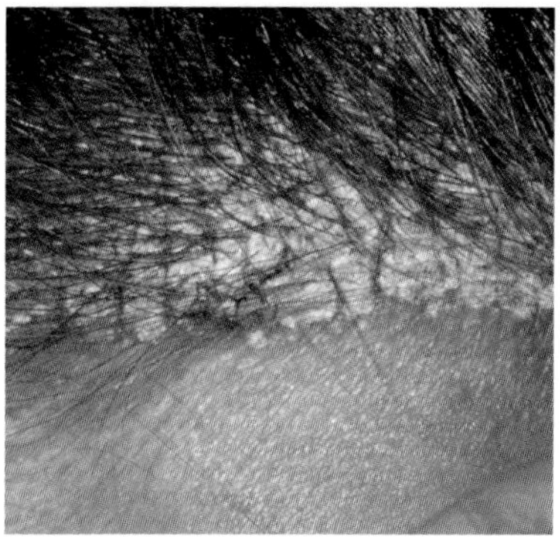	▪ Appears and feels the same as dry hair. ▪ There will be white flakes in the hair and on the shoulders.	The hair will need regular conditioning to help achieve a smooth finish. Don't use too much heat. The condition should be treated.

Hair type	How you recognise it	Effect on the styling service
Damaged 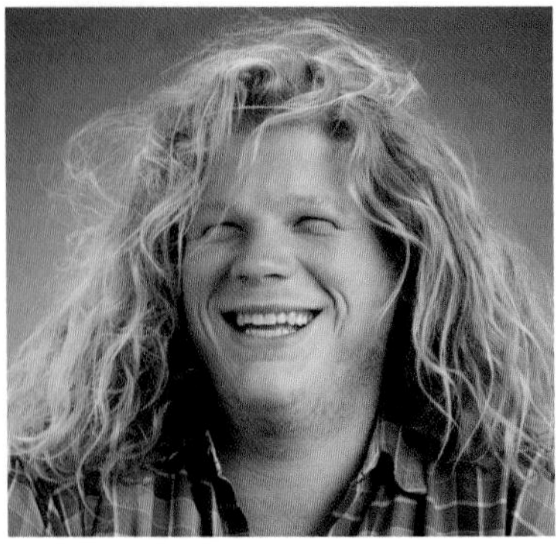	■ May look dull and straw-like. ■ Will feel rough to the touch. ■ The points of the hair may look spiky.	If the hair is damaged as a result of previous services like perming or colouring, the hair may be weak. Treat the hair carefully. Don't use too much heat or too much tension.

Determining hair condition is done by looking at and feeling the hair. You may also need to ask some questions.

ACTIVITY

Working in a group, decide what hair condition each member of the group has. Compare your answers with the others.

HAIR TYPE

The client's hair will be straight, curly or wavy. If the client has medium to long hair this can influence your choice of style. If the client has straight hair you may need to add root lift and body to your style. Straight hair tends to lie flat to the head.

With curly hair, if you want a straight, smooth style you may need to use straighteners. If your client has very wavy hair this may present some styling problems. Hair with a strong, natural wave will have a strong, natural shape which will be difficult to change. You will have to go with the natural shape when you style the hair.

HAIR LENGTH

The length of the hair will affect your choice of style and styling technique. The longer the hair the more work it will need to keep it looking nice. It will also take longer to dry so extra time may be needed. Very short hair will limit your choice of style. There may not be enough hair to do what the client would like. Long hair is heavier so the weight may cause the curl to drop sooner than it would with short hair.

HAIR GROWTH CYCLE

Each hair does not grow continuously. A single hair has a life of between 18 months and seven years. At the end of its life it will fall out and after a short while another hair will grow in its place. About 100 hairs a day will reach the end of their life and fall out. This is why you get hairs in the brush or comb when you use them.

There are three stages in the growth cycle:

- Anagen: Active or growing period – lasts for 18 months to seven years. This is the anagen stage of hair growth.
- Catagen: Breaking down stage – lasts about two weeks. This is the catagen stage of hair growth.
- Telogen: Resting stage – lasts about a month. This is the telogen growth stage of hair growth.

HANDY HINTS

See the images of the anagen, catagen and telogen stages on page 127.

Hair grows on average 1.25 cm a month. Some people's hair grows more each month than the average; some people's hair grows less than the average. Some people can grow their hair very long. Others will not be able to and will say that their hair gets to a certain length and then stops growing. How long the hair grows is determined by how much it grows every month multiplied by its life cycle.

ADVERSE SKIN, SCALP AND HAIR CONDITIONS

Any disease or condition of the hair and scalp can affect your choice of styling technique and the style you decide to do. Some diseases and conditions may be contagious. This may prevent you from carrying out any service on the client.

You should look at the hair and scalp when you are consulting with your client. Look for the following conditions:

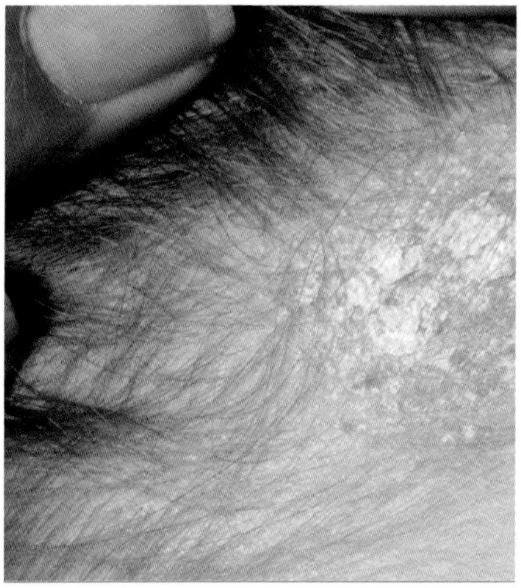

Scaly patches or rough areas on the scalp

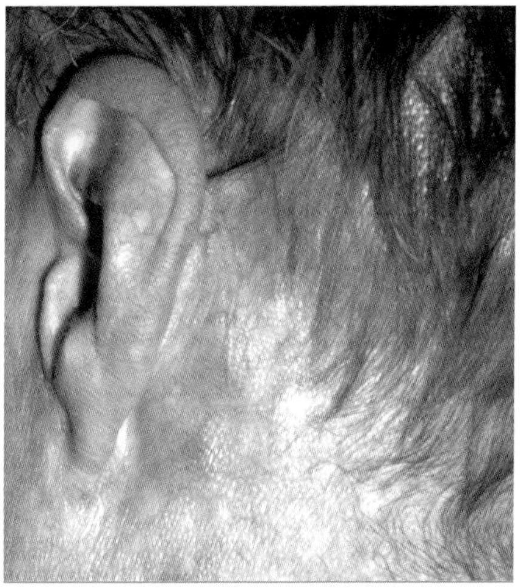

Red inflamed patches

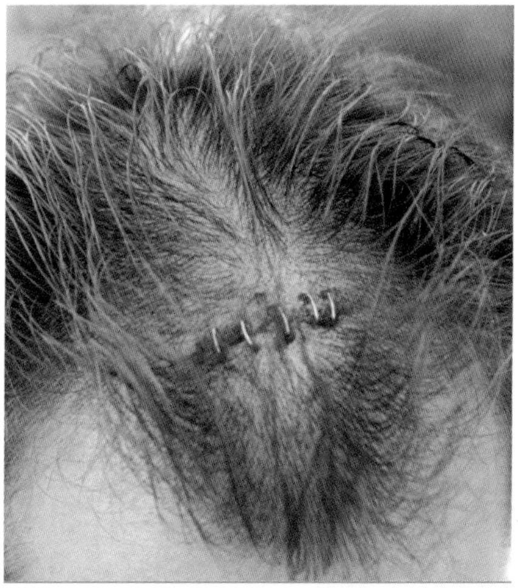

Cuts and abrasions on the skin

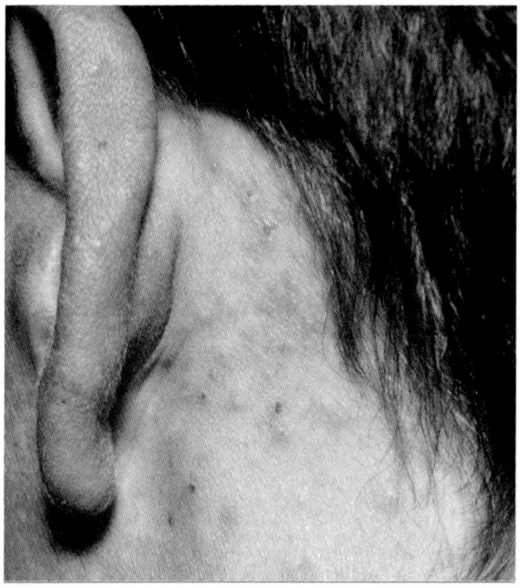

Lumps and bumps or raised areas

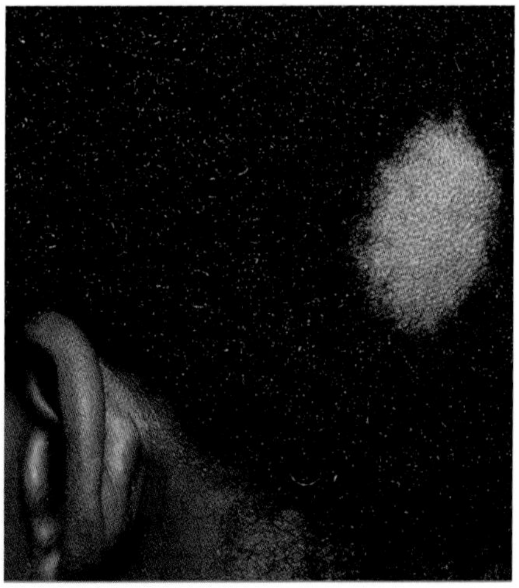

Bald patches

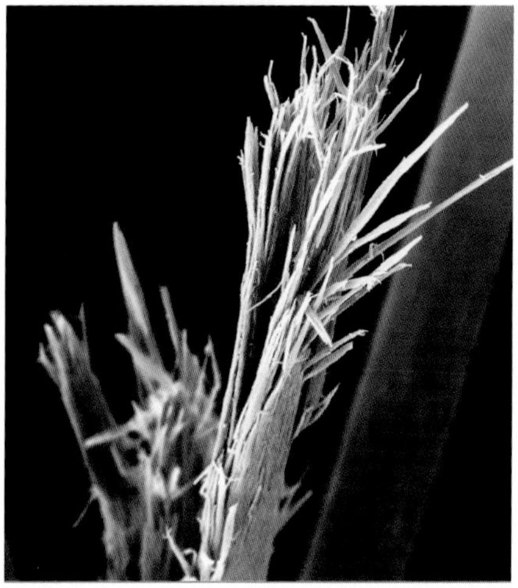

Hair breakage under the microscope

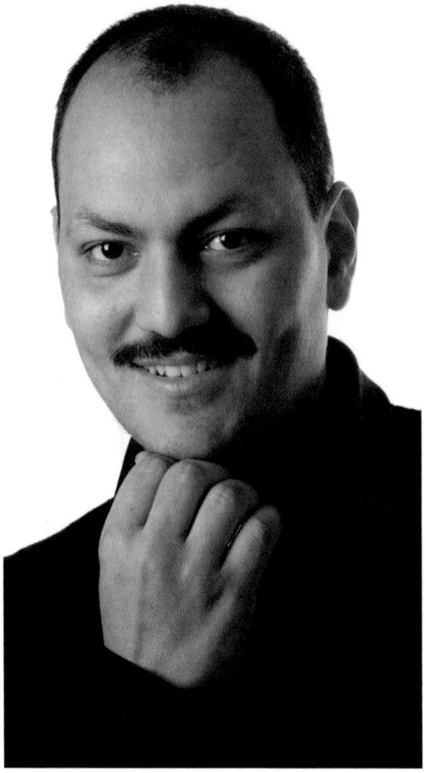

Baldness

Many male clients will suffer from baldness. This is called male pattern alopecia. The baldness often spreads across the scalp from the front to the crown. It will influence the way the hair is cut and styled.

When you check the hair and scalp, if there is anything unusual then you should ask the stylist to look and advise you. If you are unable to give the service then you may need to explain to the client that the treatment cannot go ahead. Remember that you are not medically trained. You should not name the condition in case you are wrong. Sometimes it may be necessary to advise the client to go to his doctor.

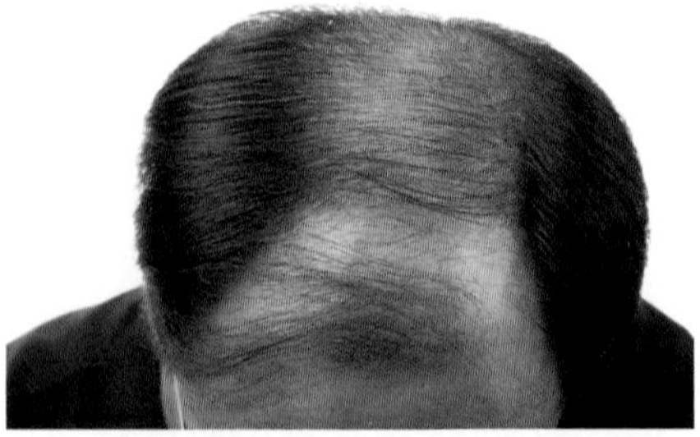

HAIR GROWTH PATTERNS

Hair growth patterns are places where the hair grows in a particular direction or directions. This may affect how the hair is styled. It can also affect how long or short the hair can be.

Look for the following when you do your consultation:

Growth pattern	How you recognise it	Effect on the styling service
Cowlick 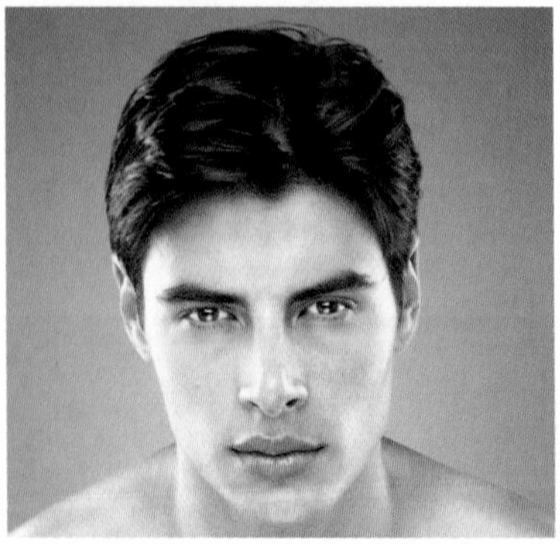	The hair falls to one side or the other at the front. It sometimes forms a natural parting.	Full fringes will be difficult to achieve as the hair will part. Work with the direction of the hair.

HANDY HINTS

Remember to look for head lice when you are checking the scalp.

Growth pattern	How you recognise it	Effect on the styling service
Nape whorl 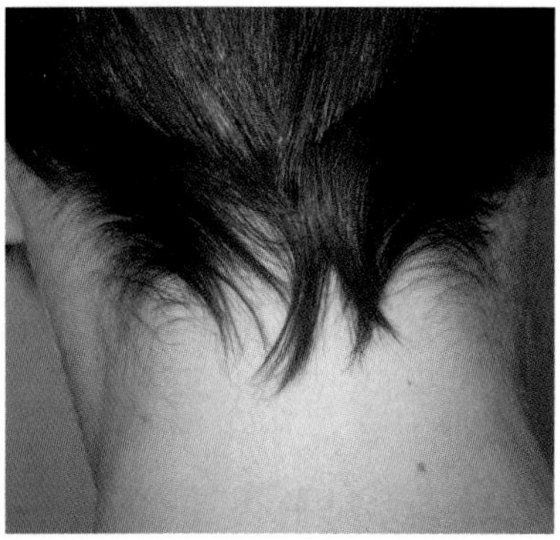	Nape whorls are found in the nape area. The hair grows upwards and inwards towards the middle. It can be on one side or both sides.	Longer styles will not be affected by nape whorls. On shorter styles dry the hair flat with no root lift.
Double crown 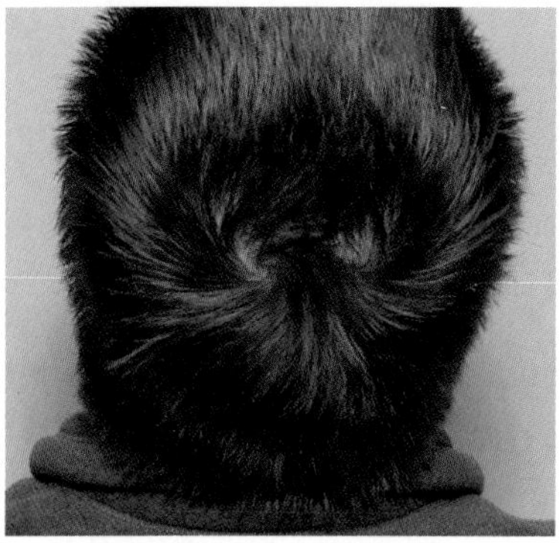	The hair forms two circles in the middle of the scalp.	If the hair is too short it may stick up. The hair should be left longer with good root lift.
Widow's peak 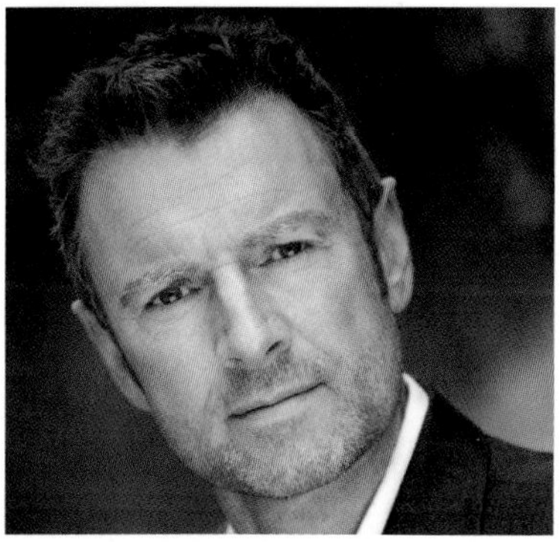	The hair grows to a defined point in the middle of the front hairline.	Fringes will difficult to achieve unless they are heavy. Styles where the hair is dressed back towards the crown are best.

FASHION TRENDS

Your client may want a hairstyle worn by their favourite pop star or celebrity. Sometimes this can be easy and sometimes difficult. The client may not have the right type of hair. It may be too short or too long. He may not have the same shape of face as the celebrity or even the right body shape.

You may need to explain to the client that it might be necessary to change the style because of his hair type or face shape.

HANDY HINTS

Remember, you must be very tactful and polite when you discuss your client's face shape and lifestyle with him.

ACTIVITY

Keep your eye on what styles and colours are popular at the moment. Keep up to date for your clients. There are many images of the latest styles in magazines or on the television. Cut out some pictures and make your own style book.

ACTIVITY

Select some pictures of your favourite pop stars or celebrities. With your group, decide which of your male colleagues could have the styles you have selected and which could not. Give reasons for your decisions and how you would tell the colleague they could not have the style.

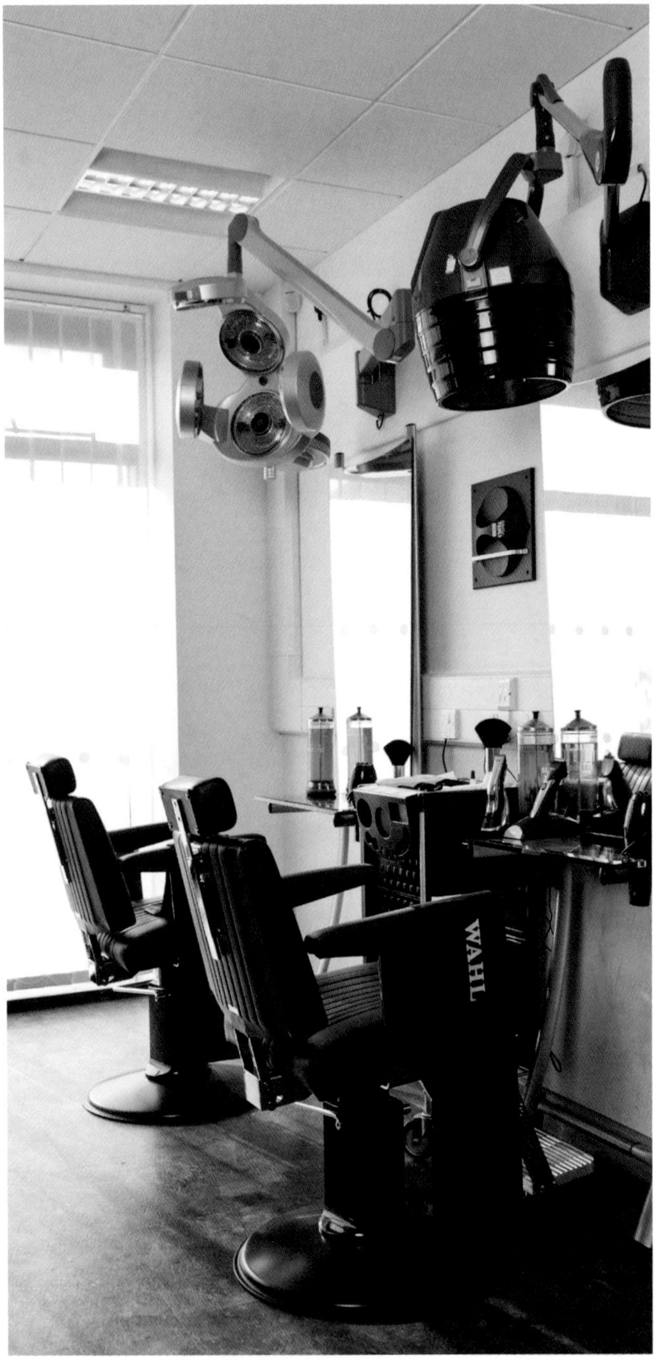

PREPARE THE WORK AREA

There are three reasons why you should prepare your work area ready to work.

1 It helps you to work safely and hygienically.

2 It looks good and gives the client the right impression.

3 It helps you to work efficiently.

- Make sure you keep work surfaces clean by wiping regularly with a suitable cleaner.
- Mirrors should be cleaned to remove smears and smudges.
- Tools and equipment should be in their proper places and always cleaned and sterilised ready for use to help prevent passing on infection from one client to another.
- Sweep and clean the floor when necessary.
- Make sure the chair is clean.

You may not be able to get all the things you need ready before the client arrives. When you have completed your consultation with the client, get the rest of the products and tools you need.

HANDY HINTS

Remember to make sure your appearance and your personal hygiene are up to standard. Read Chapter 102 to refresh your knowledge.

SAFE AND HYGIENIC WORKING PRACTICES

Working safely and hygienically is very important. It is part of every practical skill you learn; it is part of every service you give to a client; it is part of the whole of your working day.

You should keep your work area tidy and only use **hygienic** tools and equipment. This will help to reduce the risk of harm to you and your clients and help to prevent **cross-infection**. The client will also have more confidence in you and you will look more professional.

Hygienic
Clean and germ free

Cross-infection
When germs are passed from one person to another

ACTIVITY

Read Chapter 113 Following health and safety in the salon to learn about the employer's responsibilities and your responsibilities to provide a safe and healthy working environment.

When styling hair, the main safe and hygienic working practices that you need to know are:

- PPE – personal protective equipment. You may need an apron or non-latex gloves for any products you use, if the manufacturer's instructions say they should be used.
- COSHH – Control Of Substances Hazardous to Health. These regulations explain how to safely use any products that may be part of the service. They will also include using a **disinfectant** safely when cleaning tools and equipment.
- Electricity at Work Regulations. Checking all the electrical equipment you will use in the styling process is essential.
- HASAWA – Health and Safety at Work Act. You must make sure you check the work area for any hazards before you start work on the client. Make sure all the equipment, tools and products are clean and safe to use on the client
- Methods of **sterilisation**. An example in a styling service is using a disinfectant such as **Barbicide** for combs.

Disinfectant
A cleaning fluid that kills germs and helps to prevent them growing

Sterilisation
Process that kills all germs

Barbicide
A liquid disinfectant

HANDY HINTS
Go to Chapter 113 and read more about methods of sterilisation.

ACTIVITY

Go to Chapter 113 Following health and safety in the salon and list all of the health and safety laws that you should follow when carrying out a styling service.

HYGIENE WHEN STYLING MEN'S HAIR

The following is a guide for keeping your styling tools and equipment ready for use.

Towels and gowns	Machine wash on a high temperature to destroy harmful germs.
Combs	Wash in warm, soapy water. Place in the sterilising jar.
Brushes	Remove loose hair, wash in warm soapy water and dry.
Clips	Wash in warm soapy water and dry. Then place in the sterilising jar.
Disposable gloves	Throw away after use. Use a new pair for each client.

PREPARE THE CLIENT

Preparing the client for styling services will involve the following:

1 gowning the client to protect his clothes
2 carrying out a consultation with the client
3 selecting the tools, equipment and products to be used
4 shampooing and, if necessary, conditioning the client's hair.

HANDY HINTS

Read more about preparing your client in Chapter 003 Shampooing and conditioning hair.

HANDY HINTS

Check regularly that the gown is still in place and the towels are not too wet. Change the towels if you need to.

GOWNING THE CLIENT

The first part of any service will be to protect the client and their belongings. For styling services, place a gown around the client to protect his clothes and a clean towel around his shoulders.

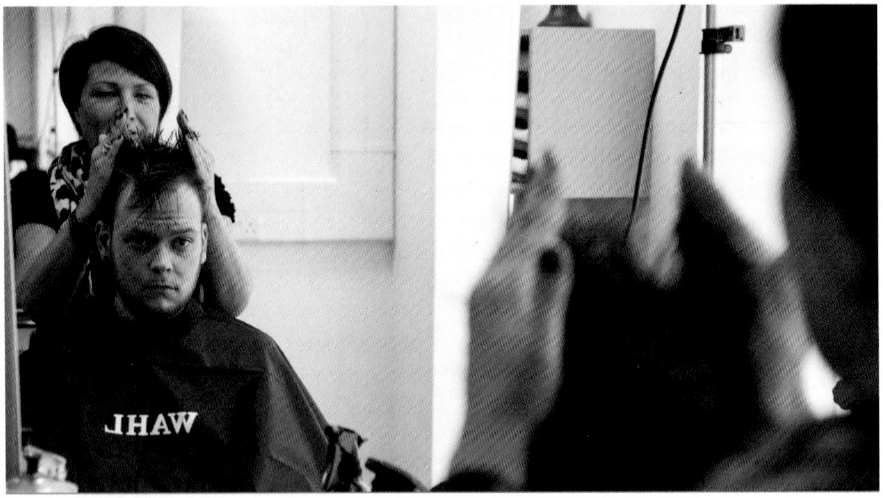

A protected client

CONSULTATION

Consulting with the client allows you to find out what the client wants. It is how you decide what you are going to do.

Chapter 003 Shampooing and conditioning hair describes how to consult with your client to find out what shampoo and conditioner you will use and how you will carry out the service. If you are going to style the client's hair then you need to find out more information from the client.

- What does the client want the finished look to be? For example, a practical eas-to-manage style or something trendy and fashionable.
- Decide which styling technique you need to consider using.
- Look at all the factors that can influence your choice of technique.
- Decide if you can achieve what the client has asked for. If you cannot then you will need to suggest something different.
- Select any products to use, such as mousse or gel, etc.
- Decide how you will carry out the technique and the tools and equipment you need to use.

HANDY HINTS

Make sure you check the hair and scalp for diseases and conditions. If the client has a contagious disease you will not be able to carry out the service.

ACTIVITY

Make a list of all the things you need to find out from your client so you can decide what you're going to do.

- Include all factors that may influence your decision.
- Write down how you will find out the information, eg asking questions, looking at and feeling the scalp.
- Make a list of questions you could ask the client.

COMMUNICATION AND BEHAVIOUR

Communication and behaviour are very important when styling men's hair. Your communication skills need to be as good as your hairdressing skills. You need to feel comfortable with clients, even if you haven't met them before. This starts with being confident about what you're doing, and thinking about the types of question you're asking. Consulting with your client will be a mixture of talking to him and looking and feeling his hair. Refer to Chapter 102 for more details about communication and behaviour.

HANDY HINTS

Don't forget to talk to the client while you are carrying out the service. For many clients good conversation is one of the reasons they visit the salon.

SHAMPOO AND CONDITION THE CLIENT'S HAIR

When you have finished your consultation, the next step is to shampoo the hair ready for the styling service. Chapter 003 Shampooing and conditioning hair describes the method of shampooing and conditioning the hair ready for other services.

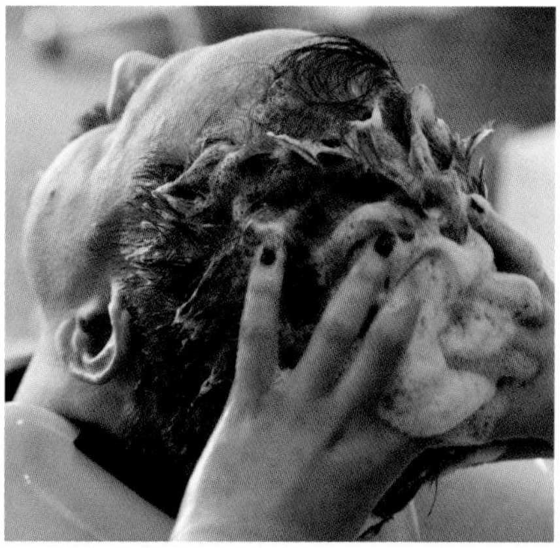

Don't forget to use conditioner if the hair needs it. Make sure the client agrees to have it.

HANDY HINTS

Read Chapter 003 Shampooing and conditioning hair, to refresh your knowledge of the procedure.

HANDY HINTS

When you towel dry after shampooing do not over dry the hair. For the styling process to work properly the hair should be moist but not dripping water. If the hair is too dry it will be difficult to get the shape you need.

PROVIDE STYLING FOR MEN

This part of the chapter looks at appropriate products, tools and equipment for styling men's hair and the basic techniques for styling men's hair safely and professionally.

TOOLS AND EQUIPMENT USED IN BASIC STYLING TECHNIQUES

Tools and equipment	Use
Wide-toothed comb 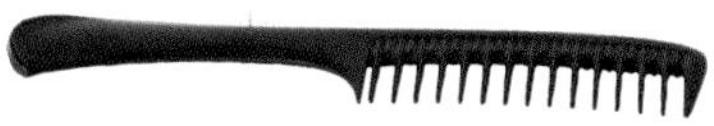	Used to detangle hair before styling.
Cutting comb 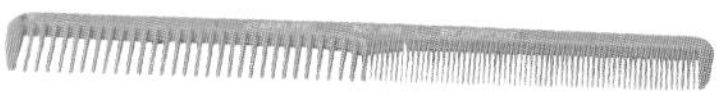	Used to split the hair into sections to keep it under control while you work.

Tools and equipment	Use
Sectioning clips 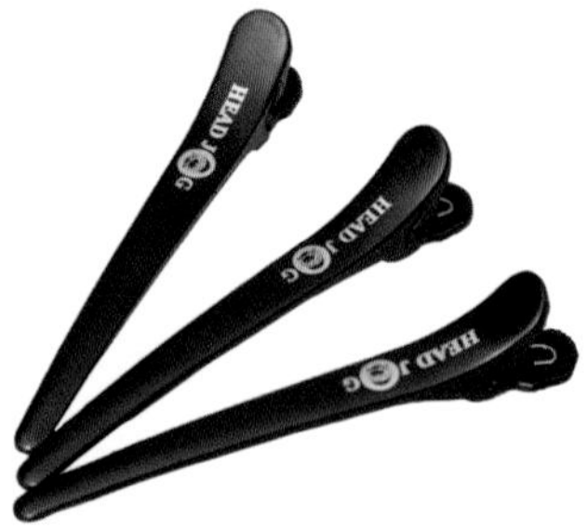	Used to secure the hair as you work.
Denman brush 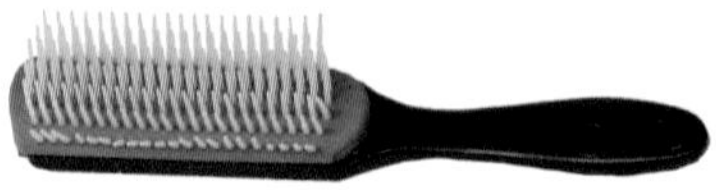	Used in blow drying to create a smooth straight finish.
Vent brush 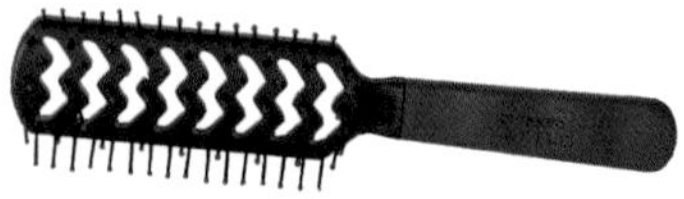	Used to create a textured, straight finish when blow drying.
Radial brush 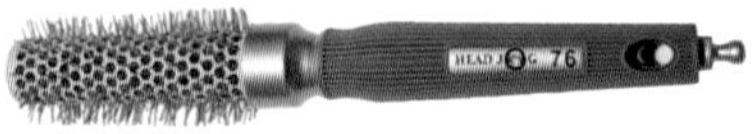	Radial brushes come in different sizes and are used to create root lift and volume in hair of different lengths.
Hand-held dryer 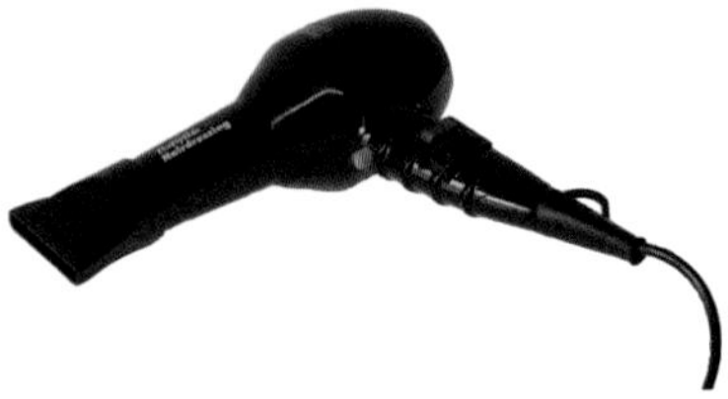	Used to dry the hair during blow drying. Has different heat settings and speeds.
Diffuser 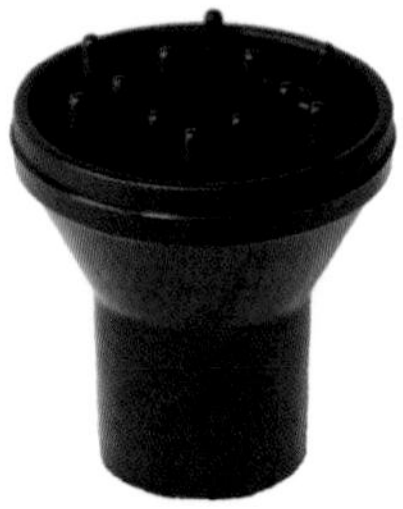	An attachment for a hand dryer used when finger drying. It spreads the airflow and decreases its force.

Tools and equipment	Use
Nozzle 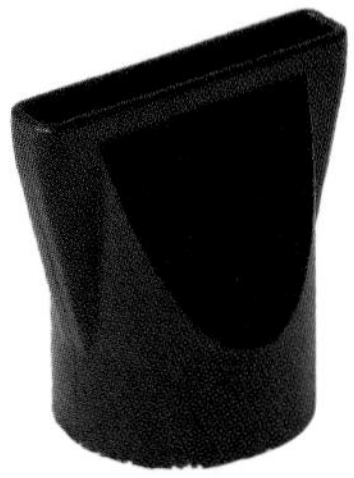	Another attachment that allows you to direct the airflow and heat more accurately when blow drying.
Straightening irons 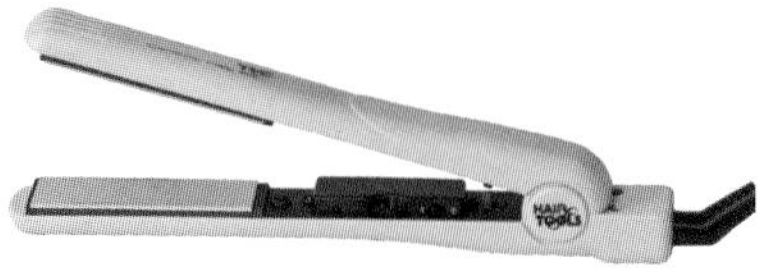	These have flat, heated surfaces that are used on dry hair to straighten and smoothe it.
Tongs 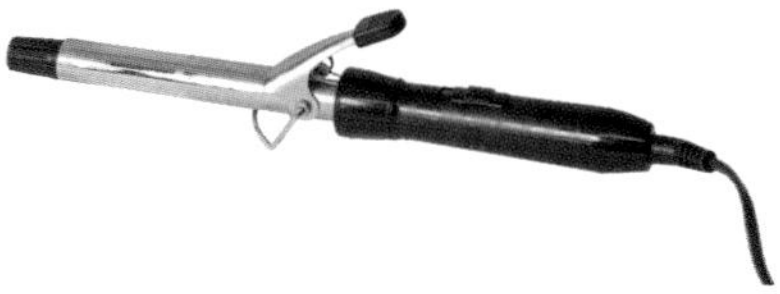	These have a round, barrel shape that is heated. Used on dry hair to create curl and body.
Gown 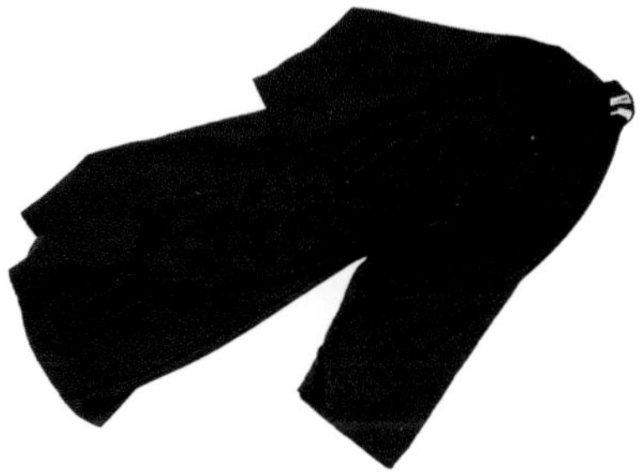	This will cover the client and help to prevent anything getting onto his clothes.
Towels 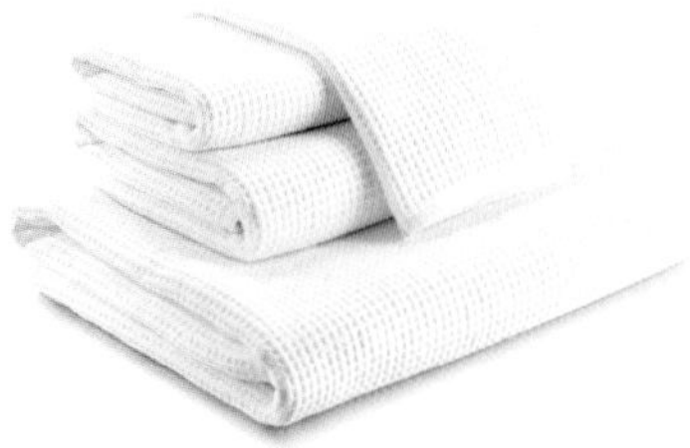	Used when shampooing and styling to prevent the client's clothing from getting wet.
Hand mirror 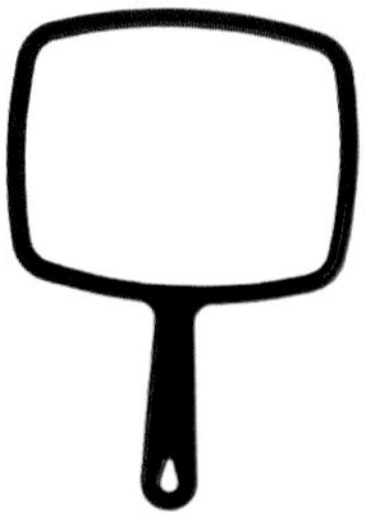	Used to show the client the back of his head so he can see the finished result.

PRODUCTS USED IN BASIC STYLING TECHNIQUES

Product	Use
Mousse 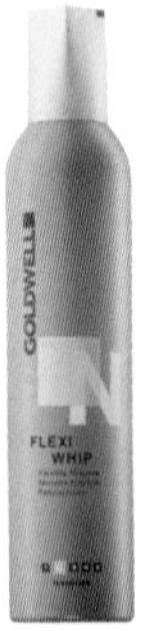	Used on wet hair before blow drying or setting. It gives support and hold to the style, making it last longer.
Gel 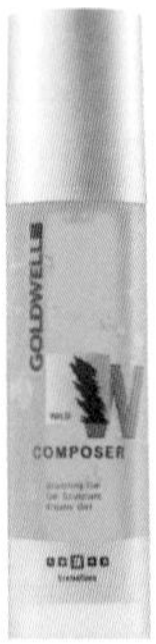	Used on wet or dry hair to provide volume and texture.
Blowdry lotion 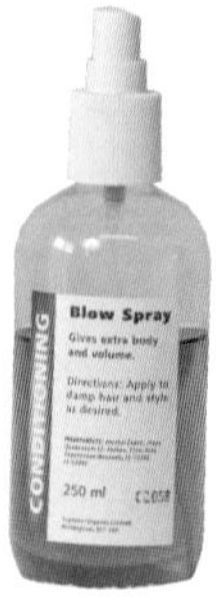	Similar to mousse but in liquid form; used on wet hair before blow drying. Gives volume, lift and support for fine hair.
Hairspray 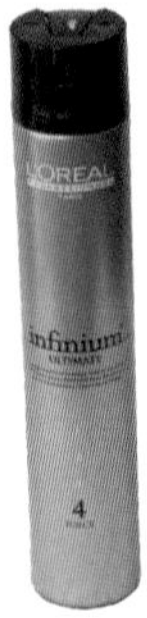	Sprayed lightly onto dry hair when dressing or drying is finished. It holds the hair in place and gives it shine.

Product	**Use**
Moisturisers 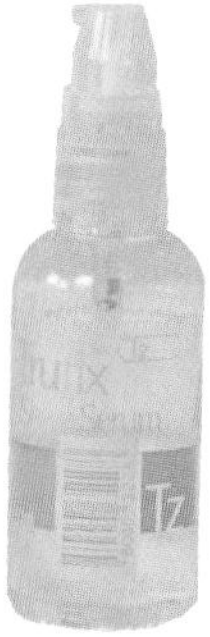	Used on wet hair when blow drying to help smoothe frizzy curly hair to get a straighter look.
Wax 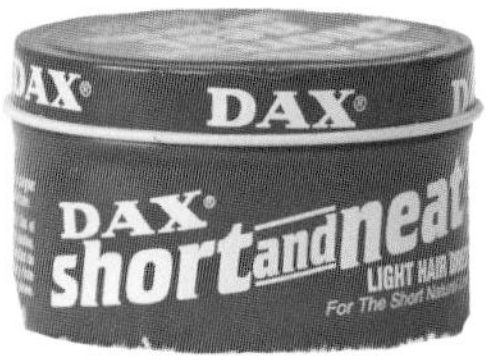 	Applied to dry hair to achieve a textured finish to the style. Often used to get a 'spiky', 'messy' look.
Dressing creams 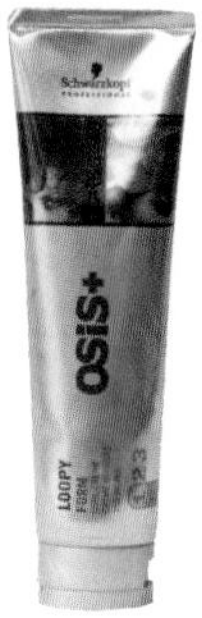 	Used on dry hair to control. Gives a slick 'wet look' finish.
Heat protectors 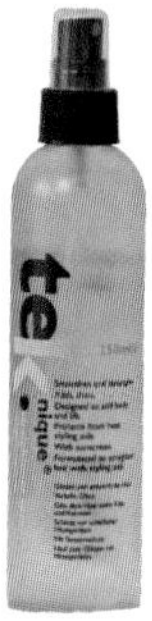	Sprayed onto dry hair before using heated appliances such as tongs, straighteners, etc. Protects the hair from the effects of the heat.

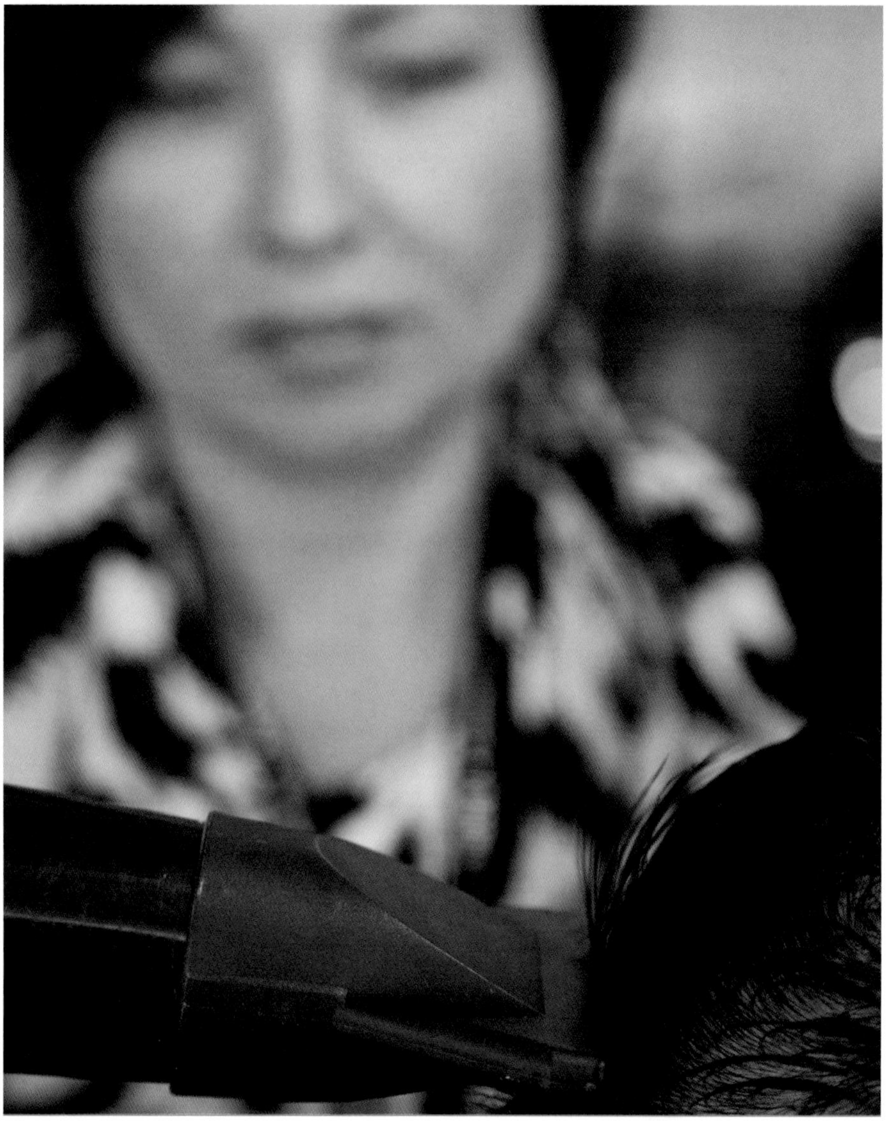
Holding the dryer still in one place or getting the dryer too close to the hair may burn the client's scalp

ACTIVITY

Find out what precautions you should take when using the styling products from the list.

BLOW DRYING THE HAIR

The most important thing to remember when you are blow drying is to have the hair under control. If the hair is not under control you will not get the shape and finish you want. Remember to work safely. You will be using heat to dry the hair. Concentrate on what you are doing all the time.

APPLYING PRODUCT

When you are ready to start your blow dry, apply any styling product that you wish to use.

Be careful to follow the manufacturer's instructions.

Do not apply too much – use only as much as you need. Always avoid waste. This costs the salon money. It can also affect the result of your blow dry, making the hair sticky and dull.

SECTIONING THE HAIR

When you are blow drying medium to long hair you should divide it into sections. Use a sectioning clip to secure them. This will keep the hair out of the way as you dry it. A simple sectioning procedure would be:

Divide the hair into four sections. Make a parting from the centre of the forehead to the centre of the nape; then from the crown to the back of the ear on each side. Secure each section with a clip.

Take one of the back sections and make a parting from the centre to the outside about 2 cm thick. (The size of the section will depend on the density of the client's hair. The more dense it is the thinner the section should be.)

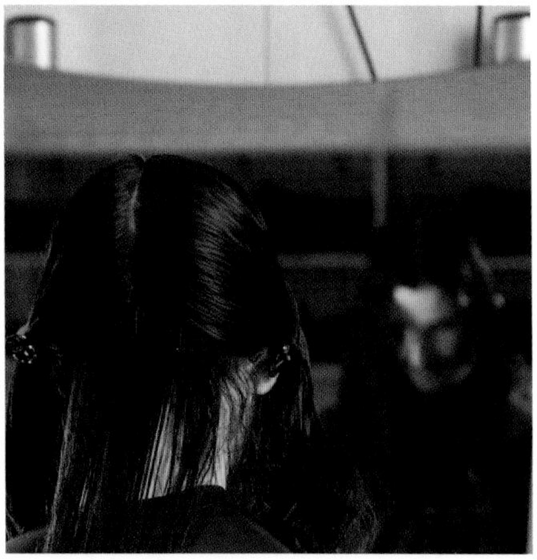

Re-secure the main section. Do the same on the other side.

You are now ready to blow the hair dry.

HANDY HINTS

Keep the hair tight so that when you put the clip in it is not loose and floppy. You will have better control and it looks more professional to the client.

USING THE DRYER

The airflow from the dryer must always be away from the client's scalp. You need to direct the airflow in the direction of the style. Hold the dryer at least 10–15 cm away from the hair as you dry it. If the dryer is too close it can damage the hair.

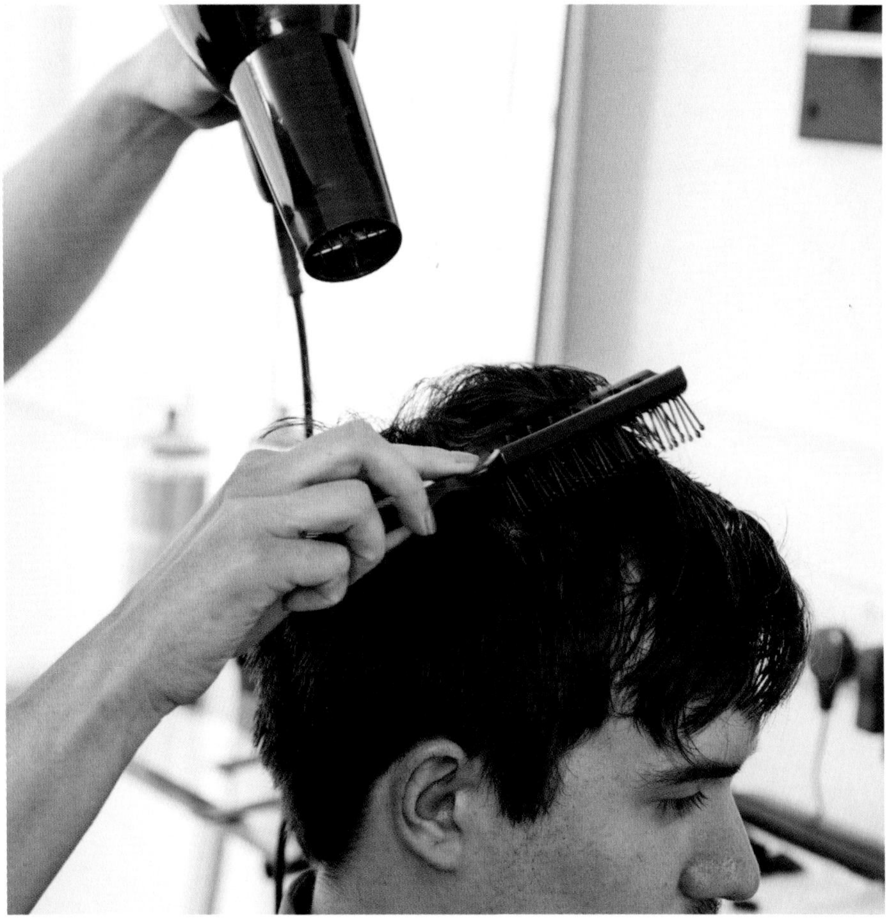

BRUSHES

Your brush choice will depend on the look you want to achieve and the hair you are working with. For shorter styles a Denman or vent brush would be used. A radial brush can be used to give lift and volume. The airflow from the dryer should follow the brush.

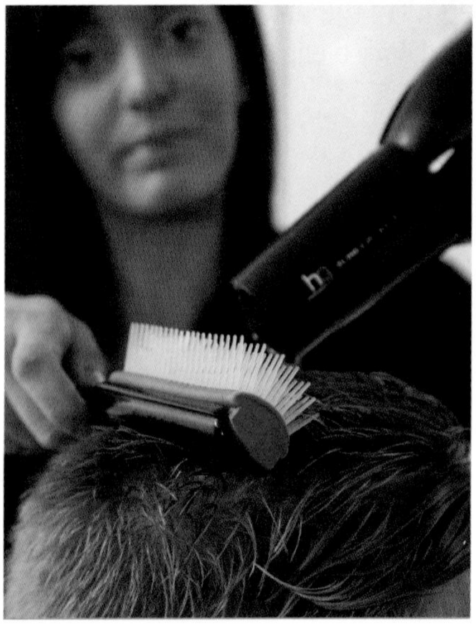

Using a Denman brush

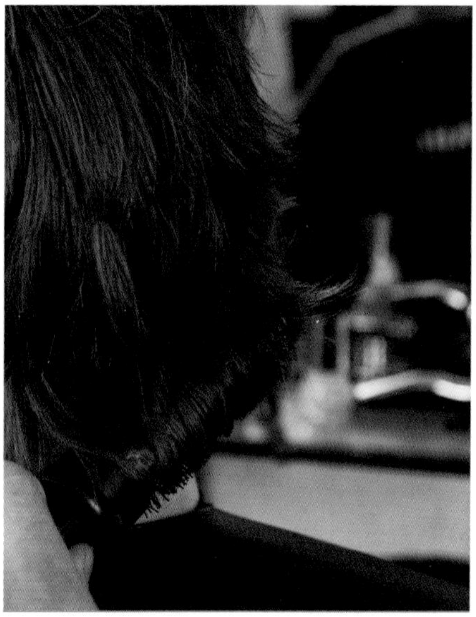

Using a radial brush

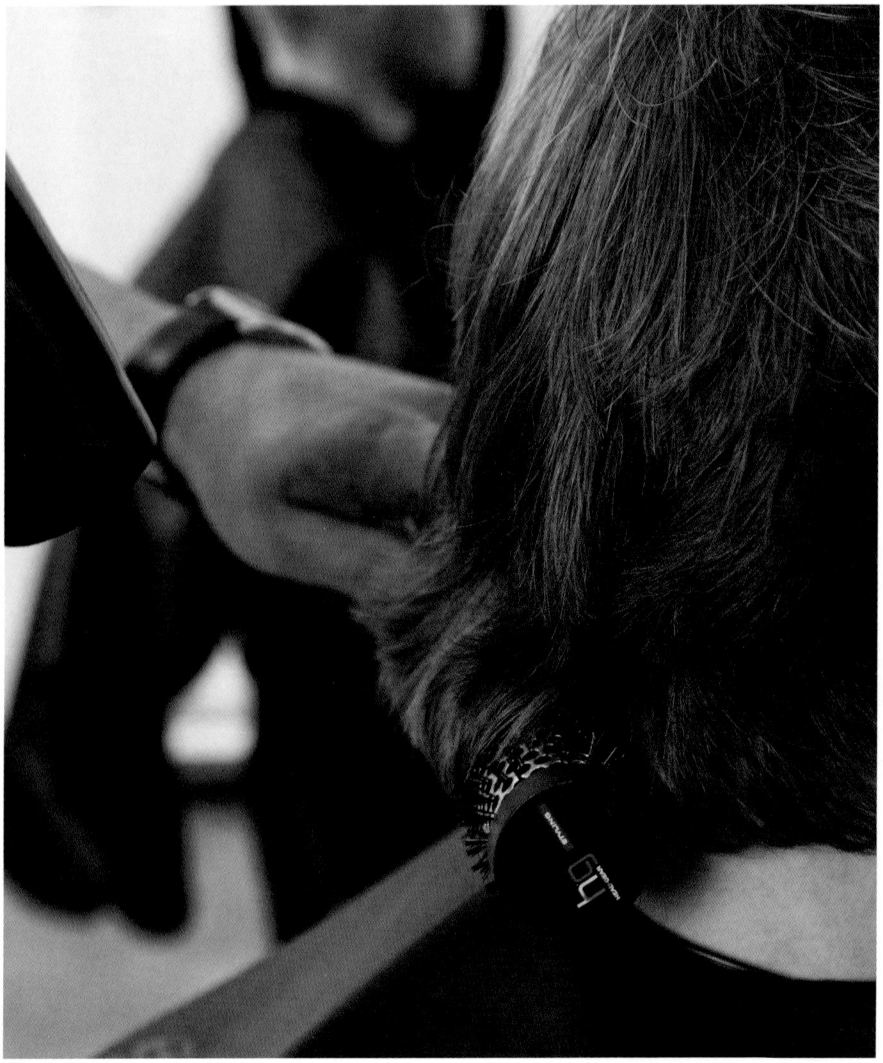

TENSION

If you are blow drying medium to long hair, keep your tension even as you dry it. This will give you a smoother finish. Do not use too much tension as this may cause discomfort to the client.

ANGLES

Changing the angle of the brush and the dryer will help you get the shape you want. You need to practise holding the dryer and brush in alternate hands. Holding the dryer and brush in different positions is necessary so you can get the result needed.

STEP-BY-STEP BLOW DRYING

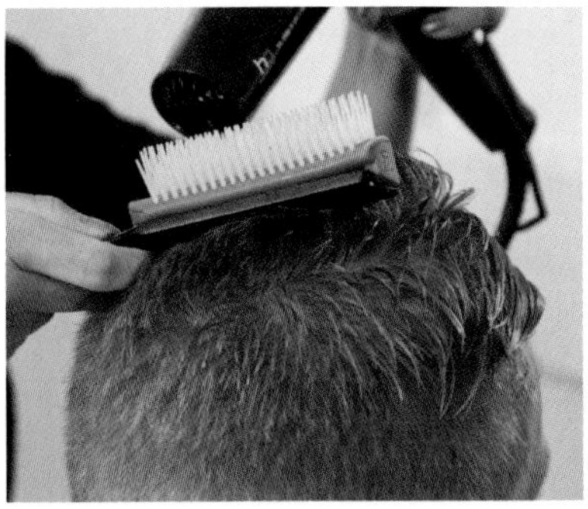

STEP 1 – Start at the front of the head and use the brush to hold the hair in the position you want as you dry.

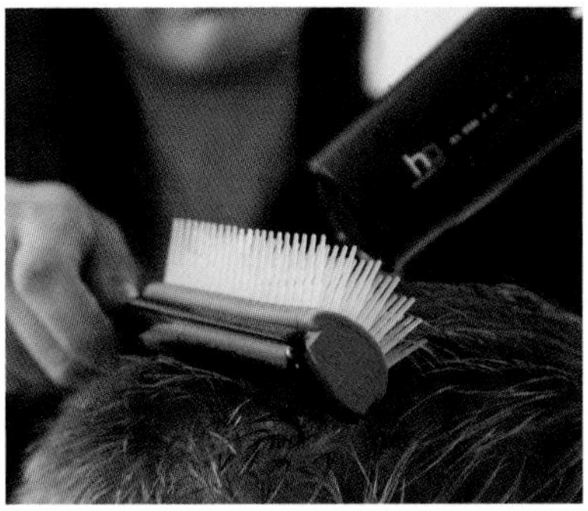

STEP 2 – Continue to the back of the head. Direct the hot air in the direction you want the hair to go.

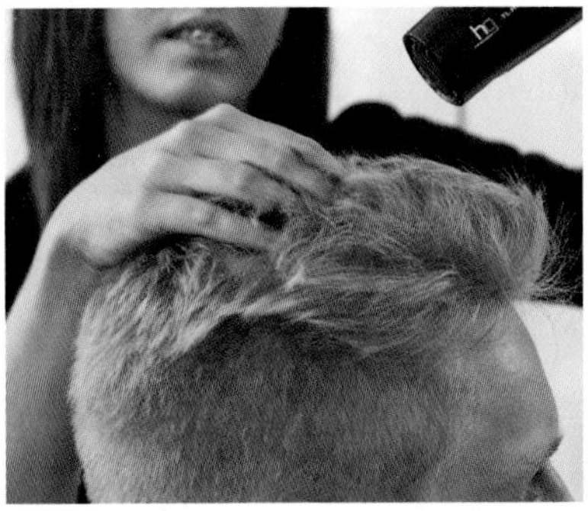

STEP 3 – Use your fingers to make final adjustments to the style.

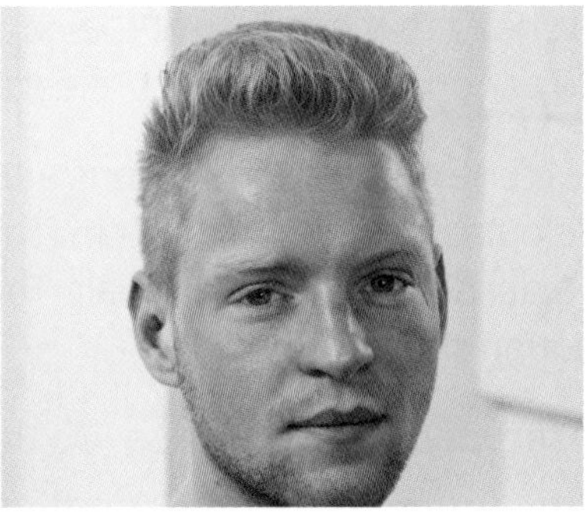

STEP 4 – Check the finish of the style and make sure the client is happy with the finished result.

FINGER DRYING THE HAIR

Finger drying can be carried out on most lengths of hair apart from very short. Like blow drying, it is important to have the hair under control. If the hair is not under control you will not get the shape and finish you want.

Remember to work safely. You will be using heat to dry the hair. Concentrate on what you are doing all the time.

When finger drying you can use a diffuser on the hand dryer. This spreads the flow of air over a wider surface, decreasing the force of the air. Even though the airflow is decreased it will still be hot; be careful not to hold the dryer in one place for too long.

APPLYING PRODUCT

When you are ready to start your finger dry, apply any styling product that you wish to use.

Be careful to follow the manufacturer's instructions.

Do not apply too much – use only as much as you need. Always avoid waste. This costs the salon money. It can also affect the result of your finger dry by making the hair sticky and dull.

SECTIONING THE HAIR

When you are finger drying medium to long hair you should divide it into sections. Use a sectioning clip to secure them. This will keep the hair out of the way as you dry a section.

A simple sectioning procedure would be:

Divide the hair into four quarters. Make a parting from the centre of the forehead to the centre of the nape; then from the crown to the back of the ear on each side. Secure each section with a clip.

Take one of the back sections and make a parting from the centre to the outside about 2 cm thick. (The size of the section will depend on the density of the client's hair. The more dense it is the thinner the section should be.)

Resecure the main section. Do the same on the other side.

You are now ready to finger dry the hair.

HANDY HINTS

Keep the hair reasonably tight so that when you put the clip in it is not loose and floppy. You will have better control and it looks more professional to the client.

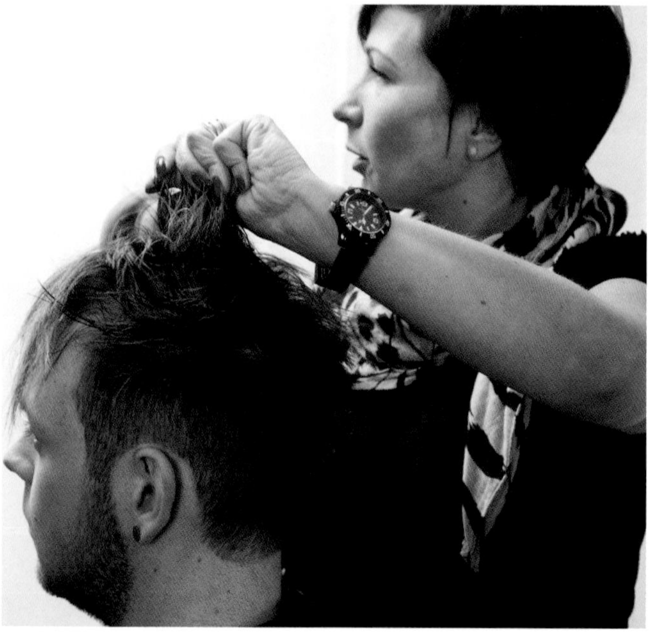

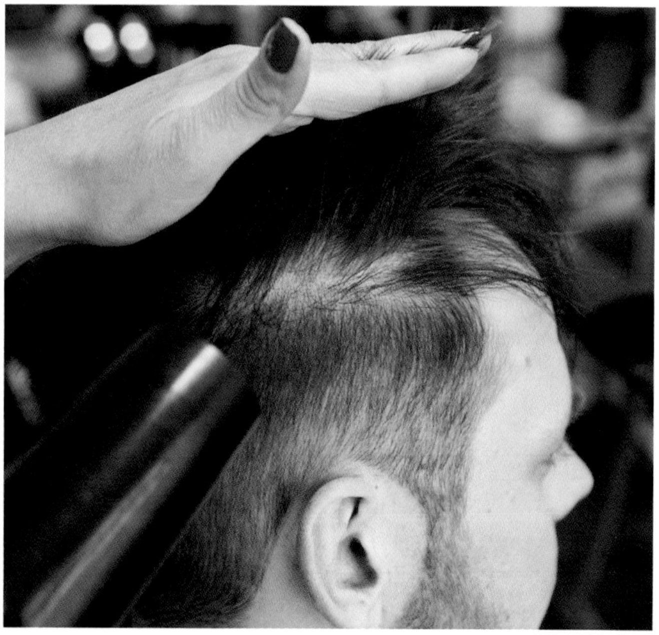

USING THE DRYER

Lift the hair with the fingers and direct the airflow through it. Lifting the hair will give root lift to the style. Use the fingers like a comb and move the hair in the direction you want. Don't keep the dryer in one place for too long.

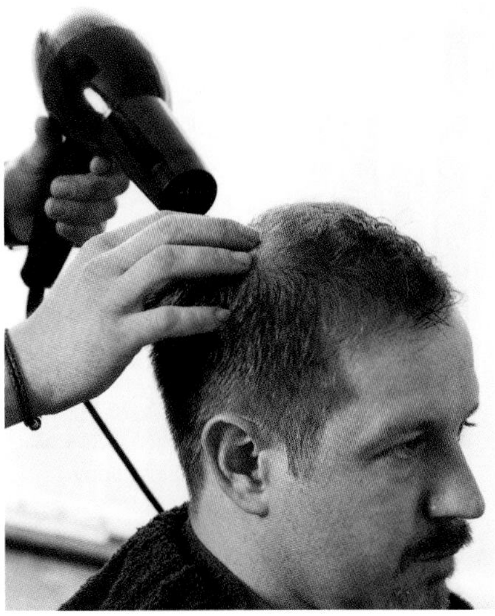 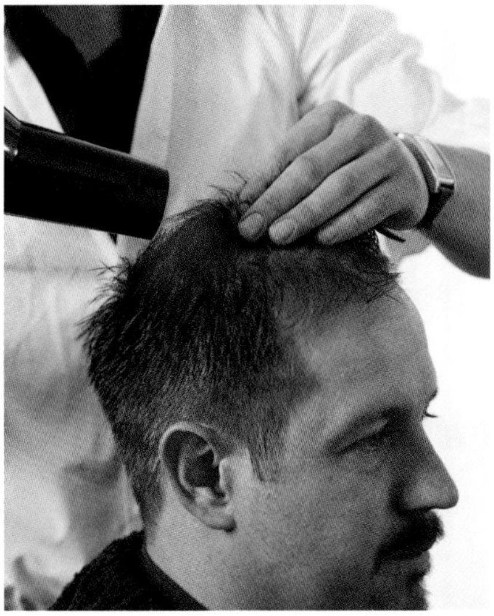

TENSION

With finger drying, keep the hair under control. You do not need too much tension. Use just enough to keep the hair in the direction you want it to go.

ANGLES

Like blow drying, you need to change the angle of the dryer according to the direction you want. Use your hands to finger dry the hair and to hold and direct the dryer.

STEP-BY-STEP FINGER DRYING A SHORT HEAD OF HAIR

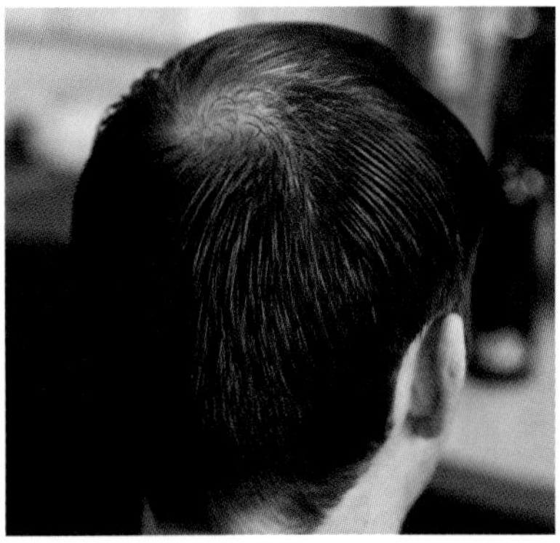

STEP 1 – Comb the hair into the direction of the finished style.

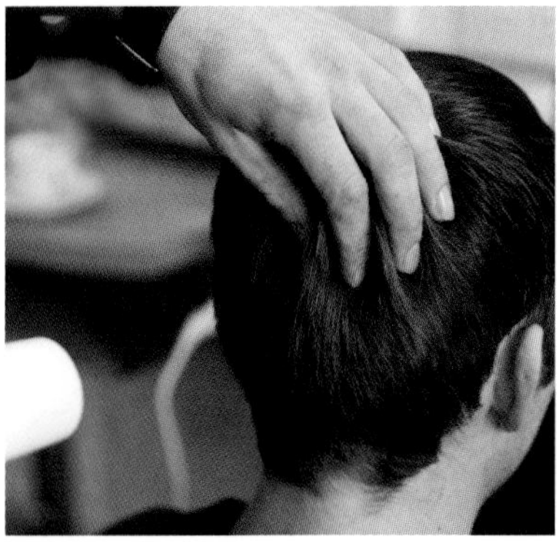

STEP 2 – Use the fingers to lift and guide the hair as you dry it.

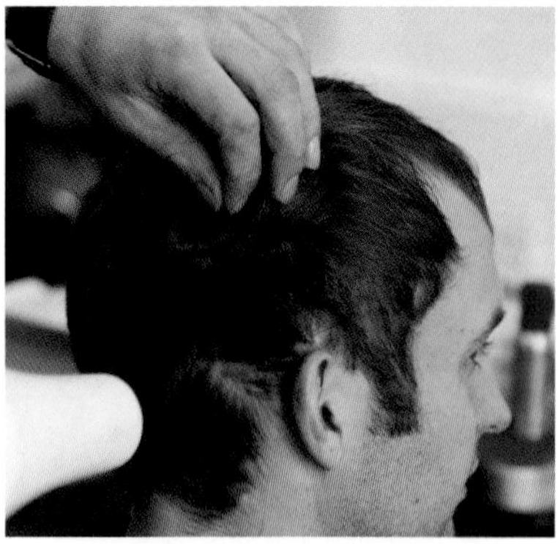

STEP 3 – Lift the hair with the fingers to add height.

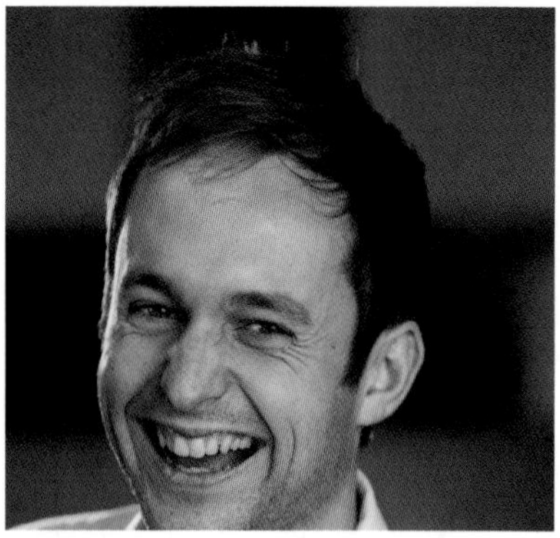

STEP 4 – Check that the client is happy with the finished result.

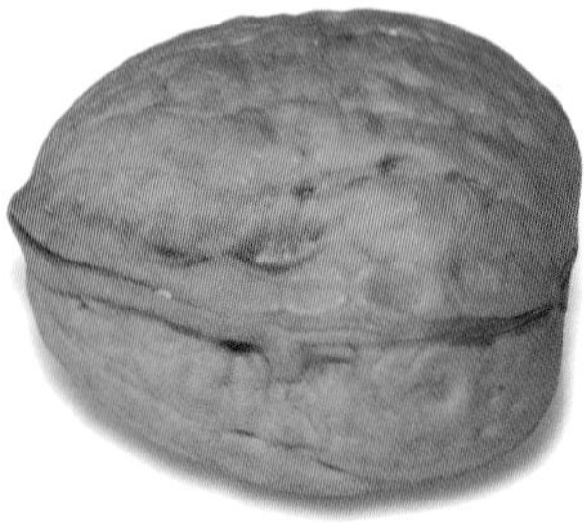

IN A NUTSHELL

You are now at the end of the chapter. Before you test your knowledge with the revision activities, check the following list to see if you feel confident in all the areas covered. If there are still any areas you're unsure of, go back over them in the book and ask your tutor for extra support:

- the basic techniques for styling men's hair
- the factors that can influence your choice of techniques
- how to prepare for styling men's hair
- the tools, equipment and products that are used in styling men's hair and selecting them
- following safe and hygienic working practices
- the importance of good communication, behaviour and attitude when styling men's hair
- styling men's hair using basic techniques.

REVISION ACTIVITIES

Use the questions below to test your knowledge of Chapter 104 to see just how much information you've gained. This can help you to prepare for your assessments. Turn to pages 498–499 for the answers.

CROSSWORD

See if you can answer the questions and write them in the crossword.

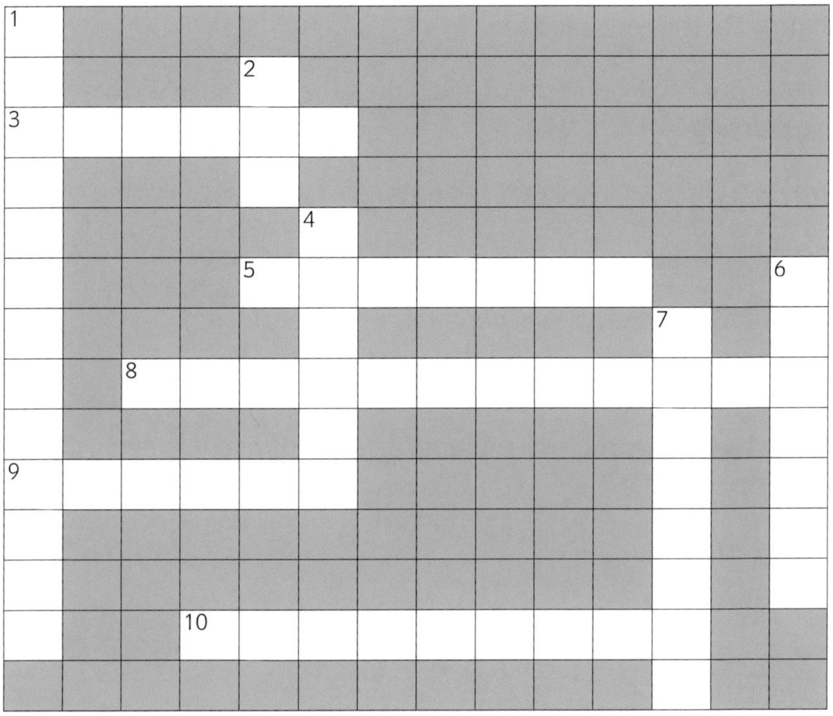

Across

3 A brush used to create root lift and volume

5 When the hair grows to one side at the front of the hairline

8 A discussion with the client before the service is carried out

9 An attachment that helps direct the airflow when blow drying

10 A liquid disinfectant

Down

1 A flat heated surface used on dry hair to help smoothe it

2 A styling product used on dry hair to add texture to the finished style

4 A styling product used on wet hair to help the style last longer

6 A word to describe the number of hairs on the head

7 An attachment for the hairdryer, which is sometimes used for finger drying

TEST YOUR KNOWLEDGE FURTHER

1 Name **three** basic styling techniques that can be used to style men's hair.

2 Name **four** factors that can influence your choice of technique.

3 Why is it important to prepare your work area before you start work on the client?

4 Name **three** styling products that can be used during styling and state what they are used for.

5 Name **four** tools or pieces of equipment that can be used for blow drying.

6 Why is it important to listen when you are consulting with the client?

7 What PPE would you use for your client when styling?

8 Why should the hair be sectioned when finger drying?

9 What would wax be used for when styling men's hair?

10 Name **two** things that will promote a good atmosphere and image in the salon?

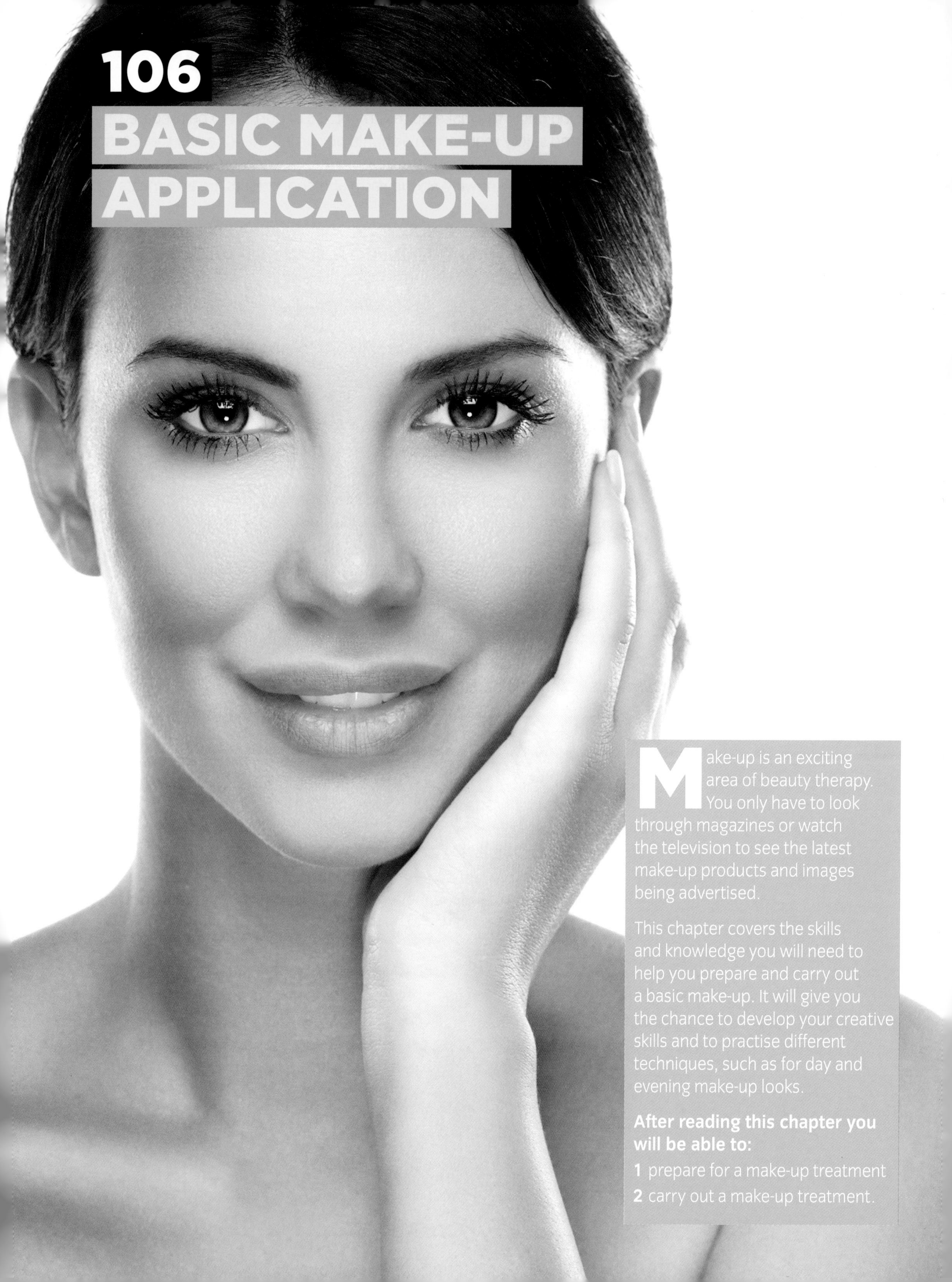

106 BASIC MAKE-UP APPLICATION

Make-up is an exciting area of beauty therapy. You only have to look through magazines or watch the television to see the latest make-up products and images being advertised.

This chapter covers the skills and knowledge you will need to help you prepare and carry out a basic make-up. It will give you the chance to develop your creative skills and to practise different techniques, such as for day and evening make-up looks.

After reading this chapter you will be able to:

1 prepare for a make-up treatment

2 carry out a make-up treatment.

PREPARE FOR A MAKE-UP TREATMENT

Before you begin the make-up treatment, it's important to be prepared. Health and safety requirements should be carried out for every treatment, but knowing how to set up your treatment area, carrying out a proper consultation and knowing about warm and cool colours are also musts for make-up treatment.

HANDY HINTS

Read back over Chapter 113 to refresh your knowledge of health and safety.

SAFE AND HYGIENIC WORKING PRACTICES

It is important that you work in a safe and clean way. You should keep your treatment area tidy and use only hygienic tools and equipment. This will help to reduce the risk of harm to you and your clients and help to prevent cross-infection. The client will also have more confidence in you and you will look more professional.

It is your responsibility to be aware of health and safety legislation to protect yourself, your clients and your colleagues. The main safe and hygienic working practices that you need to know for a make-up treatment are:

- PPE – personal protective equipment. Examples in a make-up treatment are a gown, towels and headband. These help to stop the make-up getting onto the client's clothes and hair.
- COSHH – Control Of Substances Hazardous to Health. Examples in a make-up treatment are using a disinfectant safely when cleaning tools and equipment.
- HASAWA – Health and Safety at Work Act. Examples of this in a make-up treatment are ensuring that all equipment, tools and products are clean and safe to use for each client.
- Methods of sterilisation. Examples in a make-up treatment are using a disinfectant such as Barbicide to keep spatulas in and an ultraviolet cabinet to store equipment in a hygienic way.
- Disposal of contaminated waste. Examples include placing waste (such as dirty tissues) in a lined bin.

THE SALON ENVIRONMENT

It is important that you prepare your treatment area before your client arrives for their treatment. Think about client comfort and what you will need to do your job well. The treatment area should be prepared in professional way:

- All products, tools and equipment should be clean and hygienic.
- Products, tools and equipment should be placed safely and tidily on the trolley.
- If a couch is being used, it should be covered for hygiene reasons with a couch cover and couch roll tissue.

- The client needs to be positioned so that you do not have to bend your back too much when applying the make-up. This usually means that if a couch is used, it is raised at one end so that the client is sitting upright. If a make-up chair is used, the chair should be in an upright position so that you do not have to bend over too much. This will help to stop your back from aching.

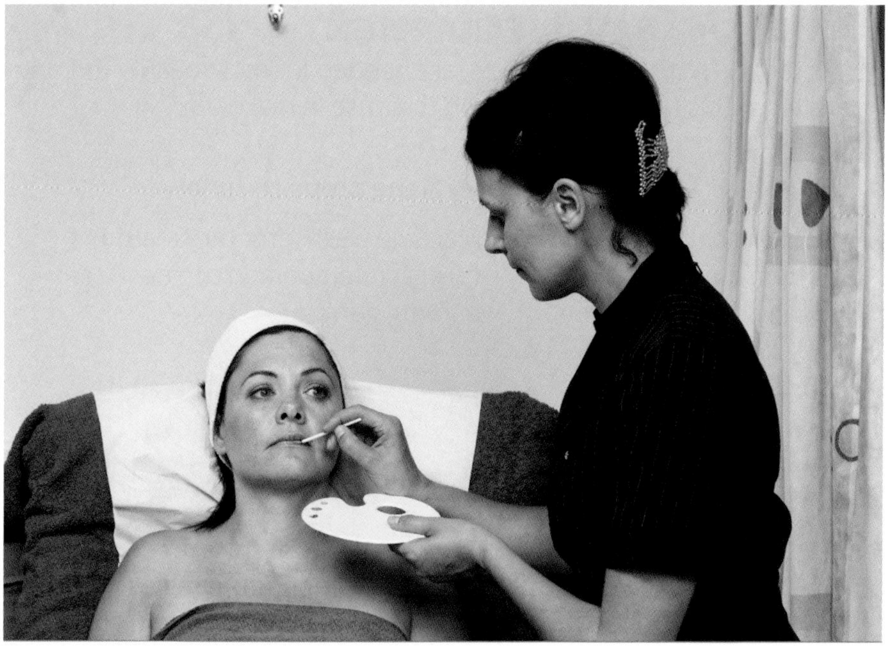

Correct positioning for a make-up treatment. Make-up can also be carried out with the client sitting on a make-up chair

HANDY HINTS

Go to Chapter 113 Following health and safety in the salon for more information on the health and safety laws that you should follow when carrying out a make-up treatment.

- The room temperature should not be too hot or too cold. The ideal temperature for a treatment room is between 16–18 degrees Centigrade.
- The air in the room should be well ventilated. This means that fresh air continually replaces stale air. It will also stop the atmosphere in the treatment room from becoming stuffy.
- It is very important that you have suitable lighting for a make-up treatment. The room needs to be well lit so that you can see clearly what you are doing.

ACTIVITY

Research on the internet how lighting affects the overall make-up look. Include examples of day and evening make-up applications.

ACTIVITY

In pairs or small groups, look at how you can work in a hygienic and safe way when carrying out a make-up treatment. You can refer to Chapter 113 Following health and safety in the salon to help you. Design a fact sheet or a poster that could be used to inform a new employee about health and safety in the salon.

SmartScreen 106 worksheet 1

PREPARING FOR THE MAKE-UP SERVICE

Before the client arrives, it is important that you get yourself and the treatment area prepared. All of the products, tools and equipment need to be ready. This will make sure that the treatment flows well and will also give the client a positive first impression. It will help the client to relax and have confidence in you.

BASIC TOOLS AND EQUIPMENT

Some items, such as couch covers, are needed for most beauty therapy treatments. This table lists them and their use in make-up.

Tools/equipment	**What is it used for?**	**Hygiene steps to follow**
Towels 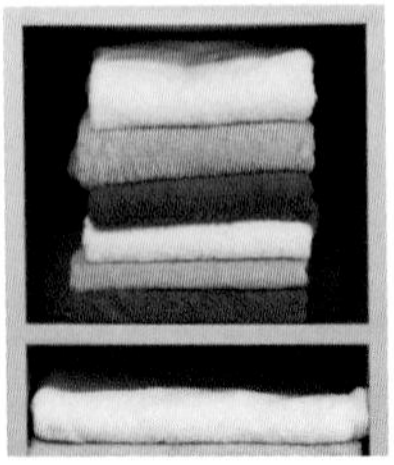	Used to cover the client and protect their clothing from make-up. Place around the client's shoulders.	Machine wash after the treatment on a high temperature to destroy harmful germs.
Headband 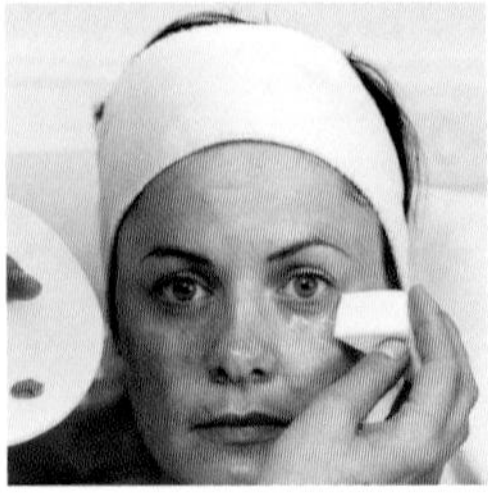	Keeps the client's hair off her face. Place around the client's head.	Machine wash after the treatment on a high temperature to destroy harmful germs.
Cotton wool 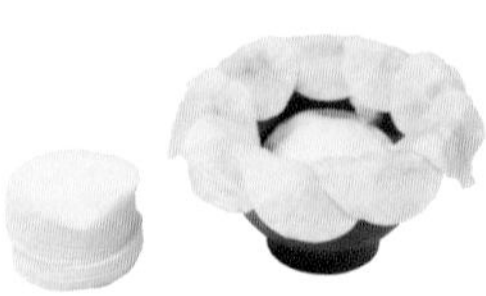	Used to remove the cleanser and help to remove surface dirt and any make-up at the start of the treatment. Also used to apply toner. Use damp.	Throw away after use.
Gown 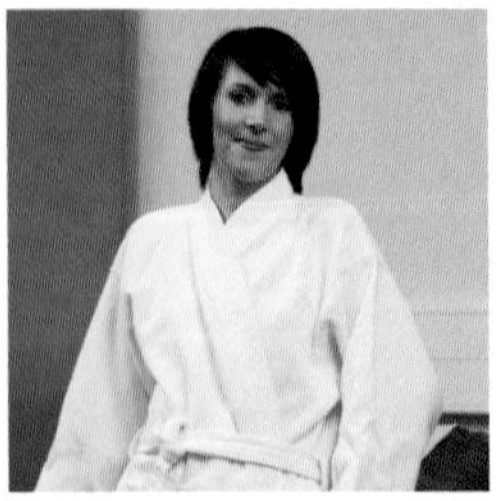	Covers the client during the treatment to protect their clothes.	Machine wash after the treatment on a high temperature to destroy harmful germs.

Tools/equipment	What is it used for?	Hygiene steps to follow
Tissues 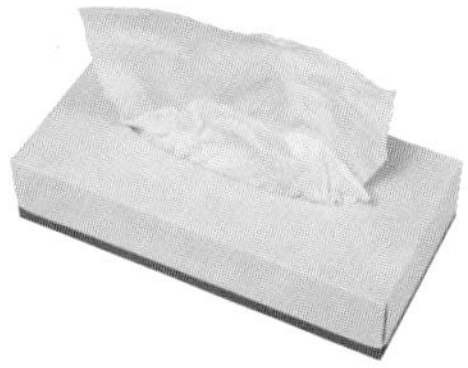	Can be used to blot the skin after toner is applied. They can also be used to blot the lips after lipstick has been applied.	Throw away after use.
Couch cover 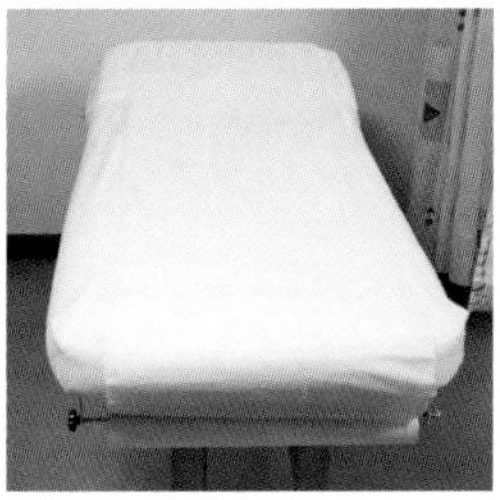	If a couch is used for the client, a couch cover is placed over the couch for hygiene reasons.	Machine wash after the treatment on a high temperature to destroy harmful germs.
Couch tissue roll 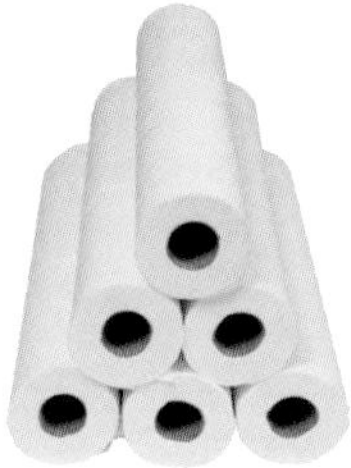	If a couch is used for the client, this is placed on top of the couch cover for hygiene reasons.	Throw away after use.
Mirror 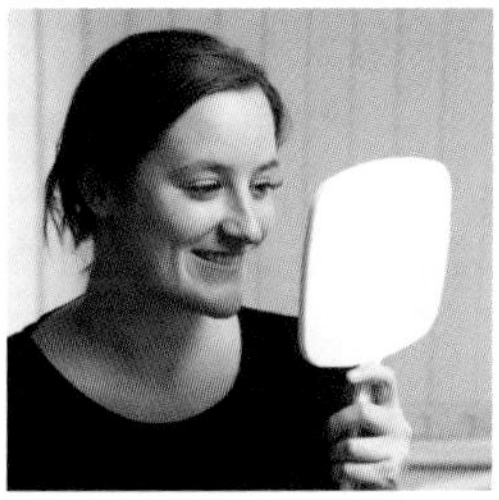	Used to show the client the finished make-up look.	Wipe over the mirror before and after the treatment to make sure that it is clean for your client to look in.
Waste bin 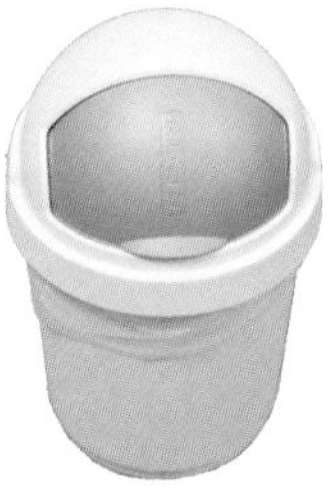	Used for throwing waste materials into, such as cotton wool and tissues.	This should be lined with a bin liner and have a lid.
Treatment plan 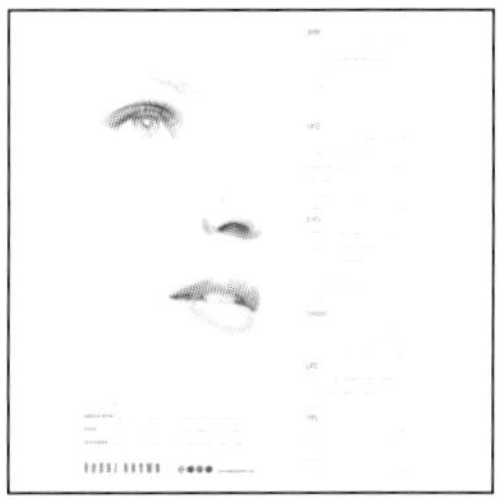	Records the treatment details, eg products used and what occasion the make-up was applied for.	Keep in a secure and **confidential** place.

Confidential
Private – not for public access

TOOLS AND EQUIPMENT USED IN A MAKE-UP TREATMENT

This table lists tools and equipment items that are not used for every treatment, but are used for make-up treatments only.

Make-up tools and equipment	What is it used for?	Hygiene steps to follow
Make-up brushes 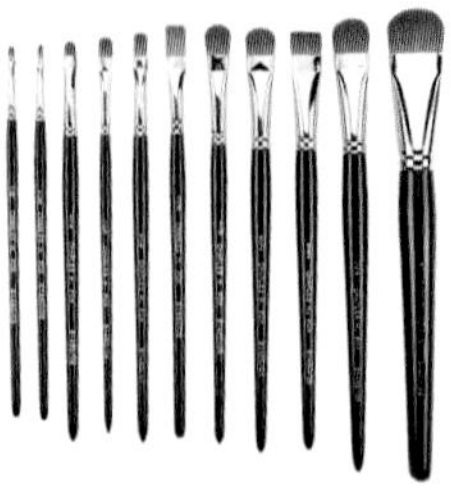	Used to apply make-up products in a professional way. A good set of brushes will include ones to apply concealer, loose powder, blusher, eyeshadow, eyeliner, lipstick and to brush the brows.	Wash the brushes after each client in warm soapy water to remove any make-up and then in a disinfectant suitable for brushes, eg Milton fluid®. Store in an ultraviolet cabinet between clients.
Palette 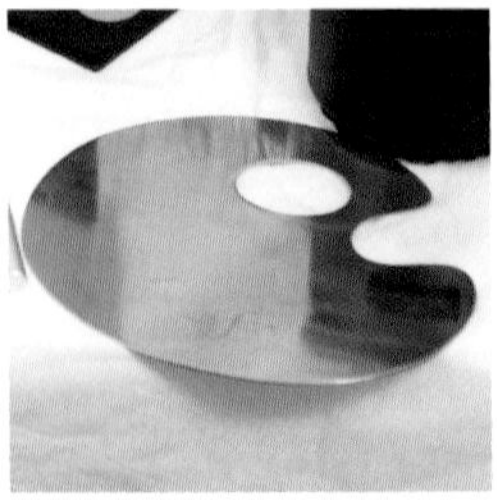	Once you have applied make-up to the palette, you can hygienically apply it to the client's face.	Apply the make-up to the palette using a damp brush or sponge. Then work off the palette with a damp sponge or brush onto the face. Wash afterwards in warm soapy water to clean.
Make-up sponges 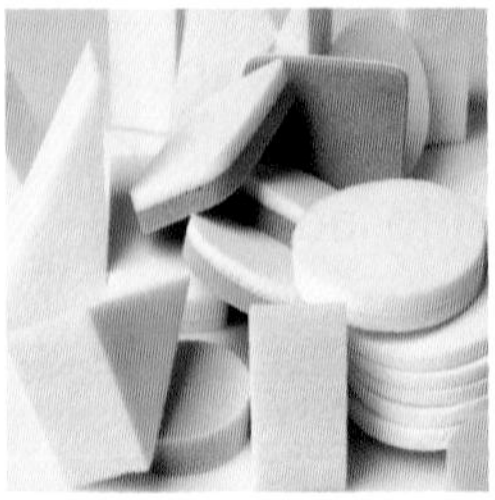	Small sponges used for applying foundation.	Wash in warm, soapy water afterwards to remove all of the foundation. Then wash in disinfectant such as Milton fluid®. Store hygienically in an ultraviolet cabinet. Make sure the brushes are totally dry before using them again.
Disposable eyeshadow sponges 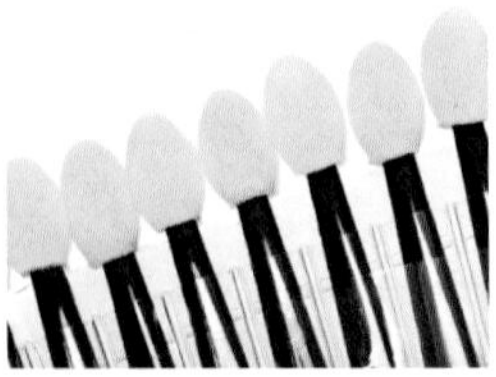	Used to apply eyeshadow in a hygienic way.	Throw away after use.
Disposable mascara wands 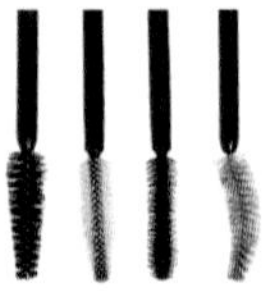	Used to apply mascara in a hygienic way.	Throw away after use.

Make-up tools and equipment	What is it used for?	Hygiene steps to follow
Disposable lip brushes 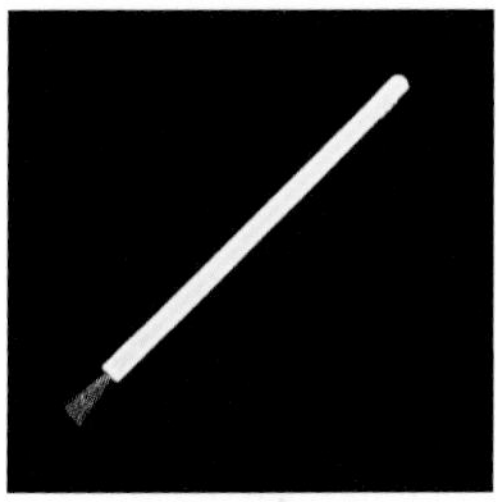	Used to apply lipstick in a hygienic way.	Throw away after use.
Spatulas 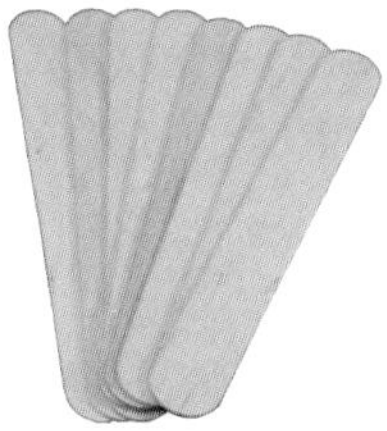	Used to scoop make-up products out from pots. These can be plastic or wooden. The wooden ones are disposable. They can also be used for scraping a small amount of lipstick onto them, before applying to the lips with a lip brush.	Wash the plastic spatulas in warm, soapy water and then disinfectant. Place in an ultraviolet cabinet to store them hygienically. Throw away the wooden spatulas after use.
Barbicide and jar 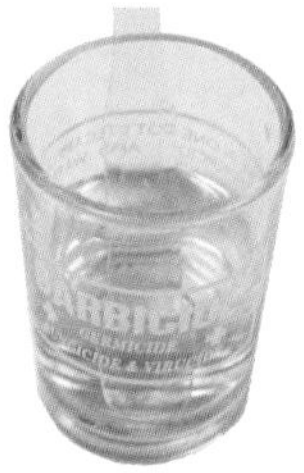	A disinfectant – the spatula can be placed in this during the treatment.	After use, pour the Barbicide down the sink. Rinse the jar with warm, soapy water and dry.

PRODUCTS USED IN A MAKE-UP TREATMENT

There are many products you need to learn about for a make-up treatment. This table will help you.

SmartScreen 106 handouts 6, 7, 8, 10, 15, 16 and 18

SmartScreen 106 worksheet 3

Make-up product	What is it used for?	Hygiene steps to follow
Cleanser 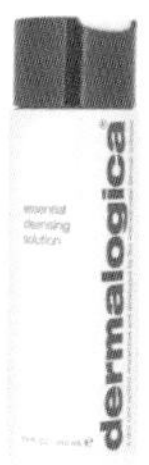	To remove make-up and surface dirt from the skin before the treatment.	Usually applied to the face using the fingertips. Then gently massaged in. Removed using warm cotton wool pads.

Make-up product	What is it used for?	Hygiene steps to follow
Toner 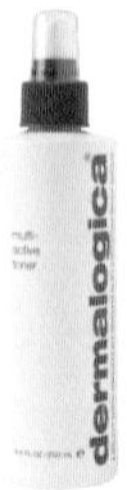	Refreshes the skin. Removes the last traces of the cleanser.	Applied onto damp cotton wool pads. These are then gently wiped over the skin.
Moisturiser 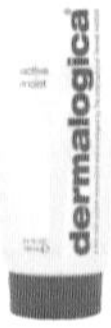	Helps to stop the skin from drying out. Makes the skin feel soft and supple. Apply only a small amount onto the client's skin. If too much is used then the skin will feel greasy and the make-up will not go on very well.	First it is applied into the palm of the hand, then applied to the fingertips and gently tapped over the skin. It is then lightly massaged into the skin until it has been absorbed.
Concealer 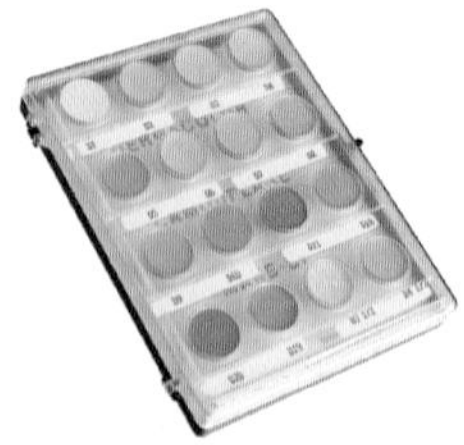	Used to cover: ▪ redness (use green-coloured concealer) ▪ **sallow skin** (use lilac-coloured concealer) ▪ **skin blemishes** (use cream-coloured concealer).	Apply on to a palette, then apply to the face using a brush or a sponge.
Foundation 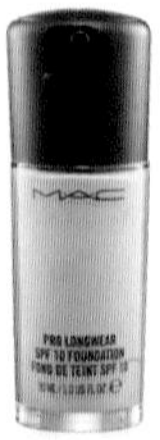	Helps to give the skin an even colour.	Apply onto a palette, then apply to the face using a brush or sponge.
Face powder 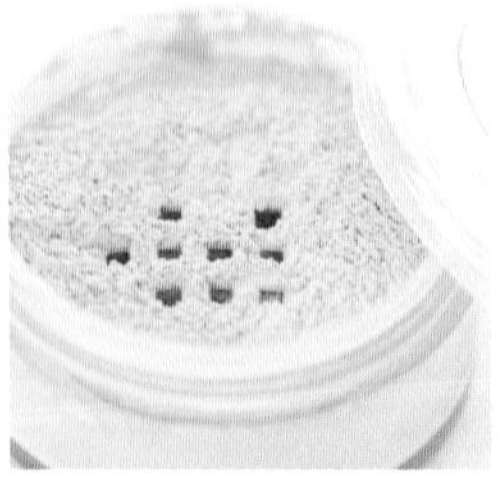	Helps to set the foundation. This will make the foundation last longer.	Apply onto a tissue and then apply to the face with a large brush.

Sallow skin

Skin that has a yellow colour; oriental and Asian skins can be sallow in colour

Skin blemishes

Marks on the skin such as spots and scars

Make-up product	What is it used for?	Hygiene steps to follow
Blusher 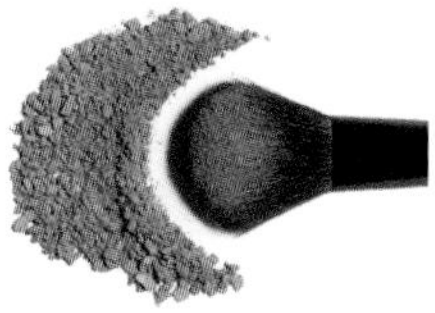	Adds warmth and colour to the cheeks.	Apply to the cheeks using a medium-sized brush. Wipe over the top of the blusher with a tissue afterwards to avoid cross-infection.
Eyeshadow 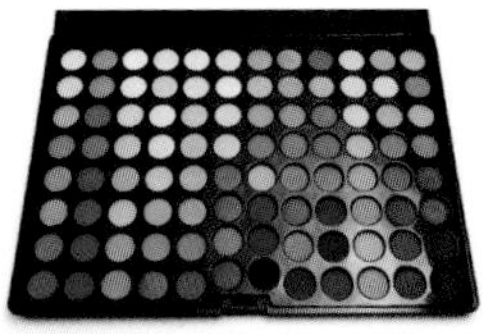	Helps to give the eyes shape. Adds colour to the eyelids.	Apply using a disposable make-up applicator. Wipe over the top of the eyeshadow with a tissue afterwards to make sure it is hygienic for the next client. Throw away the disposable make-up applicator after use.
Mascara 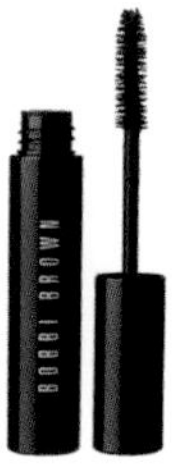	Adds thickness, colour and length to the eyelashes. It may also help to curl the eyelashes.	Apply using a disposable mascara wand. Throw away the disposable mascara wand after use.
Eye pencils 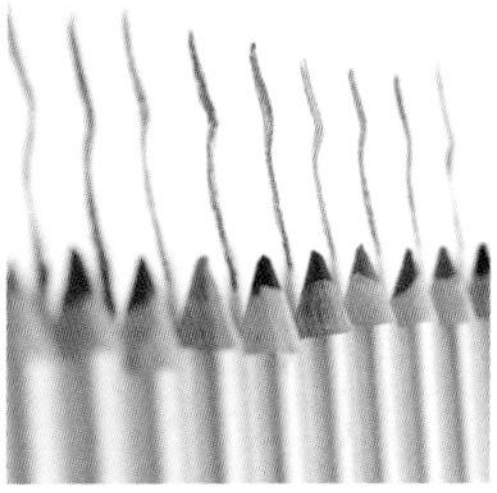	Eyebrow pencil: makes the eyebrows stand out. Eyeliner: makes the eyes stand out.	Sharpen using a pencil sharpener before using. Apply using light strokes. Sharpen afterwards using a pencil sharpener to make sure it is clean for the next client.
Lip products 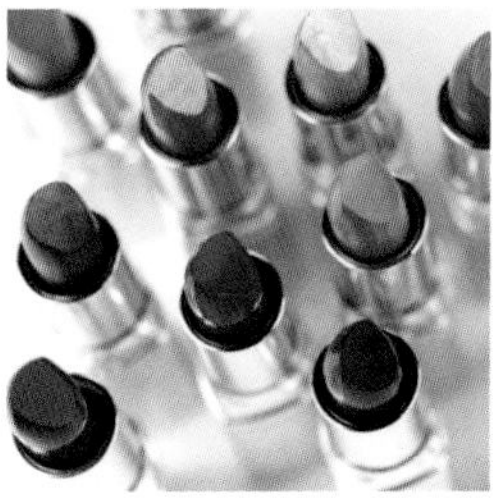	Lip liner pencil: helps to outline the lips before the lipstick is applied. Lipstick: adds colour to the lips and makes them stand out. Lip gloss: adds shine to the lips or lipstick.	Sharpen using a pencil sharpener before using. Apply to outline the lips. Sharpen afterwards using a pencil sharpener to make sure it is clean for the next client. Apply on to a palette, then apply to the lips using a disposable lip brush. Throw away the disposable lip brush after use.

HANDY HINTS

Go to Chapter 006 Skin care and read more detailed information about the different skin-cleansing products, which skin types they are used for and how to use them.

SmartScreen 106 handouts 2, 4 and 5

SmartScreen 106 worksheets 2 and 3

You will need to have the following products, tools and materials on your trolley:

- skin care products (cleansers, toners and moisturisers), suitable for oily, dry, combination and normal skin types
- make-up products (concealers; foundations; powders; blushers; lip products: lipstick, lip liners, lip gloss; eye products: eyeshadow, eyebrow pencil, eye pencil, mascara)
- make-up tools and equipment (applicators, brushes, cotton wool, tissues, make-up palette)
- a mirror
- a treatment plan and pen.

You will also need a treatment couch or make-up chair and suitable coverings for your client (headband, couch covers, couch tissue, towels and gown).

HANDY HINTS

Shaders are like blushers but are usually slightly darker. They are used to make areas look less noticeable, such as a wide jaw line.

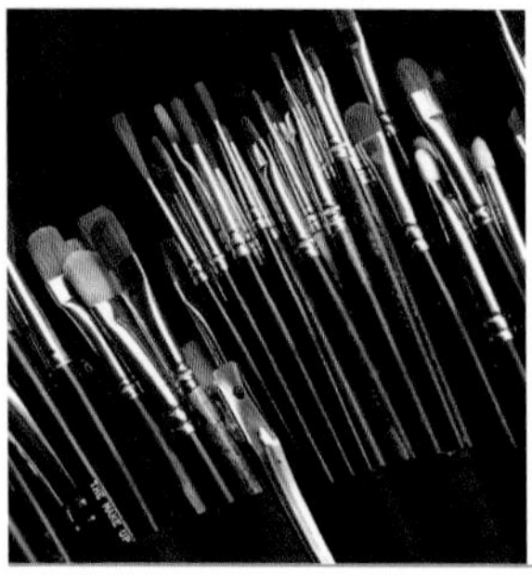

Professional make-up brushes

HANDY HINTS

Highlighters are lighter than blushers and are used to draw attention to areas such as a narrow jaw line.

HANDY HINTS

Remember, do not blow on the brushes to remove excess make-up as this is not hygienic. Instead, gently tap the brush on the back of your other hand.

SmartScreen 106 handouts 1 and 2

BASIC ANATOMY FOR MAKE-UP

Before you can carry out a consultation for make-up services, you need to have an understanding of the basic anatomy of the bones of the face and the structure and function of the skin.

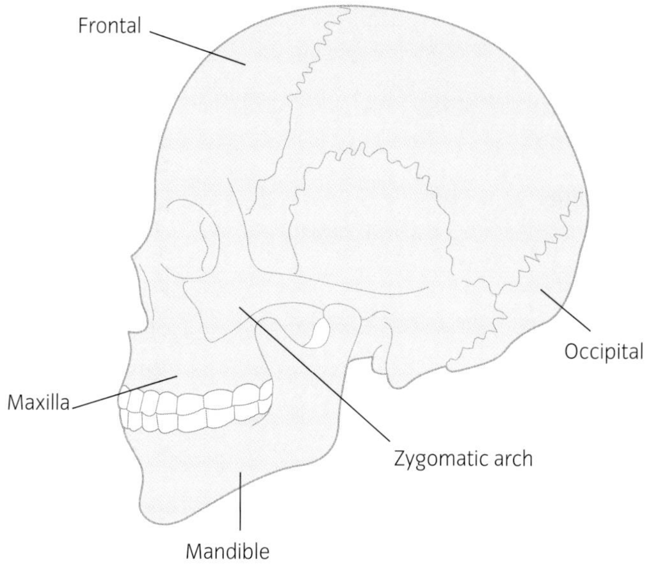

Bones of the skull

BONES OF THE FACE

- Mandible – this bone forms the lower jaw. It is the only moveable bone in the skull. It allows us to talk and chew. The mandible contains the lower set of teeth.
- Maxilla – this bone forms the upper jaw. The maxilla contains the upper set of teeth.
- Zygomatic arches – these bones form the cheekbones.
- Frontal – this bone is found at the front of the skull and forms the forehead.

HANDY HINTS

The skull is made up of 22 bones.

SmartScreen 106 worksheet 7

SmartScreen 106 handout 4 and worksheet 4

THE BASIC STRUCTURE OF THE SKIN

The skin is our largest organ and is made up of two main layers. We need to know about the basic structure and function of the skin so that we know how to improve its appearance and also understand how to care for it. These are the main parts of the skin that you need to know about:

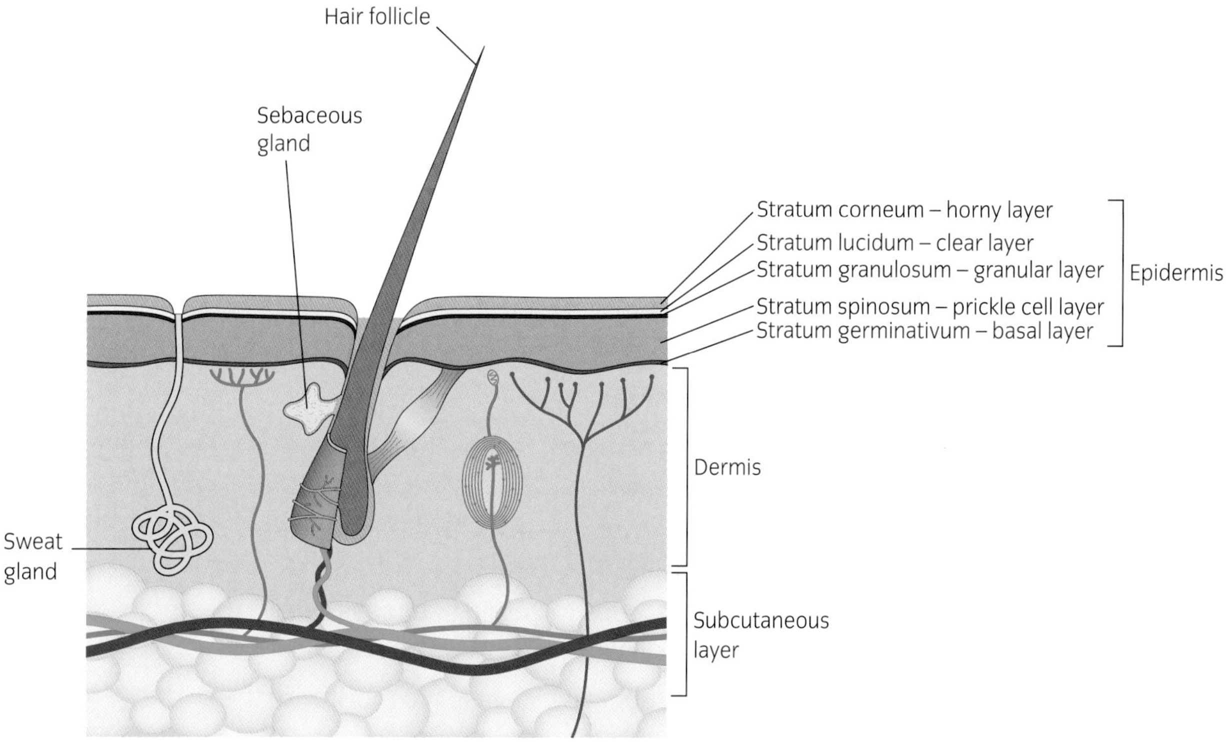

The basic structure of the skin

HANDY HINTS

The skin constantly sheds dead cells from the surface of the epidermis. Excess shedding can be seen as dandruff on the scalp.

HANDY HINTS

About 80 per cent of house dust is skin which has been shed!

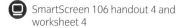

Melanin
A substance that gives skin its colour

Contract
Tighten

Antiseptic
A substance that stops bacteria growing

Supple
Flexible; in skin this means staying healthy and not ageing

Excess
Too much of something

Stimulate
To cause activity

- Epidermis – this is the outer layer of the skin (the part we touch when we stroke the surface of our skin). It is made up of five layers. The very outer layer that we can touch is constantly shedding skin cells from the surface. As skin cells are shed, new ones are produced in the deeper layers to replace them. The main functions of this layer are to:
  - protect the body from harmful substances (such as bacteria)
  - provide a waterproof coating
  - produce **melanin**, which helps to protect our skin from the sun's rays.
- Dermis – this lies below the epidermis and is a thicker layer. It contains lots of structures such as nerves, hair follicles, sweat glands, sebaceous glands and a blood supply. These are the ones you need to know about:
  - Sweat glands have an opening onto the skin's surface. They produce sweat, which is pushed out onto the skin's surface when we get hot. This helps to cool us down.
  - Hair follicles are like pockets in the skin. Hairs grow in the hair follicle.
  - Sebaceous glands are attached to the hair follicles. They produce an oily substance called sebum. This helps to keep the skin moisturised.
- Subcutaneous layer – this lies below the dermis. It contains fat cells, which help to keep us warm and also provide protection to the organs underneath.

HANDY HINTS

The skin has eight main functions. Use the word 'SHAPES' to help you remember them.

THE BASIC FUNCTIONS OF THE SKIN

Function		Description
S	Sensation	Nerves send messages to the brain. They react to touch, pressure, cold and heat.
H	Heat regulation	In the dermis there are special nerve endings that react to heat and cold. The normal average body temperature is 36.8°C. The body is kept at this temperature through the blood supply and the production of sweat. If you get too hot, sweat glands make sweat to cool you down and the blood vessels in the skin get larger to release more heat from the body (making you look red). If you get too cold the blood vessels in the skin get smaller to keep the heat in (making you look pale). The muscles can also **contract** quickly to give off heat, making you shiver and helping to warm you up.
A	Absorption	Although the skin acts as a barrier to harmful substances, it absorbs small amounts of water with nutrients and minerals.
P	Protection	The skin protects the body and helps prevent bacterial infection. It produces oil called sebum, which is an **antiseptic** and keeps the skin **supple**. It also produces melanin which protects against UV light. Sensory nerve endings in the skin mean we can feel and react to pain, heat and touch.
E	Excretion	The skin produces sweat which helps to get rid of **excess** salts in the body as well as helping to cool the skin when we are warm.
S	Secretion	The skin secretes an oil called sebum which helps to moisturise the skin and hair and stops them drying out.
Vitamin D production		Ultraviolet light **stimulates** a chemical in the skin to produce vitamin D, essential for healthy bones.
Melanin (colour pigment) production		Melanin is formed by cells in the dermis called melanocytes. It protects the deeper layers of the skin from sun damage.

ACTIVITY

To test your knowledge further, log into SmartScreen and complete the revision activities.

SmartScreen 106 handouts 13 and 14

CONSULTATION

Before you start the treatment you will need to carry out a **consultation** with the client for the following reasons:

- to find out why they are having the make-up. Is it for a special occasion, such as a party, a wedding or a photograph? This will make sure that the make-up applied is suitable for their purpose
- to check what skin type the client has so that the correct products are used
- to discuss what make-up colours the client would prefer
- to check for any skin conditions that may prevent or restrict the treatment from taking place.

Whatever the reason may be, there are many different make-up looks that you can achieve, from a natural day make-up to a more creative evening look.

Consultation
Discussion with and examination of the client before the treatment starts

HANDY HINTS

The acid mantle is the term given to the combination of sweat and sebum which creates an acidic film on the skin. This helps to prevent the growth of bacteria and fungi.

HANDY HINTS

Your skin colour is determined by the amount of melanin produced in the skin.

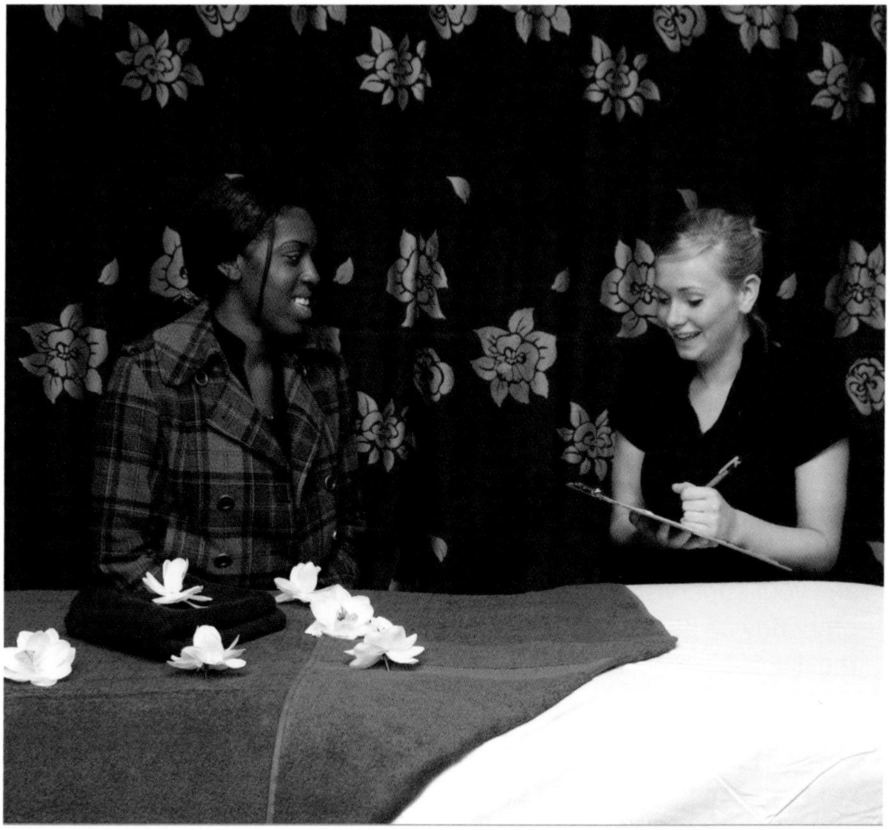

A consultation with a client

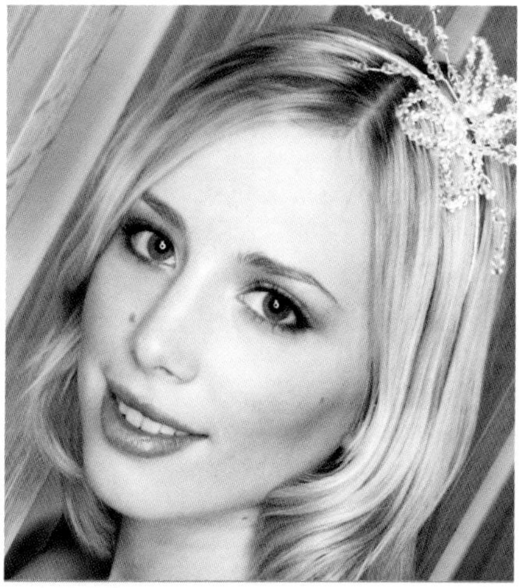

Make-up for a wedding

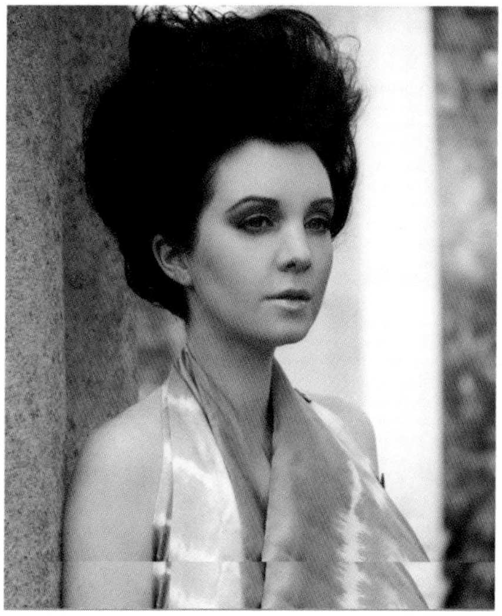

A special occasion make-up

ACTIVITY

Pair up with each other and carry out a consultation role play. One of you is the client and the other one is the therapist.

SmartScreen 106 handout 17

COMMUNICATION AND BEHAVIOUR

You must use your communication and behaviour skills at all times, but they are particularly important in a consultation.

HANDY HINTS

A thorough consultation is important. It will help to make sure that the client is happy with the treatment.

Communication skills are used to pass on information from one person to another. Positive communication can be achieved by:

- Speaking clearly and with confidence; making sure the information is correct and well explained. An example of this is explaining to the client how to apply the make-up products correctly.
- Listening to what is being said; helping to make sure that the information has been understood. This is particularly important when you are carrying out the consultation with the client. You need to make sure that you have got the correct information. If you are unsure, ask your client again. Your tutor will also help you.
- Having a positive body language; such as a relaxed, open posture, a smile and good eye contact. This will make the client feel more relaxed with you.
- Recording information clearly and correctly; such as treatment information on the client's record card. Examples of information to include are the make-up products and colours that you have used.
- Using correct **terminology** linked to the make-up treatment; this will show the client how professional you are and that you are fully trained. Examples of terminology used in a make-up treatment are the correct names for the tools, equipment and materials that you will use such as cosmetic sponges, blushers, make-up palette, cleansers, toners and moisturisers.

Terminology
Technical terms

HANDY HINTS

When using make-up terminology for products with your client (such as 'concealers' or 'shaders') remember to fully explain what they are. Your client may not know this.

SmartScreen 106 handout 12

It is important to behave in a professional manner at all times. This will make the client feel more comfortable and they will also have more confidence in you. The following are also ways in which you can make your behaviour more positive:

- Follow instructions; this will make sure the treatments are carried out professionally and correctly. Examples of this are wearing the correct salon uniform, speaking politely to work **colleagues** and clients and making sure that you work safely and hygienically with all of the products, tools and equipment.
- Work co-operatively with others; this includes your work colleagues and your supervisor (tutor or boss). This may mean helping each other tidy up between clients and also cleaning the salon throughout the day.
- Follow salon requirements; your salon may have certain rules that you will need to follow such as a dress code, eg a uniform.

Colleagues
People that you work with

HANDY HINTS

Refer to Chapter 102 Presenting a professional image in the salon, for more detailed information on communication and behaviour.

SmartScreen 106 worksheet 6

FACTORS THAT MAY INFLUENCE THE MAKE-UP TREATMENT

There are certain **factors** that you will need to think about when planning your make-up treatment. This will make sure that the make-up you apply is suitable for the client.

FASHION TRENDS

Clients may want a make-up look like their favourite pop star. There are many images of the latest make-up looks shown in magazines or on the television. It is important that you keep up to date with the latest fashion trends so that you know what make-up looks are popular. This will mean that your clients have up-to-date make-up looks

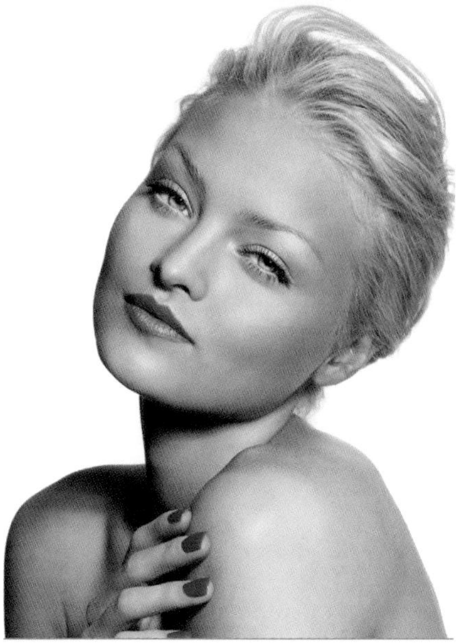

A professional make-up image

Factors
Things to consider before beginning the treatment

ACTIVITY

Keep your eye on what make-up looks and images are popular at the moment. Research on the internet, magazines, books, etc and find out what make-up looks are popular at the moment. Save the images and print them off. Practise the make-up on your class mates.

Cultural factors

It is important that we respect other people's **cultures**. The make-up chosen may need to be **adapted** to suit a client's culture (such as how the make-up is applied and also what colours are used).

An example of how culture may affect how make-up is applied is in the Asian culture. The main focus for the make-up is usually on the eyes. Both eyeliner and eyeshadows are used to make them look more **defined**.

A brighter colour can normally be used on African skins (such as bright green, blue, silver or yellow/gold) as these colours look better on a darker skin **tone**.

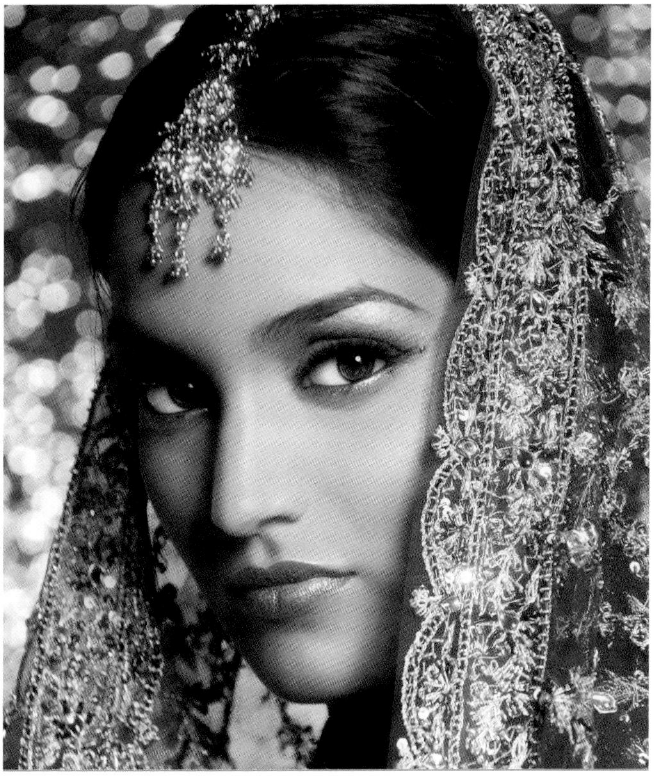

An example of an Indian bridal make-up

ACTIVITY

Research on the internet to find out how make-up is worn in different cultures such as India and Japan.

Culture
The beliefs and behaviours of a certain group of people. These might be influenced by race, religion or amount of money

Adapt
To change something

Defined
To stand out

Tone
How tight the skin feels; if the skin tone is poor this can lead to wrinkles

Portfolio
A collection of creative work and ideas to show to a client

SmartScreen 106 worksheet 8

SmartScreen 106 handout 17

ACTIVITY

Research different make-up looks on the internet. Create a **portfolio** of different images. Try to include day and evening make-up ideas. You can then use this portfolio with your clients when you are deciding what make-up they would like.

Face shape

Your client's face shape is an important factor in make-up application. The table below tells you where to apply make-up to suit every face shape.

Face shape	Where to apply the blusher, shader and highlighter
Oval 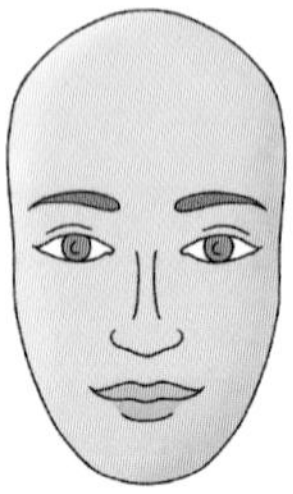 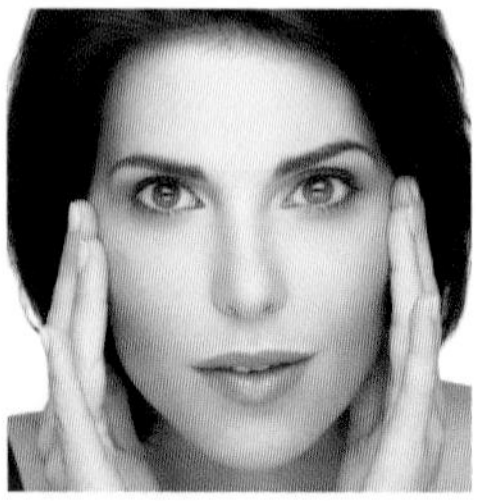	This face shape does not need any correcting – it is the ideal face shape. Blusher and highlighter can be used to make the most of the facial features as they define cheekbones. ▪ Apply blusher under the cheekbone. ▪ Apply highlighter above the blusher, on top of the cheekbone.
Square 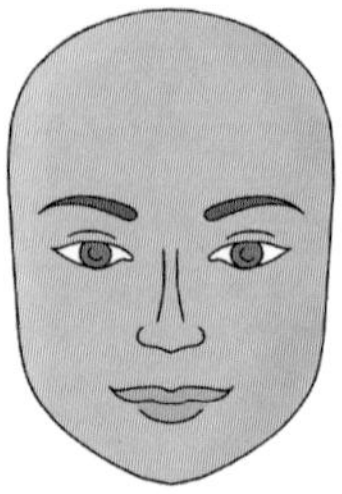 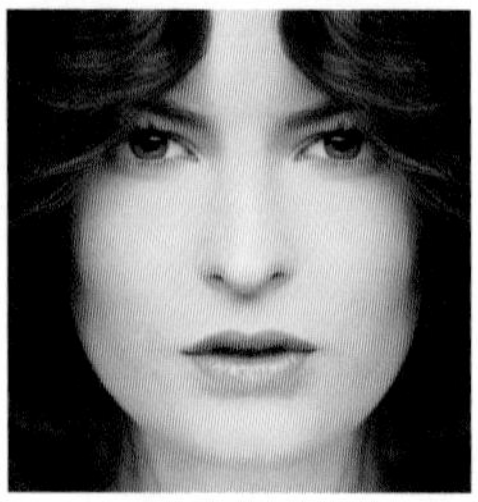	This face shape needs to be softened on the sides of the jaw and forehead. ▪ Apply blusher under the cheekbone. ▪ Apply highlighter above the blusher, on top of the cheekbone. ▪ Apply shader to the sides of the jaw and forehead to make large features look smaller.
Long 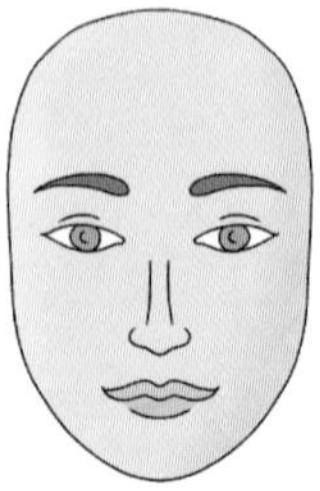 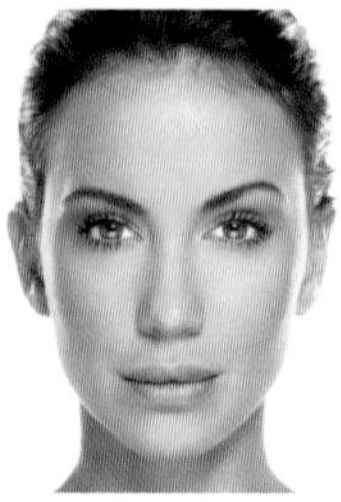	This face shape needs be made to look shorter and wider. ▪ Apply blusher under the cheekbone. ▪ Apply highlighter above the blusher, on top of the cheekbone; also at the sides of the forehead. ▪ Apply shader to the top of the forehead and tip of the chin.
Round 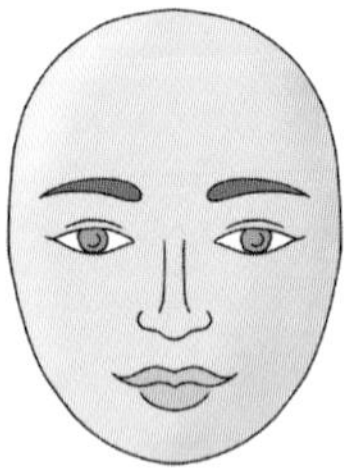 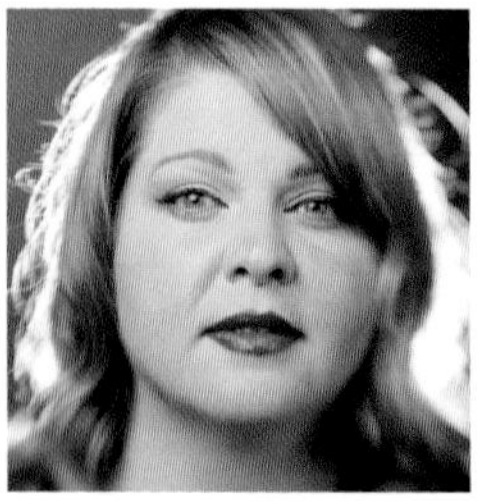	This face shape needs to be made to look slimmer. ▪ Apply blusher under the cheekbone. ▪ Apply highlighter above the blusher, on top of the cheekbone; also down the centre of the face. ▪ Apply shader below the blusher; also at the sides of the jaw and forehead.

ACTIVITY

Look at photos of famous people in magazines and on the internet. Try to work out which face shape they have. Collect examples of each of the face shapes mentioned above and stick them onto a sheet of paper for each face shape. Show these to the rest of the group.

Nose shape

The table below tells you where to apply make-up to flatter your client's nose shape.

Nose shape	Where to apply the blusher, shader and highlighter
Long 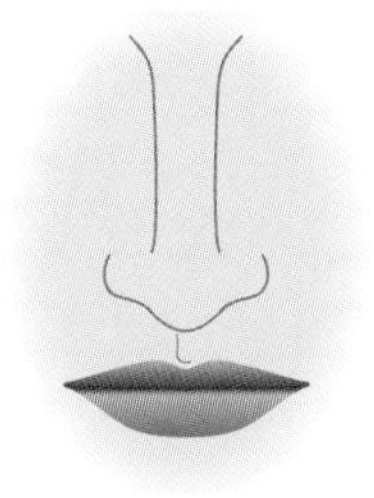	This nose shape needs to be made to look shorter: ▪ Apply shader to the tip of the nose. ▪ Apply highlighter to the sides.
Short 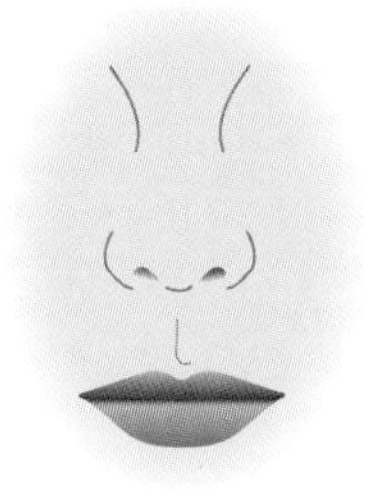	This nose shape needs to be made to look longer: ▪ Apply highlighter down the centre of the nose and onto the tip.
Wide 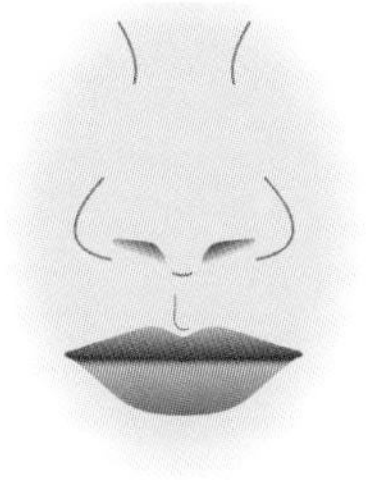	This nose shape needs to be made to look narrower: ▪ Apply shader to the sides of the nose.

Eye shape or position

There are a variety of techniques you can use to flatter your client's eyes. The table below tells you all about them.

Eye shape/position	Eye shape/position	How to correct this eye shape/position
Round 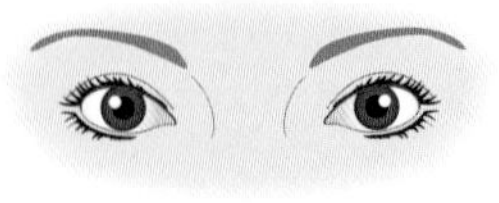	Round 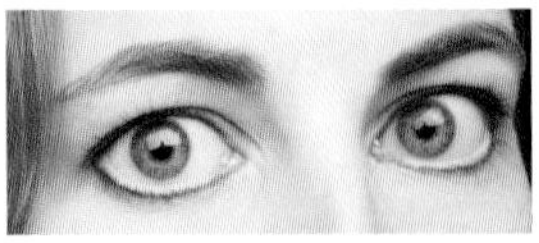	To make them appear less round: ▪ Apply darker shadow to the outer corners. ▪ Apply eyeliner to the outer corner to make the eye look wider at the edges.
Small 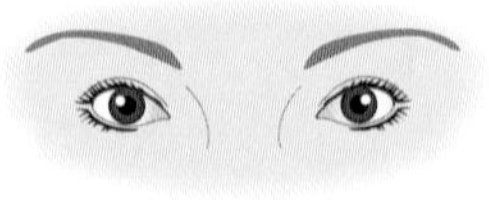	Small 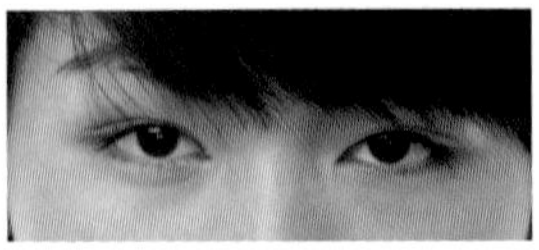	To make them look bigger: ▪ Use light colours on the lid. ▪ Use white pencil on the inner rim of the eye.
Wide apart 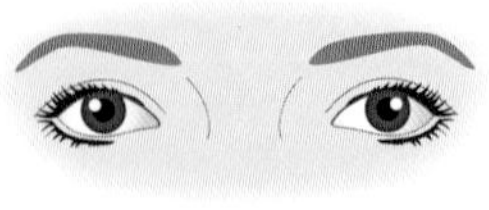	Wide apart 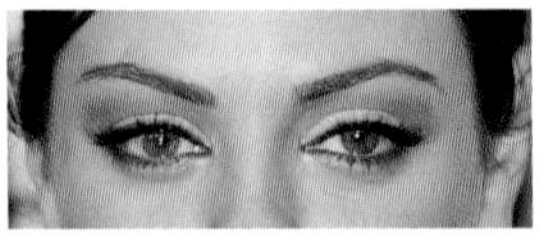	To make them look closer together: ▪ Use darker shadow on the inner part of the lid (nearest the nose). ▪ Use lighter colours on the outer part of the lid.
Close together 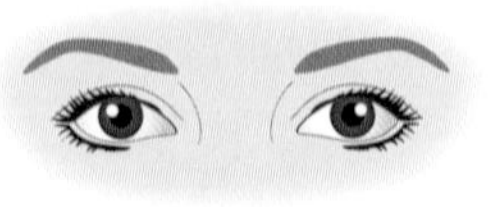	Close together 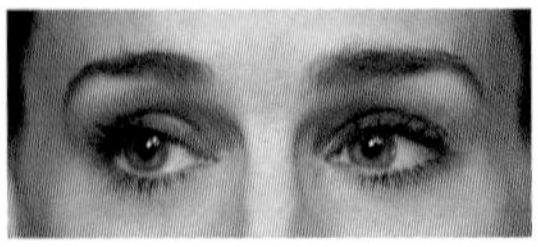	To make them look wider apart: ▪ Use lighter shadow on the inner part of the lid (nearest the nose). ▪ Use darker colours on the outer part of the lid.
Deeply set 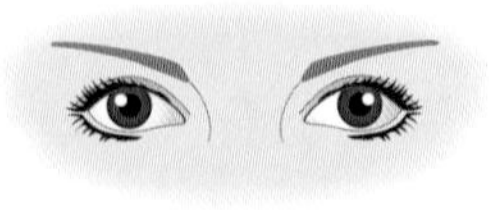	Deeply set 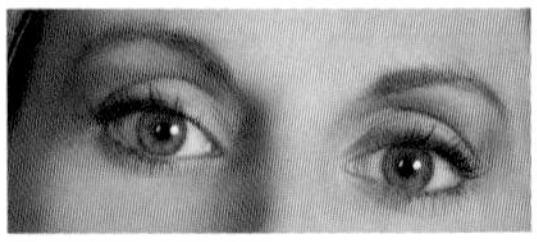	To make them look more **prominent**: ▪ Use lighter shadows on the eyelid.
Prominent 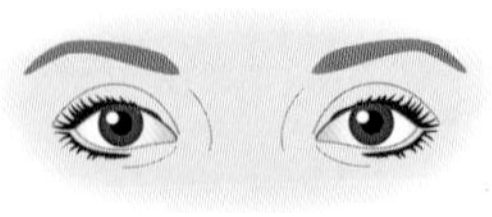	Prominent 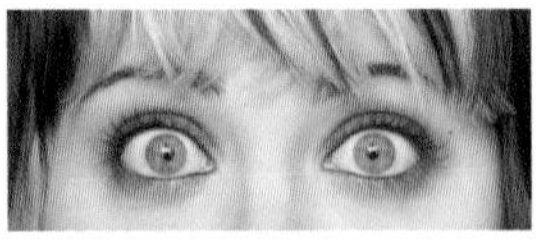	To make them look less prominent: ▪ Use darker shadows on the eyelid.

Prominent
Stands out or bulges

Lip shape

The table below tells you what make-up techniques to use to flatter your client's lip shape.

Lip shape	How to correct this lip shape
Large 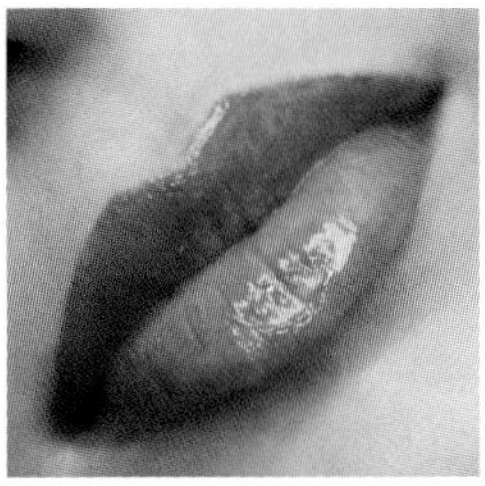	To make them appear smaller: ▪ Apply lip pencil slightly inside the natural lip line. ▪ Use darker, deeper colours.
Thin 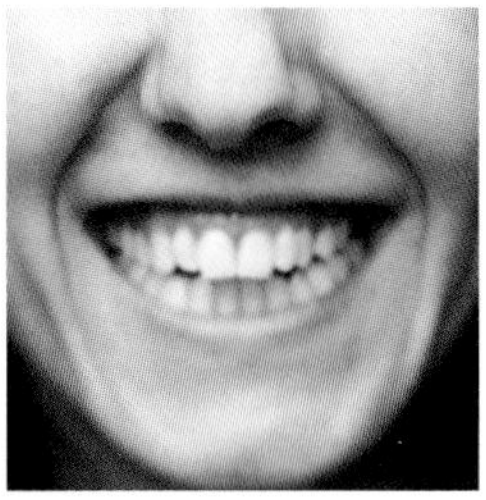	To make the lips look fuller: ▪ Apply lip pencil slightly outside the natural lip line. ▪ Use light-coloured lipstick.

SmartScreen 106 handout 3 and worksheet 2

HANDY HINTS

Clients who suffer from herpes simplex (cold sores) should avoid ultraviolet light (sunlight) as this can make it worse.

Adverse skin conditions

As part of the consultation you also need to identify whether or not the client has any contra-indications that will prevent or restrict the treatment.

Conditions that prevent a make-up treatment

Certain skin and eye conditions prevent you from carrying out a basic make-up treatment. All the skin and eye conditions described below are **contagious**, which means they can be passed from one person to another. For this reason you must never treat a client with these conditions.

If you see any of these you need to refer to your tutor/salon manager or senior therapist and they will make the decision as to what it is and if you may go ahead with the treatment.

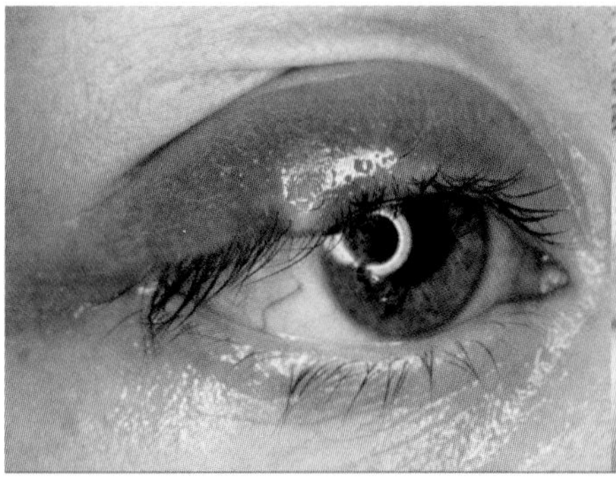

A stye

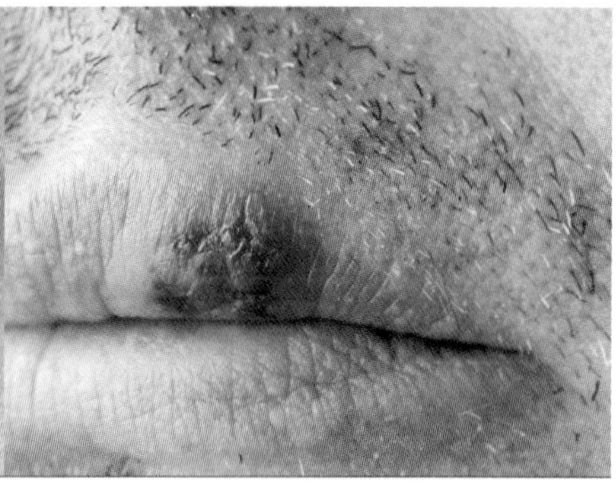

A cold sore

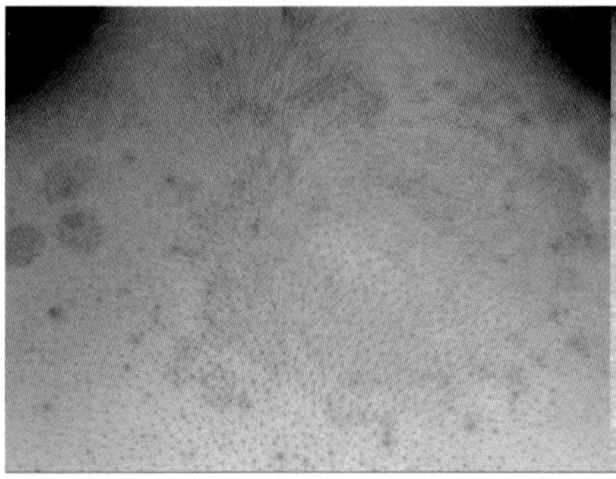

Ringworm

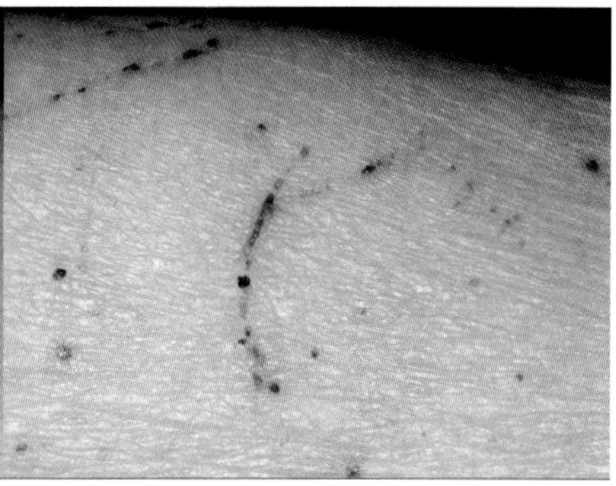

Scabies

Contagious

Describing a condition that can be passed from one person to another

Conditions that may restrict a make-up treatment
The following conditions may restrict the treatment in some way. They are not contagious but you may have to adapt your treatment.

Condition	What is it?	How may it affect the treatment?
Recent scars 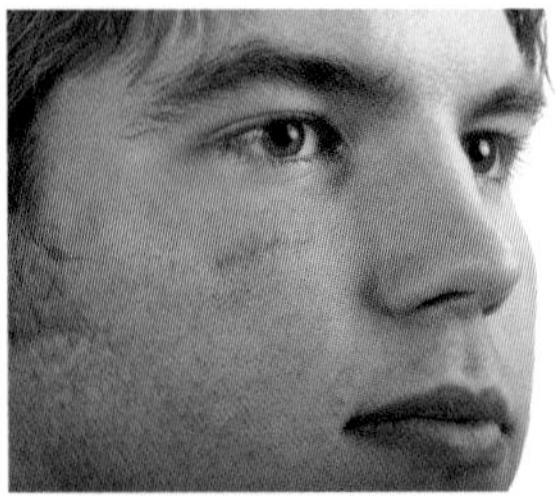	Damage to the skin; may be sensitive	Do not work over this area.
Eczema 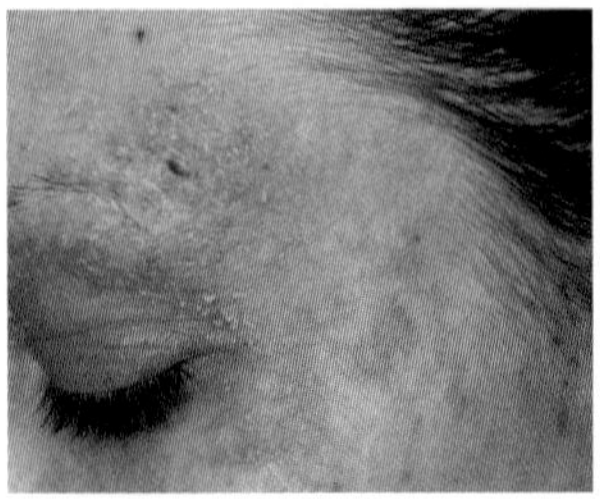	Dry, flaky skin which may be cracked	If the skin is broken and sensitive, do not work over this area. If the skin is not broken and sensitive, use cream products to help with the dryness.
Psoriasis 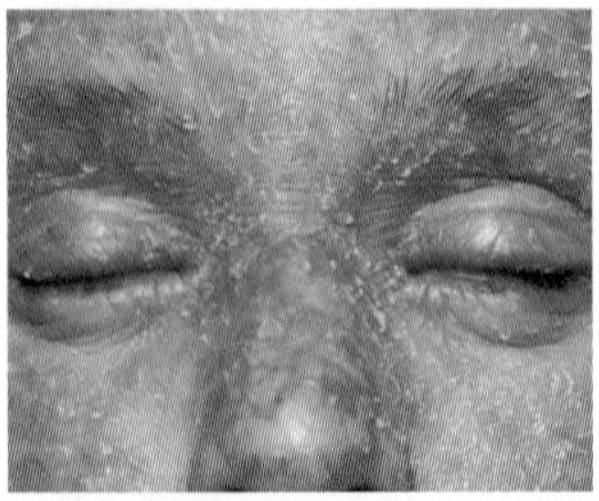	Dry silvery scales on red skin	As for eczema.
Bruising 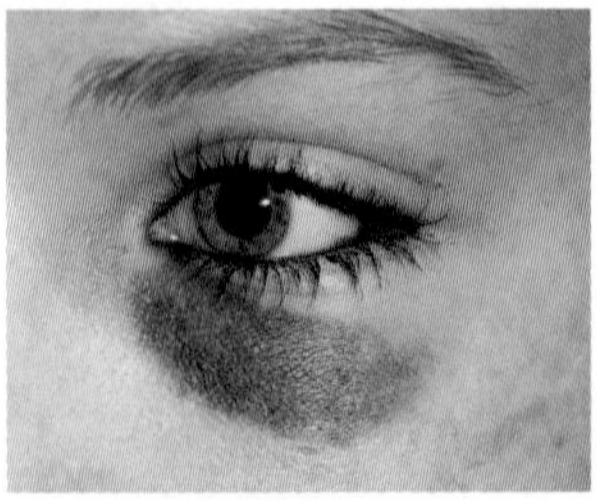	Damage to the skin	Avoid the area as it may be sensitive.
Watery eyes 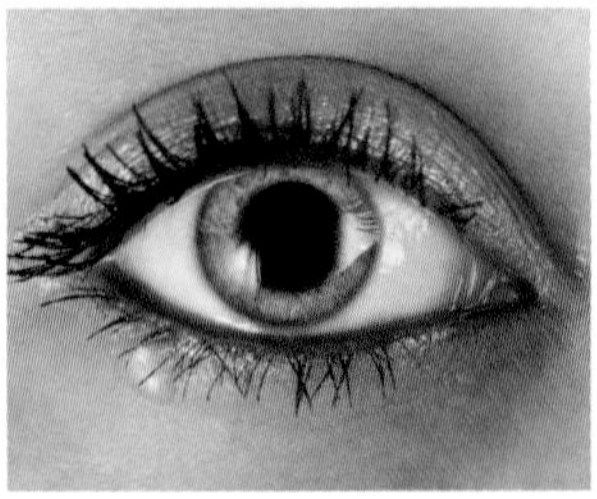	The eyes produce too much tear fluid	Use a tissue to blot the eyes. Be careful when using powder products.

HANDY HINTS

If your client has an allergic reaction to the make-up (such as redness or itching) remove the make-up immediately and refer them to their GP.

Skin type

During the consultation, you will also need to find out what skin type the client has. This will affect the make-up products and techniques that you use. You will need to discuss this with your client as well as looking at their skin to find out which skin type they have. You will then be able to choose the most suitable products for them.

HANDY HINTS

Not many people are lucky enough have a normal skin type.

Skin type	What causes it?	How would you spot it?	How may it affect the make-up treatment?
Normal 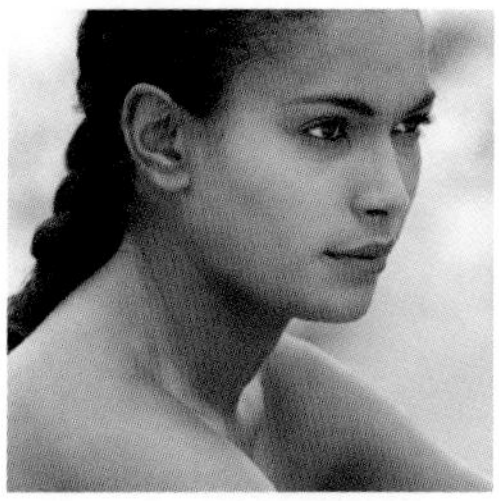	Good skin care routine. This skin type has a good balance of oil (sebum) and water (sweat).	▪ Even **skin texture** ▪ Feels soft ▪ Skin colour is even ▪ Does not feel tight ▪ Feels firm to touch	Make-up can be applied in the normal way as no corrections are needed.
Oily 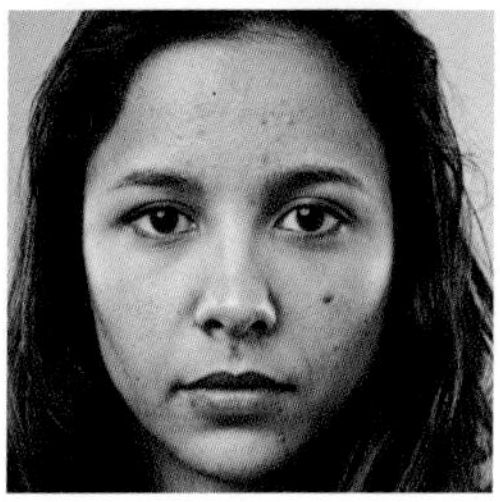	Too much of the skin's oil (sebum) is produced	▪ Shiny ▪ Spots ▪ Blackheads ▪ Large pores	Use concealer to cover the spots and powder to blot the shine.
Dry 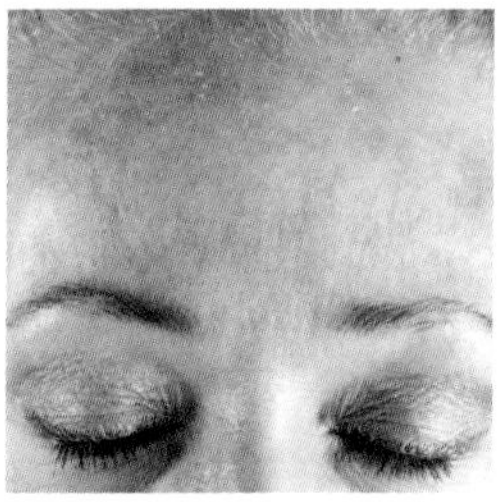	Not enough of the skin's oil is produced	▪ Flaky patches ▪ Dull ▪ Feels tight ▪ Small pores ▪ Whiteheads	Avoid too much powder as this will make the dry areas look more noticeable.
Combination 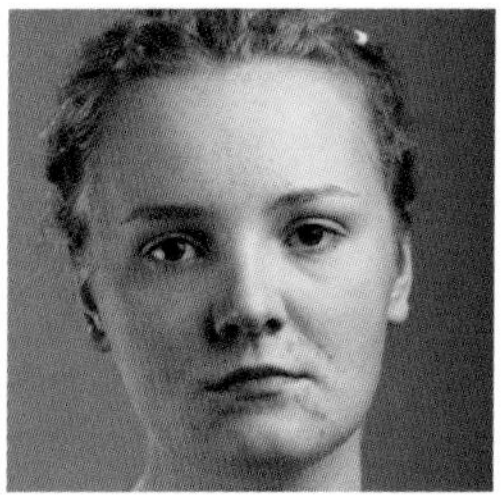	A combination of any of the above skin types	▪ Usually dry cheeks and oily skin on the forehead, nose and chin	Use concealer to cover any spots and powder to blot shine. Avoid too much powder on dry areas.

HANDY HINTS

Oily skin is sometimes referred to as 'greasy skin'.

HANDY HINTS

Refer back to Chapter 006 to remind yourself of the different skin types and conditions you are likely to come across, as well as skin care routines and products.

Skin texture

How rough or smooth the skin is

Pigmentation

The natural colouring found in the skin

SmartScreen 106 handouts 5 and 11

SmartScreen 106 worksheet 5

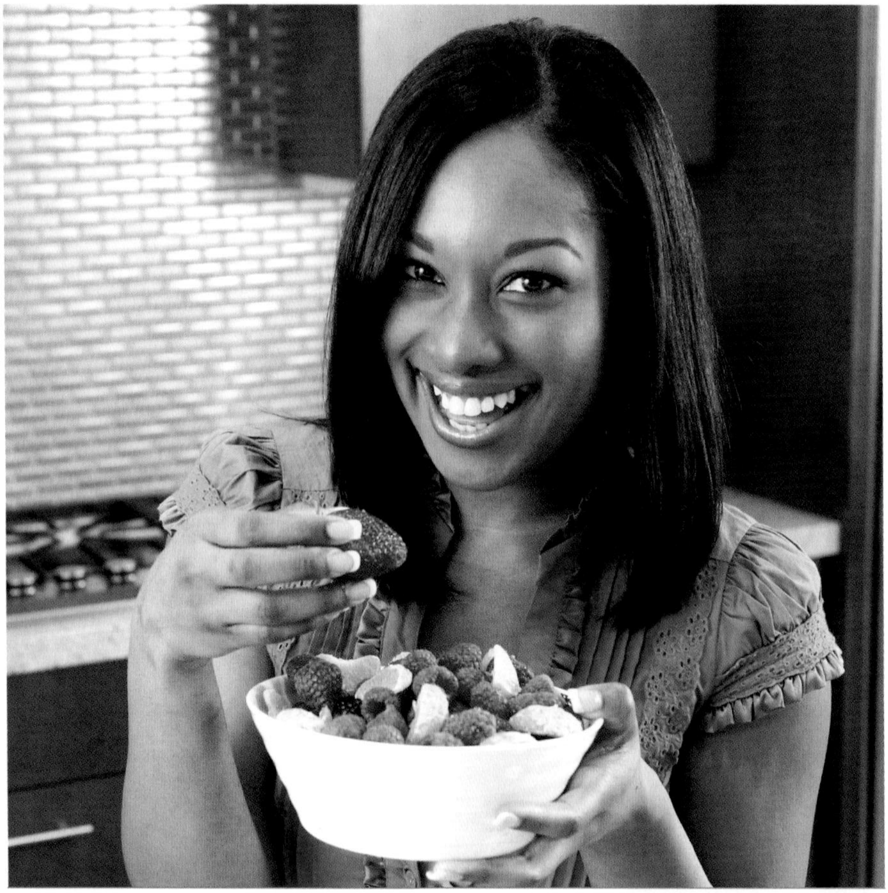

Eating healthily will make your skin look healthy too.

HANDY HINTS

Go to Chapter 006 (Skin care), and read up on how you would spot different skin types.

HANDY HINTS

As a general rule, when choosing the foundation colour, try to match the shade to the client's natural skin colour. Only go one shade lighter or darker, as anything else will stand out and look false on their skin.

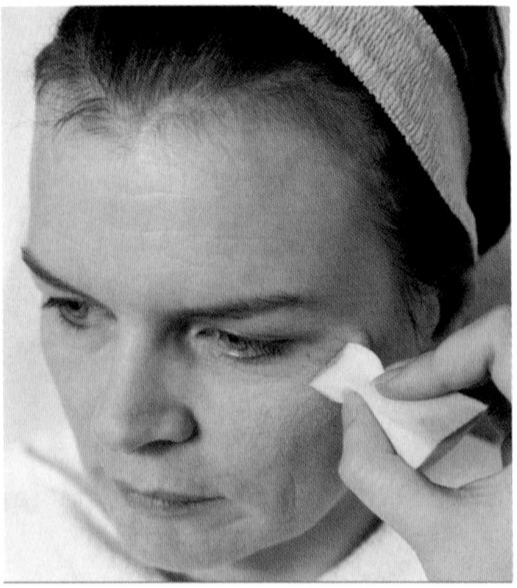

Applying the correct foundation colour

ACTIVITY

Work in pairs. Look at each other's skin and see if you can work out which skin types you and your partner have.

Skin, eye and hair colour

The choice of foundation will depend on the client's natural skin colour. It is important to make sure that it is as close to the natural skin colour as possible so that it blends well. The colours chosen for the eyeshadow and blusher should also suit her eye and hair colour.

It can sometimes be difficult to know which make-up colours are the right ones – there is so much choice out there. The most important thing about choosing the make-up colours for your client is knowing whether their skin is **cool** or **warm**. Using the wrong shades of colour for the foundation, eye and lip make-up will not **enhance** the client's **natural features**.

Cool colours
Colours that have more of a blue tone to them such as green, purple and blue

Warm colours
Colours that have more of a yellow tone to them such as orange, red and yellow

Enhance
Improve.

Natural features
Facial characteristics (eg shape, colour, etc)

Examples of cool colours
Blues, greens, and purples are cool colours.

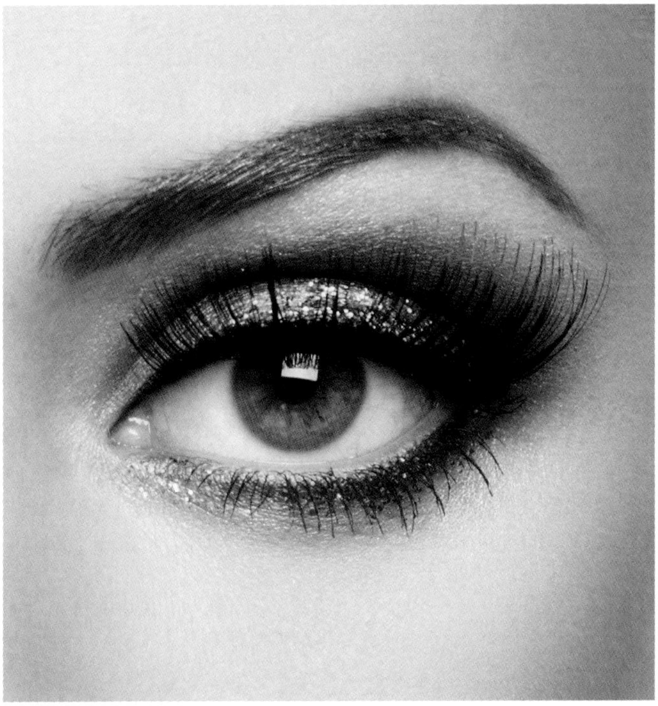

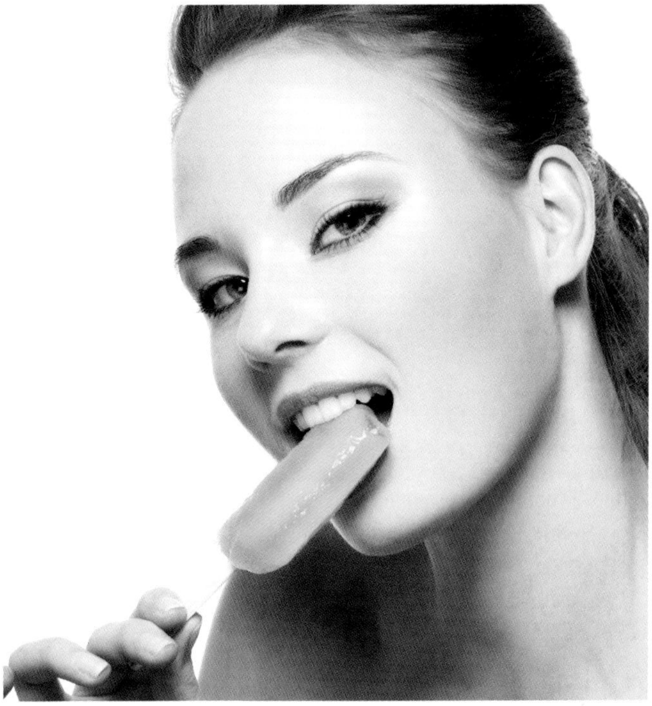

Examples of warm colours
Reds, oranges, and yellows are warm colours.

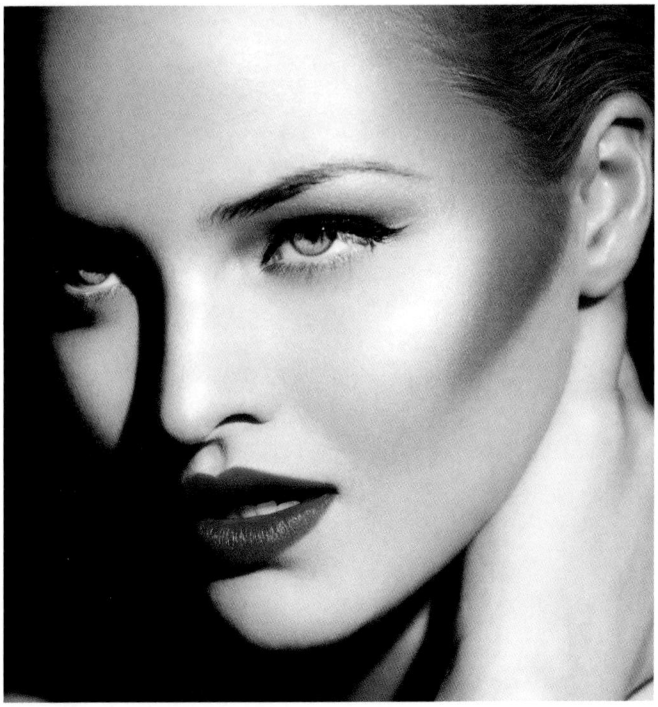

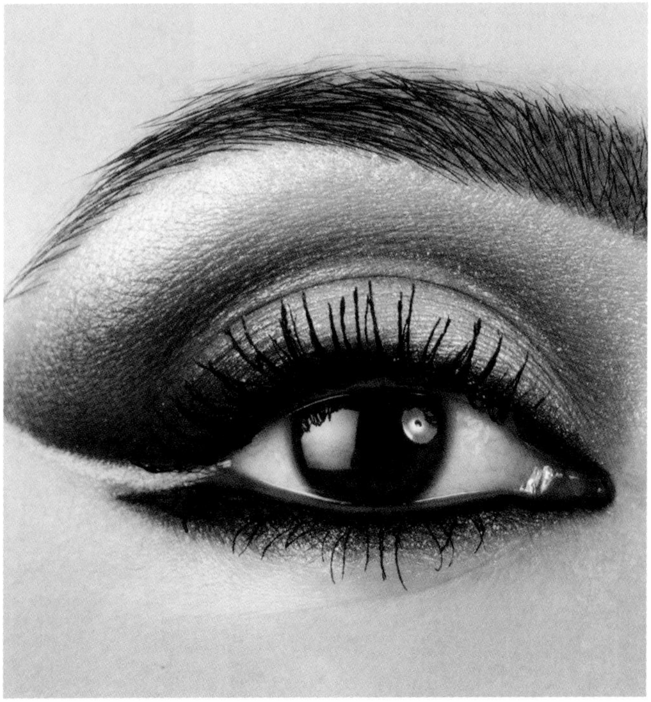

ACTIVITY

This simple activity will help you to find out whether cool or warm colours suit you. Try these tests on yourself or a partner.

1 Find a piece of silver fabric and a piece of gold fabric. Hold each fabric next to your face. If your skin looks better next to the silver fabric, then cool colours suit you. If your skin looks better next to the gold fabric, then warm colours suit you.
2 If you can easily wear black, cool colours suit you. If you look washed out wearing black, warm colours suit you.
3 If you look better in pure white rather than cream, cool colours suit you. If you look better in cream, warm colours suit you.
4 Test your jewellery. Do you look better in silver or gold? Gold is warm and silver is cool.

These tests should give you a pretty good idea whether cool or warm colours suit you. This applies to the colours of the clothes that you wear as well as make-up. Try these simple tests on members of your family or your friends.

HANDY HINTS

Choose cool colours if your:

- skin tone is black, olive, rosy brown or a light rosy colour, fair/medium rosy
- hair colour is dark, black, blond, or any of the brown tones except a golden brown
- eyes are dark, blue, green or hazel.

HANDY HINTS

Choose warm colours if your:

- skin tone is black, golden or medium fair
- hair is black, golden brown, red or strawberry blond
- eyes are hazel, dark or medium brown.

HANDY HINTS

Black skins tend to suit both warm and cool colours.

ACTIVITY

Take a look on the internet or in magazines at other celebrities. Can you tell which celebrities suit cool or warm colours?

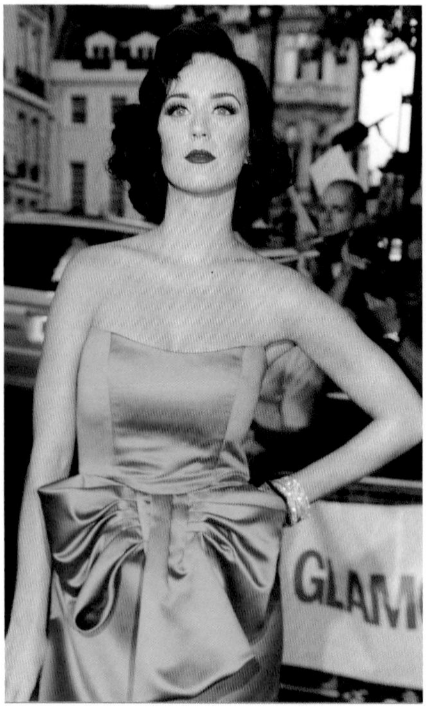

An example of a celebrity who suits cool colours is Katy Perry

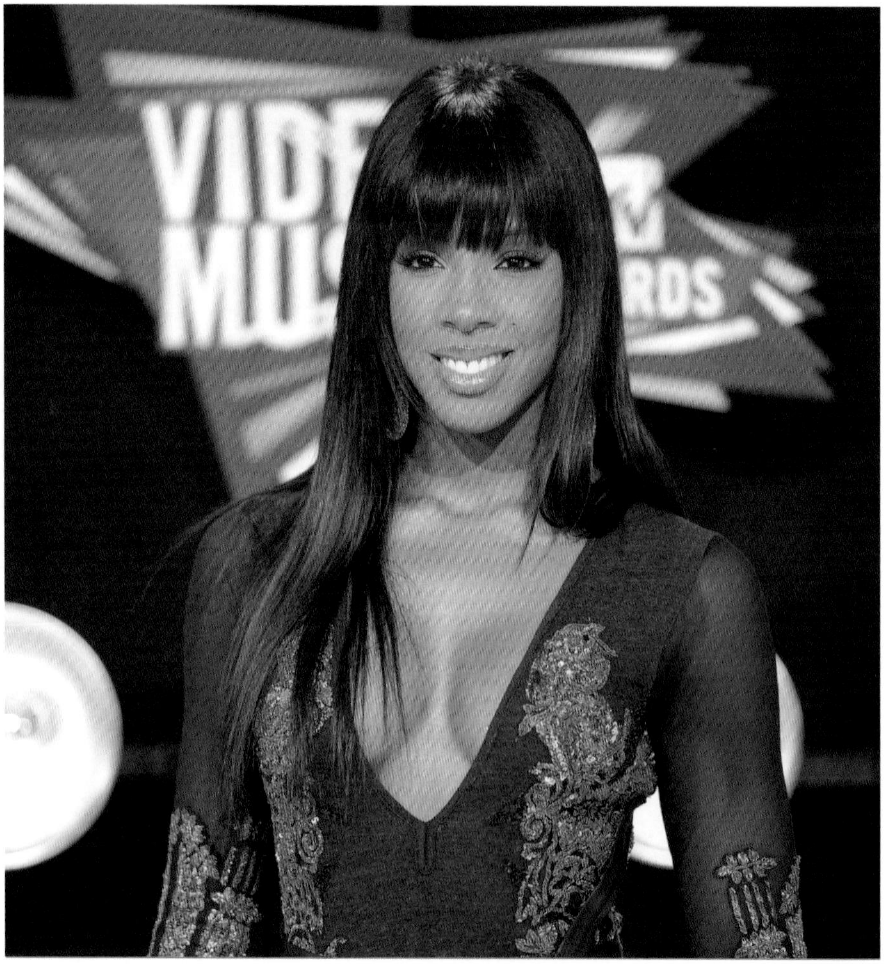

An example of a celebrity who suits warm colours is Kelly Rowland

ACTIVITY

Research on the internet or in magazines and devise a portfolio of images. Separate them out into warm and cool make-up tones.

HANDY HINTS

Read Chapter 005 Creating an image using colour for the hair and beauty sector for further information on colours.

CARRY OUT A MAKE-UP TREATMENT

You are now ready to carry out the treatment. Before you start, do a final check to make sure your client is comfortable and that you have all your tools and products ready.

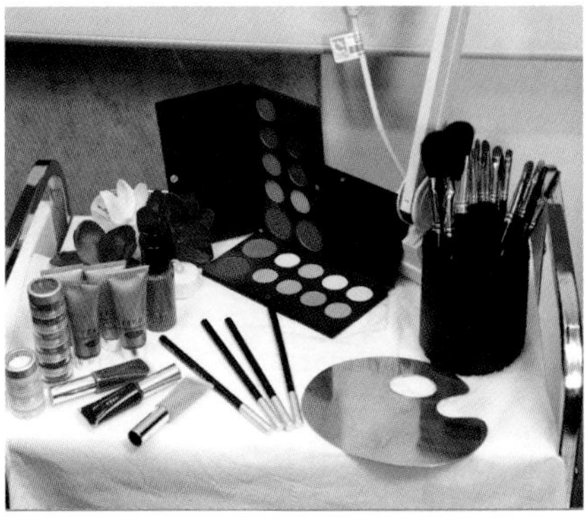

Professional set-up for a make-up treatment

HANDY HINTS

Remember to find out during the consultation what occasion the make-up is being applied for, eg for daytime or evening. Natural daylight is ideal when applying a make-up for daytime. If your make-up is for evening, you need to try to create the same lighting effect if possible.

CLEANSING PROCEDURE

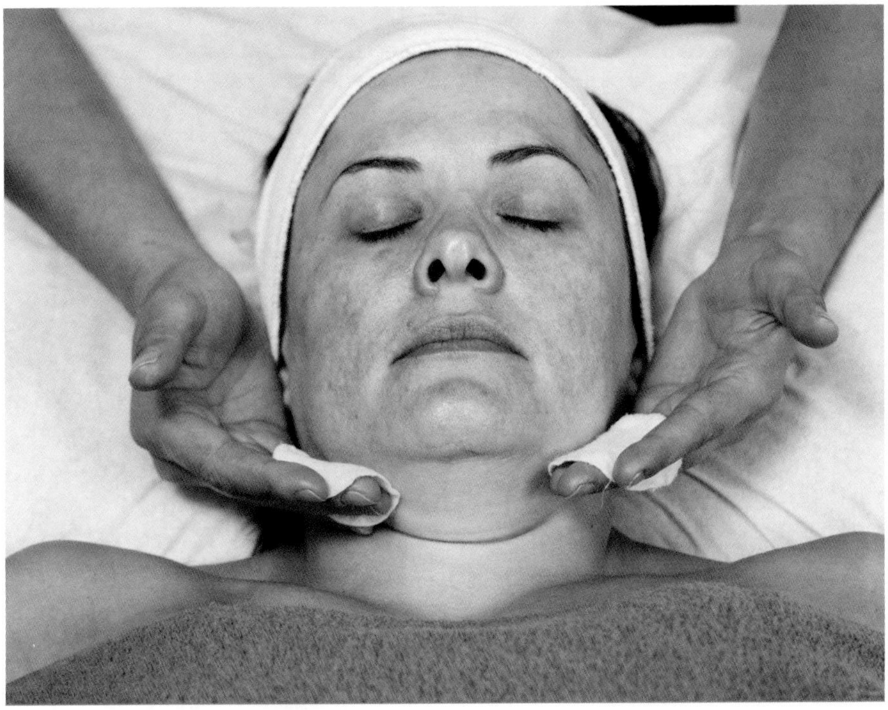

Cleansing the client's face ready for make-up

As part of a make-up treatment you need to make sure that the skin is ready for the make-up to be applied. This is done by carrying out a basic facial treatment:

- Skin cleansing – start with a gentle cleanse and remove all traces of make-up. Next, carry out a skin analysis to find out what skin type your client has. You can then choose the most suitable products for her skin type. Gently cleanse the eyes, lips and face.
- Toning – apply the toner and then blot.
- Moisturising – apply gently over the face and neck areas.

HANDY HINTS

Refer back to Chapter 006 to remind yourself of the cleanse, tone and moisturise routine.

HANDY HINTS

Remember to tone and blot the skin before applying the moisturiser.

HANDY HINTS

Remember not to apply too much moisturiser as this would make the skin too greasy for the make-up.

HANDY HINTS

It might be useful to create a mood board before you start the make-up treatment. See Chapter 112 for details.

CARRYING OUT THE MAKE-UP TREATMENT

After you have carried out a gentle basic facial routine, you are ready to carry out the make-up procedure. All products must be applied in a hygienic way to avoid cross-infection.

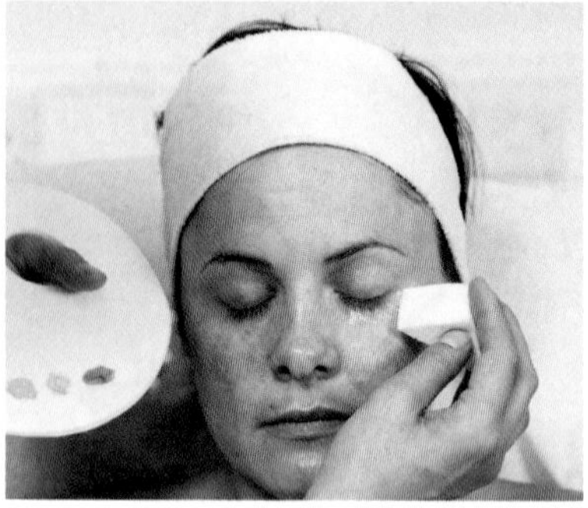

STEP 1 – Begin by applying the concealers if needed.

- Green concealer will help to cover redness on the skin.
- Lilac concealer will help to offset a yellow skin.
- Cream concealer will help to cover dark circles and spots.

Apply onto a spatula or palette. Blend with the fingertips or a concealer brush.

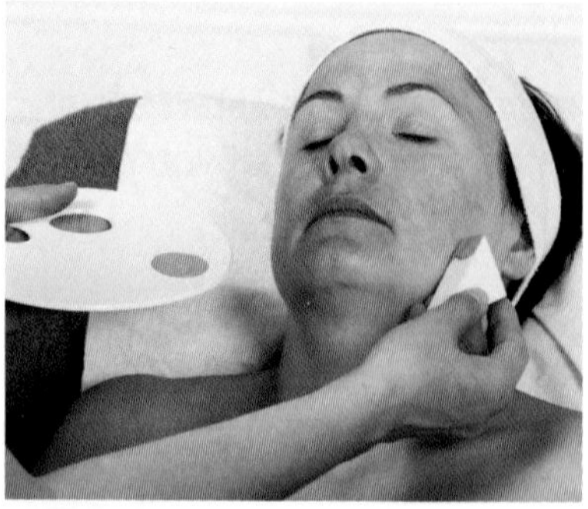

STEP 2 – Foundation. Choose the best colour by testing it on the jaw line first. Blend over the face and just under the jaw line. Apply using a sponge, taking the foundation from the palette.

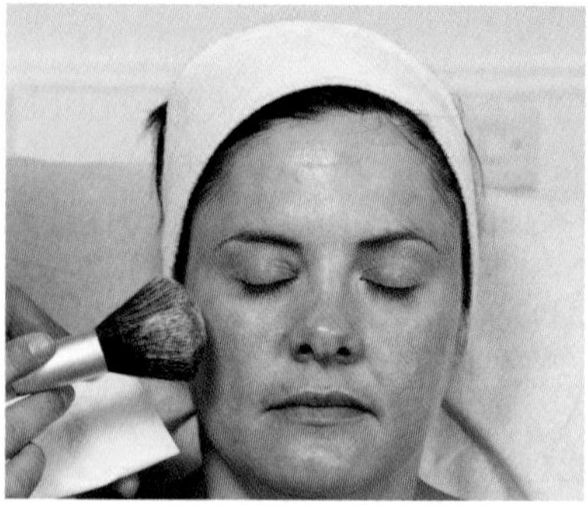

STEP 3 – Loose powder. Used to set the foundation; this will make the foundation last longer. Apply from a tissue using a powder brush.

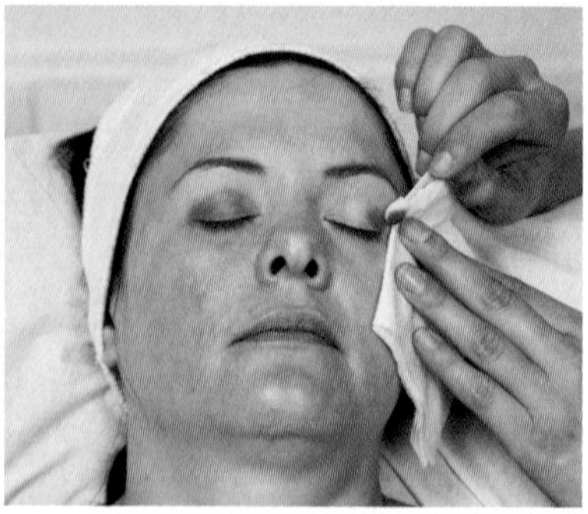

STEP 4 – Eyeshadow. Make sure the colours you have chosen suit the client's skin colour, eye colour, personality, age and the occasion. Apply using a disposable sponge applicator or small brush. Wipe over powders afterwards with a tissue.

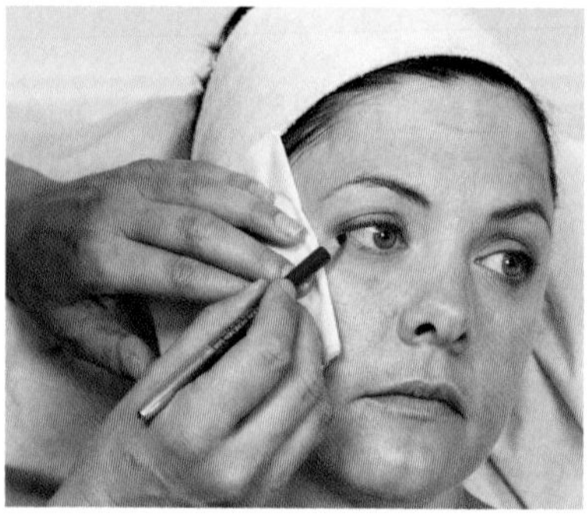

STEP 5 – Apply eyeliner to the upper and lower lids, close to the lashes. Sharpen eyeliner pencils before and after use.

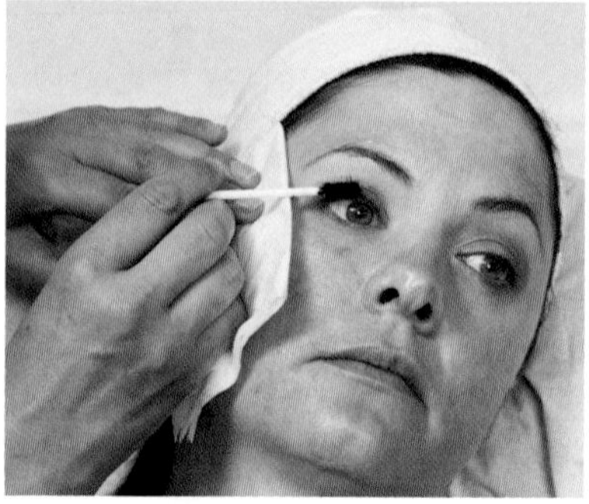

STEP 6 – Apply mascara to the upper and lower lashes. Use a disposable mascara brush.

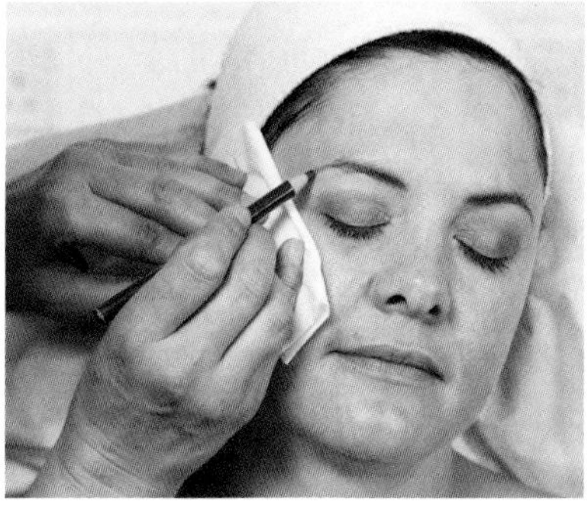

STEP 7 – Apply eyebrow pencil using light strokes to the brows. This will make them stand out more. Sharpen before and after use.

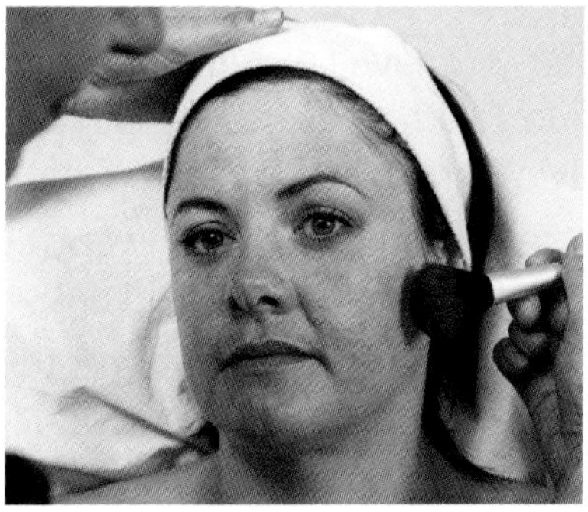

STEP 8 – Apply blusher to just below the cheekbone using a brush. Wipe over powders afterwards with a tissue.

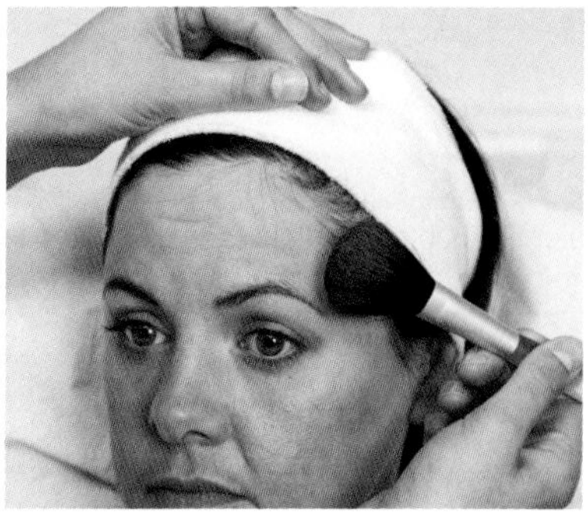

STEP 9 – Apply shader to areas you wish to make recede, eg a wide forehead or jaw.

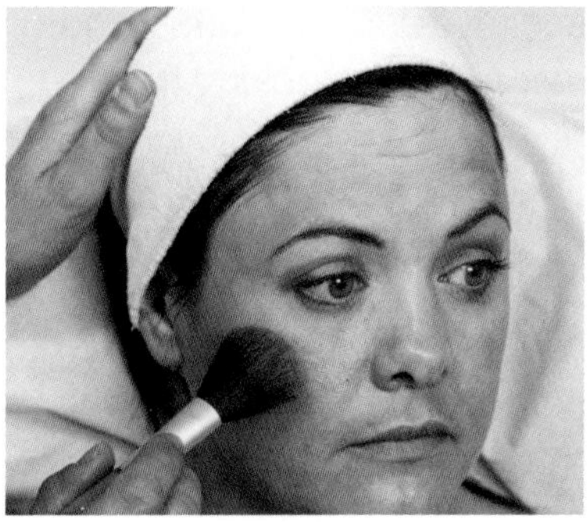

STEP 10 – Apply highlighter to the top of the cheekbone. Apply also to areas you want to make larger or more prominent, eg a short nose.

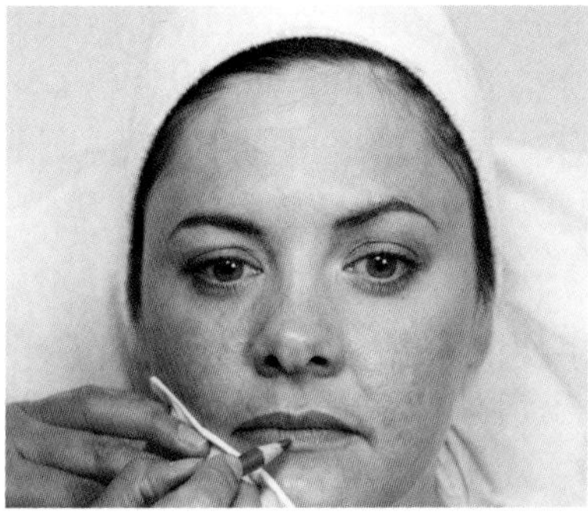

STEP 11 – Apply lip liner along the line of the lips; can be used to correct lip shapes. Sharpen lip liner pencils before and after use.

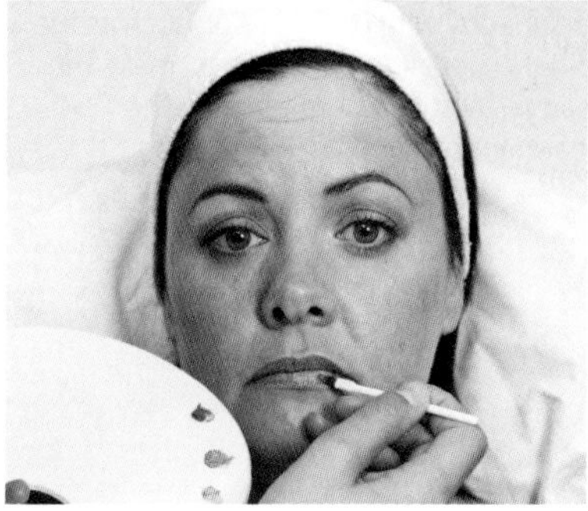

STEP 12 – Apply lipstick inside the lip liner. Apply two coats and blot on a tissue between applications. Use a new disposable lip brush for each client.

AFTER THE TREATMENT

After you have finished the treatment, make sure that you record everything you have done on the client's treatment plan. This will need to include the products that you have used as well as the colours chosen.

HANDY HINTS

Remember to include the colours that you have used on your treatment plan. This will help if the client comes in again or wants to buy any of the products.

HANDY HINTS

Remove the headband before the client looks in the mirror. This will make sure that the client gets a good first impression of the overall look.

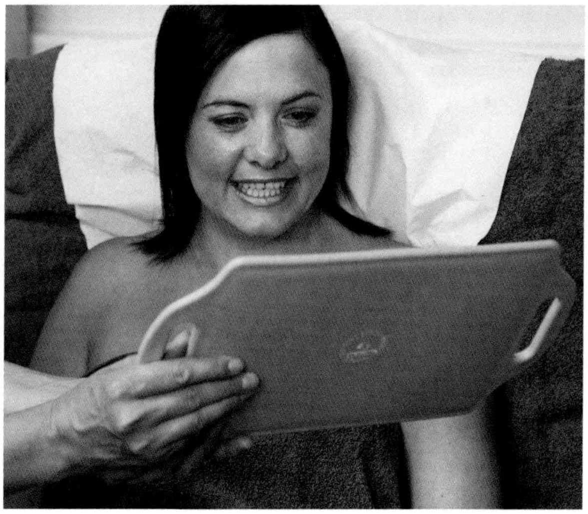

STEP 13 – Remove the headband and let the client see the finished result in a clean mirror.

SmartScreen 106 handout 19

HANDY HINTS

Refer to Chapter 006 Skin care for the correct choice of products for each skin type.

HANDY HINTS

It is important to get feedback from your client before completing the treatment so that you can change anything that she may be unhappy with or unsure of, such as the colours used. If this is the case, make the changes and also note them on the treatment plan.

AFTERCARE ADVICE

After you have finished applying the make-up to your client, it is important to make sure that you give them the correct aftercare advice. The following information should be given:

- Methods of removal: the correct cleanser, toner and moisturiser should be used for the client's skin type.
- Product recommendations: to include the correct choice and application of make-up products to suit the client's skin type, tone and colouring.
- Further treatment needs: you may suggest the client returns to you for further make-up treatment or maybe for a different treatment, such as skin care (for example if they have oily skin that needs to be treated).
- Maintenance advice: advice can be given on how to prepare and apply the products correctly for the client's face, eye and lip shapes. You may also suggest how they can keep their make-up looking fresh by reapplying face powder or lipstick.

ACTIVITY

In a group or with a partner, make a list of ways in which you can work hygienically when carrying out a make-up treatment.

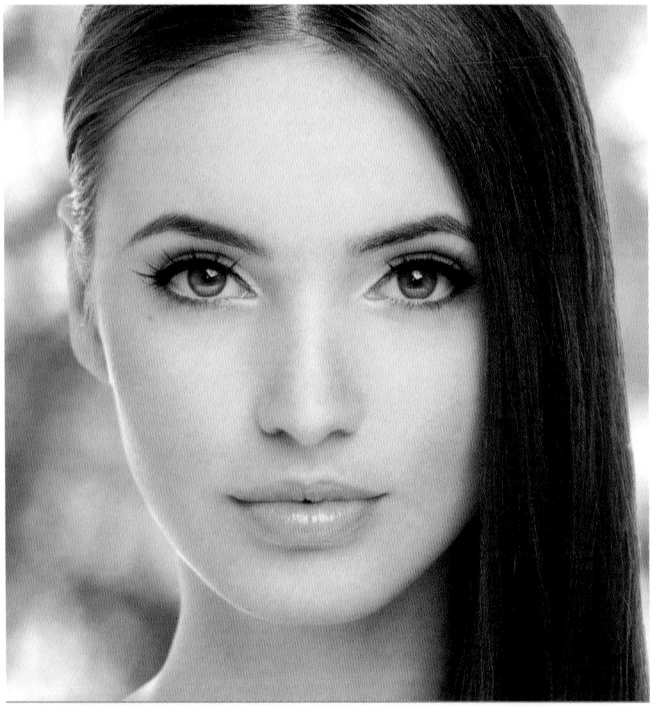

Day make-up

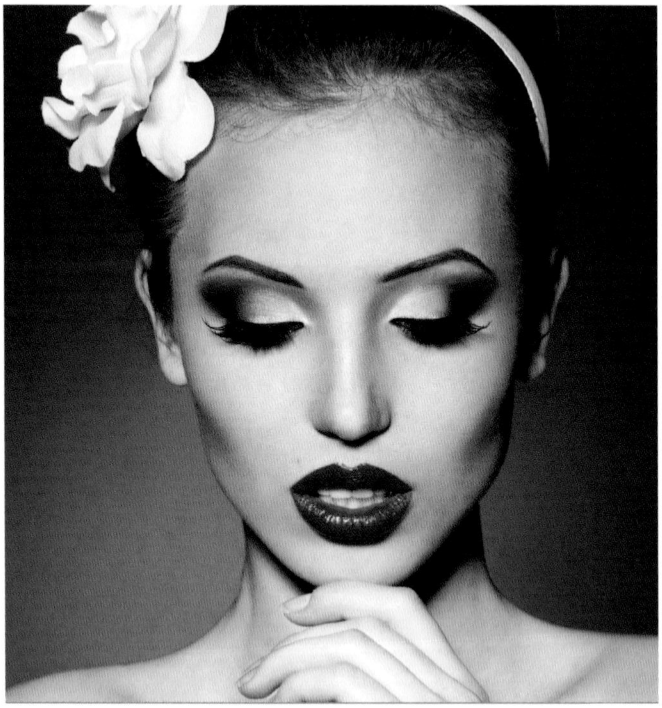

Evening make-up

IN A NUTSHELL

You are now at the end of the chapter. Before you test your knowledge with the revision activities, check the following list to see if you feel confident in all the areas covered. If there are still any areas you're unsure of, go back over them in the book and ask your tutor for extra support:

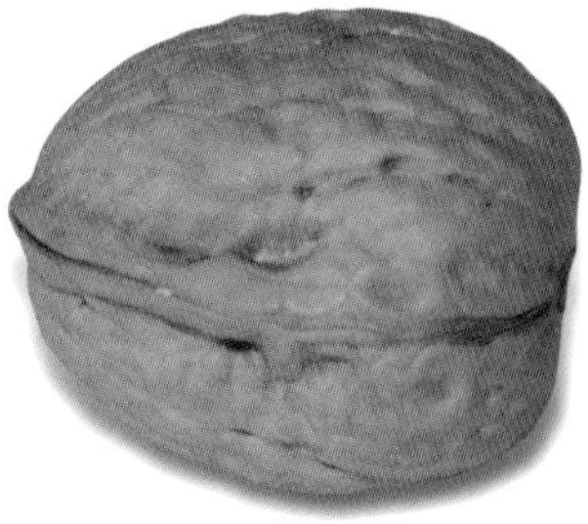

- basic anatomy of the face (the structure and function of the skin, skin types and the main facial bones)
- maintaining safe and effective methods of working when providing a basic make-up treatment
- what products, tools and equipment are required
- how to use them safely and hygienically
- what factors you need to consider
- how to communicate and behave in a positive way
- the preparation needed for applying a basic make-up treatment
- contra-indications that may prevent or restrict the treatment
- the different methods of evaluating the treatment
- the difference between daytime and evening make-up
- how to carry out a basic make-up treatment
- what aftercare to give to the client.

SmartScreen 106 sample questions

REVISION ACTIVITIES

Use the questions below to test your knowledge of Chapter 106 to see just how much information you've gained. This can help you to prepare for your assessments. Turn to pages 500–502 for the answers.

CROSSWORD

See if you can answer the questions and write them in the crossword.

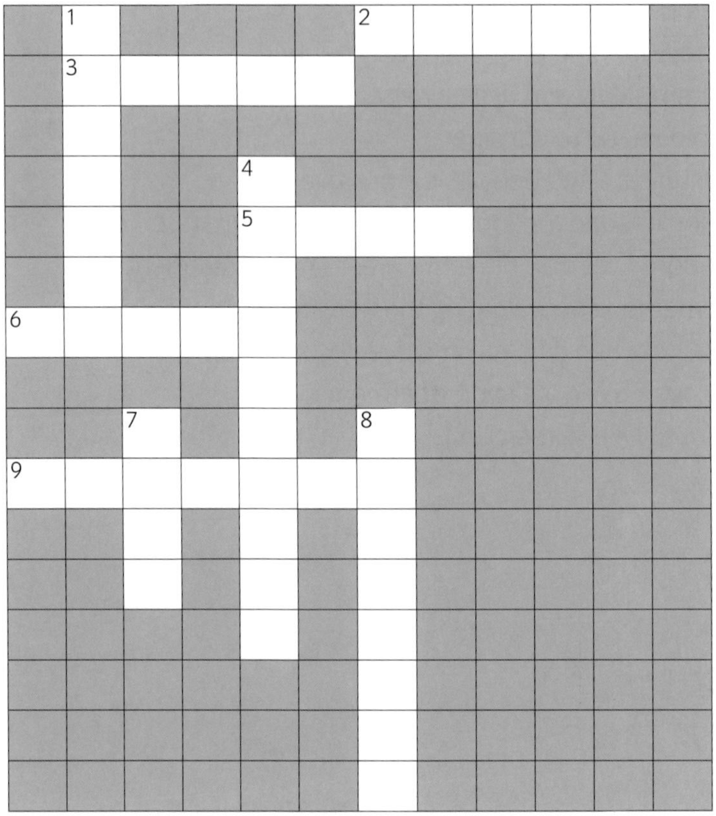

Across

2 The natural oil of the skin

3 The colour used to cover a yellow skin

5 The ideal face shape

6 The colour used to reduce redness on the skin

9 This is used to mix colours on

Down

1 A product that adds warmth and colour to the cheeks

4 This is applied after the concealer and before the face powder

7 A cool colour

8 This is used to keep the client's hair off their face during the treatment

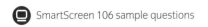

WORDS TO FIND

Copy and complete the sentences below. Use these words to help you fill in the gaps.

make-up	toner	shader	stye
headband	concealer	blusher	brushes
foundation	communication	palette	oily
cleanser	dry	eye pencil	hygiene

1 A green ______________ is used to cover up redness on the skin.

2 An example of good ______________ is washing your hands at the beginning and at the end of a treatment.

3 ______________ adds warmth and colour to the cheeks.

4 An example of good ______________ is speaking slowly and clearly to the client.

5 ______________ is applied after the concealer and before the face powder.

6 A day ______________ usually uses lighter colours than an evening one.

7 A make-up ______________ can be used to mix colours on and also to apply make-up in a hygienic way.

8 An example of an adverse skin condition is a ______________. If a client has one of these, you will not be able to apply the make-up.

9 A ______________ is used to keep the client's hair off their face during the treatment.

10 The make-up ______________ should be thoroughly cleaned between each client to avoid cross-infection.

Read the sentences below and state whether they are true or false.

11 An ultraviolet cabinet is used to store brushes in a hygienic way. True or false?

12 Towels, gowns and headbands should be machine washed at a low temperature. True or false?

13 Foundation is applied onto the face with a tissue. True or false?

14 A treatment plan has details of the client's name and address only. True or false?

15 Green concealer is used for covering redness in the skin. True or false?

16 A toner is used to cleanse the face of make-up and surface dirt. True or false?

17 A shader is used to draw attention to areas or make them look more obvious. True or false?

18 Mascara adds thickness, colour and length to the lashes. True or false?

19 An oval-shaped face does not need any correcting with a shader. True or false?

20 A good therapist will ensure that the treatment area is prepared after the client has gone. True or false?

21 Conjunctivitis is a contra-indication to a make-up treatment. True or false?

22 It is better to use cream make-up products for a photographic make-up. True or false?

23 Examples of warm colours are orange, yellow and cream. True or false?

TEST YOUR KNOWLEDGE FURTHER

1 How do you clean your eye pencils between clients?

2 Why do you use face powder? What does it do?

3 What does mascara do?

4 How can you correct a square face shape?

5 What is the main difference between a day and an evening make-up?

6 Give an example of how a therapist can behave in a positive way.

7 When would you apply face powder?

8 How do you apply lipstick in a clean and hygienic way?

9 What is the natural oil of the skin called?

10 Name the bone found in the forehead area.

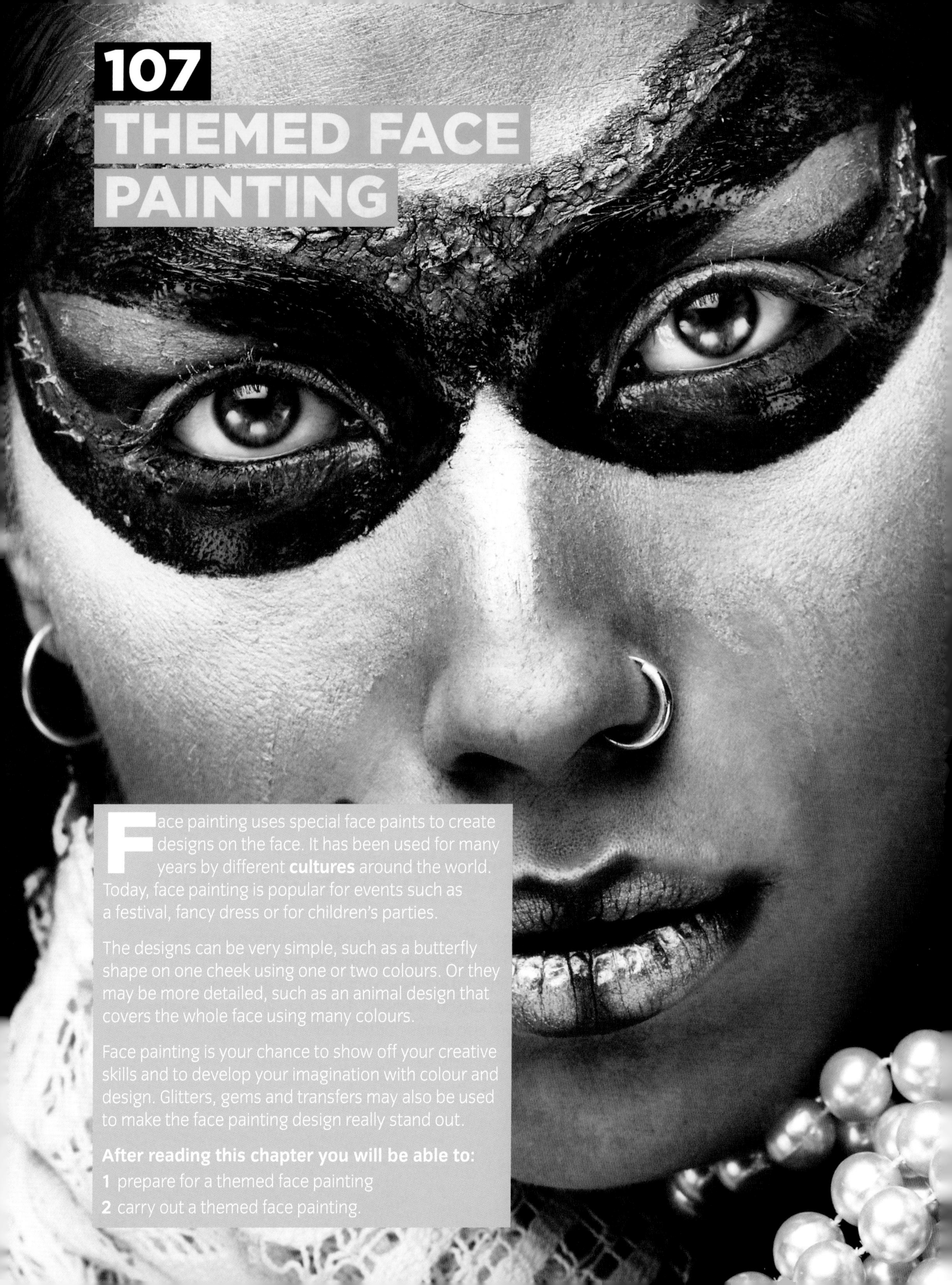

107 THEMED FACE PAINTING

Face painting uses special face paints to create designs on the face. It has been used for many years by different **cultures** around the world. Today, face painting is popular for events such as a festival, fancy dress or for children's parties.

The designs can be very simple, such as a butterfly shape on one cheek using one or two colours. Or they may be more detailed, such as an animal design that covers the whole face using many colours.

Face painting is your chance to show off your creative skills and to develop your imagination with colour and design. Glitters, gems and transfers may also be used to make the face painting design really stand out.

After reading this chapter you will be able to:

1 prepare for a themed face painting
2 carry out a themed face painting.

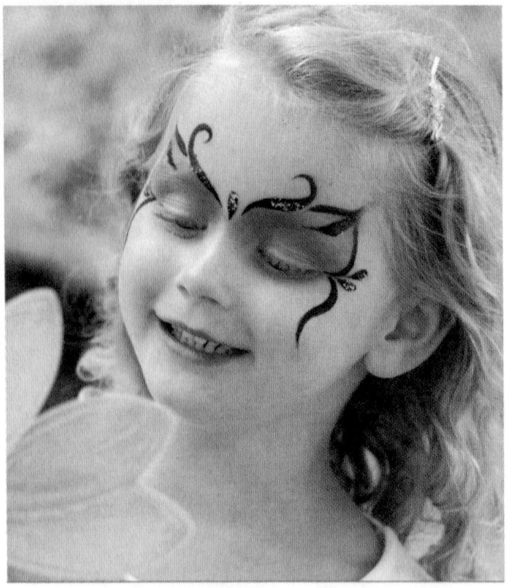
Butterfly face painting

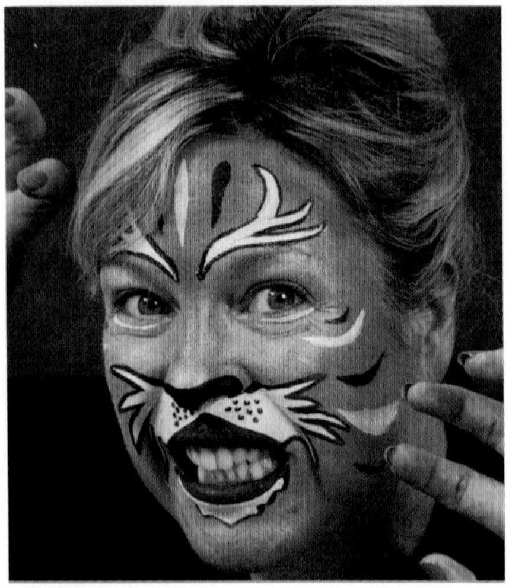
Tiger face painting

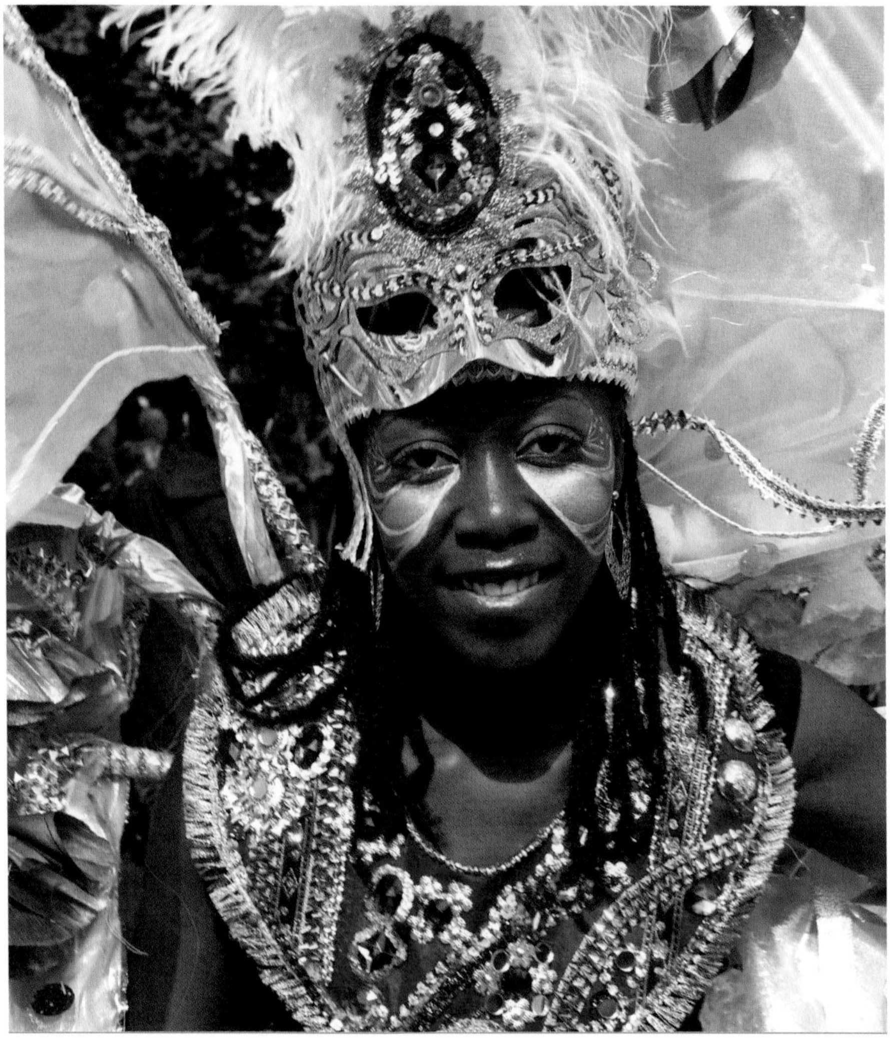
An African style face painting

Culture
How people live in different countries

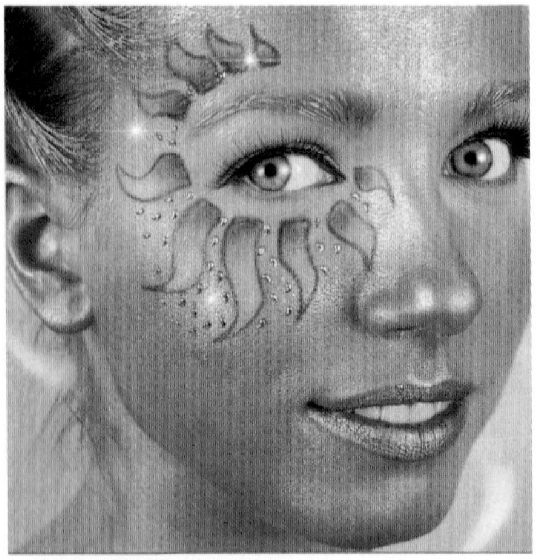
Fantasy face painting

Requirement
Something that must be done

HANDY HINTS

Go to Chapter 112 Creating a hair and beauty image for more information on how to create a mood board.

ACTIVITY

As an introduction to this topic, look on the internet and find out how face painting is used in different cultures around the world. Display your pictures on a mood board, then show and discuss these with the rest of your group.

PREPARE FOR A THEMED FACE PAINTING

Before you begin the face-painting service, it's important to be prepared. Health and safety **requirements** should be carried out for every treatment, but knowing your products and tools, factors that can affect the service, choosing the design and preparing the treatment area are also a must for themed face painting.

SAFE AND HYGIENIC WORKING PRACTICES

It is important that you always work in a safe and clean way. You should keep your treatment area tidy and only use hygienic tools and equipment. This will help to reduce the risk of harm to you and your clients and help to prevent cross-infection. The client will also have more confidence in you and you will look more professional.

SmartScreen 107 worksheet 9

THE SALON ENVIRONMENT

The treatment area should be prepared in a professional way:

- Make sure all products, tools and equipment are clean and hygienic.
- They should be placed safely and tidily on the trolley.
- If a couch is to be used for the client, it should be covered for hygiene reasons with a couch cover and couch roll tissue.
- If chairs are to be used, then both chairs should be placed facing each other. Your chair should be slightly lower than the client's chair. The reason for this is to make sure you are in the right position to work on your client. This will help to stop you getting back- and shoulderache.

HANDY HINTS

Go to Chapter 113 Following health and safety in the salon and read up on more detailed information on health and safety, including PPE, COSHH, HASAWA and methods of sterilisation.

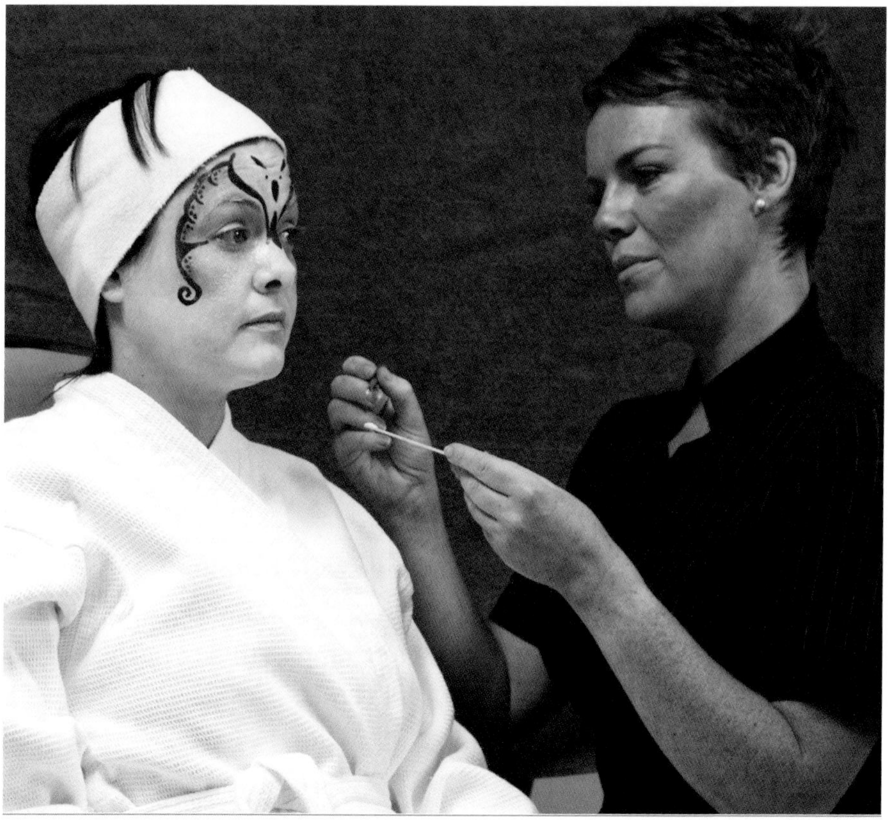

The correct posture for face-painting application

- The room temperature should not be too hot or too cold. The ideal temperature for a treatment room is between 16–18 degrees Centigrade.
- The air in the room should be well ventilated. This means that fresh air continually replaces stale air. It will also stop the air in the treatment room from becoming stuffy.
- The lighting should be suitable for a face-painting treatment. It needs to be well lit so that you can clearly see what you are doing.

HANDY HINTS

It is important that you have a good upright **posture** during the treatment. Make sure that the chair or couch is the correct height for you and the client. This will make sure that you are both comfortable. If you have to twist or bend over, it will give you backache.

Posture

How you hold your body

SmartScreen 107 handout 1

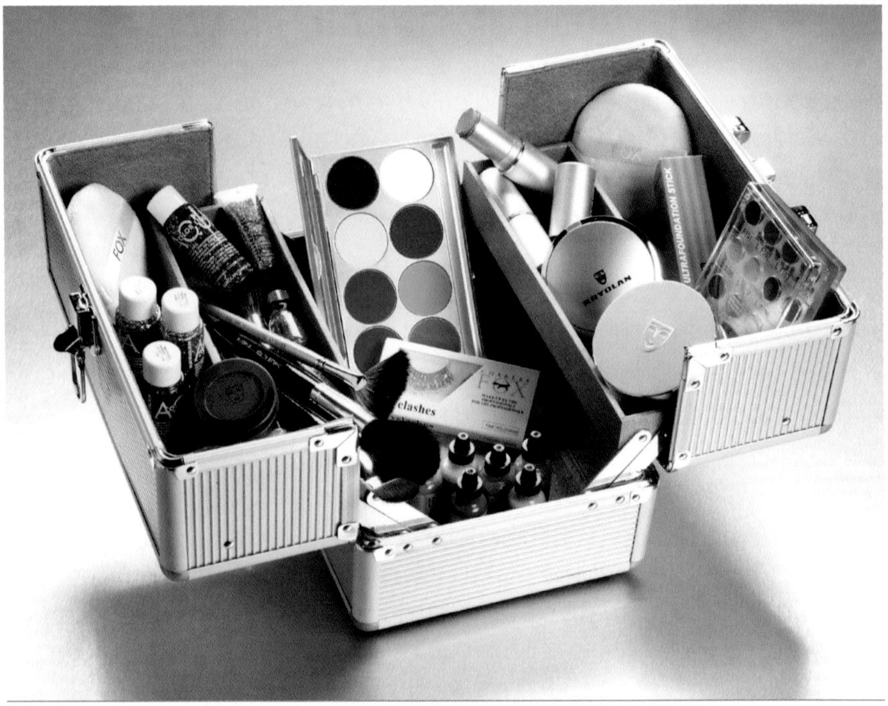

Face-painting products, tools and equipment in a carrying case

PREPARING FOR THE FACE-PAINTING TREATMENT

Before the client arrives, it is important that you get yourself and the treatment area prepared. All of the products, tools and equipment need to be ready. This will make sure that the treatment flows well and will also give the client a positive first impression. It will help the client to relax and have confidence in you.

BASIC ROOM TOOLS AND EQUIPMENT

Some items, such as couch covers, are needed for most beauty therapy treatments. This table lists them and their use in face painting.

Tools/equipment	What is it used for?	Hygiene steps to follow
Towels 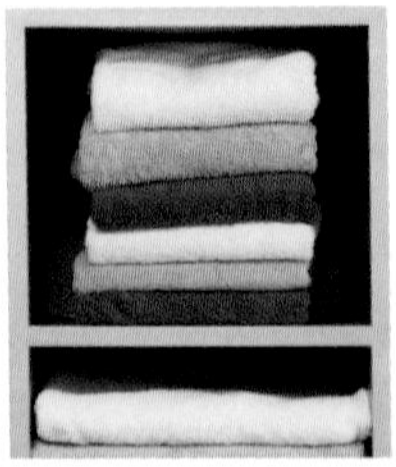	Used to cover the client and protect their clothing from the face painting. Place around the client's shoulders.	Machine wash after the treatment on a high temperature to destroy harmful germs.
Headband 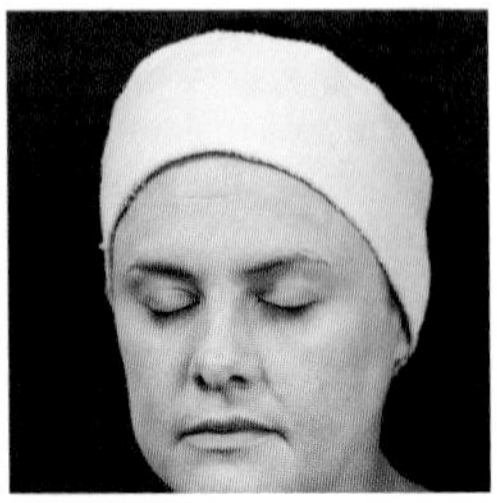	Keeps the client's hair off their face. Place around the client's head.	Machine wash after the treatment on a high temperature to destroy harmful germs.

Tools/equipment	What is it used for?	Hygiene steps to follow
Gown 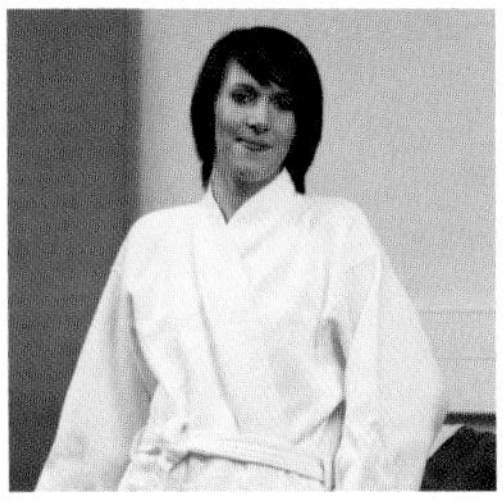	Covers the client and helps to protect their clothes from the products. It will also help to keep them warm.	Machine wash on a high temperature to destroy harmful germs and get rid of dirt and grime.
Cotton wool 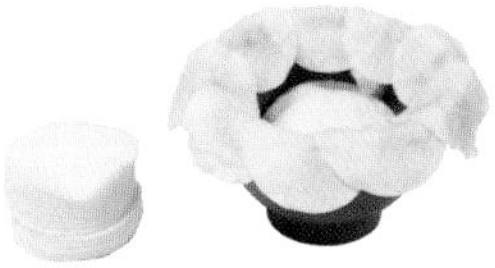	Used with the cleanser to remove surface dirt and any make-up at the start of the treatment. Can also be used during the treatment to remove mistakes made with the face painting.	Use damp with the cleanser. Use damp to remove any face painting mistakes during the treatment.
Tissues 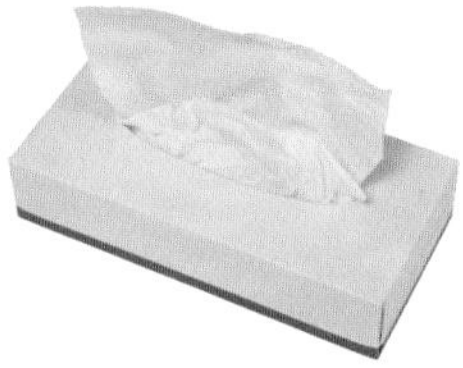	Used to blot the skin after the toner is applied. Can also be used to wipe face painting from your hands during the treatment.	Throw away after use.
Couch or suitable chair 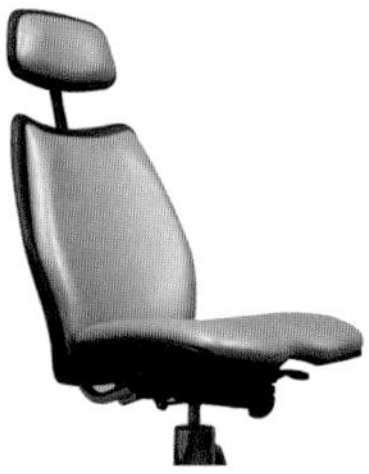	Use either a couch or a chair that is a suitable height for the client.	Cover the couch with a couch cover and tissue.
Couch cover 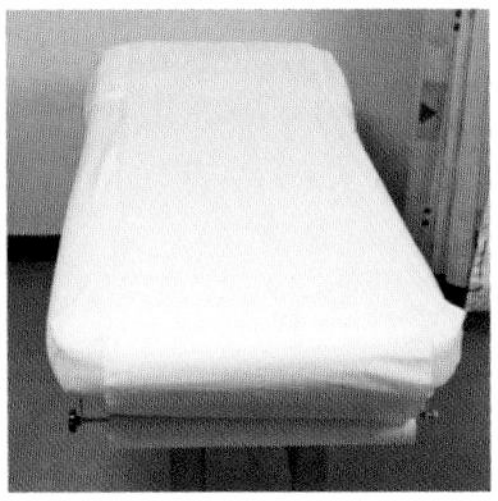	If a couch is used for the client, a couch cover is placed over the couch for hygiene reasons.	Machine wash after the treatment on a high temperature to destroy harmful germs.
Couch tissue roll 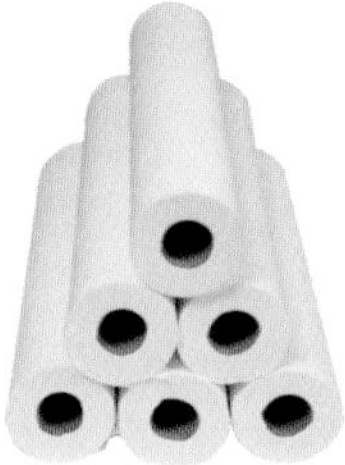	If a couch is used for the client, couch roll tissue is placed on top of the couch cover for hygiene reasons.	Throw away after use.

Tools/equipment	What is it used for?	Hygiene steps to follow
Mirror 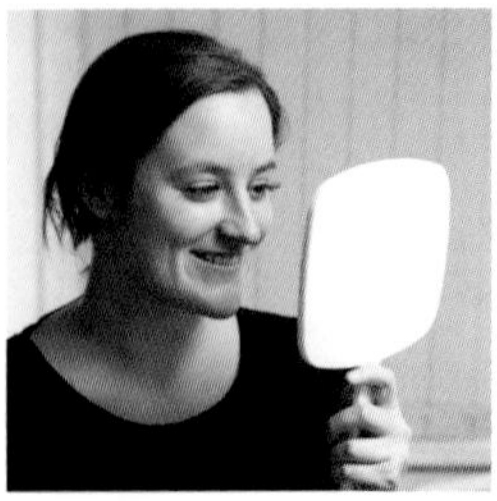	Used to show the client the finished face-painting look.	Wipe over the mirror before and after the treatment to make sure that it is clean for your client to look in.
Waste bin 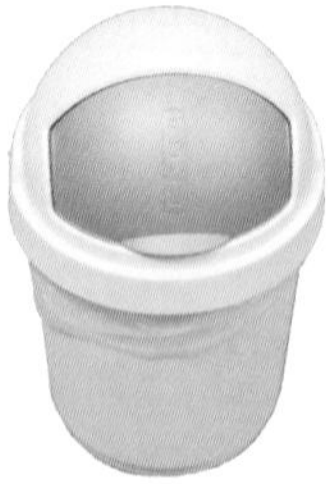	Used for throwing waste materials into, such as cotton wool and tissues.	This should be lined with a bin liner and have a lid.
Treatment plan 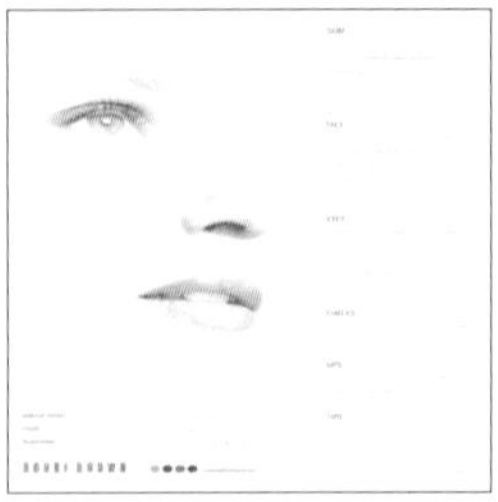	Records the treatment details, eg products used and face-painting design.	Make a note of the face-painting design that you have applied.

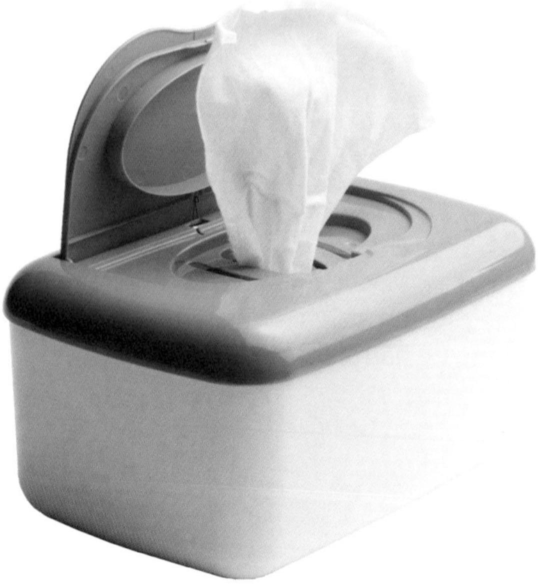

Baby wipes can also be used to clean face painting off your hands during the treatment

TOOLS AND EQUIPMENT USED IN A FACE-PAINTING TREATMENT

This table of tools and equipment lists items that are not used for every beauty treatment but are used in face-painting treatments.

Tools/equipment	What is it used for?	Hygiene steps to follow
Face painting brushes 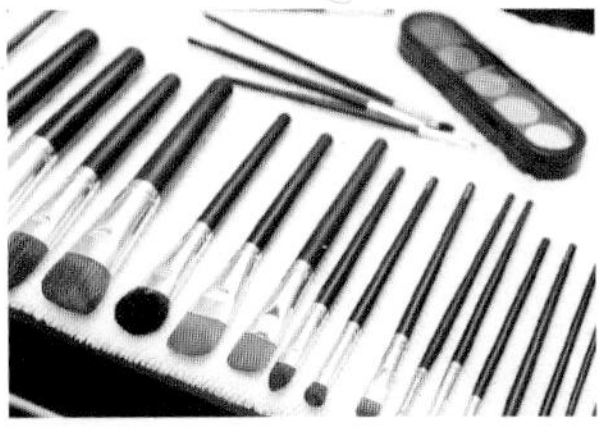 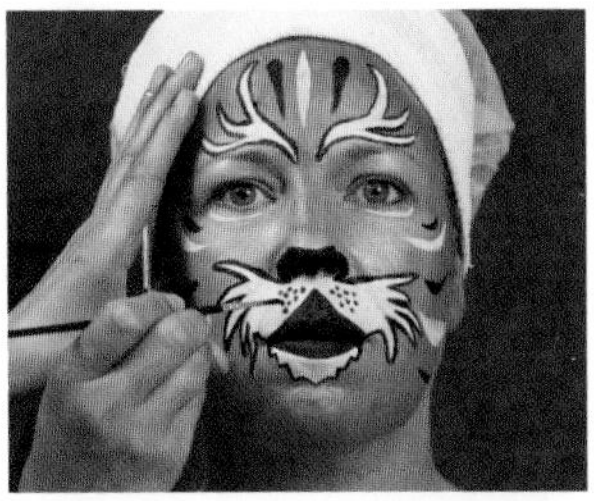 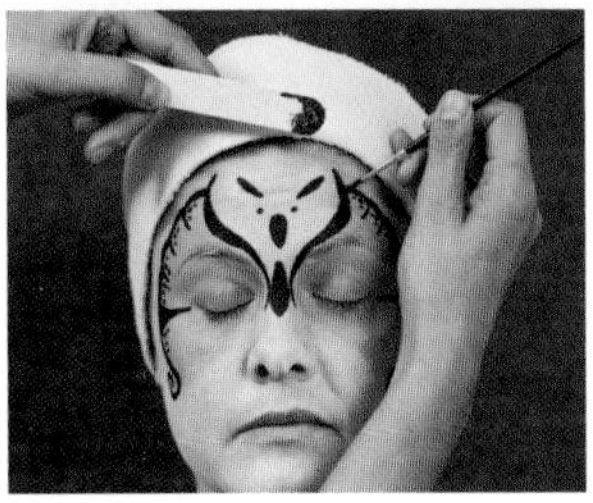	Used to apply the face paints onto the face. The type of brush used depends on the effect needed: ▪ Fine brushes give a more detailed effect, such as stripes, thin lines and dots. ▪ Medium brushes are for bolder strokes. ▪ Larger brushes are used for filling in large areas or where a thicker effect is needed. The brushes need to be soft enough to use on the face.	Apply the paint onto a damp brush and then stroke onto the skin to create the design. The brushes need to be cleaned between each colour to stop the colours mixing together. You will need to have lots of clean water to rinse them out in. Wash the brushes in warm soapy water between clients.
A suitable container for water, such as an empty Barbicide jar 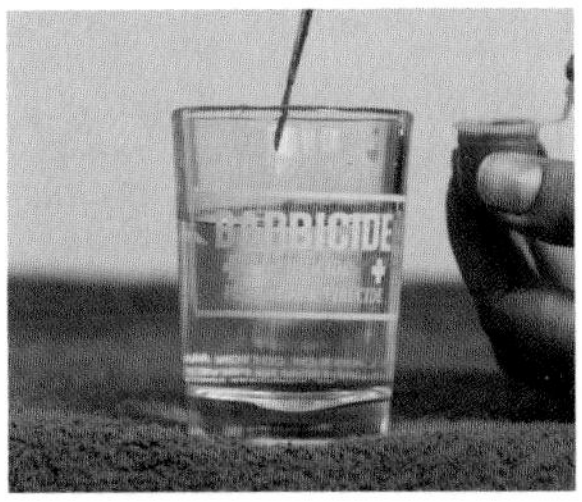	Used to rinse the brushes between the use of different coloured face paints. Water may also be added to the face paint to make it a lighter shade.	Fill the jar with clean water. You may have to change the water regularly during the treatment to make sure that a clean brush is used for each colour. Rinse the jar in warm soapy water after the treatment.
Palette 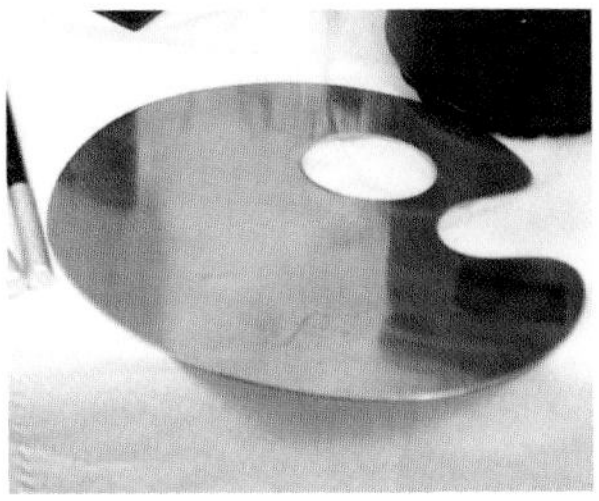	Used for putting the paint on during the treatment. This will help if you want to mix different colours together.	Apply the face painting onto the palette using a damp brush or sponge. Then work it off the palette with a damp sponge or brush onto the face. Wash afterwards in warm soapy water.

Tools/equipment	What is it used for?	Hygiene steps to follow
Face painting sponges 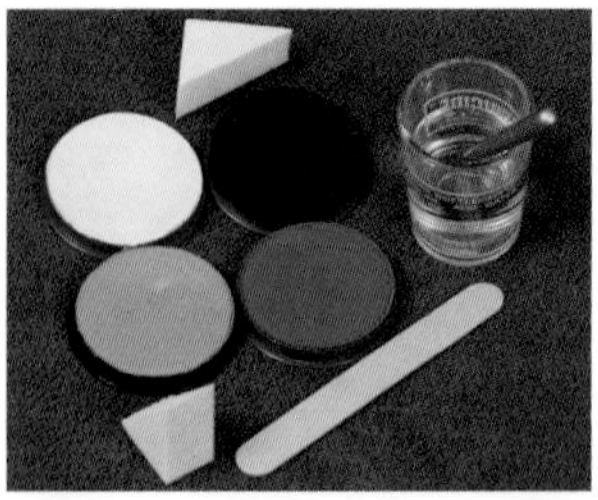 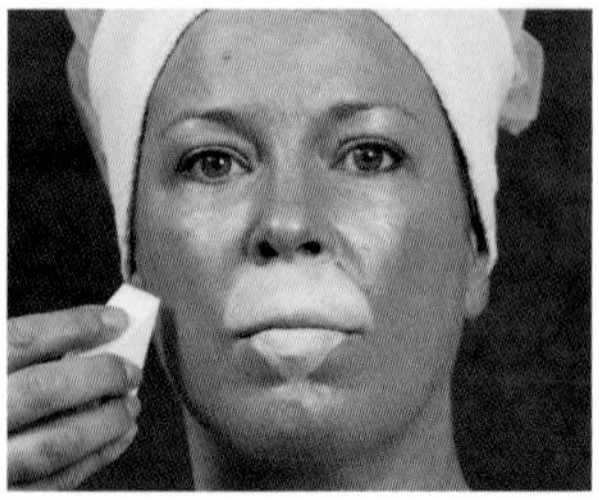	Used for applying the face painting to large areas, such as all over the face to create a base colour.	Use the sponges damp. Apply the face painting to the sponge and then gently apply to the client's face. Wash in warm, soapy water afterwards to remove all of the face painting.

HANDY HINTS

Go to Chapter 006 Skin care and read up on more detailed information about the different skin cleansing products and which skin types they are use for.

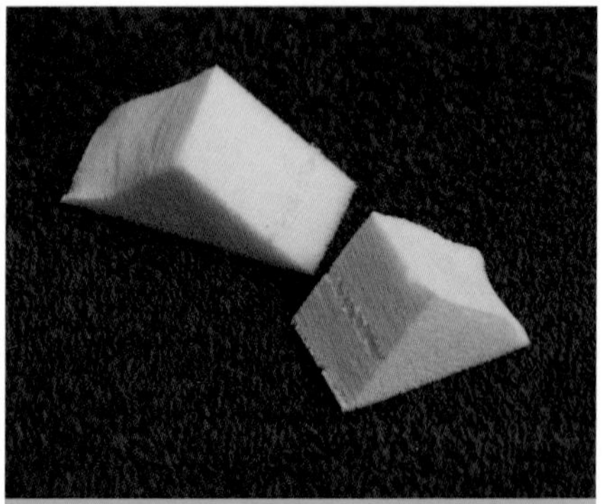

HANDY HINTS

Try cutting the sponges in half. There are two reasons for this:

1 You get twice as many sponges for your money.
2 You can use the sharp edge on the cut sponge to produce lines and clean edges if you need that effect for your design.

PRODUCTS USED IN A FACE-PAINTING TREATMENT

It's important to know the products that are used in a face-painting treatment. This table gives a useful guide.

Face painting product	What is it used for?	Hygiene steps to follow
Cleanser 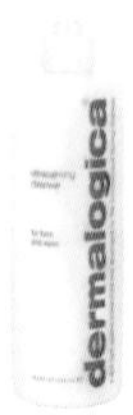	Removes make-up and surface dirt from the skin before the treatment.	Usually applied to the face using the fingertips, then gently massaged in. Remove using warm cotton wool pads.

Face painting product	What is it used for?	Hygiene steps to follow
Toner 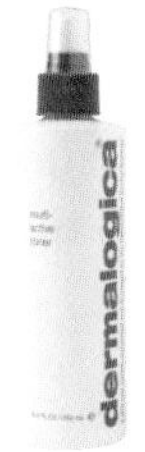	Refreshes the skin. Removes the last traces of the cleanser.	Applied onto damp cotton wool pads. These are then gently wiped over the skin.
Moisturiser 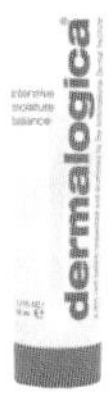	Helps to stop the skin from drying out. Makes the skin feel soft and supple. Apply only a small amount to the client's skin. If too much is used then the skin will feel greasy and the paint will not go on very well.	First it is applied into the palm of the hands, then applied to the fingertips and gently tapped over the skin. It is then lightly massaged in until it has been absorbed into the skin.
Face paints 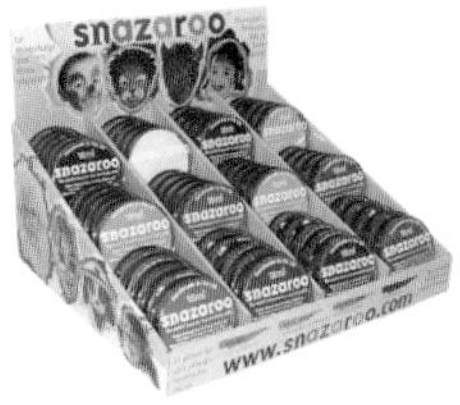	**Water-based products** that come in a wide choice of colours. They can: ▪ be plain coloured ▪ contain glitter to give a sparkle effect ▪ have a **pearlescent** effect. The choice of face painting will depend on what effect is needed.	Apply using a damp cosmetic sponge to cover large areas. Apply using a wet brush for a more detailed effect.
Transfers and stencils 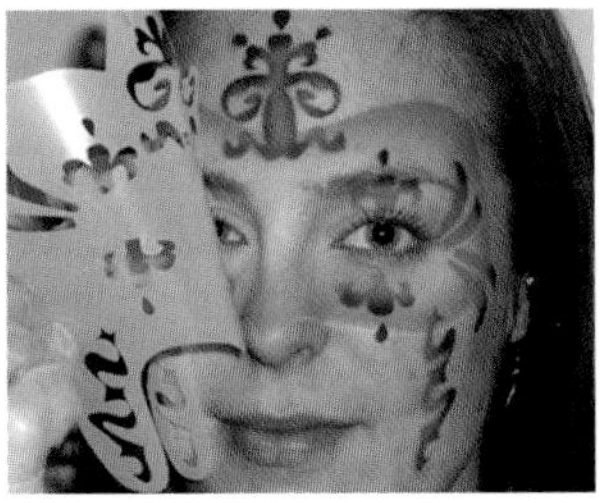	Used to add more detailed designs to a face-painting image. They come in lots of different designs and are easy to use.	Transfers: ▪ Apply to the skin with the transfer facing downwards. ▪ Add a few drops of water to the backing paper until it is completely wet. ▪ Gently press down, making sure that every part of the transfer has been pressed onto the skin. ▪ Very carefully peel back the backing paper, leaving the transfer on the skin. Stencils: these are usually made of thin plastic and have the pattern cut into them. ▪ Place them flat onto the skin where you want the design to be. ▪ Carefully paint into the area that is cut out. ▪ Gently peel the stencil off. The design will then be painted onto the skin.

Water-based products
Products that can be used with water and also easily washed off with water

Pearlescent
Having a shiny and glossy finish

Face painting product	What is it used for?	Hygiene steps to follow
Face glitters 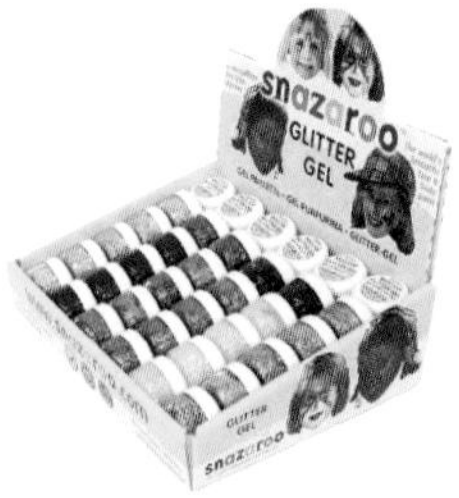	Used to give sparkle to the face-painting design. They come in lots of different colours – often in containers that you have to gently shake to get the glitter out. You can use them with a stencil to create patterns and shapes.	▪ Apply a small amount into a tissue or palette. ▪ Gently dab onto the skin using your fingertips or gently apply using a brush. If using with a stencil: ▪ Place the stencil flat onto the skin. ▪ Apply a small amount of glue through the stencil onto the skin. ▪ Gently shake the glitter onto the glue. ▪ Carefully peel off, leaving the glittery pattern.
Gems 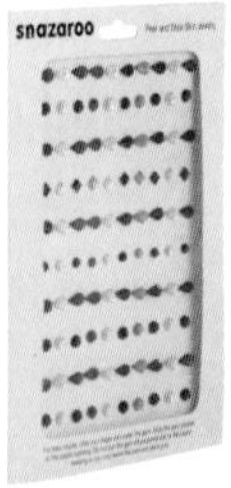	Small jewels that can be stuck onto the skin to give sparkle and create a more imaginative effect. Used a lot in fantasy face-painting designs.	To apply, peel off the backing from the gems and press them against the skin. Hold them in place for a few seconds to make sure they are stuck firmly in place.

ACTIVITY

Have a go at mixing the face-painting colours together by colouring in a diagram of the colour star. There is a blank handout for you to print off and use on SmartScreen 005 worksheet 3.

You will need red, yellow and blue face painting colours to do this. (These are known as the primary colours). Mix the primary colours together to make secondary colours (orange, violet and green).

SmartScreen 107 handouts 2, 4 and 5

SmartScreen 107 worksheet 5

HANDY HINTS

Go to Chapter 005 Creating an image using colour for the hair and beauty industry and read up on the colour star, and also primary and secondary colours.

HANDY HINTS

At first, it is best to start out with maybe five basic colours of face paints (eg white, black, red, blue, yellow). This will help you to get used to working with them.

ACTIVITY

Experiment with face paints on paper. Keep adding water to the paints. You will find that the more water you add to the paints, the lighter the shade of colour becomes and the lower the **intensity**.

CONSULTATION

Before you start the treatment you will need to carry out a consultation with the client. This is carried out for the following reasons:

- to find out why they are having the face painting and what theme they want
- to discuss what colours to use
- to check for any skin conditions or allergies to the products that may prevent the treatment from being carried out.

Communication and behaviour

Communication is important in the hair and beauty industry as you are working with clients. You need to be able to talk to people and this is very important during the consultation. These might be people that you have not met before. In order for clients to feel happy about coming to you for treatments, you will need to feel comfortable with them. This starts with being confident about what you are doing.

ACTIVITY

Copy the diagram below and fill in the boxes with examples of positive communication and behaviour. You can use Chapter 102 to help you.

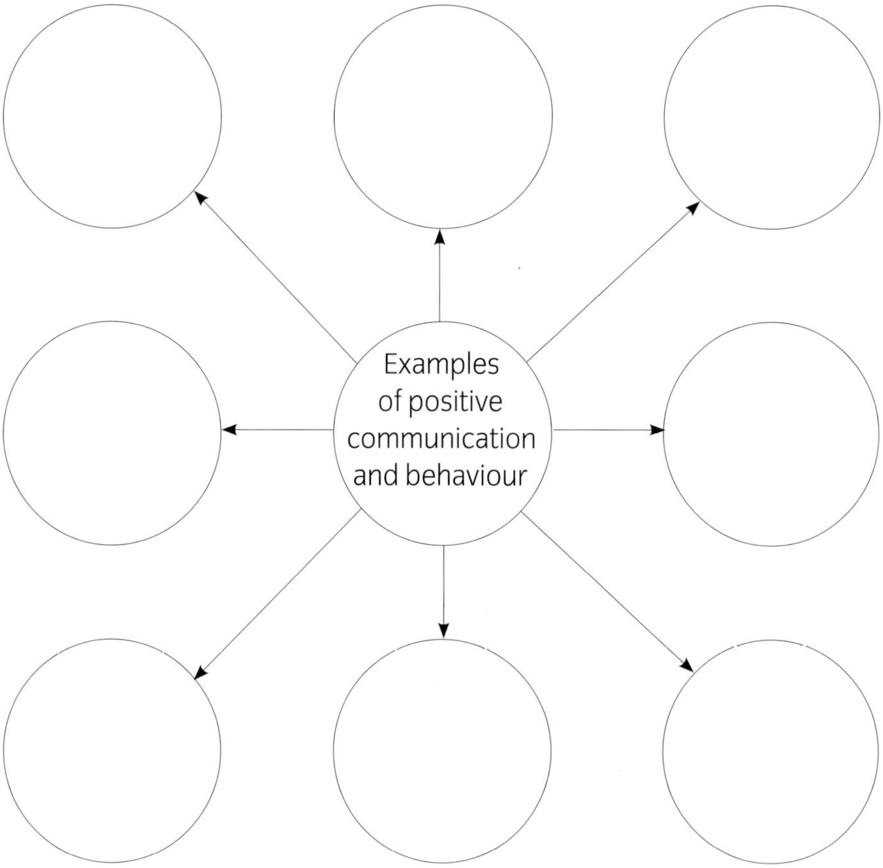

Check your answers with your tutor and discuss with your group.

HANDY HINTS

Use this checklist to help you set up for the treatment:

- ✓ towels
- ✓ headband
- ✓ gown
- ✓ cotton wool
- ✓ tissues
- ✓ couch cover (if a couch is being used)
- ✓ couch tissue roll (to cover the couch cover)
- ✓ couch or suitable chairs
- ✓ mirror
- ✓ waste bin (lined and with a lid)
- ✓ face-painting brushes
- ✓ a suitable container for water (such as an empty Barbicide jar)
- ✓ palette
- ✓ face-painting sponges
- ✓ cleansers
- ✓ toners
- ✓ moisturisers
- ✓ face paints (selection of colours)
- ✓ transfers and stencils
- ✓ face glitters
- ✓ gems
- ✓ treatment plan and pen
- ✓ portfolio of different designs to help your client choose a design.

Intensity
How dark or pale a colour is

SmartScreen 107 handout 11

HANDY HINTS

Make sure the client is not allergic to any products. If in any doubt, carry out a patch test by applying a small amount of the product behind their ear, 24 hours before the treatment. If the skin becomes sensitive to the product (red, itchy or swollen) do not carry out the treatment. If you are unsure, ask your tutor for help.

HANDY HINTS

Refer to Chapter 102 Presenting a professional image in the salon, for more detailed information on communication and behaviour.

SmartScreen 107 handout 10

SmartScreen 107 worksheet 4

HANDY HINTS

Look back at Chapter 106 to refresh your knowledge on face shapes. This chapter will also tell you how to apply make-up to flatter each face shape.

Factors
Things you have to think about during the service; a factor such as age or gender may require you to change the service

Hollow
A dark space

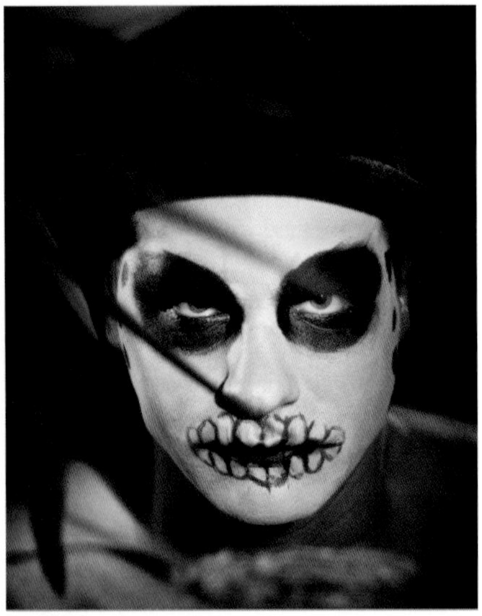

Fantasy face painting

HANDY HINTS

Use the information in Chapter 006 Skin care to refresh your knowledge on skin types and to help you with the activity.

SmartScreen 107 handouts 3 and 11

SmartScreen 107 worksheet 1

FACTORS THAT MAY INFLUENCE THE FACE-PAINTING TREATMENT

During the consultation, there may be certain **factors** that you need to find out about so you can plan your face-painting treatment.

Face shape

Use light and dark colours to help create the shape you need for your total look. A lighter colour will make areas look more noticeable. A darker colour will make an area appear less noticeable or create a **hollow** effect.

The use of colours in this way will help to create the look you are trying to achieve on different face shapes, such as with the skull face painting in the photo on page 331.

Skin type

You will need to look at the client's skin before you start. The reason for this is to:

- make sure that you choose the correct skin care products
- check that the client does not have any skin conditions that would affect you carrying out the face painting.

Choose the correct cleansing products for your client's skin. This will help to prepare the skin for the face-painting products.

ACTIVITY

Copy and complete the table below. Choose from the following skin types, showing which skin care products are suitable for each skin type: dry, oily, combination, normal.

Skin care product	Skin types used for
Cleansing face wash	
Cleansing lotion	
Cleansing milk	
Cleansing cream	
Freshener	
Toner	
Astringent	
Moisturising lotion	
Moisturising mousse	
Moisturising cream	

Adverse skin conditions

Certain **adverse** skin conditions will stop you from carrying out a face-painting treatment. It is important to check that the client does not have any of these conditions:

- bruising (as the area will be too painful to work over)
- allergy to the products (as the skin may become red, swollen, itchy)
- open sores, cuts or **abrasions** (as the area will be tender to work over).

Ask your tutor for help if your client has any of these, or you if are not sure.

Adverse
Something bad

Abrasion
A scraped area

Age

Face painting is very popular for children's parties, as well as for older clients for events such as fancy-dress parties and festivals. The designs you choose should be suitable for the age of the client and the purpose of the event.

Gender

Gender means whether someone is a female or male. Face painting can be applied to both male and female clients. This may make a difference to the colours chosen. For example, you would probably not use pink colours on a male client. The face-painting design and colours should be suitable for the gender and event.

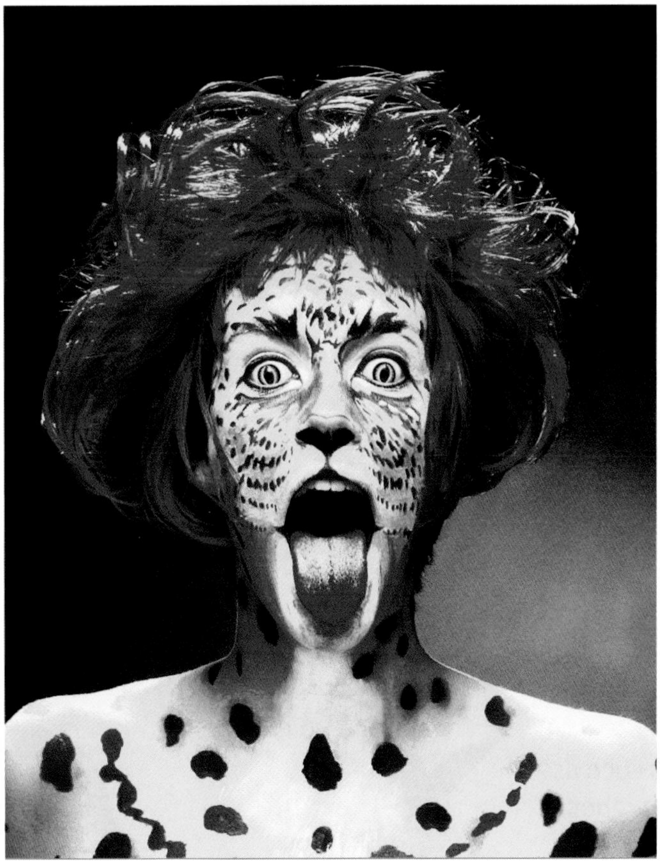

Face painting on a man

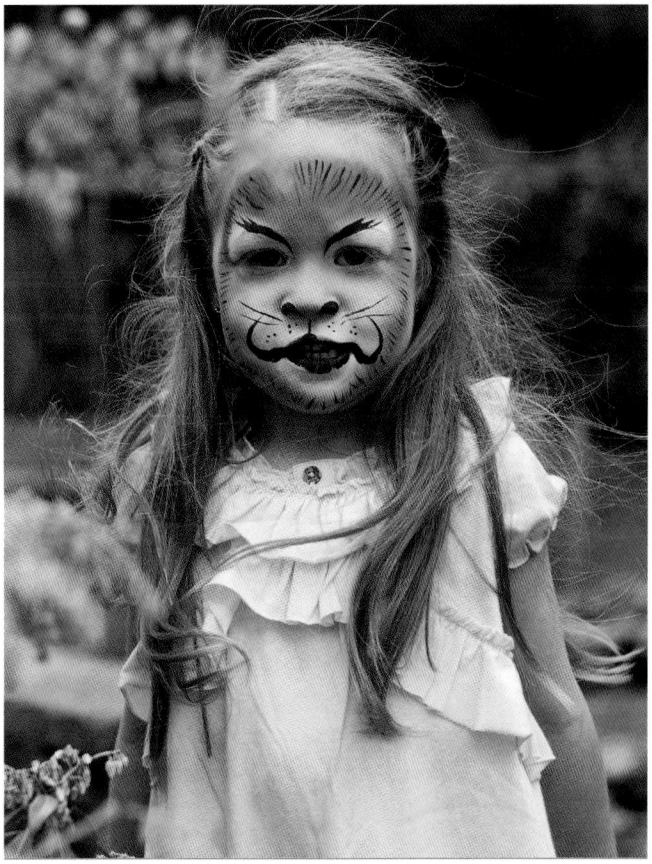

A lion face painting on a child

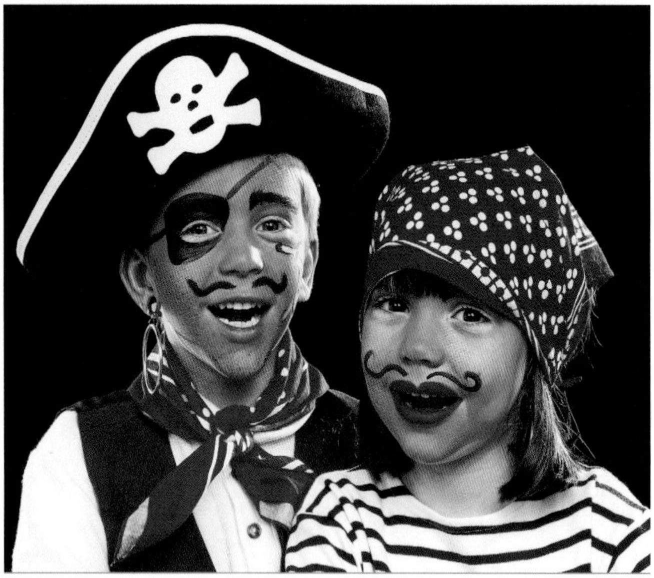

Pirate face painting

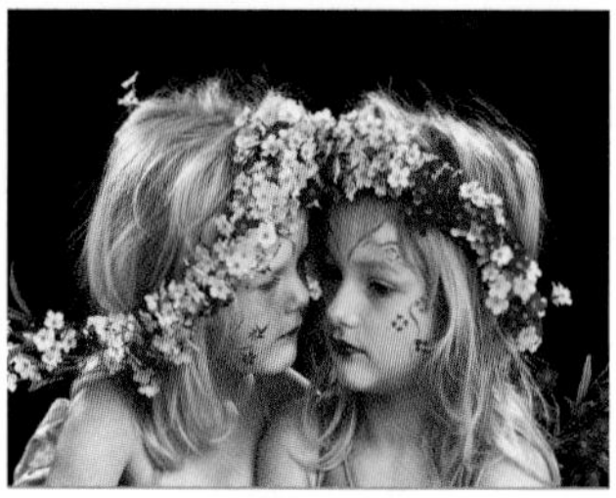

Flower girl face painting

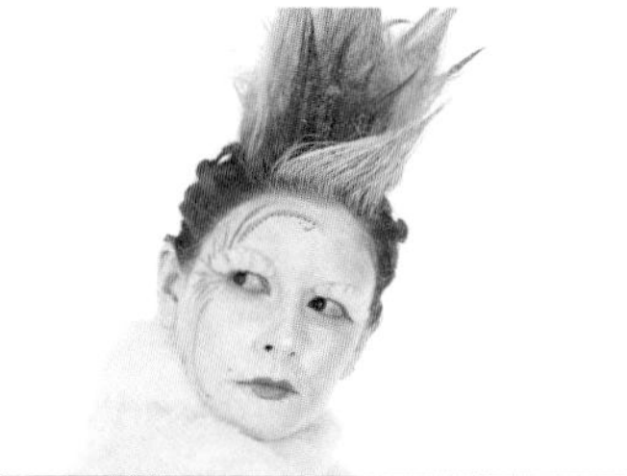

A Stephenson college photoshoot entry: ice theme face painting

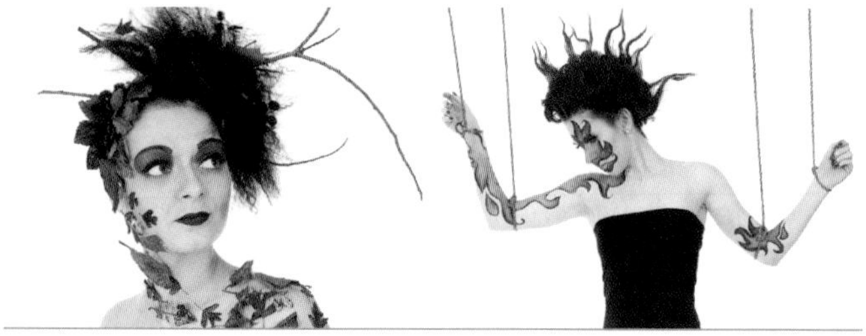

Stephenson College photoshoot entries: autumn and fire themes

HANDY HINTS

You must also think about the culture that your client belongs to when face painting. Refer to Chapter 106 for how to take cultural factors into account.

SmartScreen 107 worksheet 8

Occasion

There are many reasons why a client may want their face painted, such as for a festival or a party. It is important to discuss this at the start of the treatment and decide on what design and colours the client would like.

Topical themes

A topical theme is a theme based on a certain topic or subject. There are many different themes that could be chosen for a face-painting design. Examples include:

- animal images such as butterflies, tigers, dogs and rabbits
- fantasy images – here is your chance to be creative. Glitters, gems and transfers can also be used to make the designs stand out
- nature images such as flowers, water, earth, fire
- character images such as witches, vampires, ghosts.

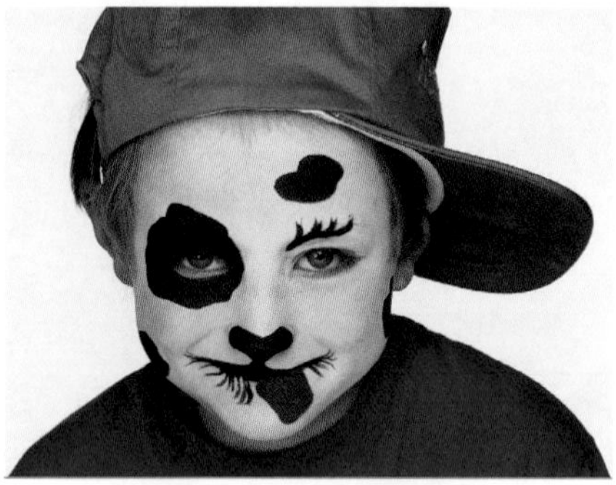

An animal-themed face painting: a dog

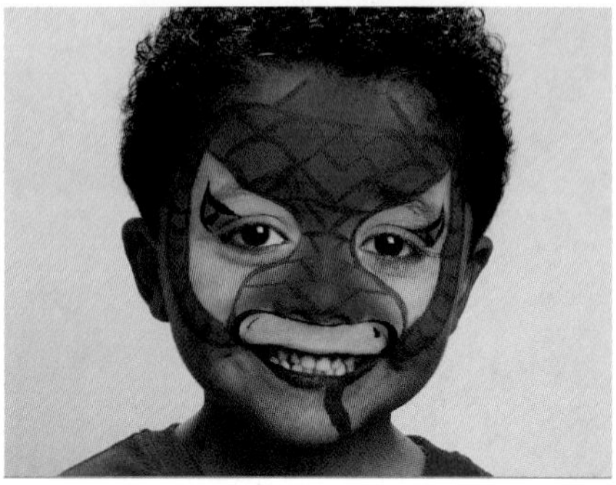

An animal-themed face painting: a snake

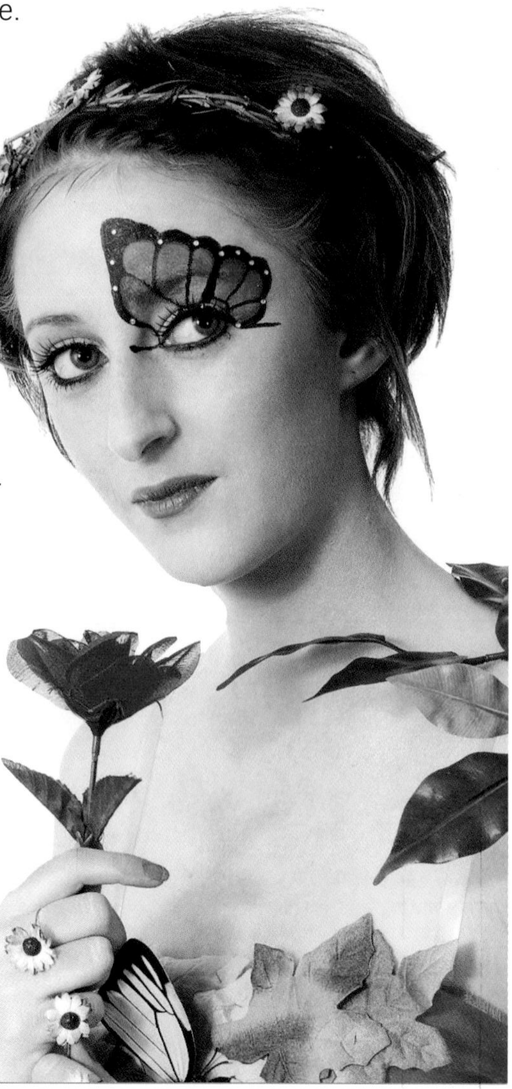

A Stephenson College photoshoot entry: a nature-themed face painting

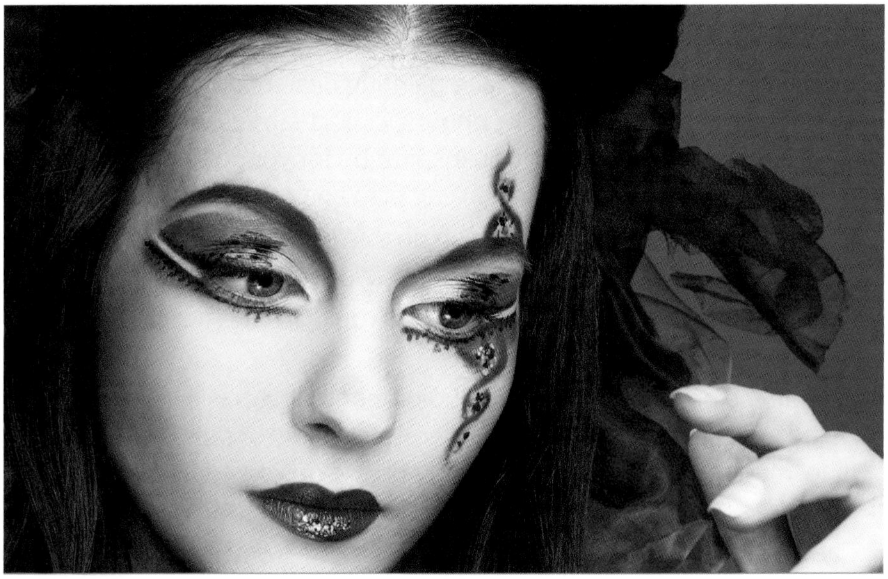

Fantasy-themed face paints (top left, middle and bottom right)

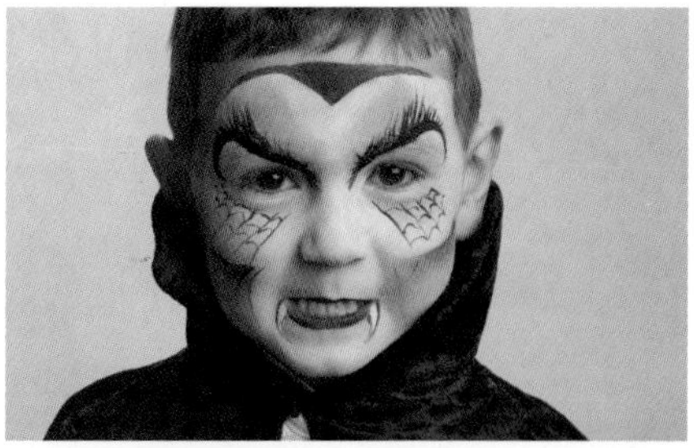

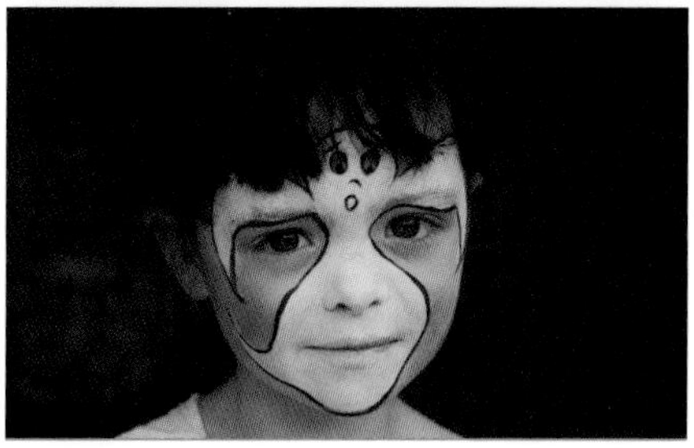

Character-themed face paints: a vampire and a ghost

CHOOSING YOUR FACE-PAINTING DESIGN

Now that you have all the information from the client, you can choose your face-painting design. To be a good face painting artist, you will need to be able to apply a few different designs. You will build up your different designs and skills with time and practice.

FINDING INSPIRATION

The first step in learning to do face-painting designs is research. You can find **inspiration** in the following places:

- The internet – google 'face painting' for design ideas, or search for 'face painting' in image libraries such as iStock. Many websites also give you step-by-step instructions on how to carry out face-painting designs.
- Magazines – fashion magazines such as *Vogue* may include face painting in their make-up looks.
- Sketches or photographs – you might have your own ideas, which you can put on paper as a reference point, or practise a look on a friend and take a photo of it.
- In books – look at the books that you have in your college library or your local library. Search for books that contain face painting and step-by-step guides.
- Media such as theatre, TV, DVDs and films – shows such as 'Cats', 'The Lion King' and 'The Rocky Horror Picture Show' are good for getting ideas. Try to find the DVD recordings.
- Hair and fashion shows – for more dramatic make-up looks.
- Craft shops – these are great places for getting ideas for designs. You may find colours, patterns and different textures that you like from fabrics and beads – all of which may be useful in your face-painting design.
- From outside – for example the flowers and leaves that are in your garden. These are good inspiration for nature-themed face-painting designs.

Once you have collected lots of face painting ideas you will find it much easier to come up with your own designs.

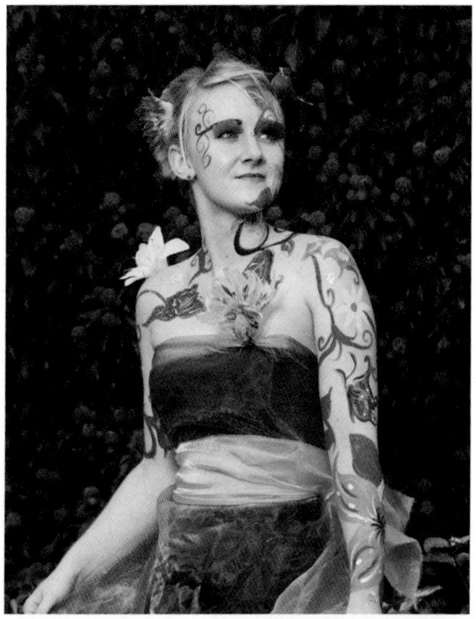

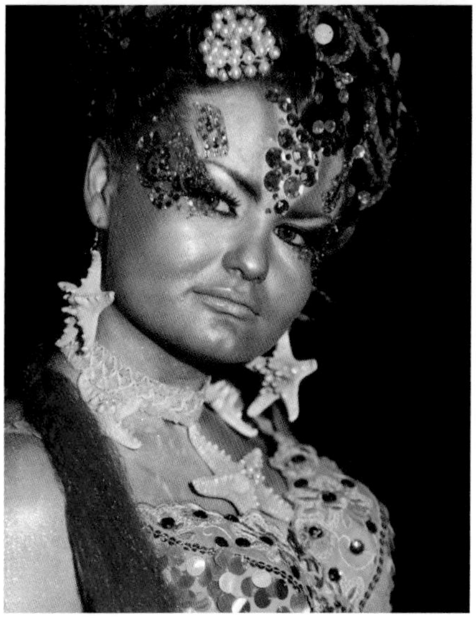

Inspiration

Places you can go to to find ideas for your designs, eg films and magazines

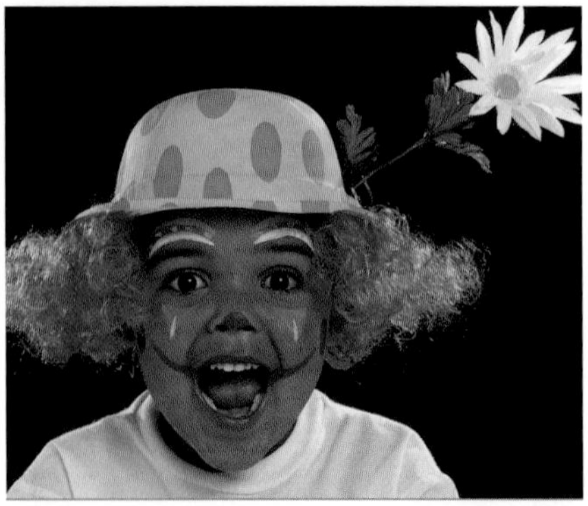

A face painting for a children's party

HANDY HINTS

You could do this activity as a competition within your group.

ACTIVITY

Collect some ideas for a nature face-painting design from as many different places as you can. Take photos, collect fabrics, draw pictures or print off any ideas that give you inspiration for your design. When you have collected these ideas you can plan and carry out your design:

- Plan your design on paper. You can do this by drawing a face onto the paper and then adding your design using coloured pencils.
- Remember to use the colours that you would like the finished design to be.
- Include the products, tools and equipment that you will need, such as face-painting colours, glitters, gems, transfers or stencils, brushes (fine, medium, large sizes depending on the design you want to achieve), sponges, etc.
- Carry out the face-painting design on a person from your group. Take a photo of the completed design and add it to your portfolio of images.

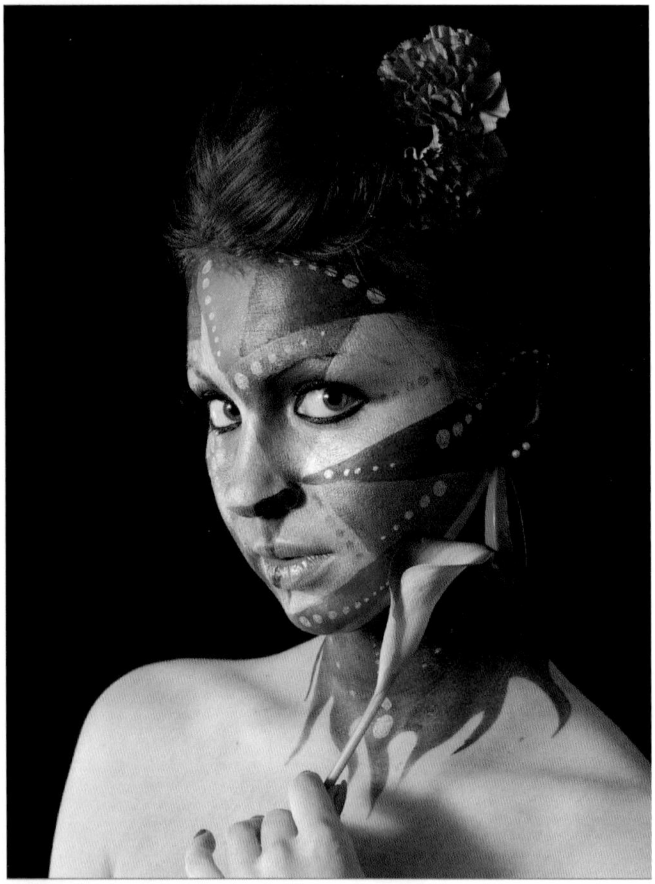

A 3D face-painting design

ACTIVITY

Put together a portfolio of different face-painting images to show your client. This can be a collection of images from the internet, magazines or photos of your own work that you have created. Try to choose designs for all ages, cultures and for different themes and occasions.

FACE-PAINTING DESIGNS ON 2D AND 3D SURFACES

Designs that have been created on paper or found in books and magazines or printed off the internet are examples of **2D** surfaces.

Designs can be **transferred** from a 2D surface to a **3D** surface by applying the face-painting design onto:

- a mannequin (a dummy)
- a client (a person)
- a mask.

The choice of 3D surface would depend on the effect that was needed and also the occasion. An example of this is applying face painting to a mask for a festival.

HANDY HINTS

Remember that you can change the colours of any of the designs that you find. This will create a different face-painting design.

HANDY HINTS

Why not practise different designs on yourself! Take a photo of the face-painting designs that you create and add it into your portfolio to show your clients.

2D

Two dimensional – a flat surface, such as a piece of paper

Transfer

To move from one place to another

3D

Three dimensional – a rounded surface, such as a person's face or a mask

ACTIVITY

Have a go at taking a design idea from a 2D surface to a 3D one:

- Draw a 2D design of a face-painting image for one of the following themes: animal, fantasy, nature, character.
- Using your 2D design as a guide, carry out a face-painting treatment and try to create the face-painting image onto a 3D surface such as a person or a mask.
- Take photos of your finished designs and add them to your portfolio.

SmartScreen 107 handout 6

HANDY HINTS

You may find Smartscreen 107 handout 11 useful as a guide for a blank face picture to draw on.

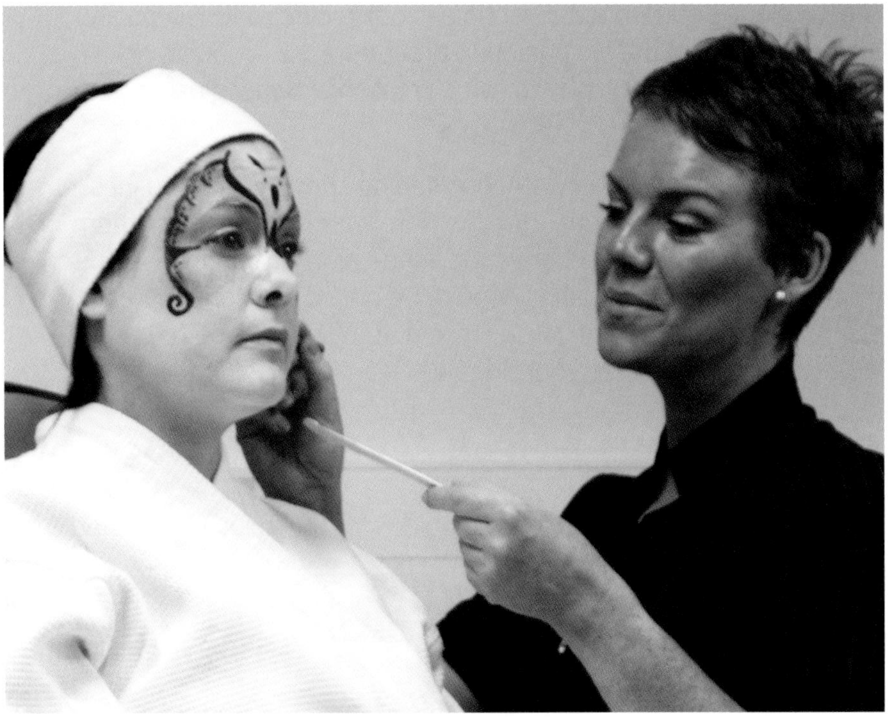

CARRY OUT A THEMED FACE PAINTING

Before starting the face-painting treatment, you must make sure your client is comfortable on either the chair or the couch. Place a headband around their head (to keep the hair off the face). Lastly, make sure that you have all your tools and products ready.

ACTIVITY

To help you remember the routines, answer the following questions:

1 Do you use dry or damp cotton wool to remove the cleanser from the face?
2 Do you apply the toning product before or after the moisturiser?
3 Which cleanser is most suitable for a dry skin?
4 Which toning product is most suitable for an oily skin?
5 Which moisturiser is most suitable for a combination skin?

Check your answers with your tutor.

HANDY HINTS

Refer back to Chapter 006 to remind yourself of the cleansing, toning and moisturising products and routines.

HANDY HINTS

Remember also to blot the skin after applying the moisturiser. The skin will need to be dry before applying the face-painting products.

FACE-PAINTING TREATMENT PROCEDURE

As part of a face-painting treatment you need to make sure that the skin is ready for the paint to be applied. This is done by carrying out a basic facial treatment:

- Skin cleansing – choose the most suitable products for your client's skin type. Gently cleanse the eyes, lips and face.
- Toning – apply the toner and then blot dry with a tissue.
- Moisturising – apply a small amount gently over the face and neck areas.

After you have carried out a gentle basic skin care routine, you are ready to carry out the face-painting procedure. All products must be applied in a hygienic way to avoid cross-infection, eg using clean brushes and sponges.

SmartScreen 107 handouts 7, 8 and 9

You will need lots of clean water for dipping sponges and brushes into. Most face paints will get thinner the more water you mix with them. This means that you can change the shade or intensity of the colour by adding water. The brushes need to be rinsed in water between each colour to stop them getting mixed up. You will need to change your water often to keep your brushes clean.

CARRYING OUT SIMPLE FACE-PAINTING DESIGNS

Here are some simple step-by-step guides for the following themed face paints:

- tiger face-painting design
- butterfly face-painting design.

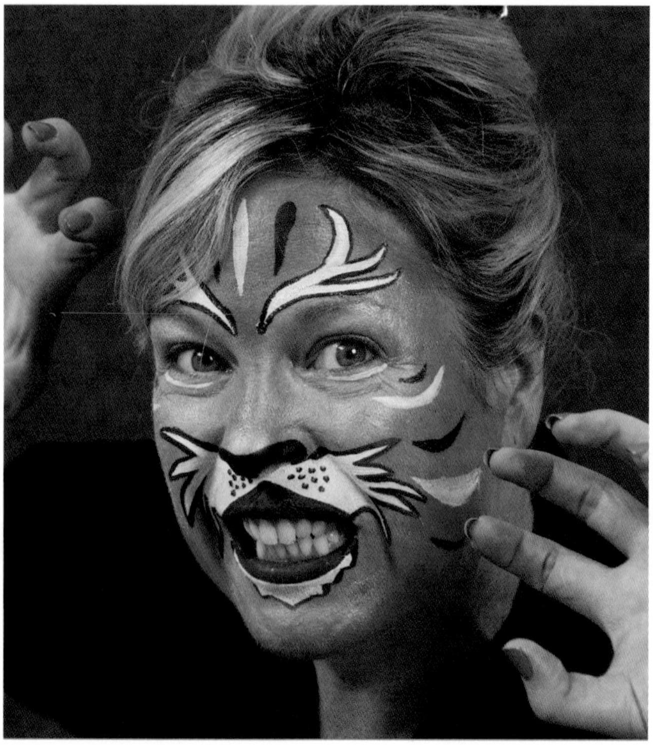

The finished tiger face painting

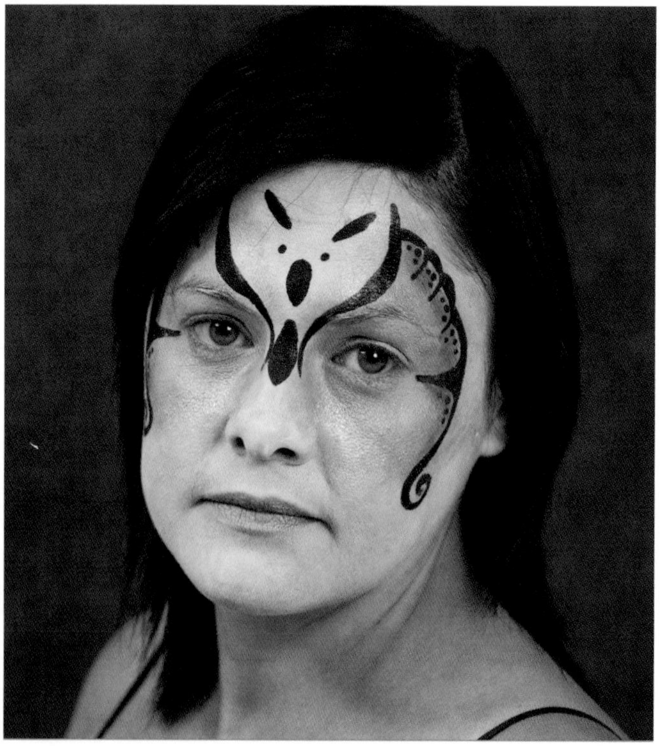

The finished butterfly face painting

TIGER FACE-PAINTING DESIGN

Face-painting colours needed: Black White Yellow Orange

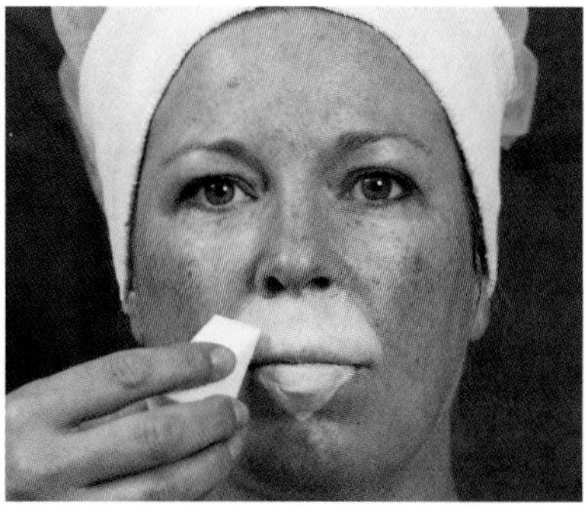

STEP 1 – Using a damp sponge, paint a white area around the mouth.

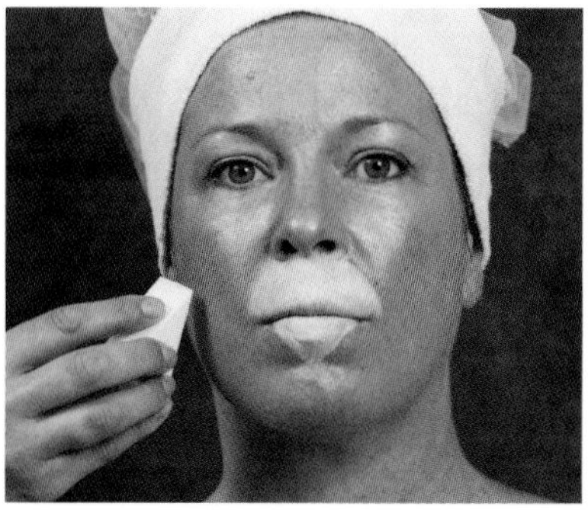

STEP 2 – Using a clean part of the sponge, paint yellow around the eyes, cheeks and chin.

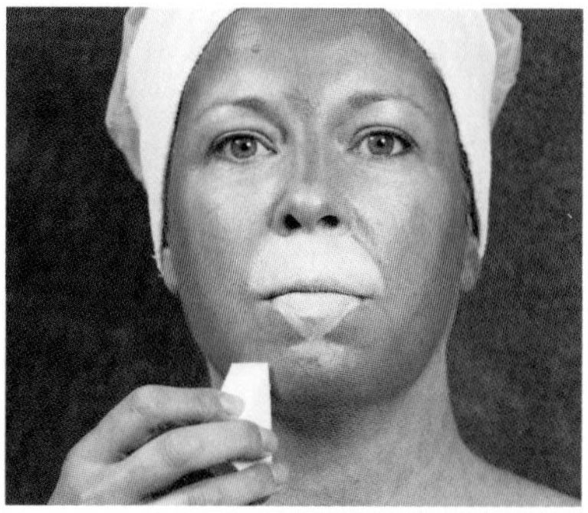

STEP 3 – Using a clean part of the sponge, add orange around the outside of the face. Blend the orange and yellow together by going slightly over the edges of the yellow paint with the orange.

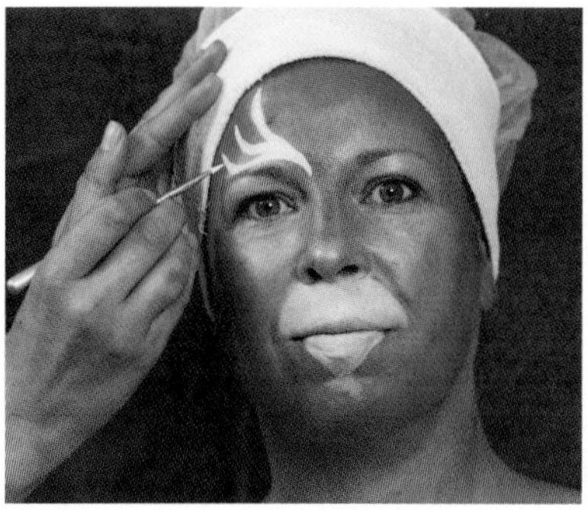

STEP 4 – Using a medium thick brush, paint white eyebrows above the eyes. Use the line of the client's eyebrows as a guide. Lift the brush at the end of the stroke to create the point at the end.

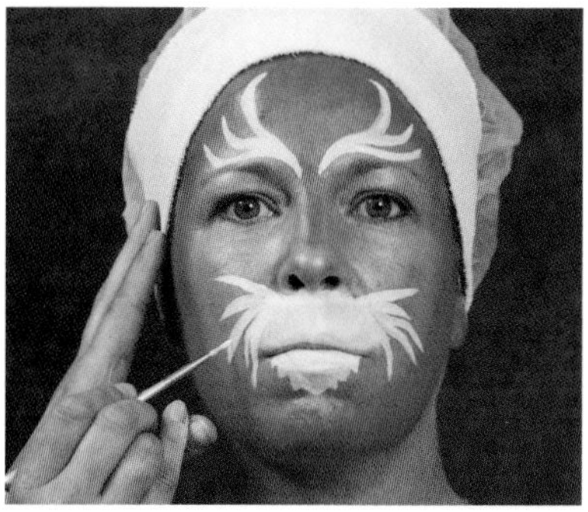

STEP 5 – Add white brush strokes around the mouth, creating the whiskers. If you lift the brush as you come to the end of the stroke and flick the tip of the brush slightly you can achieve the pointed look to your whiskers.

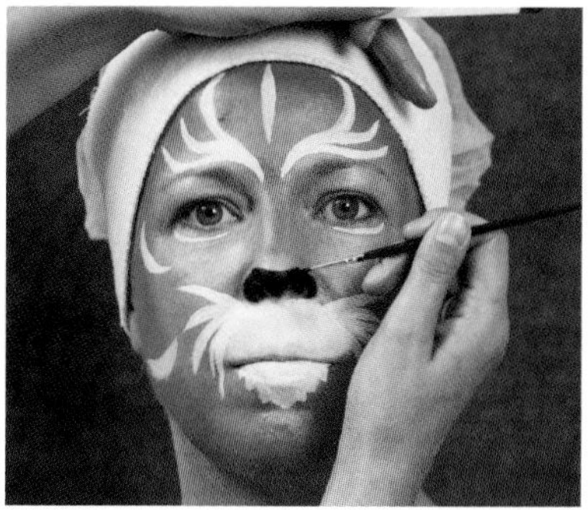

STEP 6 – Add white stripes under the eyes and at the sides of the face. Start your brush strokes at the outer edge of the orange paint and move the brush inwards. If you lift the brush as you drag it in, you will make the ends of the stripe come to a point. Add a nose by applying the blank paint to the sides of the nostrils.

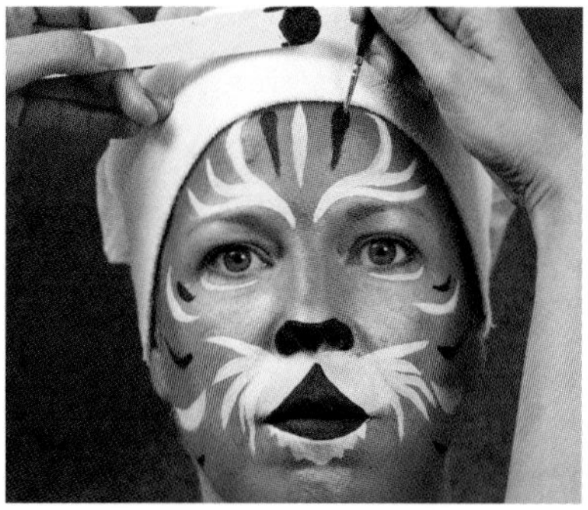

STEP 7 – Using the black face paint, add a line from under the nose to the sides of the top lip. Colour this area in and also the bottom lip. Add some black stripes to the sides of the face and forehead, as in step 6.

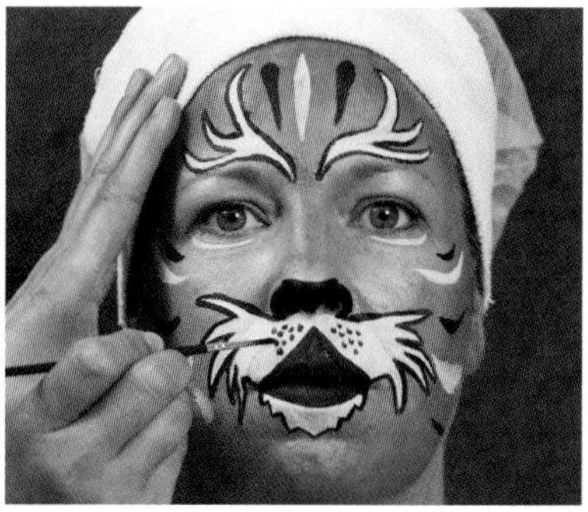

STEP 8 – Using a thin brush, add small dots above the top lip in black. Draw a thin black line around the white paint (on the mouth and forehead).

SmartScreen 107 worksheet 6

BUTTERFLY FACE-PAINTING DESIGN

Face painting colours needed: Black White Yellow Pale green

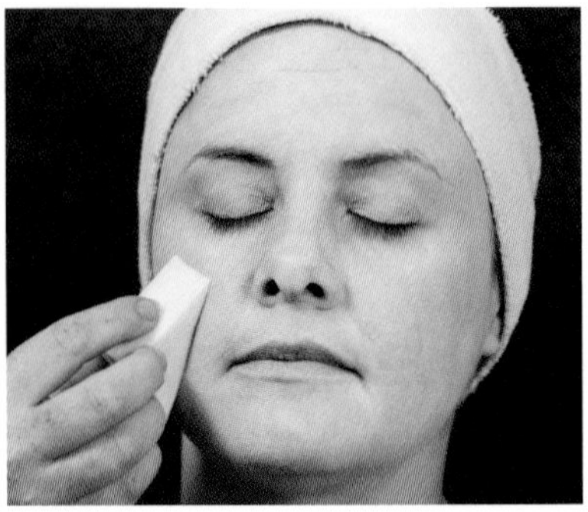

STEP 1 – Using a damp sponge, cover the whole face with white face paint.

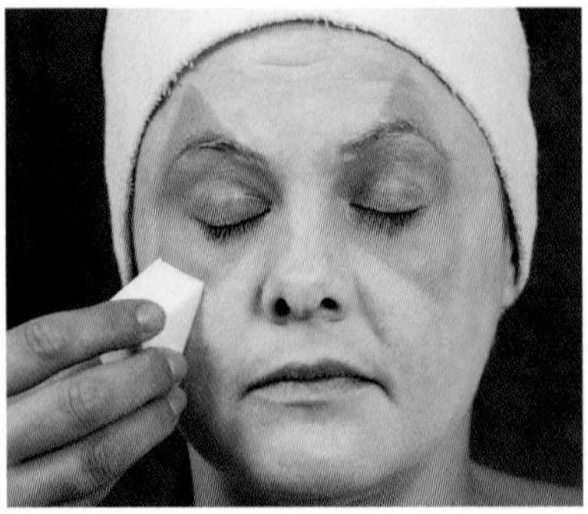

STEP 2 – Apply some yellow face paint around the eyes, using a clean side of the damp sponge. This will be the shape of the butterfly wings, so it needs to be in the shape of a triangle on each eye.

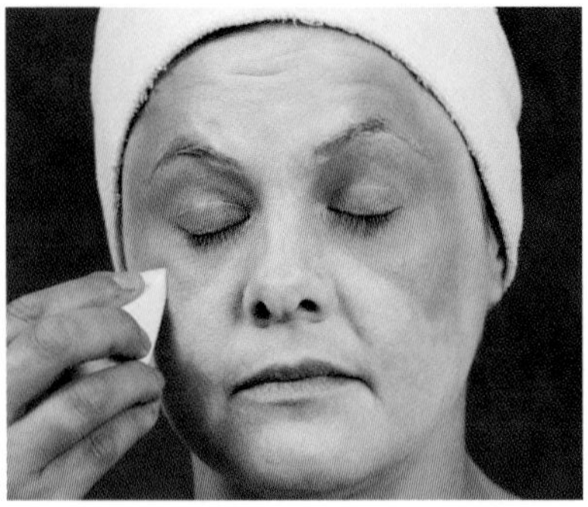

STEP 3 – Apply a small amount of pale green face paint to a damp sponge and add a little of this colour to the outer part of the wings. Blend the yellow and green colours together around the edges by dabbing gently with the sponge.

HANDY HINTS

Try to keep your butterfly shape small as this will stand out more.

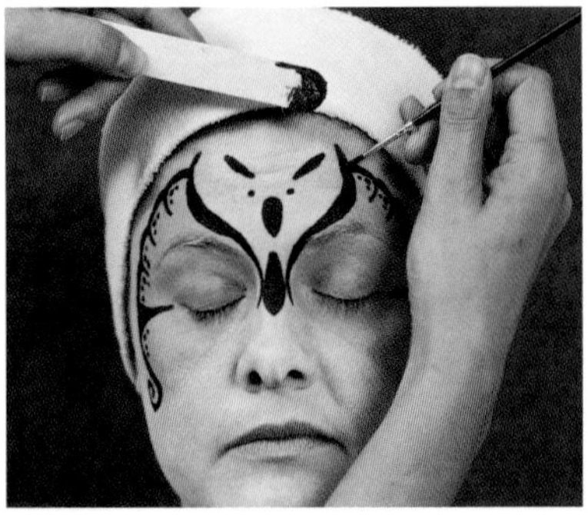

STEP 4 – With a fine brush, use the black face paint to carefully draw lines around the wings of the butterfly. Finish the design by adding the butterfly body and antenna with your fine brush as shown.

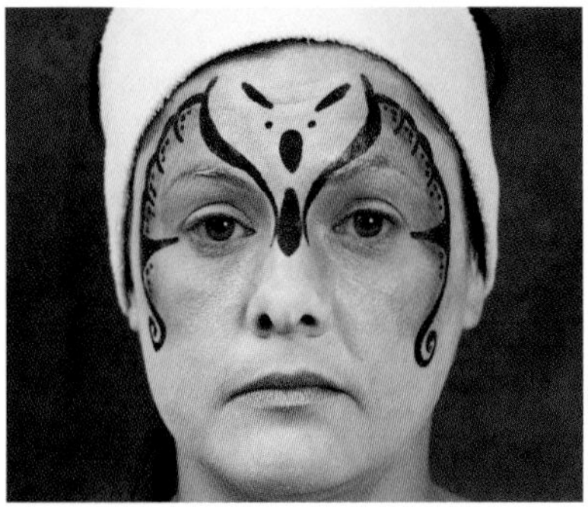

STEP 5 – To add sparkle, apply some yellow or green glitter to the butterfly wings using either a brush or your fingertips. Apply gems to the outer edges of the butterfly's wings and on the body. Remove the backing paper from each gem and gently stick in place using your finger.

HANDY HINTS

Practise these face-painting designs using different colours.

AFTER THE TREATMENT

After you have finished the treatment, remove the headband and let the client see the finished face-painting design in a clean mirror. Make sure that you record everything you have done on the client's treatment plan. This should include the products that you have used as well as the colours and design applied.

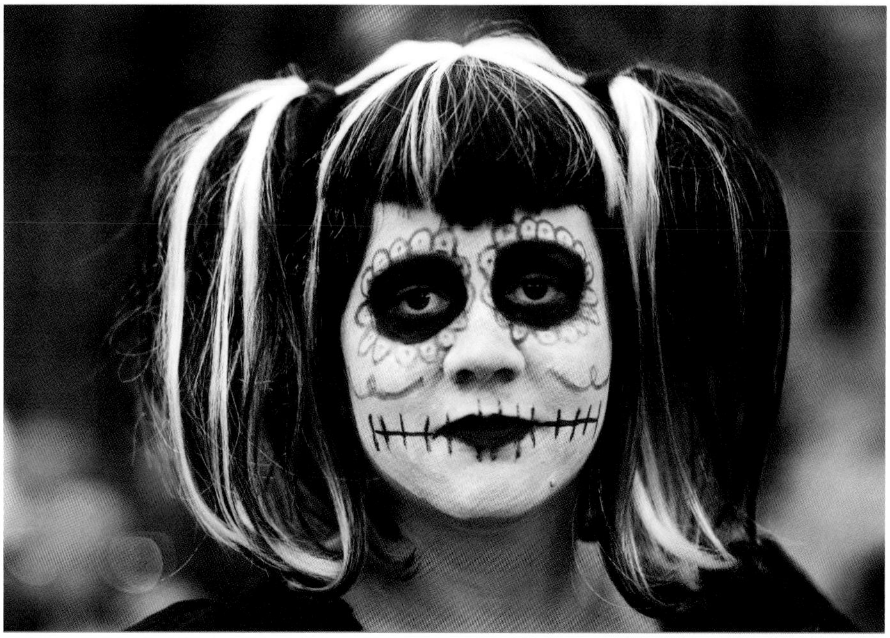

A Hallowe'en-themed face painting

HANDY HINTS

You may want to draw the design you have created onto paper or take a photo of the finished look (you will need to ask the client's permission to do this). Add the picture or photo to your portfolio of designs.

HANDY HINTS

Care needs to be taken when removing the face painting. If it gets into the eyes it may make them sting and become watery. If this happens, the eyes need to washed with cool water.

ACTIVITY

Hold a themed face-painting competition with your group. Decide on what the theme is going to be, eg Halloween, Christmas or fantasy. Work in pairs or small groups.

AFTERCARE ADVICE

Aftercare advice on the way of removing the face paints should be given to the client after the treatment. Because the face paints are water based, they should easily wash off using water. For best results, suggest that the client uses mild soap and water and then wipes the paint off with a damp flannel.

HANDY HINTS

Baby wipes may also be used to remove small face-painting designs from the face.

IN A NUTSHELL

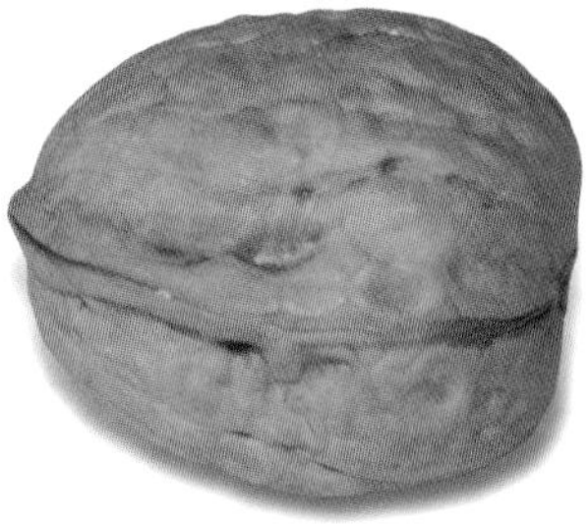

You are now at the end of the chapter. Before you test your knowledge with the revision activities, check the following list to see if you feel confident in all the areas covered. If there are still any areas you're unsure of, go back over them in the book and ask your tutor for extra support:

- what preparation is needed for a themed face-painting treatment
- how to communicate and behave in a professional manner
- how to design a themed face painting
- identify factors that could influence the treatment
- how to prepare for the treatment
- what products, tools and equipment you will need
- how to use the products, tools and equipment safely and hygienically
- how to adapt a 2D image into a 3D one
- how to carry out a face-painting treatment
- how to remove face painting.

REVISION ACTIVITIES

Use the questions below to test your knowledge of Chapter 107 to see just how much information you've gained. This can help you to prepare for your assessments.

Turn to pages 502–503 for the answers.

WORDS TO FIND

Copy and complete the sentences below. Use these words to help you fill in the gaps.

face paint	toner	posture	technique
headband	face	glitter	brushes
occasion	communication	palette	safety
cleanser	gems	sponge	hygiene

1. A ______________ is used to keep the client's hair off their face during a treatment.
2. A ______________ is used to apply face painting over large areas of the face.
3. ______________ are used to apply the face painting when more detail is needed in the design (such as a line or dots).
4. To stop you getting backache, you should have a good ______________ .
5. An example of good ______________ is smiling and listening to the client.
6. Face paints can be mixed on a ______________ before being applied to the face.
7. ______________ can be stuck onto the face to make the face-painting design look more effective.
8. You need to ask the client for what ______________ they are having their face painted. You can then choose the most suitable design.
9. ______________ ______________ is a water-based product.
10. Washing your hands before and after the treatment is an example of good ______________ .

TEST YOUR KNOWLEDGE FURTHER

Read the sentences below and state whether they are true or false.

1. Face paints are water-based products. True or false?
2. Gems are used to give sparkle to a face-painting design. True or false?
3. Face painting can be carried out on a mask, mannequin or a client. True or false?
4. An example of a face-painting design on a 3D surface is a picture on a piece of paper. True or false?
5. Examples of face-painting themes are animals and nature. True or false?
6. Face painting is an opportunity for you to be creative. True or false?
7. A consultation is carried out to find out what face-painting design the client wants. True or false?
8. Face paints come only in three colours – red, yellow and blue. True or false?
9. Face painting is popular for fancy-dress parties. True or false?

108 NAIL ART APPLICATION

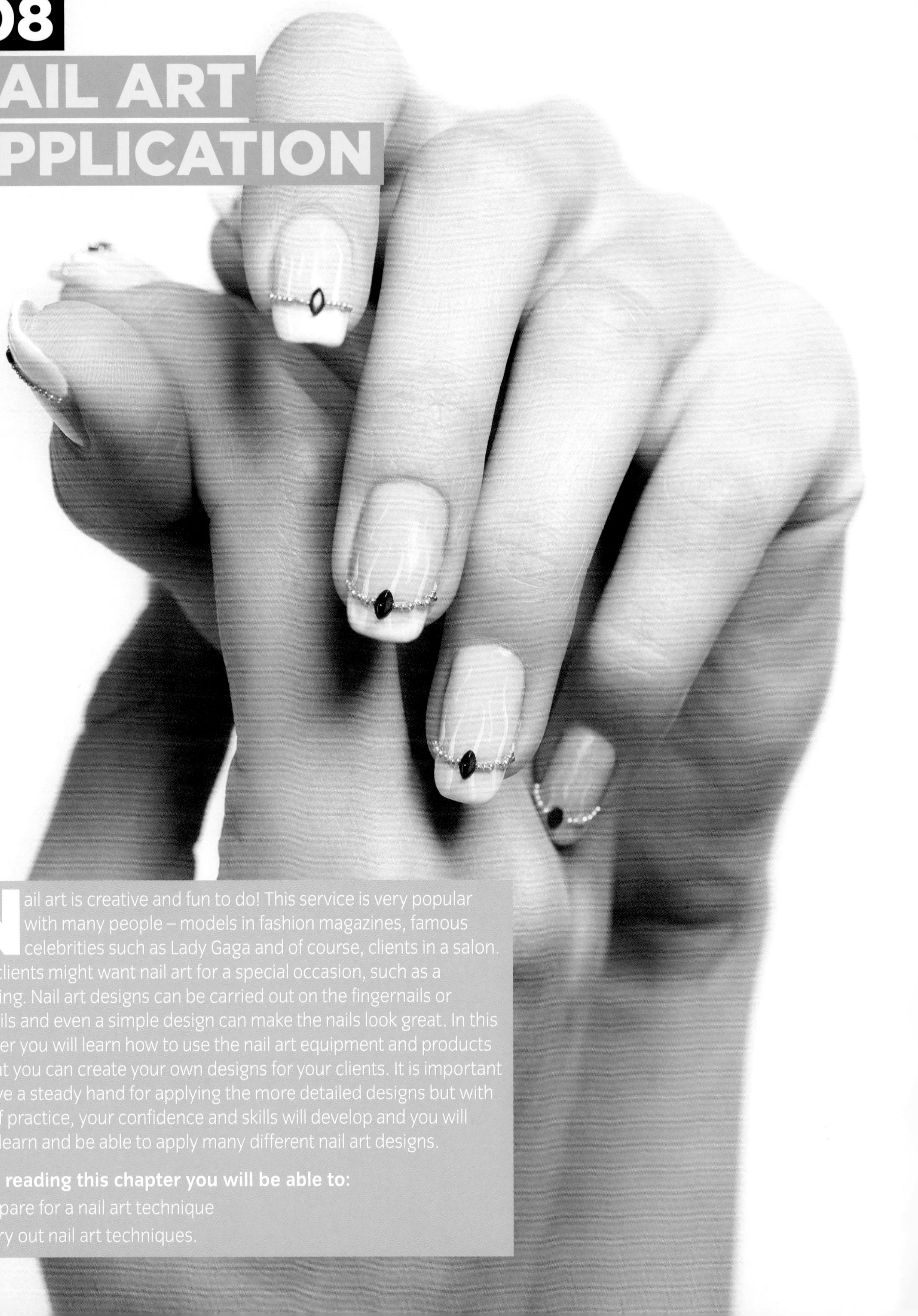

Nail art is creative and fun to do! This service is very popular with many people – models in fashion magazines, famous celebrities such as Lady Gaga and of course, clients in a salon. Your clients might want nail art for a special occasion, such as a wedding. Nail art designs can be carried out on the fingernails or toenails and even a simple design can make the nails look great. In this chapter you will learn how to use the nail art equipment and products so that you can create your own designs for your clients. It is important to have a steady hand for applying the more detailed designs but with lots of practice, your confidence and skills will develop and you will soon learn and be able to apply many different nail art designs.

After reading this chapter you will be able to:

1 prepare for a nail art technique

2 carry out nail art techniques.

PREPARE FOR A NAIL ART TECHNIQUE

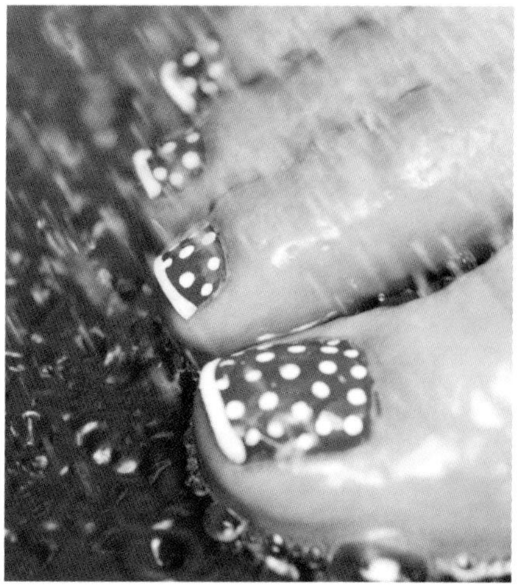

Before you begin the nail art service, it's important to be prepared. Health and safety requirements should be carried out for every treatment, but knowing how to set up your treatment area and carrying out a proper consultation are also musts for nail art services. There are also many different products available for nail art, so make sure you are familiar with these well before you start work on a client.

SAFE AND HYGIENIC WORKING PRACTICES

Keep your treatment area tidy and use only tools and equipment that have been properly cleaned, which means they are hygienic. This will help to reduce the risk of harm to you and your clients and help to prevent cross-infection. The client will also have more confidence in you and you will look more professional.

All the safe and hygienic working practices that you need to know for nail art services are the same as for manicure and pedicure treatments.

ACTIVITY

To help remind you of some of the important health and safety practices that you should follow, answer these questions:

1 Why is it important to make sure that there is suitable lighting in the nail art treatment area?
2 What is the ideal temperature for a salon?
3 What would happen if the treatment room was not well ventilated?
4 What might happen if the tools and equipment that you were using were not clean and hygienic?

Check your answers with your tutor.

THE SALON ENVIRONMENT

The treatment area should be prepared in a professional way.

- All products, tools and equipment should be clean and hygienic and should be placed neatly in the treatment area or safely and tidily on the trolley.
- If used, the couch should be covered for hygiene reasons with a couch cover and couch roll tissue.
- The chairs used should be the correct height. **Adjustable** ones are the best so that you can alter the height for different clients. Back rests will also help to make sure that the client is comfortable.

HANDY HINTS

Go to Chapters 113 Following health and safety in the salon and 007, 109, 110 Hand care and providing basic manicure and pedicure treatments, and read up on the health and safety laws that you should follow.

Adjustable
Can be changed or altered

Client comfort is also very important:

- The room temperature should not be too hot or to cold.
- The treatment room should be well ventilated.
- The lighting should be suitable for a nail art treatment so that you can clearly see what you are doing.

HANDY HINTS

Ask the client if they are seated comfortably before you begin.

PREPARING FOR THE NAIL ART SERVICE

Before the client arrives, it is important that you get yourself and the treatment area prepared. All of the products, tools and equipment need to be ready. This will ensure that the treatment flows well and will also give the client a positive first impression. It will help the client to relax and have confidence in you.

BASIC TOOLS AND EQUIPMENT

Some items, such as couch covers, are needed for most beauty therapy/ nail services. The table lists these and their use in nail art.

Tools/equipment	What is it used for?	How is it used?
Cotton buds 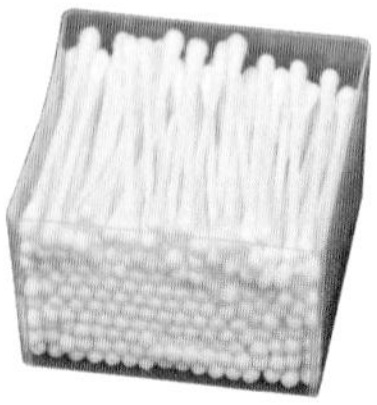	Used for rubbing foil onto the nail.	▪ Use a cotton bud to gently help the foil stick to the nail plate.
Towels 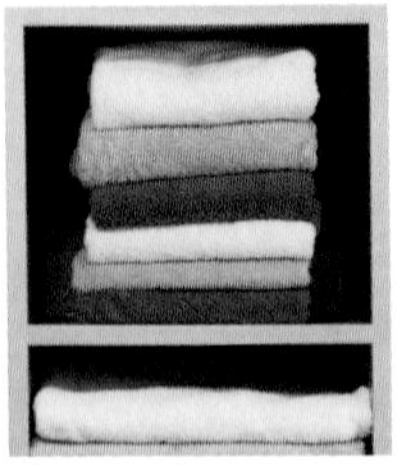	Used to cover the treatment couch. Also used to rest the client's hands on during the treatment.	▪ Place over the treatment area, then cover with couch roll tissue. ▪ Machine wash at a high temperature after each client.
Cotton wool 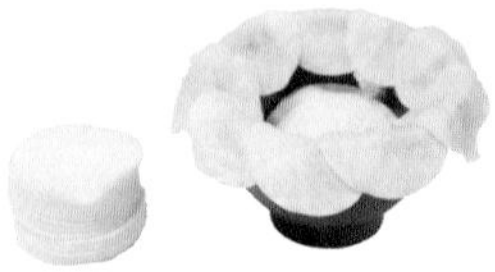	Used with nail-enamel remover. Also used with sanitising spray to wipe over the arms and hands.	▪ Apply the sanitising spray or nail-enamel remover to the cotton wool pad and wipe over the area. ▪ Throw away after use.
Treatment plan 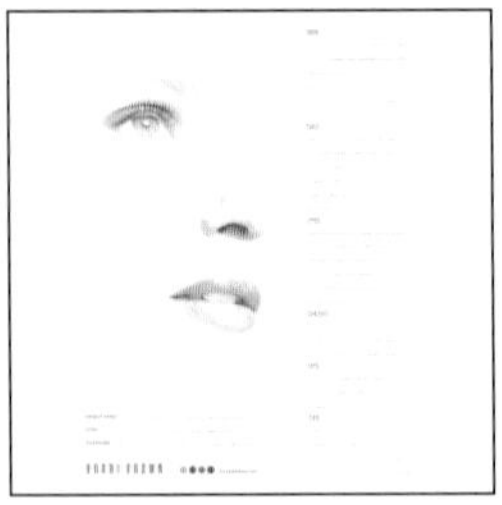	Used for recording the treatment details, eg products used.	▪ Record all details of the treatment on the plan.

Tools/equipment	What is it used for?	How is it used?
Waste bin 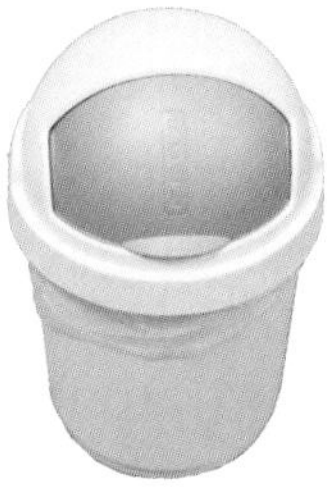	Used for throwing waste materials in (such as cotton wool and tissues).	▪ They should be lined with a bin liner and have a lid.
Couch tissue roll 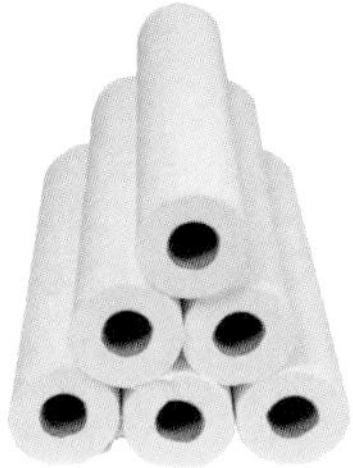	Placed over the couch cover for hygiene reasons.	▪ Throw away after each client.

TOOLS AND EQUIPMENT USED IN A NAIL ART TREATMENT

This table lists tools and equipment that are not used for every treatment, but are used in nail art treatments.

Nail art tools/equipment	What is it used for?	How is it used?
Nail table and stool 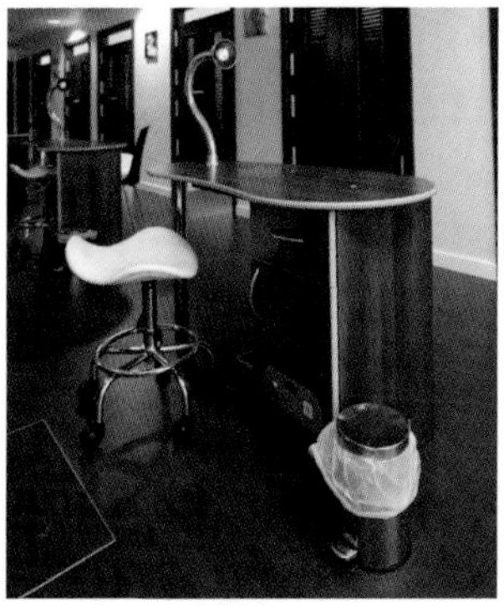	Used to sit at with the client during nail art treatment.	▪ Make sure your stool is at a comfortable height for the table. ▪ Put all your products on the table in time for the client's arrival.
Disposable nail file 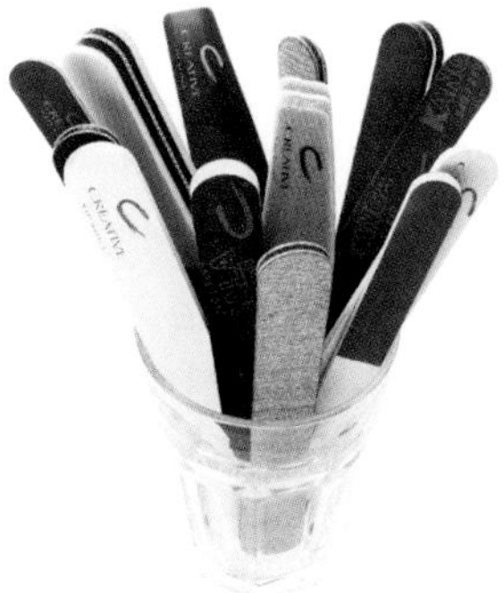	Helps to shape the free edge and prepare the nail for the nail art design. Helps to remove rough edges of the nail and smoothe it off. Can be used to reduce the length of the nail, if necessary, for the nail art design.	▪ Use the rough side for reducing the nail length. ▪ Use the fine side for finishing off and smoothing. ▪ File the nails from side to centre only. Do not use the file in a side-to-side movement across the nail edge as this can split the nail. ▪ Throw away after each client or use an antibacterial/disinfecting equipment spray.

Nail art tools/equipment	What is it used for?	How is it used?
Disposable orange stick 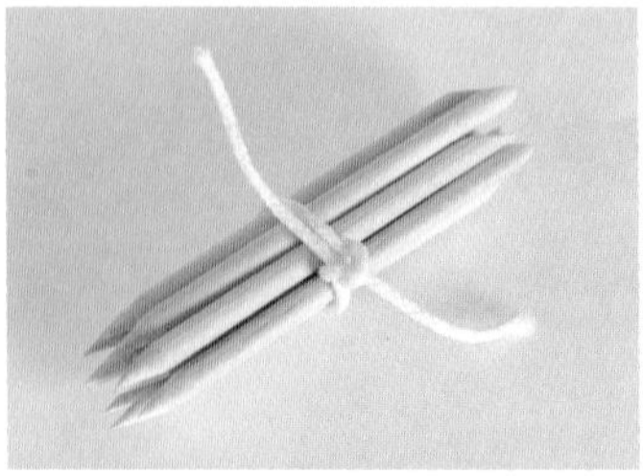	Used to remove nail enamel from the edges of the nail (tipped with cotton wool). Used to apply polish secures (tipped with Blu-Tack®). See page 340 for a description of what polish secures are. Used to make dot patterns on the nail plate (using acrylic paints).	▪ To remove nail enamel from the edges of the nail plate, tip them with cotton wool and dip into nail-enamel remover. ▪ To apply polish secures, tip them with a small ball of Blu-Tack®. This will help to pick up the polish secure before sticking it to the nail plate. ▪ Use the pointed end to make dot patterns on the nail plate. ▪ Throw away after each client.
Blu-Tack® or double-sided sticky tape 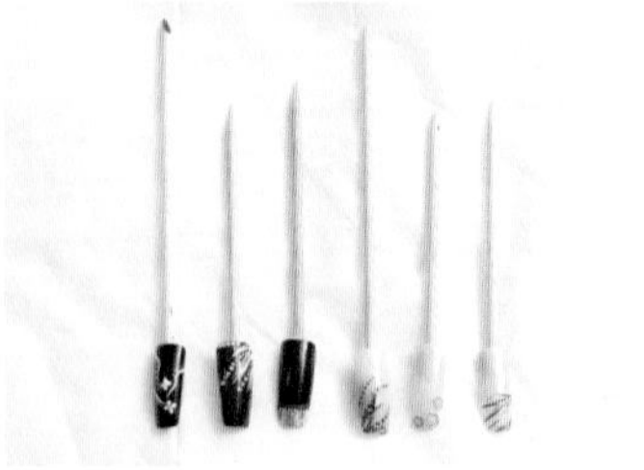	Used at the end of an orange stick to help pick up and apply polish secures. Also used to stick down artificial nail structures when you are practising your nail art designs on them.	▪ Apply a small ball of Blu-Tack® or double-sided sticky tape to the end of an orange wood stick. Press onto a polish secure to pick it up. ▪ Use a small ball of Blu-Tack® or double-sided sticky tape under the artificial nail structure to help secure it down when applying nail art to them.
Tweezers 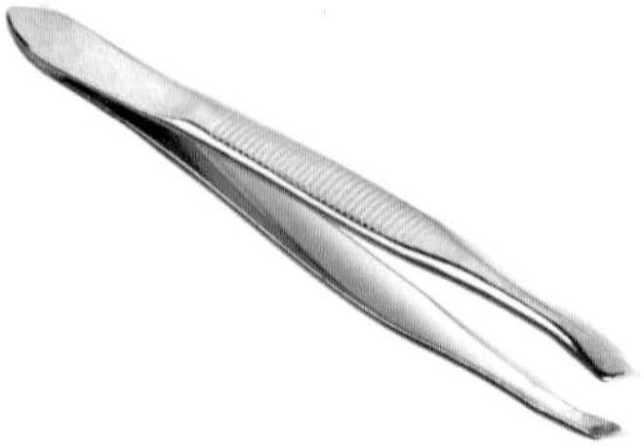	Used for peel-off transfers.	▪ Use to help peel off the transfer from the backing paper. ▪ Using tweezers rather than the fingers to do this will make sure that the transfer sticks to the nail. ▪ Wipe over with Barbicide before and after use.
Striping brushes 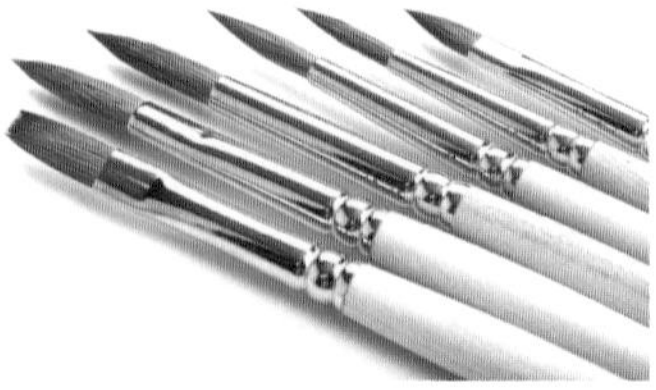	There are many different types of brush available in various thicknesses. Fine brushes will produce a finer stripe; thicker brushes will produce a thicker stripe.	▪ Choose the correct size brush for the nail art design. ▪ Use with water-based acrylic paints. ▪ Wash in water after use. The protective plastic cover should then be placed over the brush tip to help keep them in good condition.
Striping pens 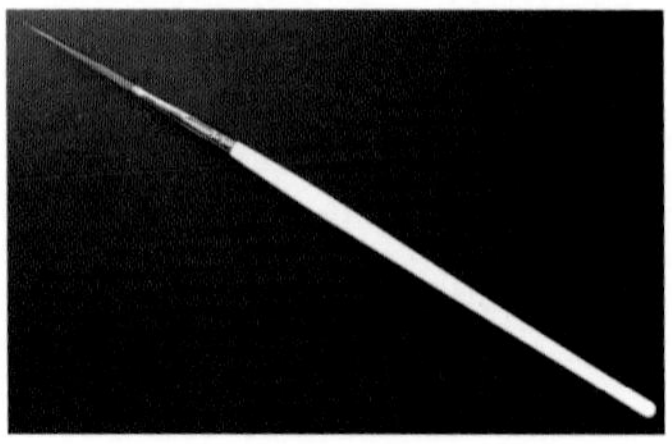	Used as an alternative to striping brushes. These come in lots of different colours and are popular because they are very easy to use. The product is used straight from the bottle, so no need for a separate brush.	▪ Remove the lid and use the product straight from the bottle. ▪ They usually come with a very fine metal pin. Place this in the end of the nozzle to stop the paint from drying up between uses.

ACTIVITY

Look on the internet at the nail art products and equipment listed above. Make a poster or mood board with pictures of all of the different types of nail art products that are available. You can work on your own, in pairs or small groups.

HANDY HINTS

Refer to Chapter 007, 109, 110 Hand care and providing basic manicure and pedicure treatments for more detailed information on the products and equipment needed.

HANDY HINTS

Make sure that you keep all of your nail art tools and products together. Make sure you also keep the lids tightly shut to prevent them from spilling or drying out.

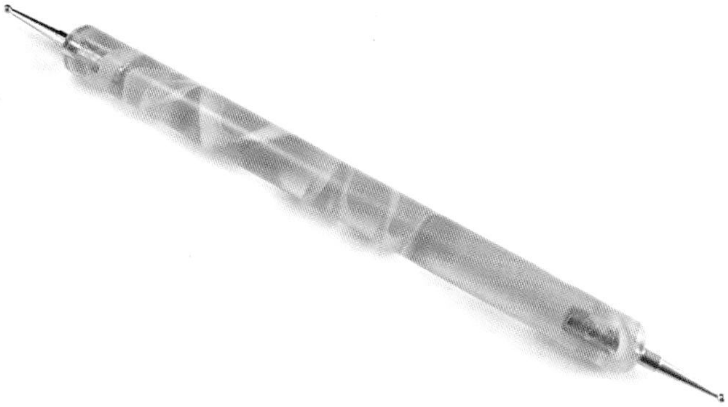

Using marbling or dotting tool is a more professional way of creating dots and also for mixing colours together. It has small circular balls at each end

PRODUCTS USED IN NAIL ART

There are many products that you need to learn about for a nail art treatment. This table will help you.

Nail art products	What is it used for?	How is it used?
Sanitiser 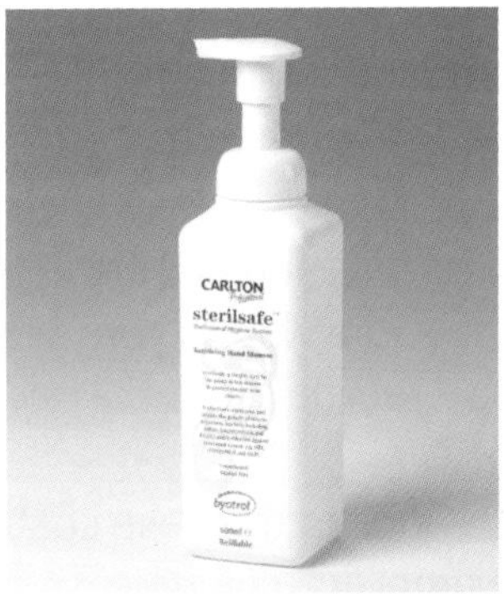 	Used to clean the client's hands or feet before you start the treatment. Helps to remove dirt and germs. Helps to prevent cross-infection. Usually in gel or liquid form.	▪ Apply to cotton wool pads. ▪ Gently wipe over the hands and fingers or feet and toes. ▪ Use a fresh piece of cotton wool for each hand or foot.
Non-acetone nail-enamel remover 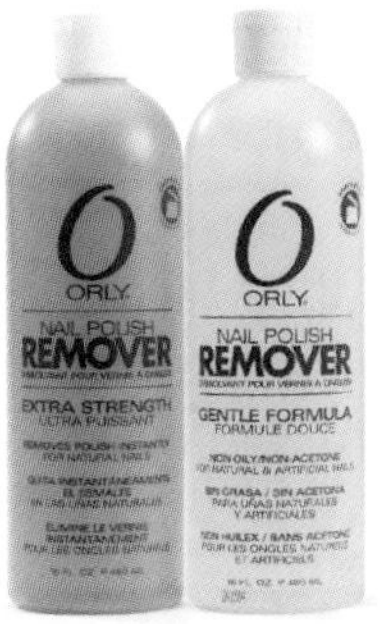 	Removes nail varnish, dirt and grease from the nail. Can also be used after the treatment to remove any nail varnish that has accidentally gone onto the skin around the nail. It can dry the nail plate if used too often.	▪ Apply to cotton wool pads. ▪ Gently press onto the nails and then wipe off. ▪ Continue until all varnish has been removed. ▪ Apply to a cotton-wool-tipped orange stick when removing nail varnish from the skin around the nail.

Nail art products	What is it used for?	How is it used?
Base coat 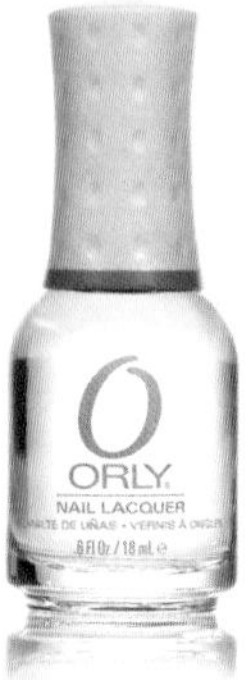	Provides a smooth base for the nail enamel and nail art products. Helps to prevent the nails from becoming stained by the nail enamel.	▪ Apply one coat to clean nails. ▪ Leave to dry before applying coloured nail enamel.
Nail enamel 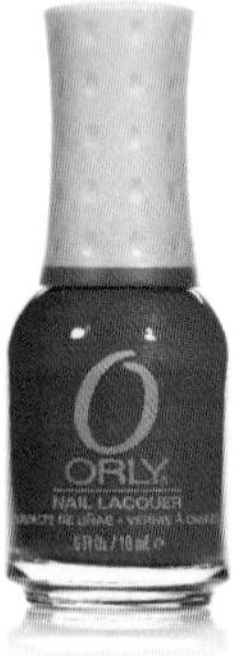	Available in lots of different colours. Gives the nail plate colour. Available in matt/cream or pearlised effects.	▪ Apply on top of the base coat. ▪ Apply two coats if using matt/cream enamel. ▪ Apply three coats if using pearlised enamel.
Artificial nails 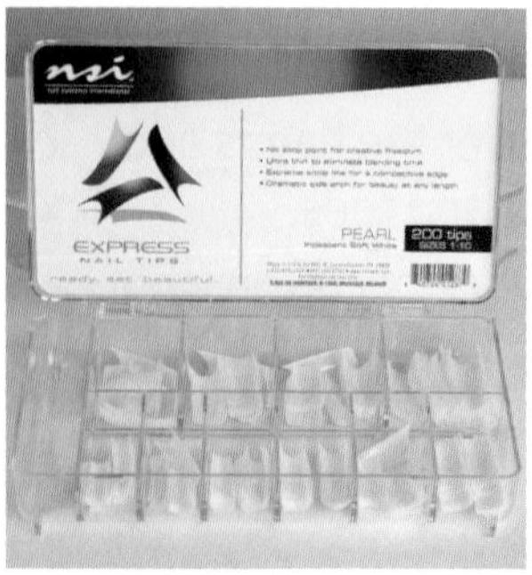	Used to practise your nail art designs on.	▪ When using them to practise designs, it will help if you attach them to the end of an orange stick or to the side of a box. ▪ Use a small amount of Blu-Tack® or double-sided sticky tape to attach them. ▪ Apply your varnishes and nail art products in the same way as you would if it was a real nail.
Polish secures 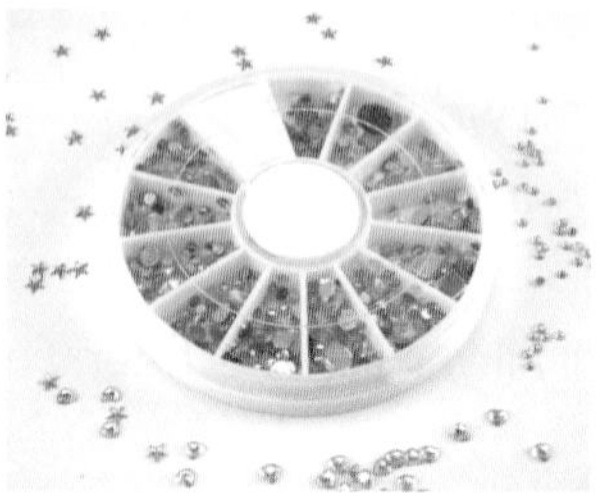	These are little gems that can be placed on the nail plate. Examples are rhinestones, pearls and flatstones.	▪ After you have applied the base coat and colour enamel (if a colour is required), apply a top coat. ▪ Using a small amount of Blu-Tack® on the end of an orange stick, carefully pick up the polish secure. ▪ Place the polish secure onto the wet top coat. ▪ Once you have all the polish secures in place, apply one to two coats of top coat over them. This will help to keep them in place.

HANDY HINTS

Make sure that you have a wide range of different coloured nail enamels.

HANDY HINTS

The tiny stones are sometimes called 'rhinestones' (if they are slightly raised) or 'flatstones' (if they are flat).

Nail art products	What is it used for?	How is it used?
Acrylic paints 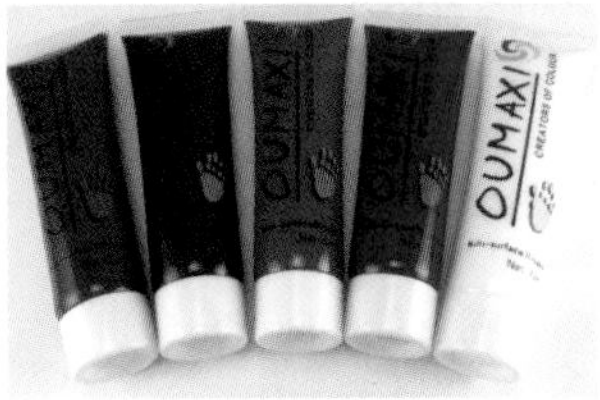	Water-based products that are used with nail art brushes. They are very cheap to buy and come in a wide variety of colours. They are not toxic so are safe to use.	▪ Use with nail art brushes. ▪ If they are too runny, you can leave the lid off for a short while and they will thicken up. ▪ If they are too thick, you can add a small amount of water to them.
Foils and **adhesive** 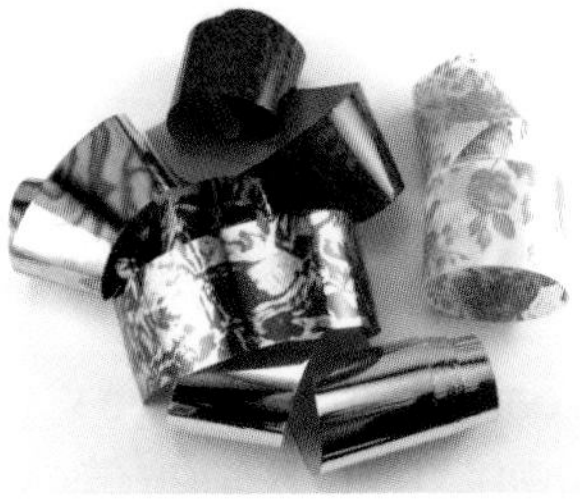	Sometimes called metallic wrap. A very easy but effective form of nail art. The very fine foils are supplied on a roll. They are available in coloured and patterned designs. The foil comes with a glue called metallic foil adhesive. There is also another product called metallic wrap sealer. This is applied after the foil has been applied to the nail. It helps to fix the foil on the nail and stops it from peeling off.	▪ Apply a base coat. ▪ Apply nail enamel (if needed). It is best to use a colour that matches the colour of the foil. ▪ Apply a thin, even coat of metallic foil adhesive over the area that you want the foil to stick to. ▪ The adhesive will be white in colour to start with, but will dry clear. ▪ Make sure that the adhesive is clear, then apply the foil with the shiny side facing upwards. ▪ Using a cotton bud, gently rub the foil onto the adhesive. ▪ Gently peel the foil strip away from the nail. ▪ Apply 'metallic wrap sealer'.
Transfers 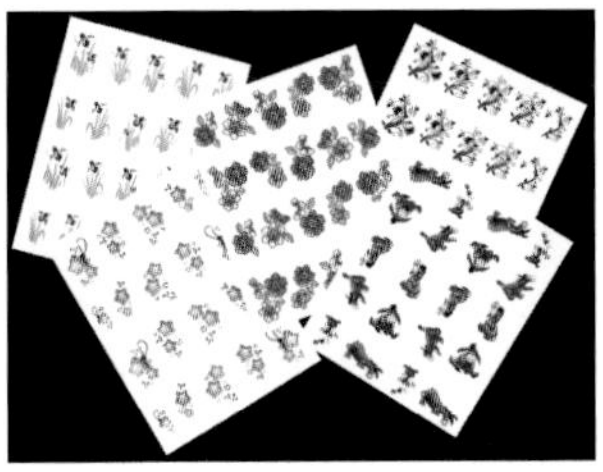	Transfers are ready-made designs that can be applied to the nail. They come in two types: ▪ soak off – you soak them in water to remove the backing paper ▪ peel off – the backing paper peels off. They are excellent for quick and easy, but effective, nail art designs.	Soak-off transfers: ▪ Cut around the transfer and place it in some water. ▪ Leave for a few seconds and then lift it out using tweezers. ▪ Slide the transfer off the backing paper between your fingers. ▪ Apply it to the nail. Peel-off transfers: ▪ Peel the transfer off the backing paper using tweezers. ▪ Take care not to touch the sticky side as this may stop it sticking to the nail properly.

HANDY HINTS

Practise using soak-off and peel-off transfers. See which ones you prefer using.

Adhesive

Glue

Nail art products	What is it used for?	How is it used?
Glitter 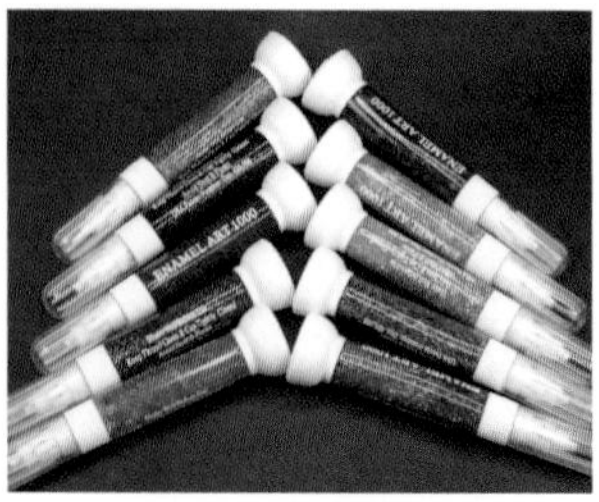 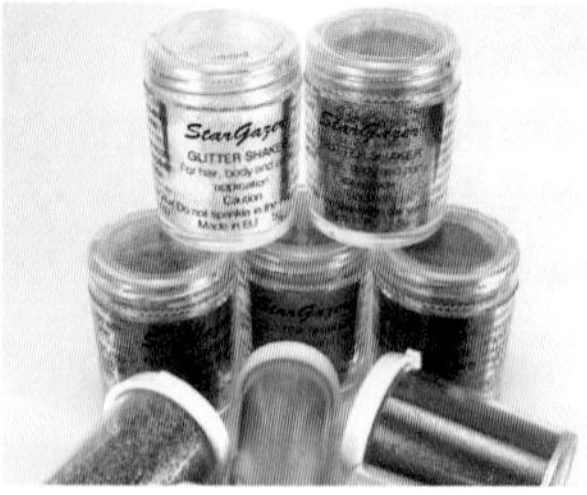	Can be applied to all or part of the nail. Comes either already mixed in a clear polish or loose in a pot. Adds shine to the nail art design and can make it look more exciting.	▪ If you are using ready-mixed glitter polish, paint onto the area just like nail enamel. ▪ If you are using loose glitter, either sprinkle it onto wet enamel (coloured or clear), or dip the nail into the pot. ▪ For larger areas, it can be painted straight from the bottle using the brush. ▪ For smaller areas where stripes are needed, a fine nail art brush can be used. ▪ For smaller areas where dots are needed, the point of an orange stick can be used.
Top coat/nail art sealer 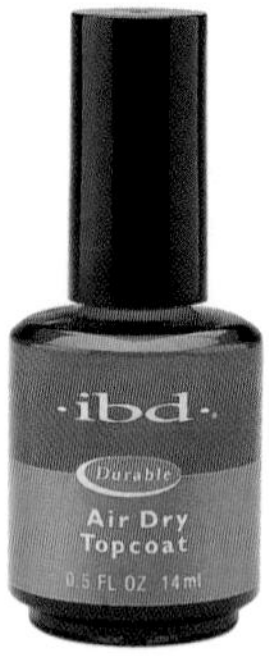	Provides an extra glossy finish to the nails and also makes sure that the nail art stays in place. Helps to protect the nail art designs from chipping. This will also make them last longer. Also helps to secure 3D designs in place such as polish secures (rhinestones, flatstones, pearls).	▪ Apply one coat once the nail enamel is dry to the touch. ▪ Apply one coat before attaching polish secures. This will help stick them to the nail plate. ▪ Apply another coat after the polish secures are attached. This will help to keep them on the nail.

HANDY HINTS

If you are using loose glitter, make sure that you cover the treatment area with tissue paper. This will catch any loose glitter that falls and will keep the treatment area clean and tidy.

HANDY HINTS

Practise using glitter polish and loose glitter. See which ones you prefer using.

ACTIVITY

To help get you started, find out about the different nail art designs that can be produced. Use different resources, such as the internet, magazines and books to look up more information.

You may find the following websites useful:

- www.thenaildirectory.com
- www.nailartgallery.com
- www.creativeten.co.uk
- www.salongeek.com
- www.scratchmagazine.co.uk

If you like any of the nail art designs that you see, print them out. You will be able to use these designs later when you are putting together a portfolio of designs.

ACTIVITY

Plan some simple colour designs on paper. Then, using your brushes, some water and your paints, try to copy your designs onto some artificial nails. See what different colours you can create when you mix the colours together.

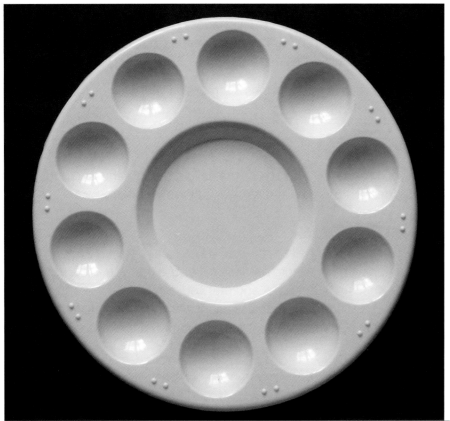

A mixing palette can be used for mixing the paints together

HANDY HINTS

If the foil is very flaky when you have peeled it away, you have not left the adhesive to dry long enough. If this happens, apply some more glue and follow the steps in the table on page 341.

HANDY HINTS

Make sure that you apply the metallic wrap sealer around the edges of the foil. This will help to stop it from peeling off.

HANDY HINTS

Loose glitters will only stick to wet polish, so apply either a coloured or clear enamel to the nail first before applying the glitter.

HANDY HINTS

Have a cup of clean water in your treatment area to rinse the acrylic paint from the brushes between different colours.

ACTIVITY

Practise some nail art using the striping pens or striping brushes and acrylic paints. You can work on each other or use artificial nails for your designs. You may choose to use coloured nail enamel as a base colour before you apply the paints or keep the nail's natural colour.

ACTIVITY

Practise some nail art using foils. You can work on each other or use artificial nails for your designs. You may choose to use coloured nail enamel as a base colour before you apply the foil or keep the nail's natural colour.

HANDY HINTS

Make sure you put the paint lids on tightly after use. This will stop them from drying out and spilling.

CREATING YOUR DESIGNS

A good way for you to plan and then create your nail art designs is to first of all draw some ideas onto a piece of paper. This is known as a **2D design**. There are several ways in which you can do this, for example:

- Research some ideas from the internet, magazines or books. Print them off or make sketches of some design ideas.
- Draw some pictures of large nail shapes onto a piece of paper. Use coloured pencils to colour in the nail shapes that you have drawn to create some nail art designs.

You can then use these drawings to create nail art designs on artificial nails or on each other's nails. This is known as a **3D design**.

2D design

A two-dimensional design on a flat surface. An example of this is drawing a nail art design on a piece of paper

3D design

A three-dimensional design on a rounded surface. An example of this is carrying out a nail art design on an artificial nail or a real nail

ACTIVITY

When you have learnt how to use the nail art equipment and products, practise designs on your own nails to improve your skills.

CONSULTATION

Before you start your nail art service, you will need to carry out a consultation with the client. This will make sure that you know what nail design to choose for her nails, and that you don't use any products they might be allergic to. Good communication is important in making sure that both you and the client are clear on what the finished design will look like.

HANDY HINTS

To help your client decide on the nail art design they want, you could show some examples of nail art designs that you have done already, eg in a portfolio of photos showing your designs, or examples that you have done on some artificial nails. You could even draw a design on paper before you go ahead with the service.

HANDY HINTS

Refer to Chapter 102 Presenting a professional image in the salon, for more detailed information on carrying out a consultation and on communication and behaviour.

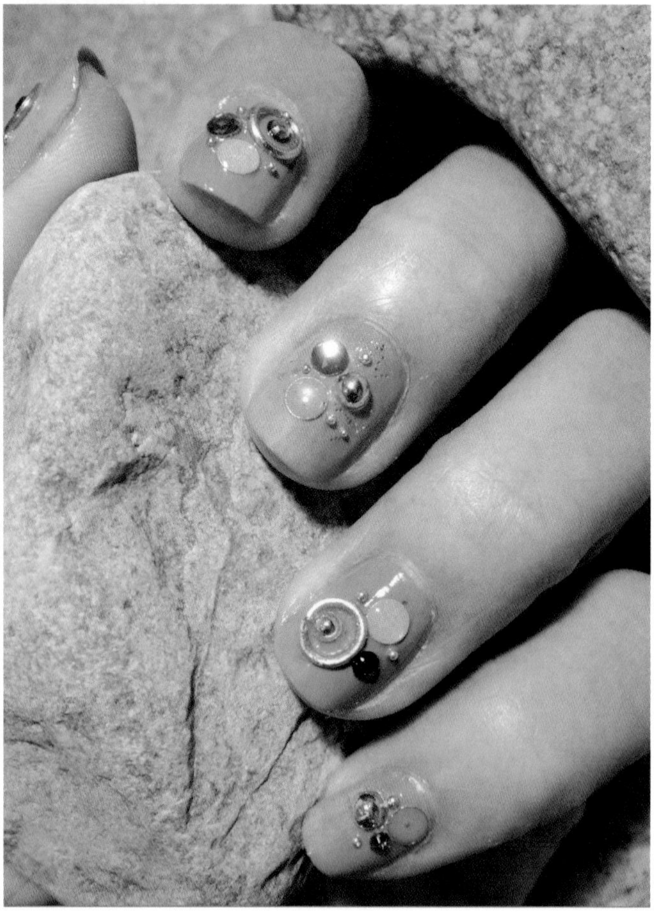

Polish secures will help to give a 3D effect on the nails

FACTORS TO CONSIDER

During the consultation, there may be certain factors that you need to find out about so you can plan your nail art treatment.

Factor	How might it affect the treatment?
Length 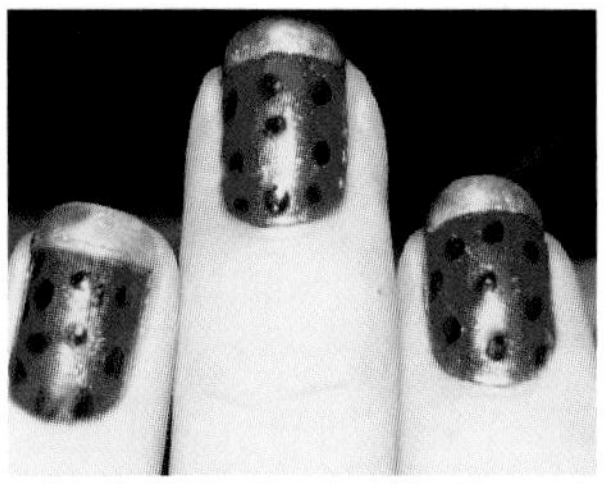 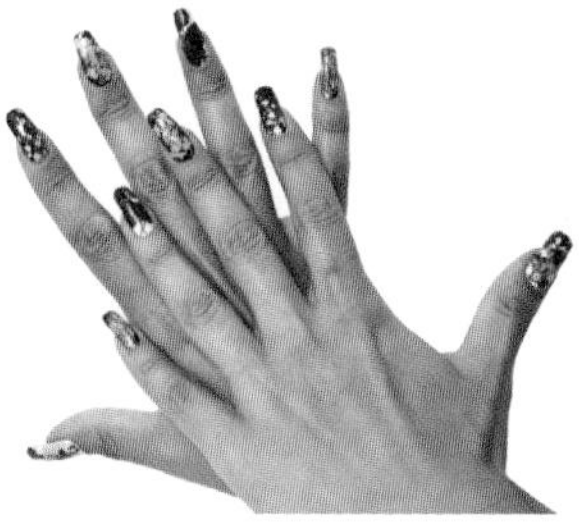	Think about the length of your client's nails when choosing the nail art design. If the nails are short, then there will be less room on the nail for the design. This means that for shorter nails, the design will need to be more simple. If the nails are longer, then you will have more room for the design. You can be more creative in the techniques that you use.
Strength 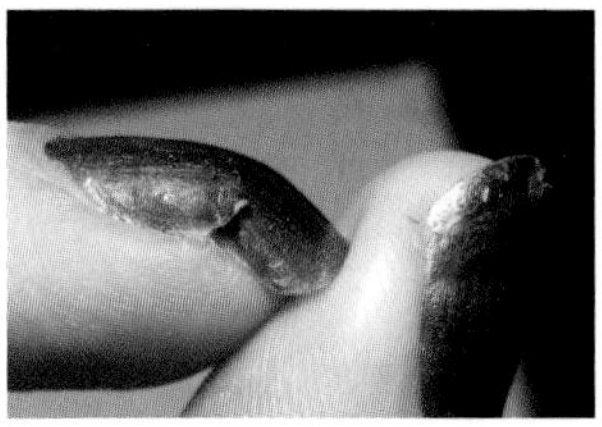 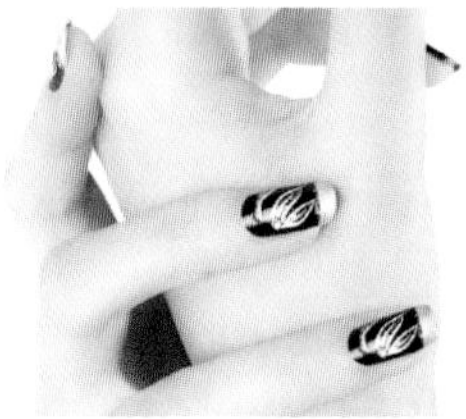	Each client will have a different nail strength. Some clients may have weak nails that bend easily. Other clients may have strong, thick nails that do not bend easily. ▪ Thin, weak nails – suggest your clients keep their nails shorter. ▪ Strong, thick nails – clients may be able to have their nails longer. Adapt your nail art designs to the strength and length of the nails. For example, for a weaker nail, choose a more simple design that can fit on a shorter nail. For a stronger nail you can choose a detailed design that can fit on a longer nail.

ACTIVITY

Practise some nail art using glitter. You can work on each other or use artificial nails for your designs. You may choose to use coloured nail enamel as a base colour before you apply the glitter or keep the nail's natural colour.

Factor	How might it affect the treatment?
Shape 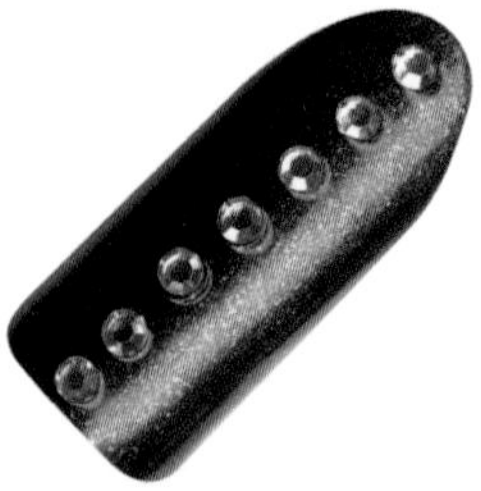 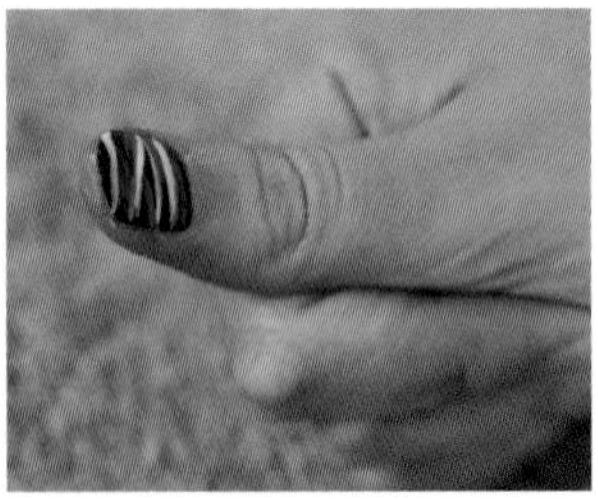 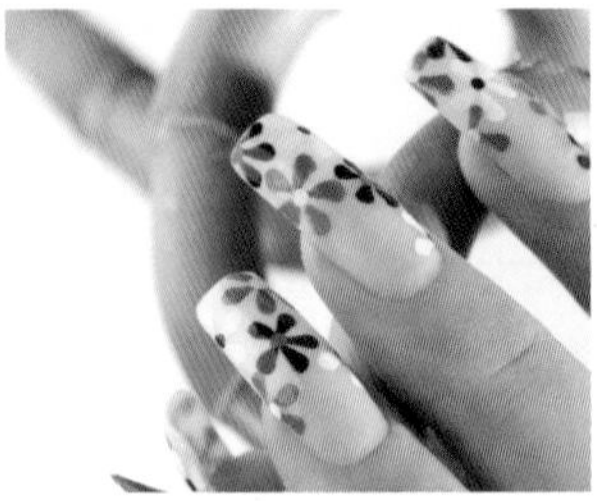	A client's nails may be one of several different shapes. Different nail shapes will suit different nail art designs: ▪ Oval – the nail art design may need to be more simple as oval nails tend to be smaller. ▪ Rounded – the nail art design may need to be shorter as this nail shape is not particularly long. ▪ Square – the nail art design can be more detailed on this nail shape as the nail is longer.
Adverse skin and nail conditions 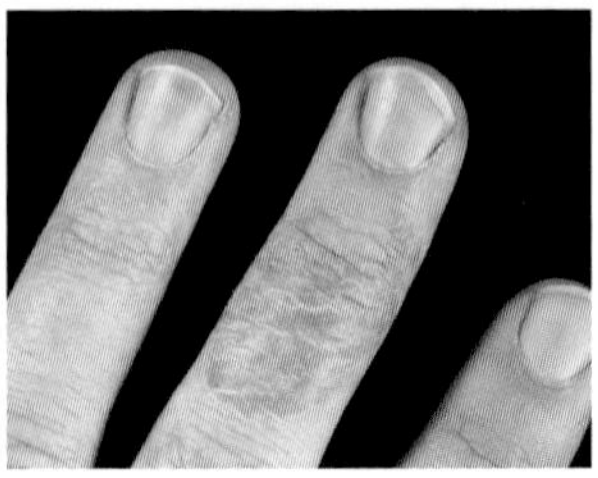	You will need to check the condition of the client's skin and nails before you start to make sure that it is safe to carry out the treatment. Examples of possible adverse skin and nail conditions are: ▪ Allergies: this is when the body reacts adversely to products. The skin may become red, itchy, swollen and feel hot. If the client is allergic to any products you must not use them. You should decide this during the consultation. If your client has an allergic reaction to the nail art products during the treatment, such as redness or itching, remove the product immediately and apply a cool, damp, cotton wool pad. Speak to your tutor who may refer them to their doctor. ▪ Cuts and abrasions around the nail area or on the hands: if the client has these around the nail or on their hands you will need to avoid this area because it may be sensitive and could make the condition worse. ▪ Bruising and swelling: bruises can appear blue, purple and sometimes yellow. They can be sensitive and painful to touch. If the client has these on their hands, fingers and particularly around the nails you will need to avoid the area because it may be sensitive and could make the condition worse. ▪ Severe nail damage: this is where the nail lifts off from the nail bed. It is usually caused by an injury to the nail, such as trapping it in a door. It is often very painful to touch. If the client has severe nail damage then you will not be able to work on this area because it may be sensitive and could make the condition worse, ie cause the nail to lift off even more.

Factor	How might it affect the treatment?
Occasion 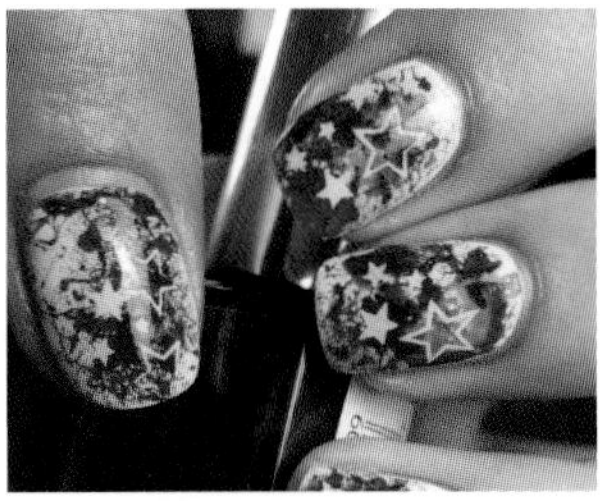	At the beginning of the treatment, you will need to ask your client why they are having a nail art treatment. This will help you to choose the best colours and design for them. It may be a special occasion such as a party, wedding, holiday or birthday treat.
Fashion trends 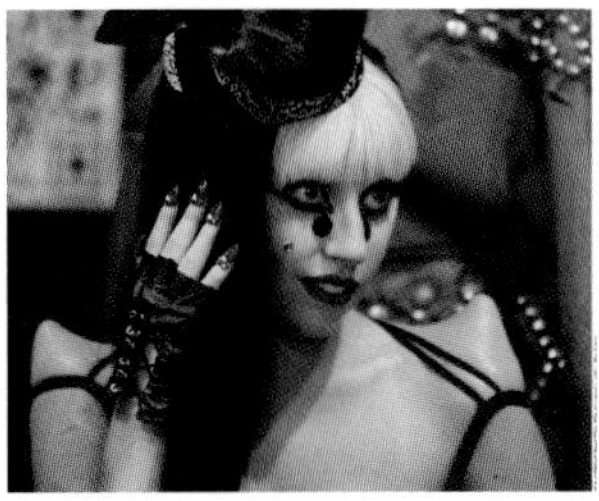	Nail art has become very popular. When you look through magazines, on the internet and at the television, you will see many celebrities and models with nail art designs on their nails. It is important for you to keep up to date with the latest fashion trends so that your client has the most current nail art designs to choose from.
Cultural factors 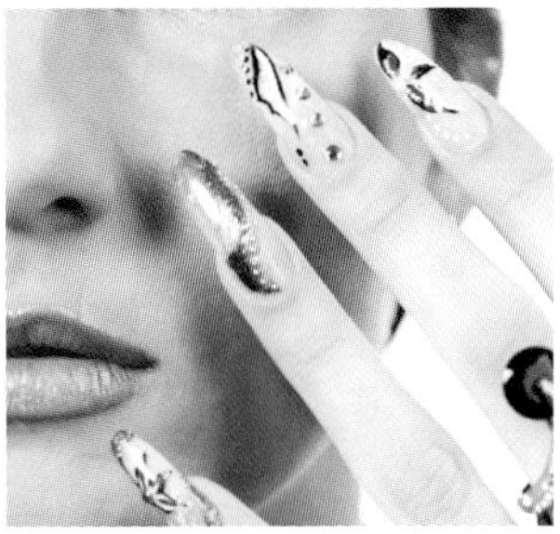	Culture can play an important part in the nail art design chosen. This can affect the colour or the design. For example, nail art in Japan is often very detailed.
Nail growth rate 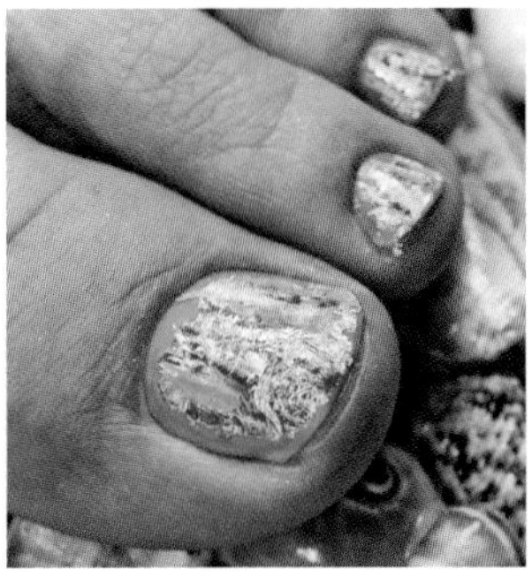	Nails grow on average about 0.5 to 1.2 mm per week. Some people's nails grow more quickly and some more slowly. It is important to explain to the client the correct way to remove the nail art design from their nails as their nails grow. They can then return to your salon for another nail art treatment.

ACTIVITY

What nail art designs would be suitable for:

- short nails
- longer nails?

Draw, print or carry out some nail art designs for the above nail types.

HANDY HINTS

Go to Chapter 007, 109, 110 Hand care and providing basic manicure and pedicure treatments and read up on different nail shapes.

HANDY HINTS

The nail art design chosen will need to be suitable for the shape of the client's nails.

HANDY HINTS

Refer to Chapter 007, 109, 110 Hand care and providing basic manicure and pedicure treatments for more detailed information on adverse skin and nail conditions.

HANDY HINTS

Remember to take photos of any nail art designs that you do and put them in a portfolio of designs. You can then use this to show your clients, which will help them choose which design they would like.

HANDY HINTS

Refer to Chapter 007, 109, 110 Hand care and providing basic manicure and pedicure treatments for more detailed information on factors affecting treatments on the hands and nails.

HANDY HINTS

Before you start the treatment, look at the client's hands and nails and discuss the above factors with her to see if any of them are relevant and need to be taken into account.

HANDY HINTS

Discuss which nail art design your client wants before you start the treatment.

ACTIVITY

- Can you think of any more reasons why a client may want a nail art service?
- Which type of nail art design would be the most suitable for each occasion?

Discuss this with your tutor and the rest of your group.

You may want to draw some designs on paper, then practise them on either artificial nails or each other.

ACTIVITY

Look on the internet at the nail art designs that are available in different countries such as Japan. Are they different in any way to nail art designs in this country?

ACTIVITY

On paper, draw some 2D nail art designs that would be suitable for each of the factors mentioned in the previous table. You can then practise these designs in 3D either on each other or on artificial nails.

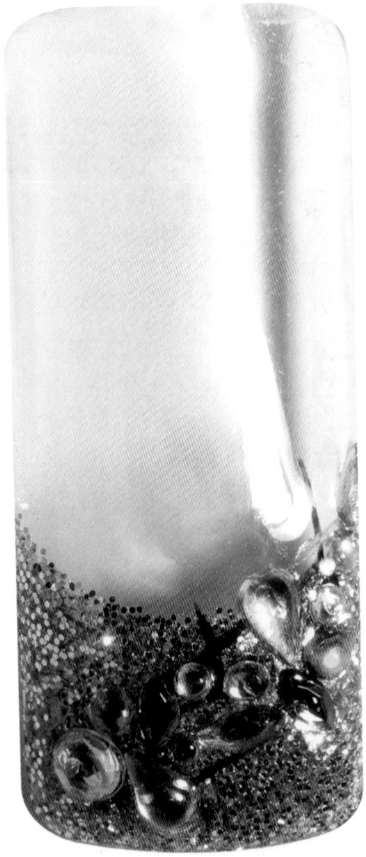

ACTIVITY

Look on the internet at the latest trends in nail art. Also look at the products that are the most popular. Discuss your findings with your tutor and the rest of your group.

Before starting the nail art treatment you must make sure your client is comfortable on either the chair or the couch. Make sure that you have all your tools and products ready.

HANDY HINTS

Refer to Chapter 007, 109, 110 Hand care and providing basic manicure and pedicure treatments for more information on how to carry out the preparation steps in more detail.

HANDY HINTS

Remember to keep any designs that you like for your display to show your clients.

PREPARING THE NAILS

You will often carry out the nail art service after a manicure or pedicure treatment. If your client is just having a nail art service you will need to prepare the nails in the following way:

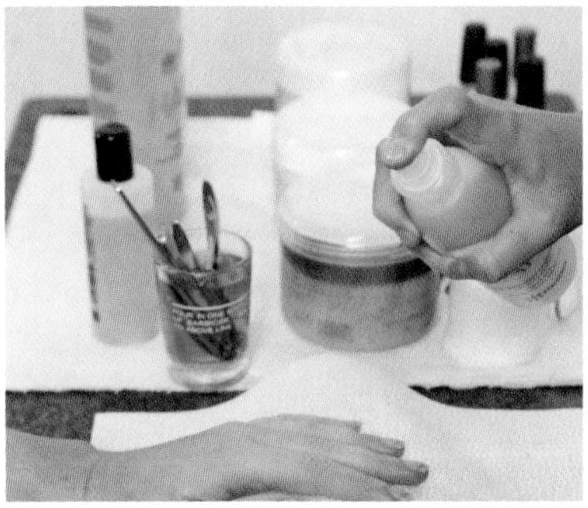

STEP 1 – Clean the hands or feet using a sanitiser.

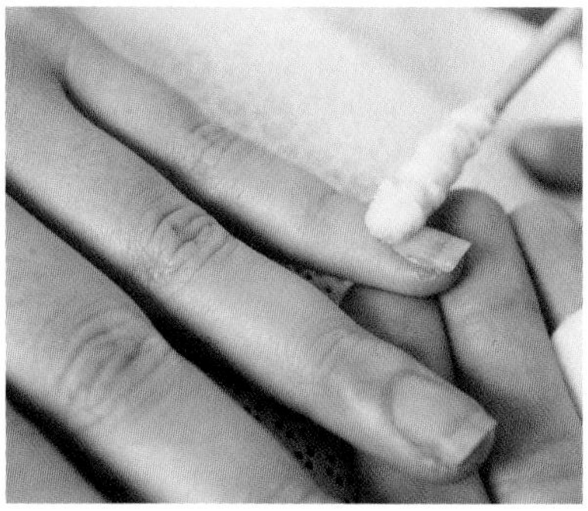

STEP 2 – Remove any nail enamel that is already on the nails with non-acetone nail-enamel remover.

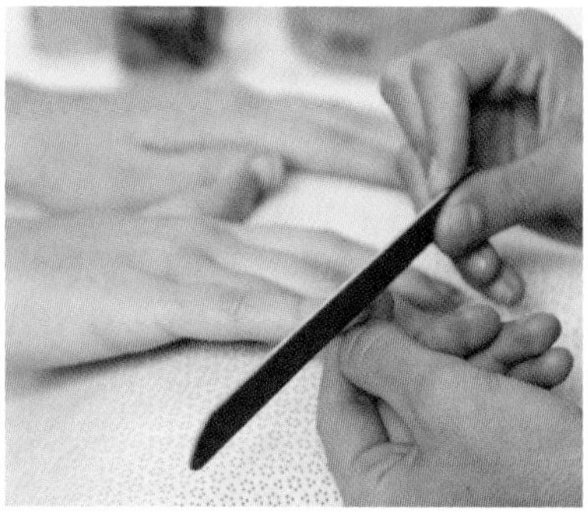

STEP 3 – File and shape the nails if necessary.

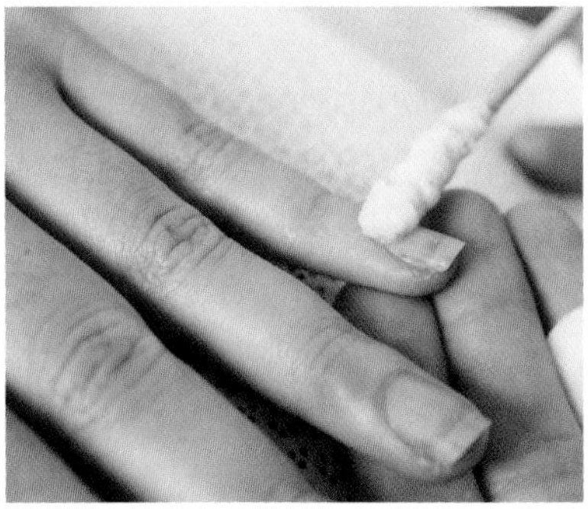

STEP 4 – Wipe over the nails again with non-acetone nail-enamel remover.

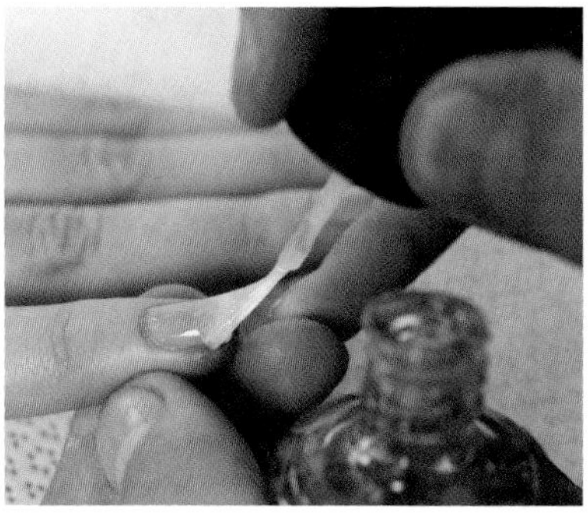

STEP 5 – Apply a base coat. If your nail art design needs colour apply coloured nail enamel once the base coat has dried.

HANDY HINTS

Recommend that your client uses a non-acetone nail enamel remover to take off the nail art designs from her nails.

You are now ready to apply the nail art design.

STEP-BY-STEP BASIC NAIL ART TECHNIQUES

TRANSFERS

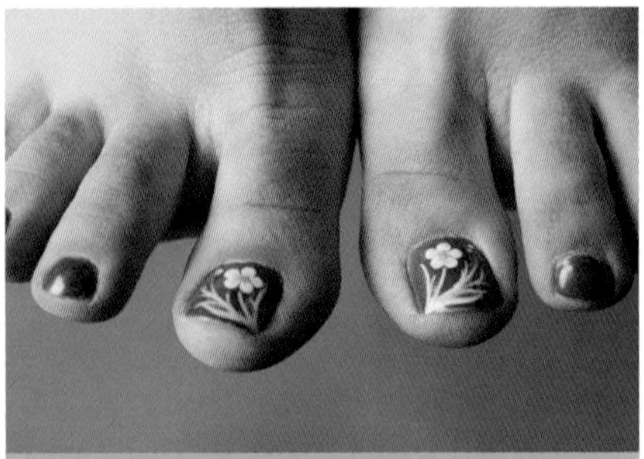

HANDY HINTS

Remember, nail art can be carried out on toenails as well as on fingernails. This is most popular in the summer when sandals are worn.

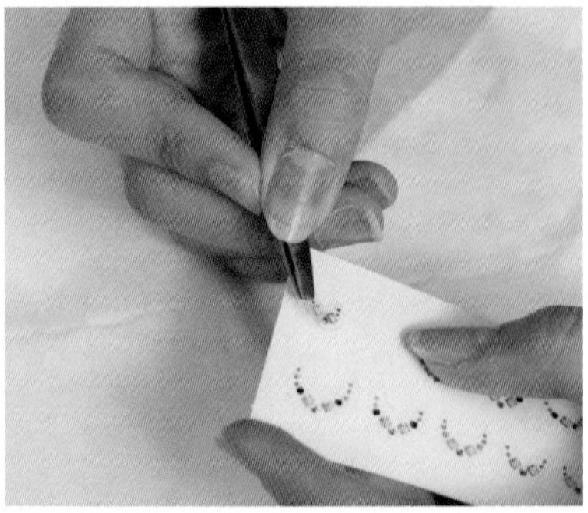

STEP 1 – **Peel-off transfers**: start by carefully lifting the transfer off the backing sheet using tweezers.

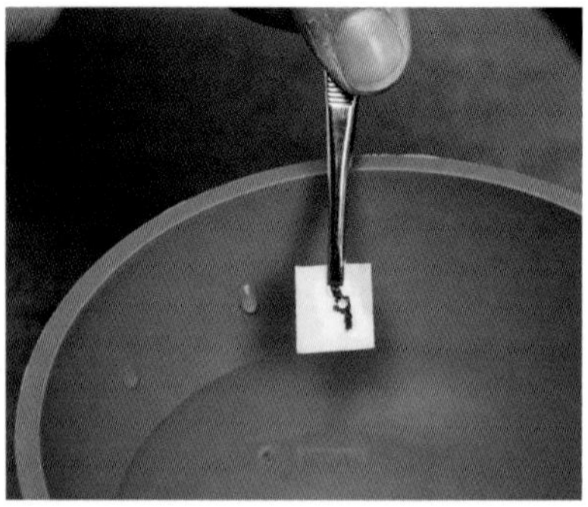

STEP 2 – **Soak-off transfers**: place the transfer into water first, then remove the backing sheet using tweezers.

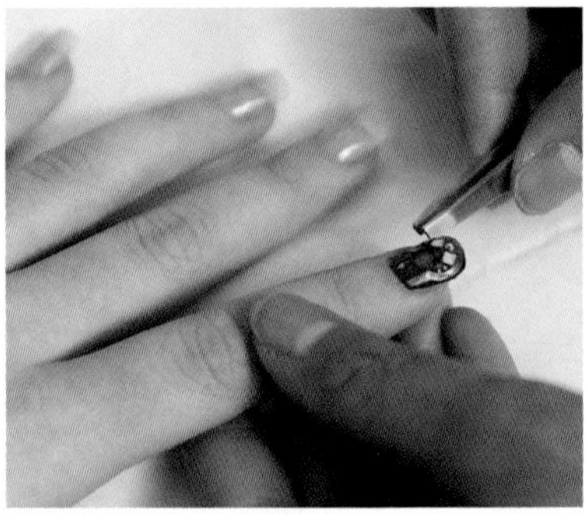

STEP 3 – Place the transfer onto the nail that has been prepared by painting it with base coat and nail enamel.

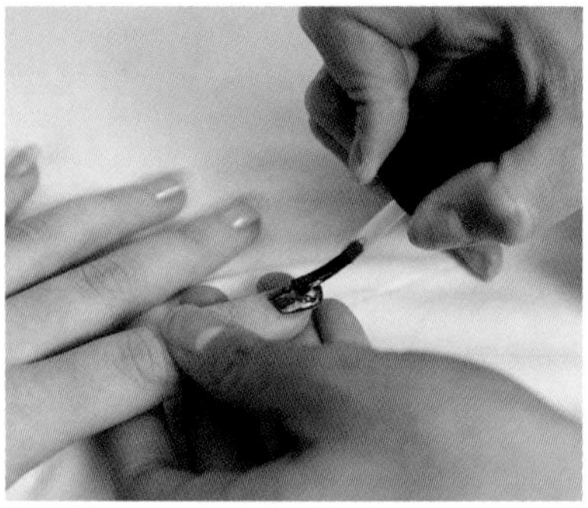

STEP 4 – Apply nail art sealant/top coat to protect the transfer and seal it on the nail.

ACTIVITY

Practise some nail art using transfers. You can work on each other or use artificial nails for your designs. You may choose to use coloured nail enamel as a base colour before you apply the transfers or keep the nail's natural colour.

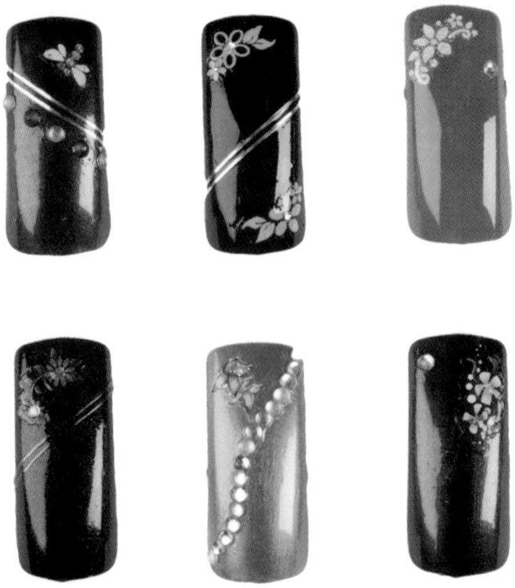

Nail art designs using transfers

GLITTERS

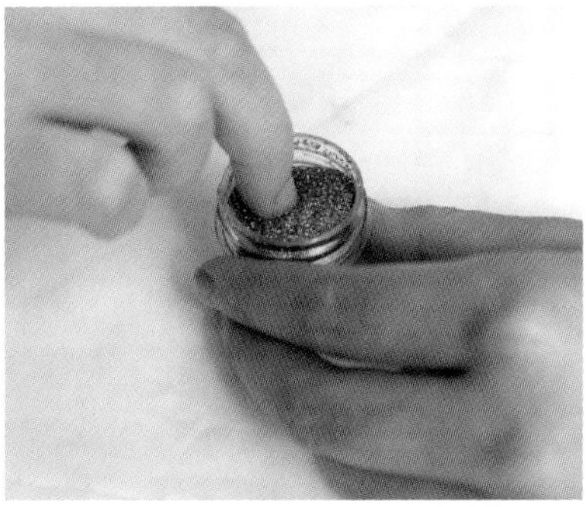

STEP 1 – Paint the nails with a base coat, then a coloured enamel (if a colour base is needed for the nail art design). Whilst the nails are still wet, dip the tips into the glitter.

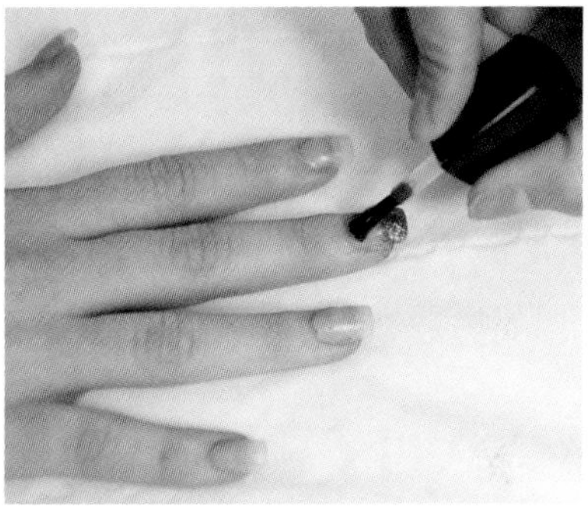

STEP 2 – Very gently, apply nail art sealant/ top coat to seal the glitter onto the nail.

HANDY HINTS

If glitter pens or varnish are used, simply paint them onto the nails.

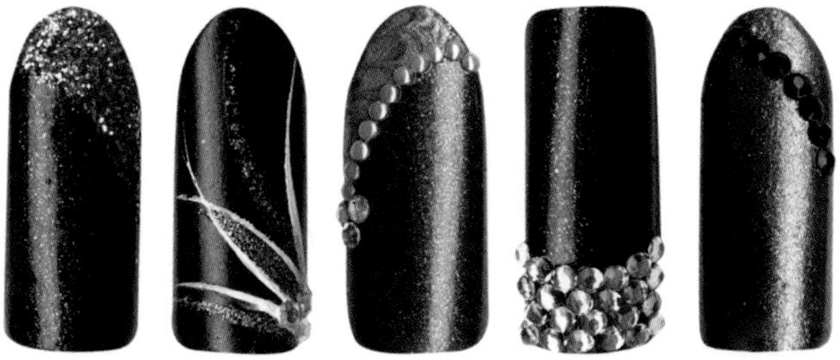

Nail art design using glitters and gems

FOILS

There are many different foil designs that you can use. To begin with, choose a silver and a gold foil as these will go with most nail art designs.

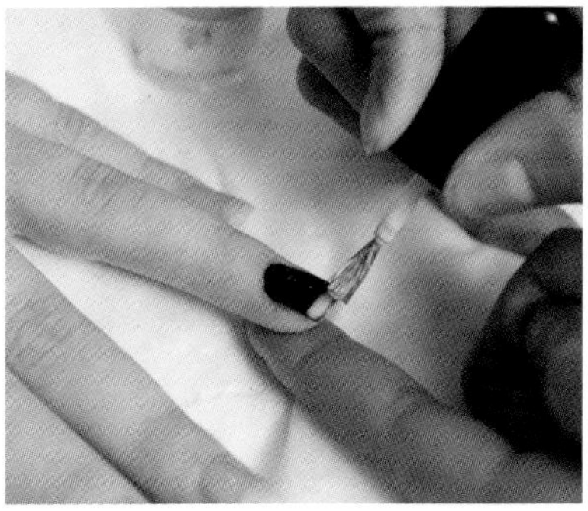

STEP 1 – Apply a thin layer of adhesive to the area that you want the foil to stick to.

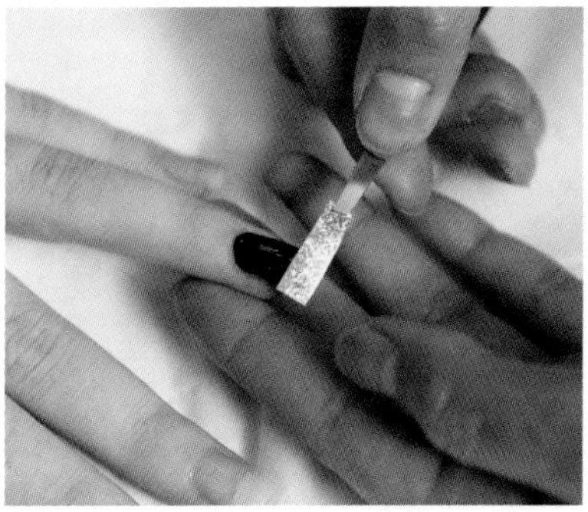

STEP 2 – When the adhesive has dried (the adhesive will go clear when it is dry), cut the foil to the size needed and with the pattern facing upwards, place it over the adhesive using tweezers to hold it. Gently rub over the foil using a cotton bud until the foil has come off the backing sheet and is on the nail.

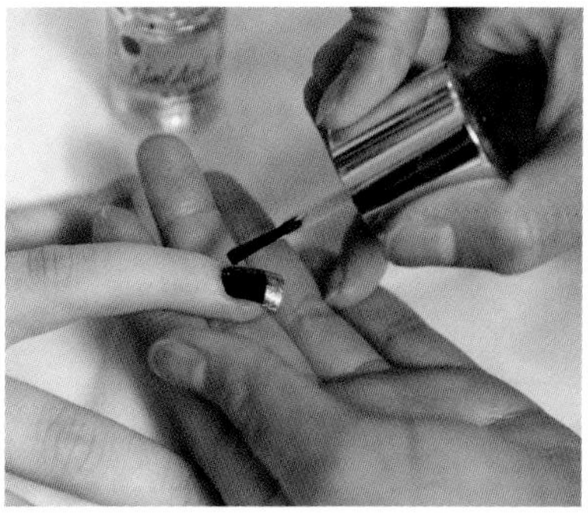

STEP 3 – Very gently, apply nail art sealant/ top coat to seal the foil onto the nail.

HANDY HINTS

Foils look very effective when applied just to the ends of the nail (the free edge).

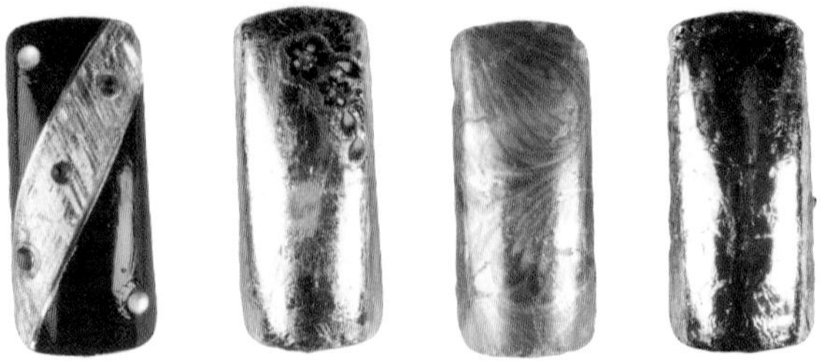

Nail art design using foils

ACTIVITY

Have a look on the internet on websites such as eBay to see what flatstones and rhinestones are available and also how much they cost.

POLISH SECURES (FLATSTONES AND RHINESTONES)

There are many different stones to choose from in lots of different colours and sizes.

HANDY HINTS

Try not to use polish secures that are too big, as these do not sit very well on the nails and may come off more easily.

HANDY HINTS

If any areas have been missed, simply apply some more adhesive to the area and repeat the process.

HANDY HINTS

You can apply some polish secures to the edges of the foil of different colours and sizes.

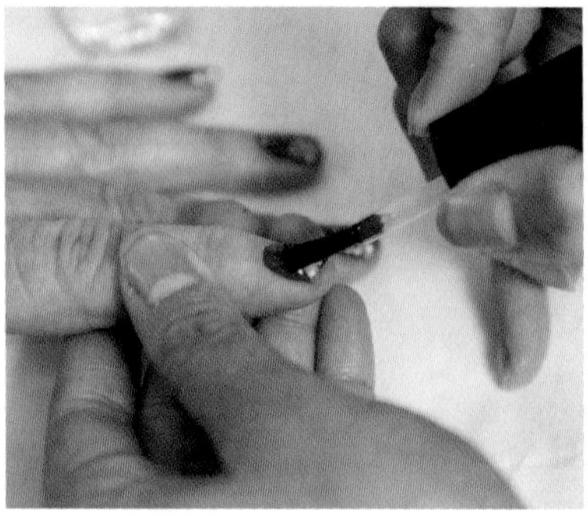

STEP 1 – Apply a top coat to the nail.

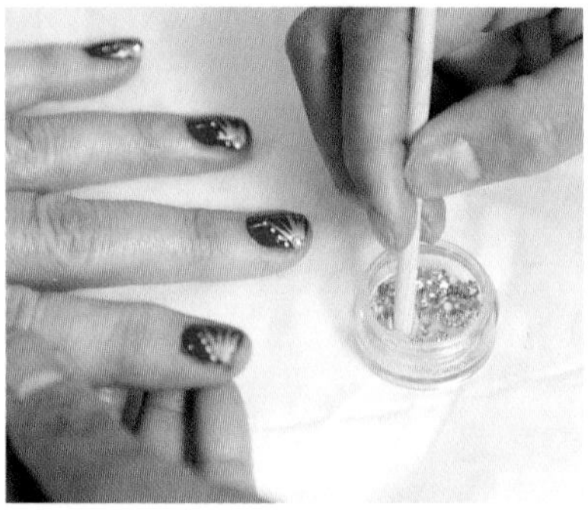

STEP 2 – Pick up a polish secure with an orange stick tipped with Blu-Tack®.

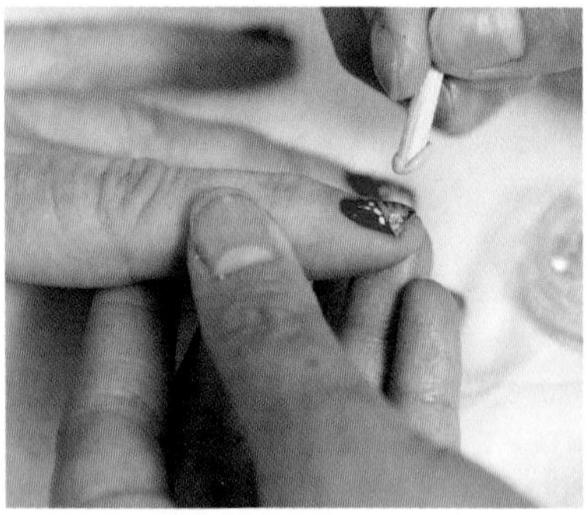

STEP 3 – Place the polish secure onto the nail and gently press it in with the orange stick.

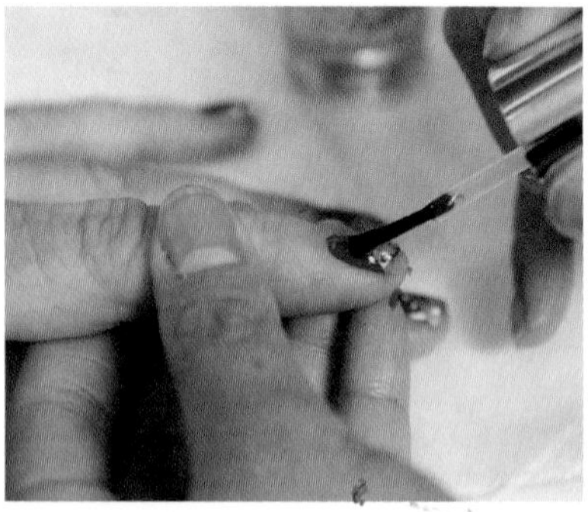

STEP 4 – Apply nail art sealant/top coat to seal the polish secure onto the nail.

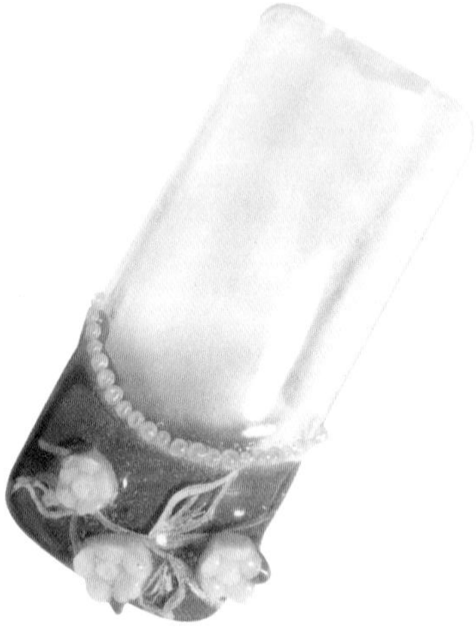

Nail art design using polish secures

ACTIVITY

Have a go at some nail art using polish secures. You can work on each other or use artificial nails for your designs. You may choose to use coloured nail enamel as a base colour before you apply the polish secures, or keep the nail's natural colour.

ACTIVITY

Look up what is meant by a 'marble effect'. You will then understand more about what this nail art design should look like. See what colours are used – this will help you when you choose the colours for your designs.

COLOUR BLENDING

This is where two or more colours are blended together to produce a marbling effect. It is achieved by using at least two different-coloured acrylic paints and dotting them onto the nail plate or artificial nail (using an orange stick or dotting tool). Next, you gently do half-circle shapes using the tip of the orange stick until a marble effect is achieved.

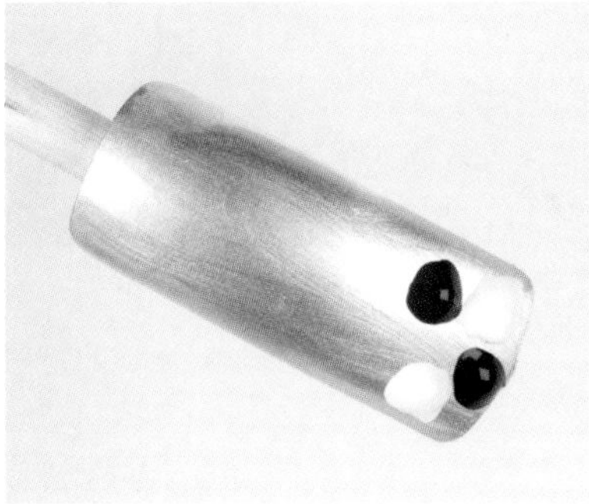

STEP 1 – Apply large dots of at least two colours to the nail tip.

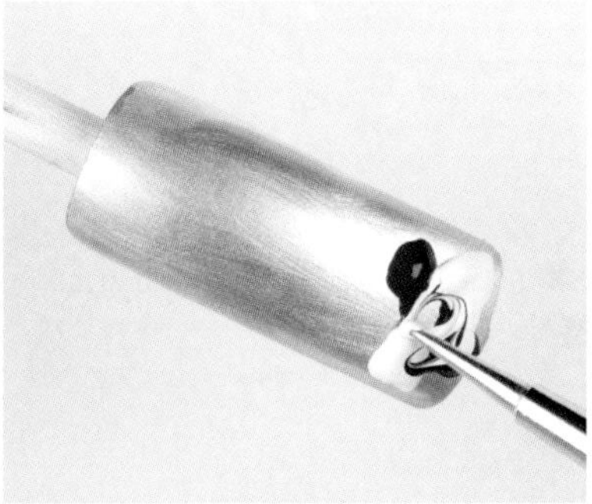

STEP 2 – Using either the tip of an orange stick or the tip of a dotting tool, make gentle half-circle movements to blend the colours together.

HANDY HINTS

When choosing which colours to use, use similar coloured nail enamels as the base colour. This will help the colours to blend well together.

HANDY HINTS

Do not blend the colours together too much. If you do, you will lose the marbling effect and end up with just one colour.

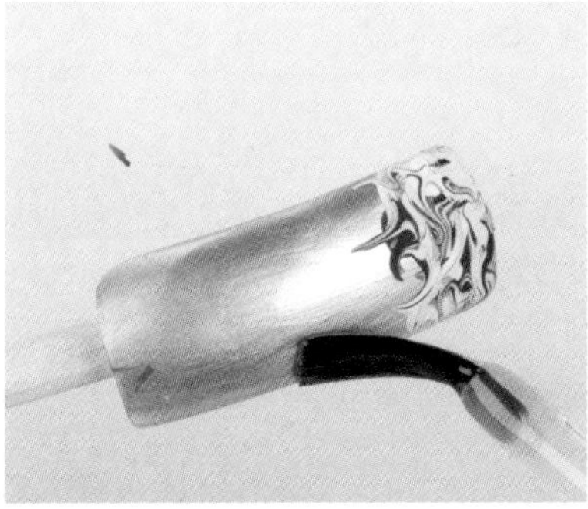

STEP 3 – Apply nail art sealant/top coat to seal and protect the marbled enamel.

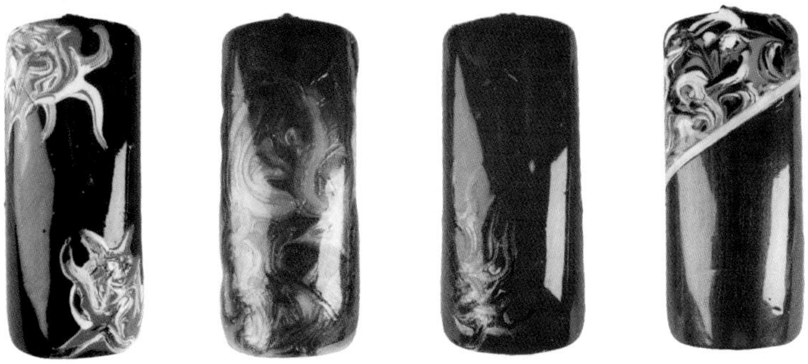

Nail art designs using colour blending

ACTIVITY

Practise this effect by using more than two colours. Keep the ones that you like for your display board, to show your clients.

DOTS

These designs are created using either the tip of an orange stick or dotting tool dipped in paint, or by using the nozzle end of a nail art pen.

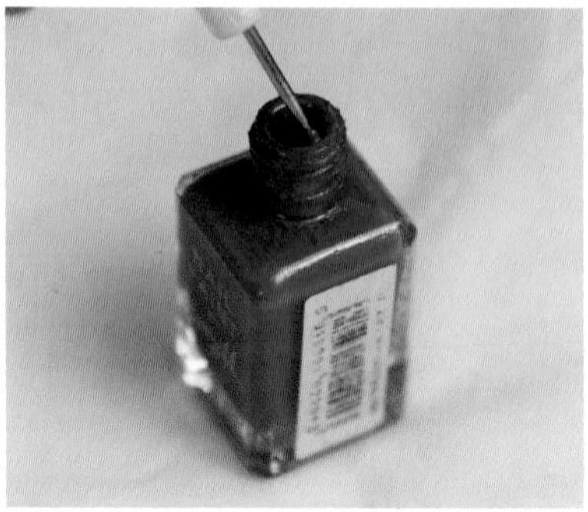

STEP 1 – Dip the end of your dotting tool or orange stick into the paint.

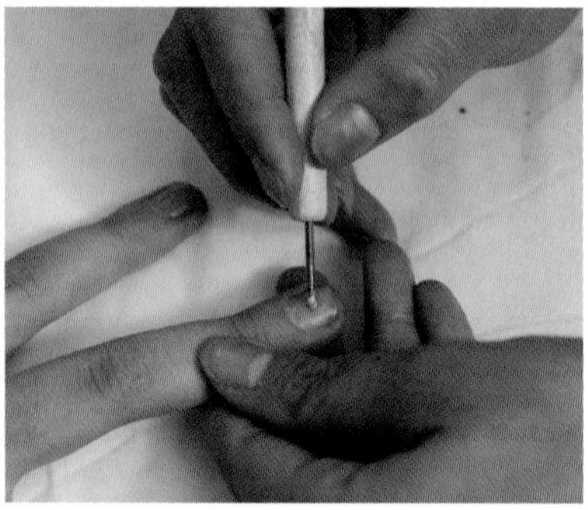

STEP 2 – Carefully dot the paint onto the nail.

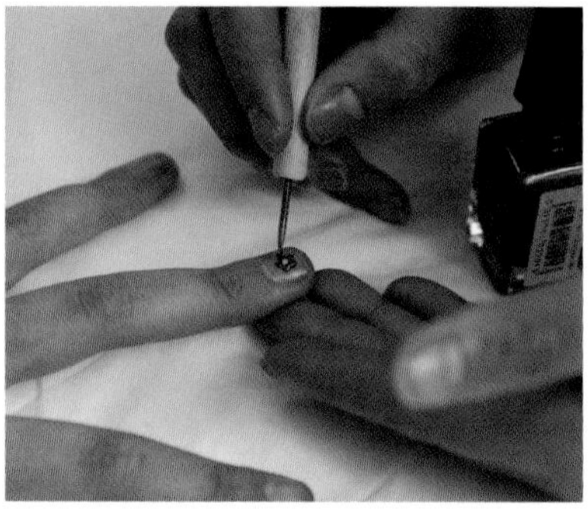

STEP 3 – Add different coloured dots around the outside of the first dot. This creates a flower design. Apply nail art sealant/top coat to seal and protect the design.

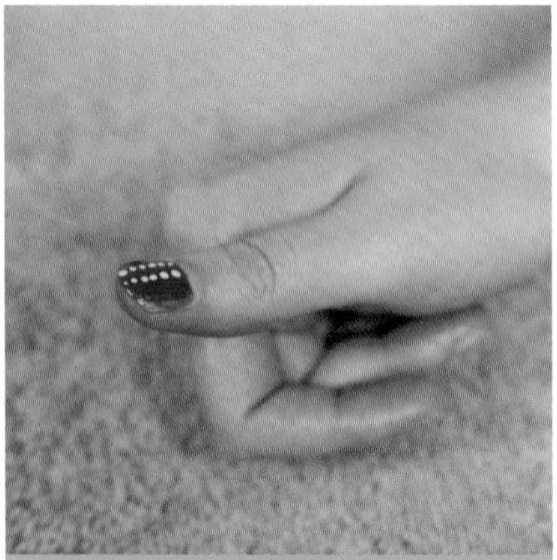

HANDY HINTS

The heavier you press onto the nail with the dotting tool, the larger the dot will be. Press lightly for small dots.

HANDY HINTS

If striping pens are used, simply paint straight from the nozzle at the top of the bottle onto the nails.

HANDY HINTS

Why not add some dots using either the tip of an orange stick dipped in paint or the nozzle of a nail art pen. You could also add a polish secure into the design to make it more attractive.

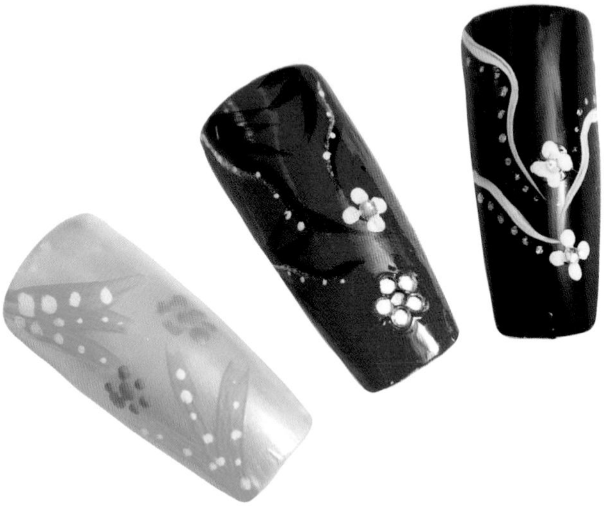

Nail art designs using the dotting technique

STRIPING DESIGNS

These designs are created using either:

- a striping brush and water-based acrylic paints
- a nail art striping pen that has the brush already in the bottle. These come in many different colours.

A simple design is achieved by putting stripes across the corners of the nail or by fanning out from one side.

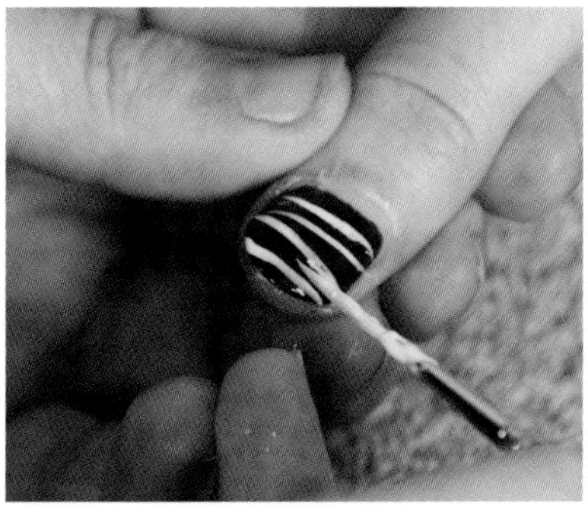

STEP 1 – Dip the striping brush into the paint. Lay the brush on the nail or pull the brush across the nail.

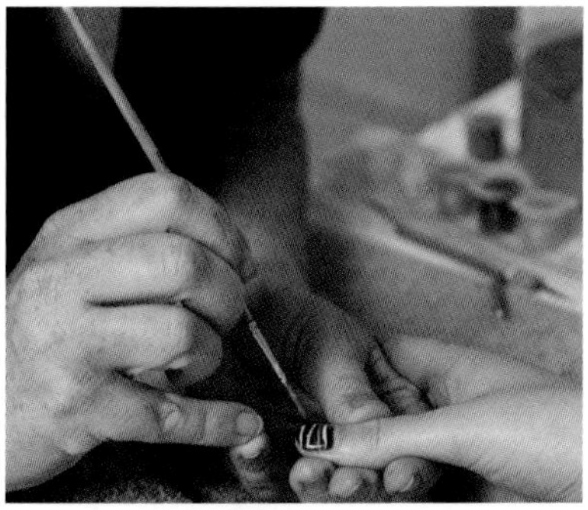

STEP 2 – Apply a different colour stripe to create a fan effect. Apply nail art sealant/top coat to seal the design.

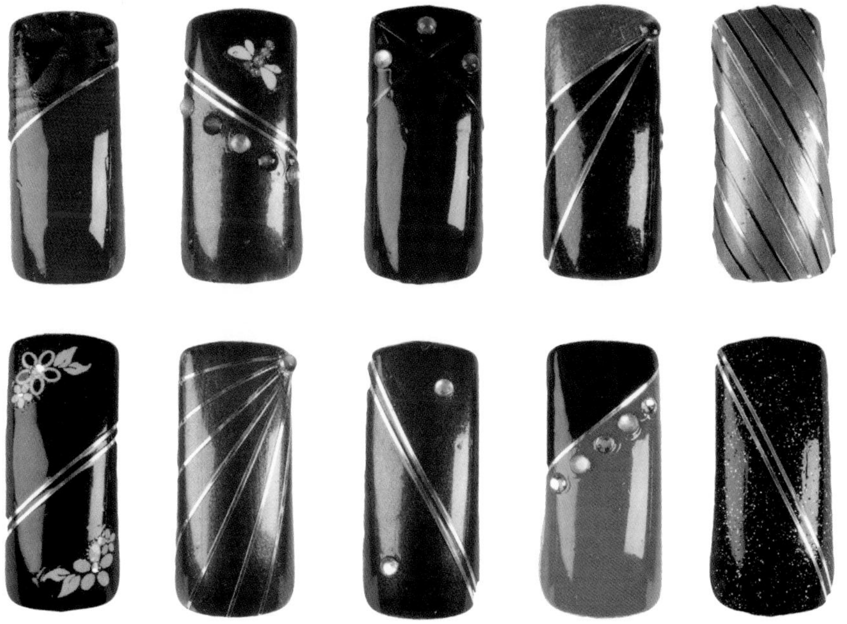

Example of nail art designs

HANDY HINTS

To start off with, have the three primary colour paints (red, yellow and blue). By mixing these colours together you can create the secondary colours (orange, green and violet). Black and white paints are also useful colours to have. Adding white will make the colour lighter. Adding black will make the colour darker.

HANDY HINTS

For more information on primary and secondary colours, go to Chapter 005 Creating an image using colour for the hair and beauty sector.

ACTIVITY

Practise different designs using different colours. Keep the designs that you like for your display board, to show your clients.

ACTIVITY

Mix the three primary colours (red, yellow and blue) together to see what colours you can create. Practise adding black and white to see how this affects the colours.

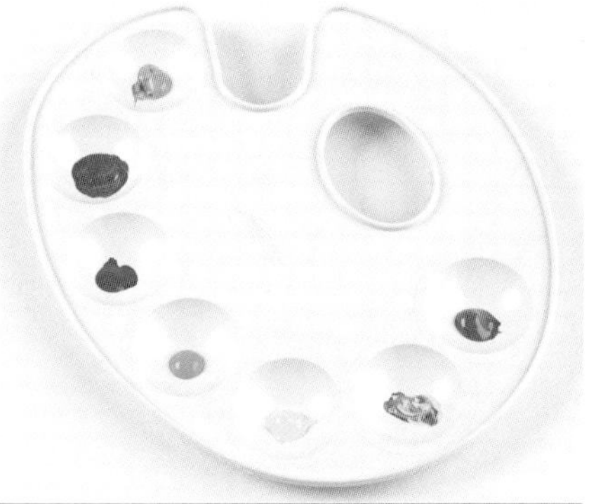

Paint palette used for mixing colours

ACTIVITY

Design a mood board of nail art designs that you could have in your salon to show to a client. Decide on a specific occasion (such as a wedding, a holiday or a party). Have a look on the internet at the latest nail art designs that are around at the moment to help you. Try to include pictures of famous celebrities and designs that use the techniques mentioned in this chapter. You can work on your own, in pairs or small groups.

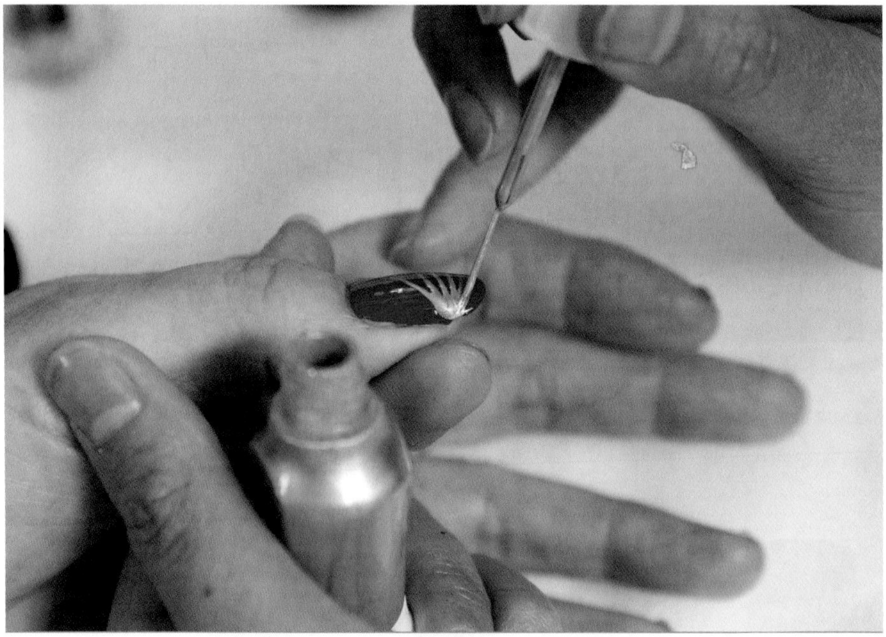

If striping pens are used, simply paint them straight from the bottle onto the nails

HANDY HINTS

If you need any help thinking of different designs, have a look on YouTube. There are lots of step-by-step guides for different nail art designs for you to follow.

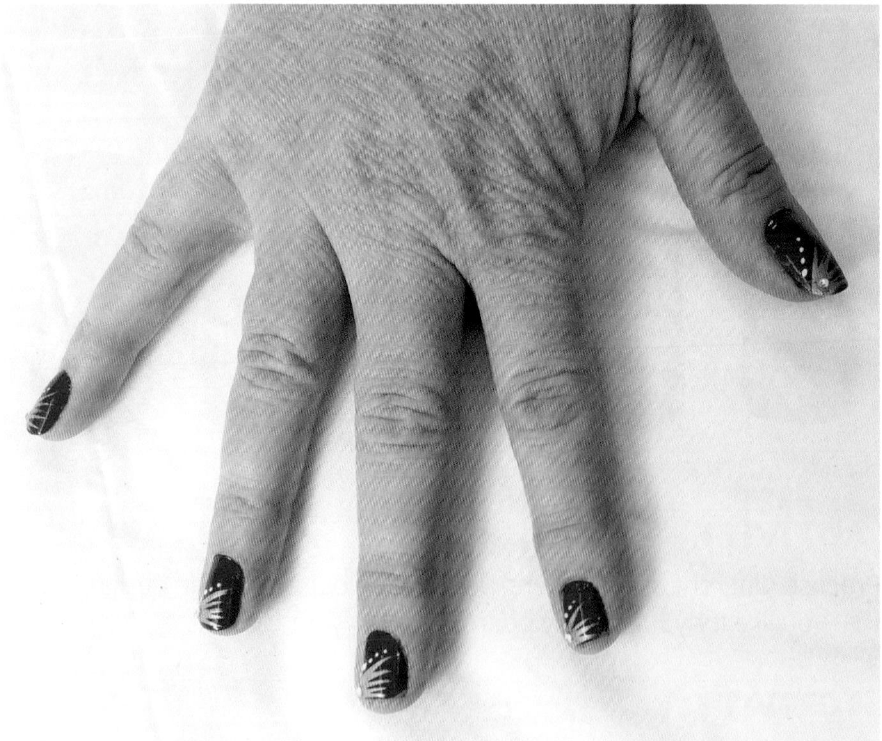

You can use more than one of these techniques together for your nail art design, so you can be as creative as you want!

ACTIVITY

Make a display board of at least ten nail art designs that have been painted onto artificial nails. This can be used to show your client what designs you can do for them.

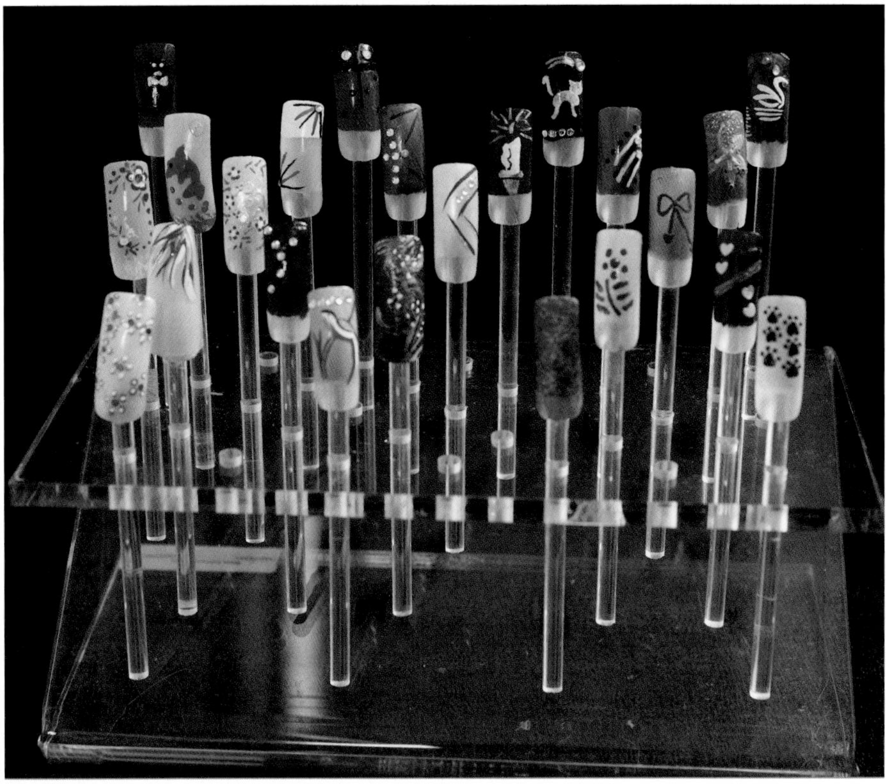

A nail art display for clients

HANDY HINTS

Make sure that your display board has examples of designs that are suitable for short nails as well as longer nails.

AFTERCARE ADVICE

After the treatment it is important to explain some simple aftercare tips to the client, which will help the nail art last longer. They should:

- apply another coat of top coat every two days
- try to be careful with their hands and nails, eg wear rubber gloves when washing up
- remove the nail art with non-acetone nail enamel remover
- return to the salon for repeat treatments.

HANDY HINTS

Most nail art designs need a base colour of nail enamel. Prepare for your nail art designs by painting a few artificial nails beforehand.

ACTIVITY

Design a leaflet that you could use to promote nail art treatment to your clients. Remember to include examples of designs that they could have and your salon name. You may want to make your leaflet into a special-offer promotion for your clients, to promote this as an additional service following a manicure or pedicure treatment.

HANDY HINTS

Design your leaflet on the computer so that it looks really professional.

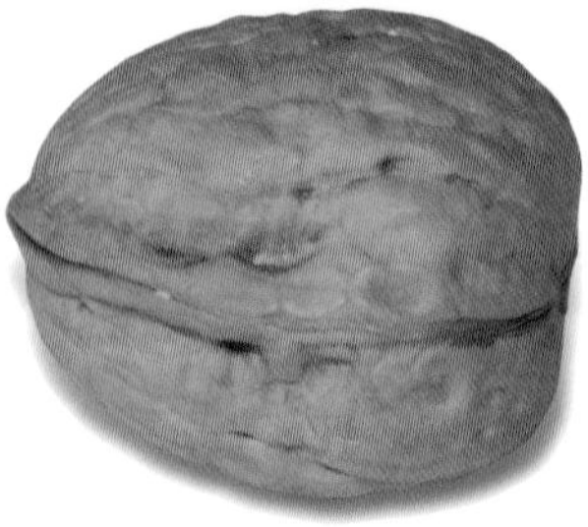

IN A NUTSHELL

You are now at the end of the chapter. Before you test your knowledge with the revision activities, check the following list to see if you feel confident in all the areas covered. If there are still any areas you're unsure of, go back over them in the book and ask your tutor for extra support:

- how to prepare for a basic nail art technique
- how to select products and tools
- how to design a 2D image
- factors that could influence the choice of techniques and products
- the importance of the preparation procedures
- the products and techniques used
- carry out basic nail art techniques
- follow safe and hygienic working practices
- communicate and behave in a professional manner.

REVISION ACTIVITIES

Use the questions below to test your knowledge of Chapter 108 to see just how much information you've gained. This can help you to prepare for your assessment.

Turn to pages 503–504 for the answers.

WORDS TO FIND

Copy and complete the sentences below. Use these words to help you fill in the gaps.

foils	transfers	glitter	enamel
occasion	nail art	factors	striping
colour	design	communication	products
fashion	blend	tools	palette

1 Nail art often needs a colour base of nail __________ before applying the nail art __________.

2 Your __________, __________ and equipment should be clean and hygienic for each client.

3 __________ come in two different types: peel off and soak off.

4 Apply a thin layer of adhesive before you rub the __________ onto the nails.

5 An example of good __________ is smiling and listening to the client.

6 Water-based acrylic paints can be mixed on a __________ before being applied to the nail using a __________ brush.

7 You need to ask the client what __________ they are having the nail art service for. You can then choose the most suitable design.

8 __________ is often applied to the nails after a manicure or pedicure treatment.

TEST YOUR KNOWLEDGE FURTHER

Read the sentences below and state whether they are true or false.

1 The salon should be well ventilated. True or false?

2 Nail art is only applied to artificial nails. True or false?

3 Polish secures produce a 3D effect on the nails. True or false?

4 It is important to choose the correct size brush for the nail art design you want to achieve. True or false?

5 Orange sticks can be used for striping designs. True or false?

6 Another name for a foil is a metallic wrap. True or false?

7 Tweezers can be used to help apply peel-off transfers to the nail. True or false?

8 Colour blending is where two or more colours are used. True or false?

9 Poor communication will help to promote a professional image for the salon. True or false?

111

COLOURING HAIR USING TEMPORARY COLOUR

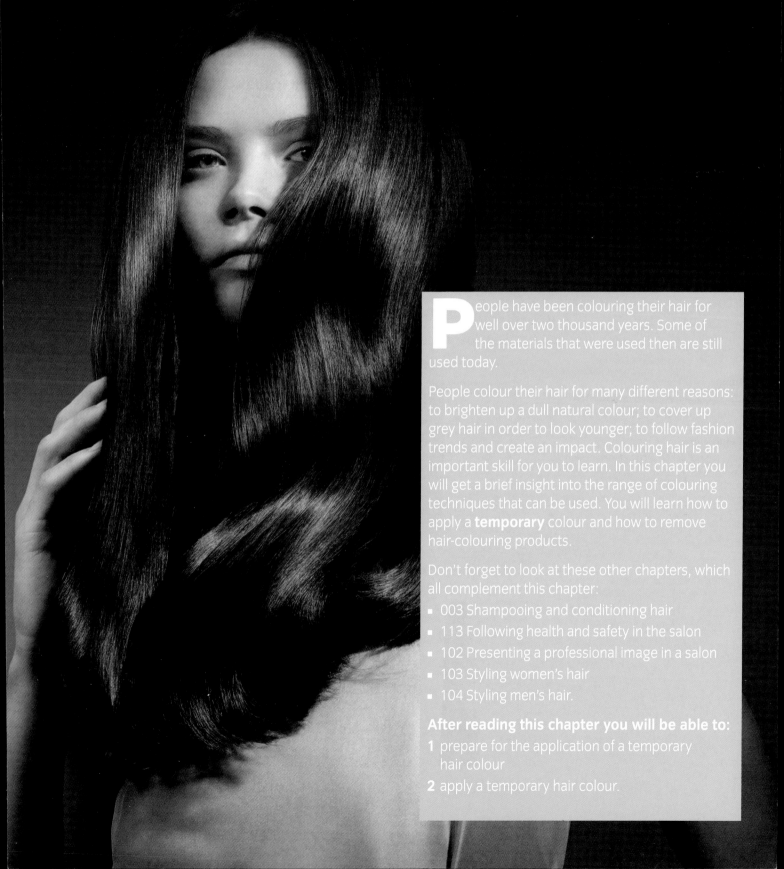

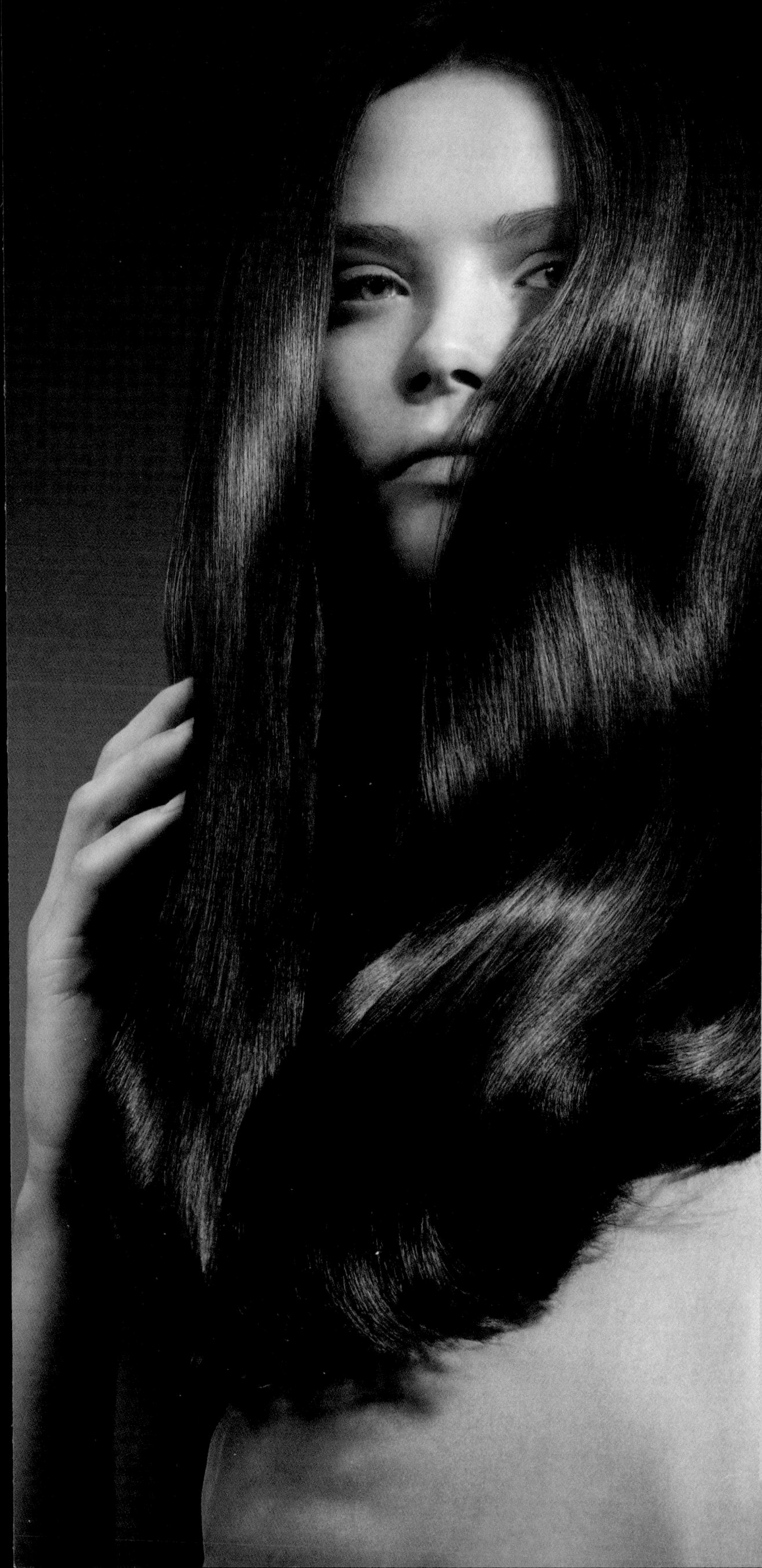

People have been colouring their hair for well over two thousand years. Some of the materials that were used then are still used today.

People colour their hair for many different reasons: to brighten up a dull natural colour; to cover up grey hair in order to look younger; to follow fashion trends and create an impact. Colouring hair is an important skill for you to learn. In this chapter you will get a brief insight into the range of colouring techniques that can be used. You will learn how to apply a **temporary** colour and how to remove hair-colouring products.

Don't forget to look at these other chapters, which all complement this chapter:

- 003 Shampooing and conditioning hair
- 113 Following health and safety in the salon
- 102 Presenting a professional image in a salon
- 103 Styling women's hair
- 104 Styling men's hair.

After reading this chapter you will be able to:

1. prepare for the application of a temporary hair colour
2. apply a temporary hair colour.

Temporary
Lasting only a short while

THE PURPOSE AND EFFECT OF HAIR COLOURS

There are five types of hair-colouring product that can be used to change the colour of the hair:

- **temporary** colour
- semi-permanent colour
- quasi-permanent colour
- permanent colour
- lighteners (hair bleach and high-lift colour).

Each type is used for a different purpose and has different effects on the hair.

Enhance
To complement or improve something

Tone
The colour of the hair, for example red, gold, brown, blonde, etc

Depth
How dark or light the colour is, for example, dark brown, light brown, very light blonde, etc

Type of colour	What it does
Temporary colour 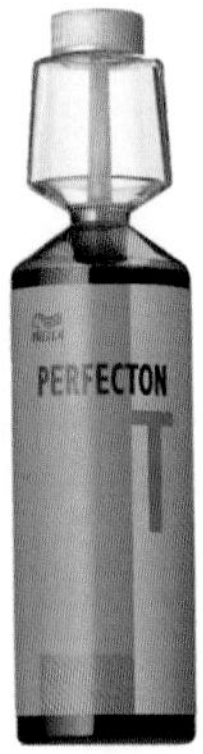	- Will last only until the next shampoo - Can be used for fashion effects - **Enhances** natural colour - Will add shine to the hair
Semi-permanent colour 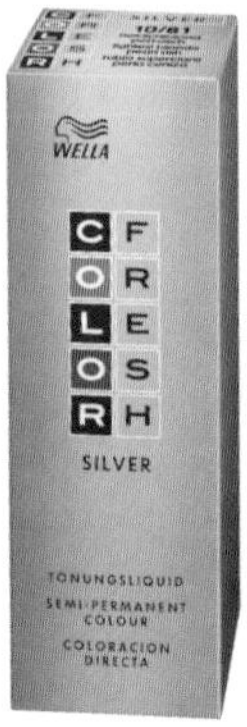	- Will last between six and eight shampoos - Adds shine, **tone** and **depth** - Blends up to 20% white hair - Enhances the natural colour - Can be used for fashion effects
Quasi-permanent colour 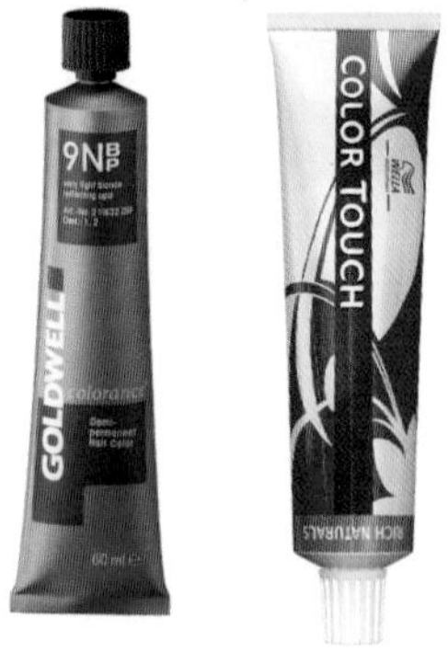	- Adds depth and tone - Covers up to 50% white hair - Lasts between 12 and 24 shampoos - Introduction to permanent colour - Weaker chemicals used - Used for colour correction - Fashion colours - Refreshes faded colours

Type of colour	What it does
Permanent colour 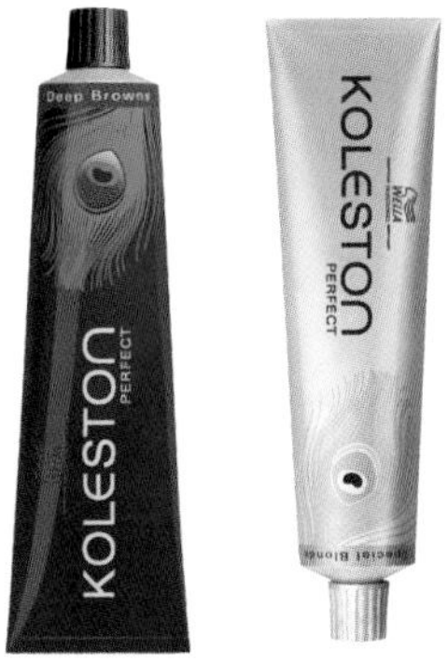 	■ Will give a permanent result ■ Adds tone and depth ■ Covers 100% white hair ■ Can lighten hair ■ Can be used for fashion effects and vibrant colours
Lightening products, eg bleach 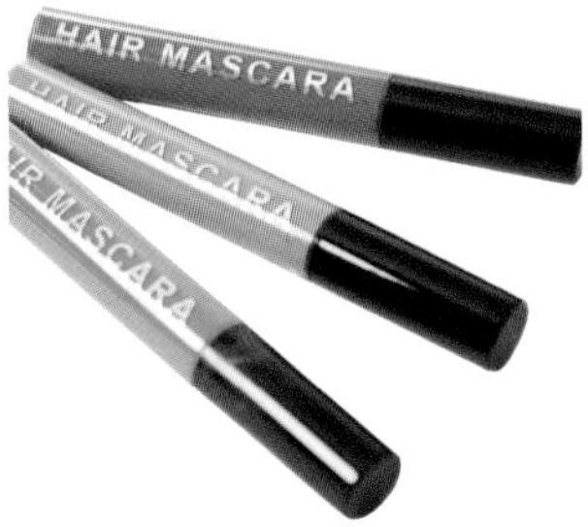 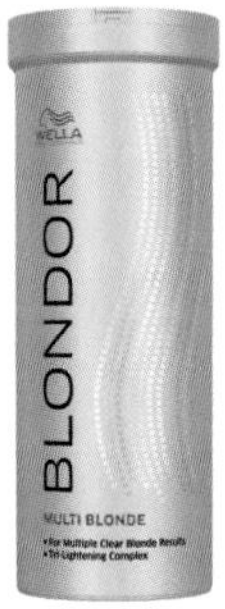 	■ Will give a permanent result ■ Will remove tone and depth ■ Enhances the natural colour ■ Can be used for fashion effects ■ Can lighten hair by five to six shades

ACTIVITY

Collect some pictures of people who have had their hair coloured. Find examples of each type of colour.

Try to find a range of effects that can be achieved with colour. Make notes about each one you find. These will be useful for your assignment.

PREPARE FOR THE APPLICATION OF A TEMPORARY COLOUR

Factors
Things to consider about a subject

This part of the chapter looks at the choice of different temporary colouring products, the preparation procedures for, and the effects of, applying them. It investigates the **factors** that influence the choice of temporary colouring products and their method of application.

FACTORS THAT CAN INFLUENCE YOUR CHOICE OF TEMPORARY COLOURING PRODUCTS AND THE METHOD OF APPLICATION

Like all hairdressing and beauty services there are many factors that you will need to take into account when choosing a temporary colouring product. They will also help you decide how the colour should be applied to the hair.

Molecules
Very small pieces that something is made of

ACTIVITY

Any temporary colour service will also include a styling service. Read Chapter 103 Styling women's hair, or Chapter 104 Styling men's hair, to learn more about the factors that may influence your choice of product and method.

HOW TEMPORARY COLOURS WORK

Temporary colour will coat the cuticle layer of the hair with a film of colour **molecules**. These stay on the hair when it is dried. The film of coloured pigments is washed off when the hair is next shampooed.

Understanding the structure of the hair is important when you are giving a colouring service, as it can affect the result you get.

ACTIVITY

Read Chapter 003 to refresh your knowledge of the structure of the hair.

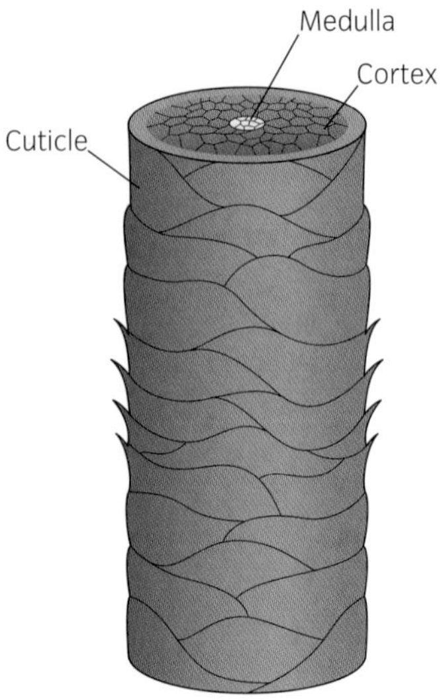

The structure of the hair

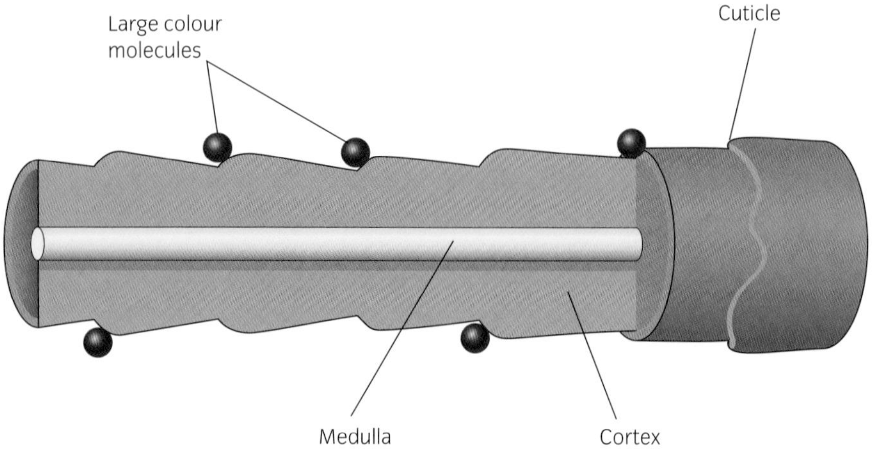

Effects of temporary colour molecules on the hair

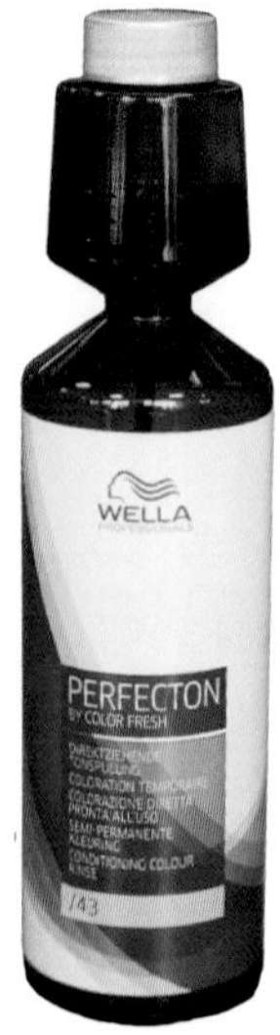

A temporary colour (water rinse)

THE FINISHED LOOK

Whenever you are carrying out a colour service, the first thing you need to find out is what colour hair your client wants to have. Finding this out will be a major factor in deciding:

- which temporary colour product you need to use
- what shade of colour will give the best result

It may also help you to decide whether you can achieve what the client is asking for.

THE CONDITION OF THE HAIR AND SCALP

The hair

The condition of the client's hair is very important when you are deciding if you can use a temporary colour. It will affect the colour you are going to use to get the finished result. It is also important when you are deciding which method to use. These are the things you need to look for:

- Dry hair: looks dull and straw-like; feels rough to the touch.
- Damaged hair: looks dull and lifeless; feels rough to the touch; the points of the hair may be split; there may be some breakage of hair.
- **Porous** hair: occurs as a result of damage; the hair feels rough to the touch when you run your fingers over it.

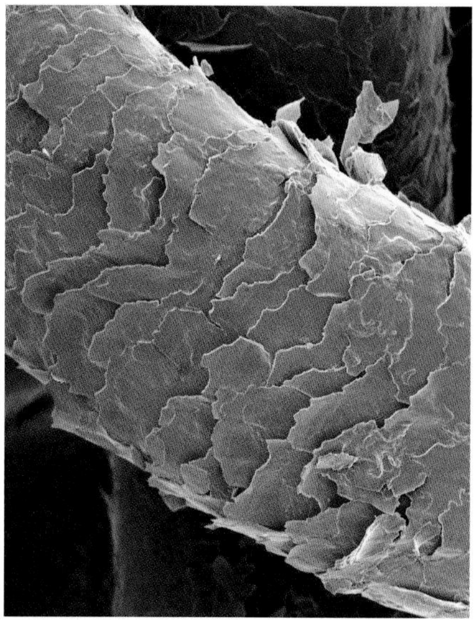

Porous
Lets in water or other liquids

With both dry and damaged hair the cuticle is rough and will not lie flat. This makes the hair porous. The colour can get under the cuticle. If the hair is damaged the colour can also get into the cortex. This can affect the result you will get. The colour could turn out to be patchy and uneven. It may also be difficult to remove when the hair is next shampooed.

It is a good idea to do a porosity test when you consult with the client. Take a few strands of hair and run your fingers from root to point gently. If the hair feels rough this is a sign of cuticle damage. The hair will be porous and might soak up your colour. The rougher the hair feels the more porous it is.

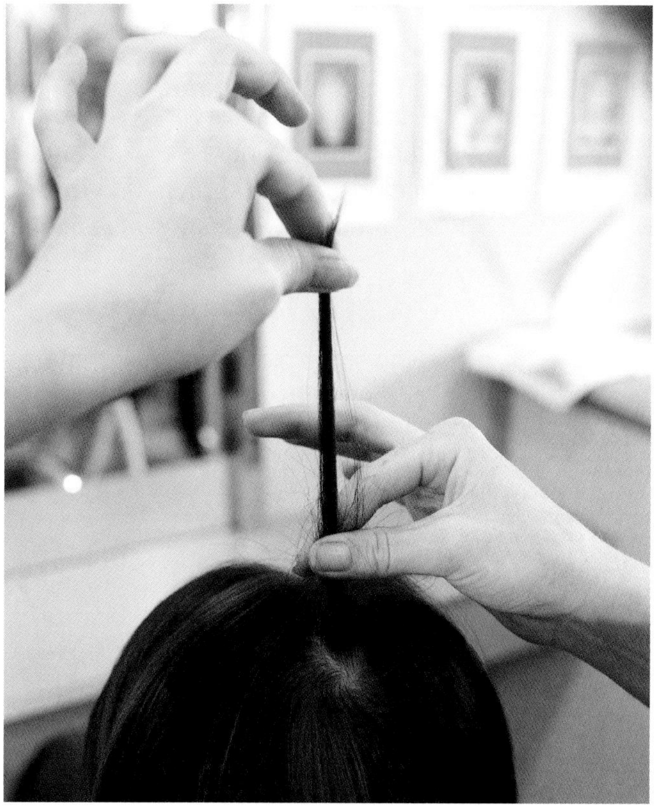

ACTIVITY

With other members of your group, carry out a porosity test on each other. Make notes on what you think the porosity is. Compare your decisions with the others.

The scalp

Check the scalp carefully for any signs of possible conditions and diseases. Make sure you look for contagious diseases like head lice. Remember to look for:

- scaly patches or rough areas on the scalp
- red inflamed patches
- cuts and abrasions on the skin
- lumps and bumps or raised areas
- bald patches.

ACTIVITY

Read Chapter 003 to refresh your knowledge of how to recognise head lice and what other signs to look for when you check the scalp.

NATURAL HAIR COLOUR

The client's natural colour will be a key factor in choosing a temporary colour. Remember, temporary colours **enhance** the natural colour, they do not change it. The client's natural colour will help you choose the colour you need to use. It will also give you the range from which you can choose. For example:

Enhance
Intensify; improve

- If the client's hair is quite dark, temporary colours that are light will not show up on the hair.
- If the client's hair is light, then darker temporary colours may show up too much and give the wrong result.
- If the client has a lot of white hair, temporary colours can show up brighter than you want them too.

HANDY HINTS

If your client has a lot of white hair then you must be very careful about what colour you choose to use. It may be better to advise the client to have a different type of colour which will cover the white hair.

FASHION TRENDS

Colouring the hair will always be affected by fashion trends. Some temporary colours are used after the hair has been styled. This group includes glitter sprays and **vibrant** colour sprays. These can be used to create a wide range of fashionable effects.

Vibrant
Brightly coloured

HANDY HINTS

Keep your eye on what colouring techniques are currently popular. It is important to keep up to date for your clients. Magazines and the internet are good places to find examples.

ACTIVITY

Find some pictures of hair that has been coloured with temporary colour. With your group, decide which of your colleagues could have the colour you have selected and which could not.

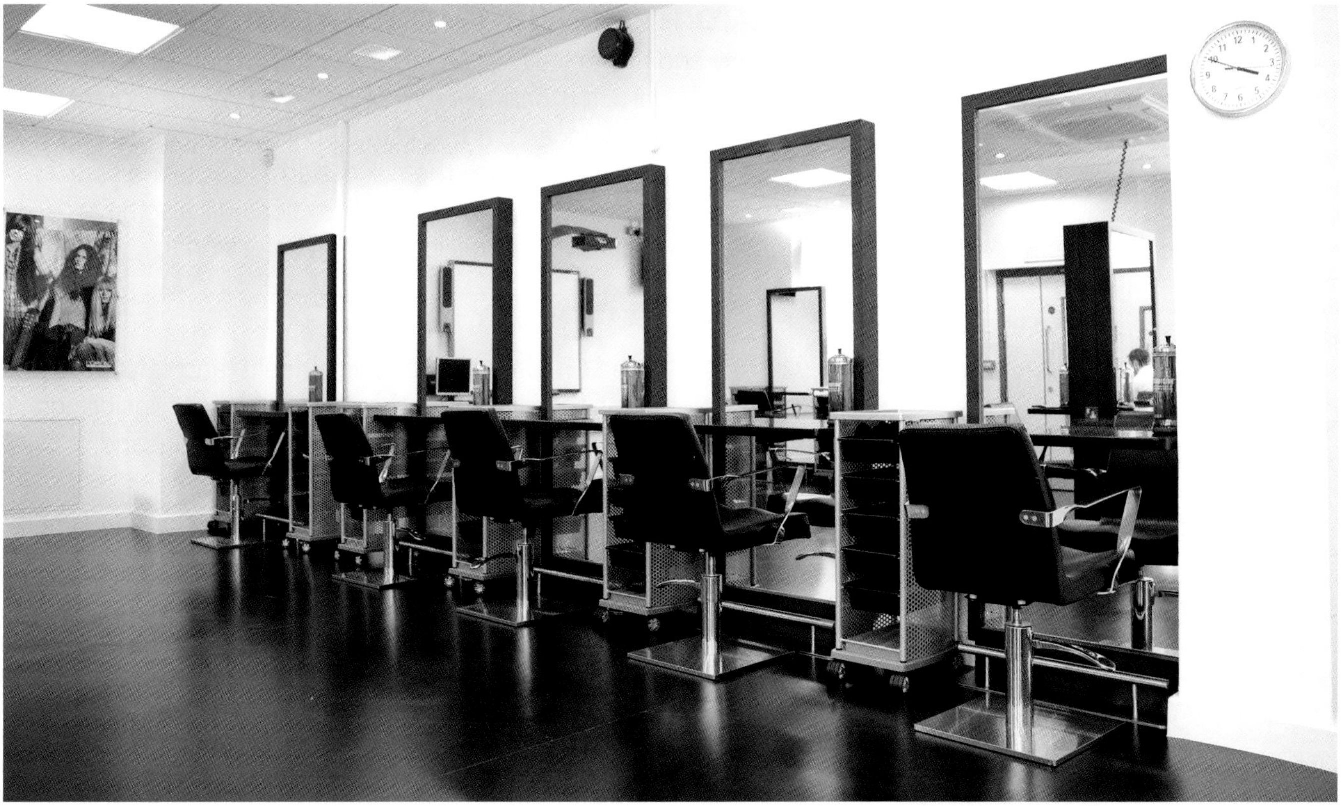

PREPARE THE WORK AREA

There are three reasons why you should prepare your work area ready for work:

1 It will help you to work safely and hygienically.

2 It will look good and give the client the right impression.

3 It will help you to work efficiently.

Before your client arrives, prepare in the following ways:

- Make sure you keep work surfaces clean by wiping regularly with a suitable cleaner.
- Mirrors should be cleaned to remove smears and smudges.
- Tools and equipment should be in their proper places and always cleaned and sterilised ready for use to help prevent the transfer of infection from one client to another.
- Sweep and clean the floor when necessary. Make sure the chair is clean.

You may not be able to get all the things you need ready before the client arrives. When you have completed your consultation with the client, get the rest of the products and tools you need.

HANDY HINTS

Remember to make sure your appearance and your personal hygiene are up to standard. Read Chapter 102 to refresh your knowledge.

SAFE AND HYGIENIC WORKING PRACTICES

Working safely and hygienically is very important. It is part of every practical skill you learn. It is part of every service you give to a client. You should keep your work area tidy and use only hygienic tools and equipment. This will help to reduce the risk of harm to you and your clients and help to prevent cross-infection. The client will also have more confidence in you and you will look more professional.

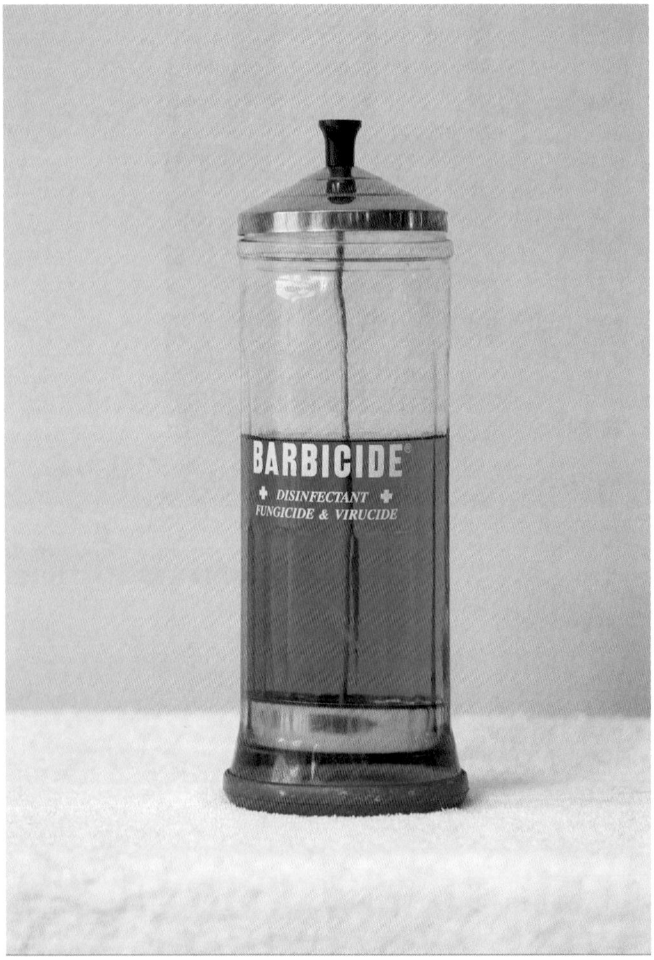

Barbicide

ACTIVITY

Read Chapter 113 Following health and safety in the salon to learn about the employer's responsibilities and your responsibilities to provide a safe and healthy working environment.

- **PPE** – personal protective equipment. You will need non-latex gloves and an apron for yourself. Make sure you follow the manufacturer's instructions.
- **COSHH** – Control Of Substances Hazardous to Health. This tells you how to safely use any products that may be part of the service. It will also include using a disinfectant safely when using it to clean tools and equipment.
- **HASAWA** – Health and Safety at Work Act. Check the work area for any hazards before you start work on the client. Check that all the equipment, tools and products are clean and safe to use on the client.
- **Electricity at Work Regulations** – Check all the electrical equipment you will use in the styling process before you start.

Don't forget to check that all the tools are sterilised ready to start work. A method of sterilisation used in a colouring service is using a disinfectant such as Barbicide for combs.

HANDY HINTS

Read Chapter 113 for more information about methods of sterilisation.

ACTIVITY

Go to Chapter 113 Following health and safety in the salon and list all of the health and safety laws that you should follow when carrying out a styling service.

HYGIENE WHEN USING TEMPORARY COLOUR

The following table is a guide for keeping your tools and equipment ready for use.

Disposable
Something that you throw away after you have used it

Tools and equipment	How to clean and store ready for use
Towels and gowns	Machine wash on a high temperature.
Plastic cape and apron	Wash in hot soapy water; rinse and dry.
Combs and brushes	Wash in warm, soapy water; place in the sterilising jar.
Clips	Wash, dry, then place in the sterilising jar or the UV cabinet.
Disposable gloves	Throw away after use. Use a new pair for each client.

PREPARE THE CLIENT

When you are carrying out temporary colouring services you will also be doing a styling service. You will need to prepare the client for shampooing first. Once the shampoo and conditioning is completed you will need to prepare the client for the colouring service.

HANDY HINTS
Check regularly that the gown is still in place and the towels are not too wet. Change the towels if you need to.

GOWNING THE CLIENT FOR SHAMPOOING

Place a gown around the client to protect her clothes and a clean, freshly laundered towel around her shoulders.

HANDY HINTS
Read more about preparing your client in Chapter 003 Shampooing and conditioning hair.

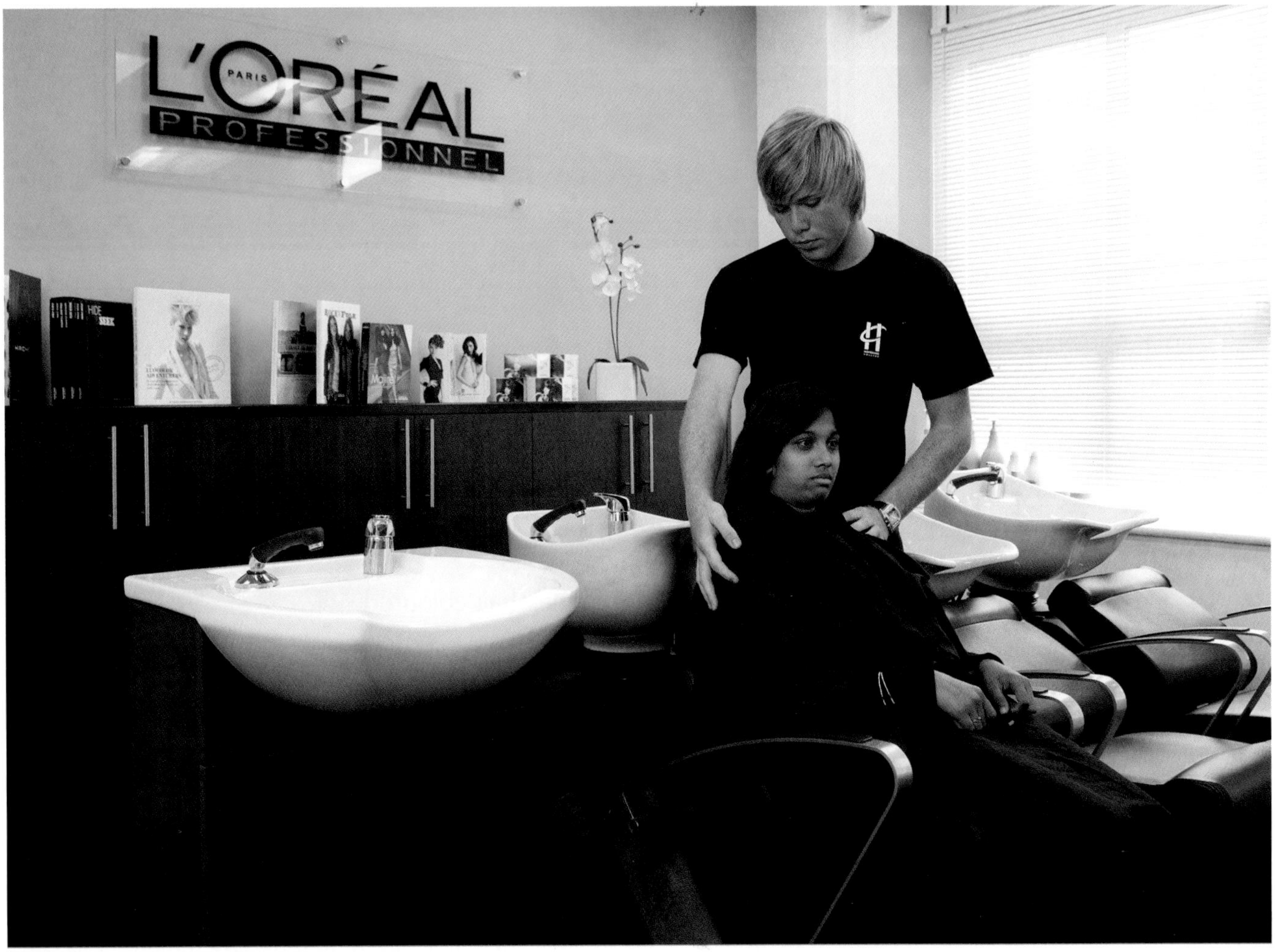

Guide your client to the sink

CONSULTATION

Consulting with the client helps you to find out what the client wants and decide what you are going to do. When you consult with the client about the colour service you will also consult with them for the styling service and the shampoo.

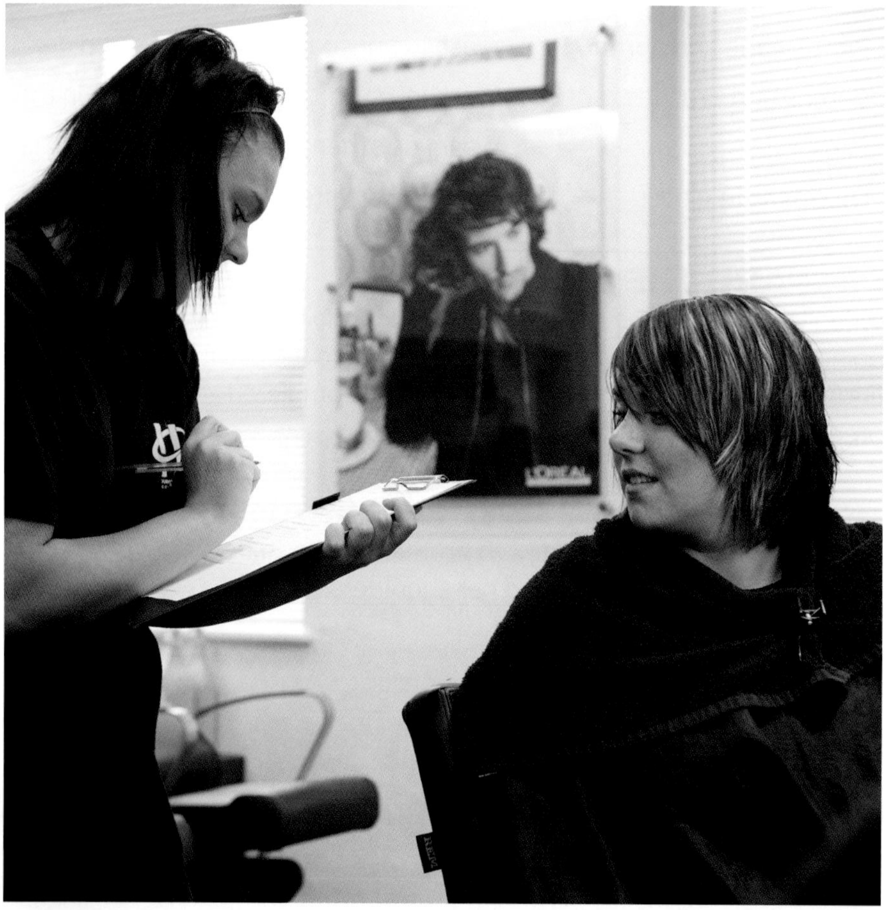

HANDY HINTS

The colour the client wants should complement the style that you will create. It should also complement the client's lifestyle and job.

ACTIVITY

Refresh your knowledge about consulting with the client for shampooing and styling services. Read Chapter 003 Shampooing and conditioning hair and Chapter 103 Styling women's hair or Chapter 104 Styling men's hair.

If you are going to carry out a temporary colour, you need to find out more information from the client. You must find out:

- what effect the client wants
- why the client wants their hair coloured
- the style they want.

Now look at all the factors that can influence your choice of colour and technique.

When you have looked at all the factors you need to decide if you can achieve what the client has asked for. If it is obvious that you cannot, then you will need to suggest something else.

Next, select your colour, shampoo, conditioner and finishing products. Finally, decide how you will carry out the technique and which tools and equipment you need to use.

COMMUNICATION AND BEHAVIOUR

Communication and behaviour are very important before and during a colour service. If you can't communicate with clients properly, they may end up with a colour result that is different from what they were expecting. Think carefully about the types of question you should ask. Refer to Chapter 102 for more detail about communication and behaviour.

HANDY HINTS

Don't use technical words or jargon that the client does not understand. Keep it simple.

ACTIVITY

Make a list of all the things you need to find out from the client concerning the colour service. Include all the factors that may influence your decisions. Write down how you will find out the information. Make a list of the questions you could ask the client. Working in pairs, try out your questions and observations on each other to see if you get the information you need.

SHAMPOO AND CONDITION THE CLIENT'S HAIR

When you have finished your consultation, the next step is to shampoo the hair ready for the colouring and finishing service. Chapter 003 Shampooing and conditioning describes the method of shampooing and conditioning the hair ready for other services.

HANDY HINTS

Put the colour towels in the laundry basket and carefully wash the colour bowls and brushes.

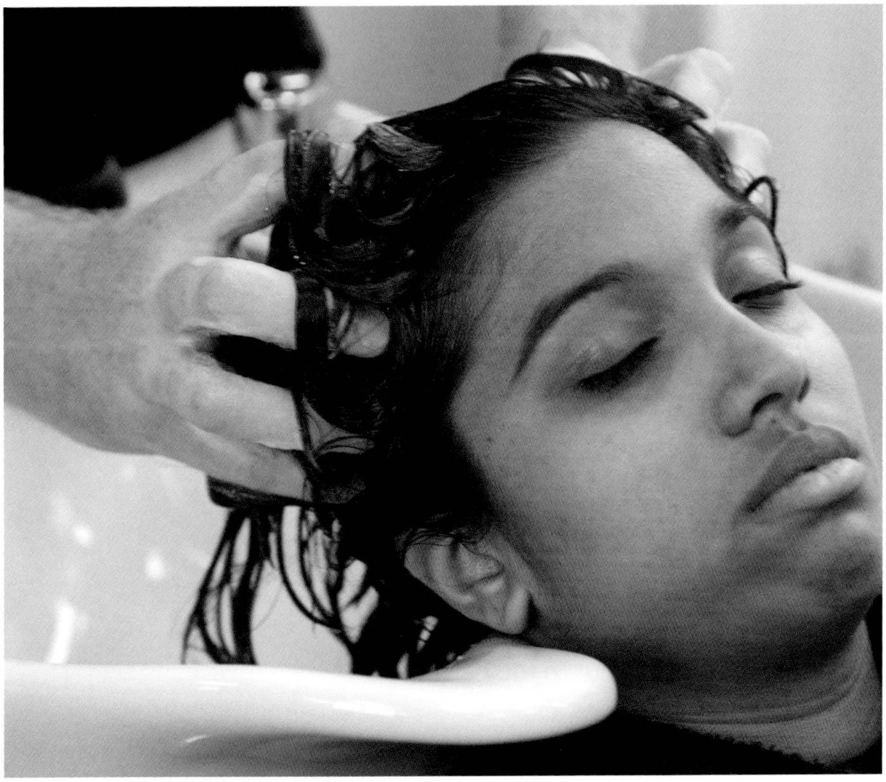

Don't forget to use conditioner if the hair needs it. Make sure the client agrees to have it. Using conditioner will help smoothe the cuticle.

TOOLS AND EQUIPMENT USED IN TEMPORARY COLOURING

Tools and equipment	Use
Wide-toothed comb 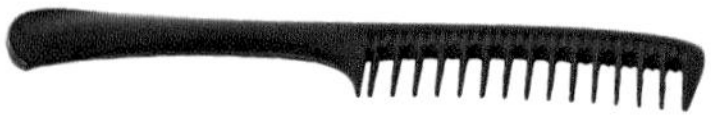	Used to remove tangles from the hair before shampooing and to prepare the hair for the colour after it has been shampooed.
Tail comb 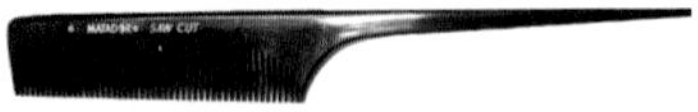	Used to make sections in preparation for colouring.
Sectioning clips 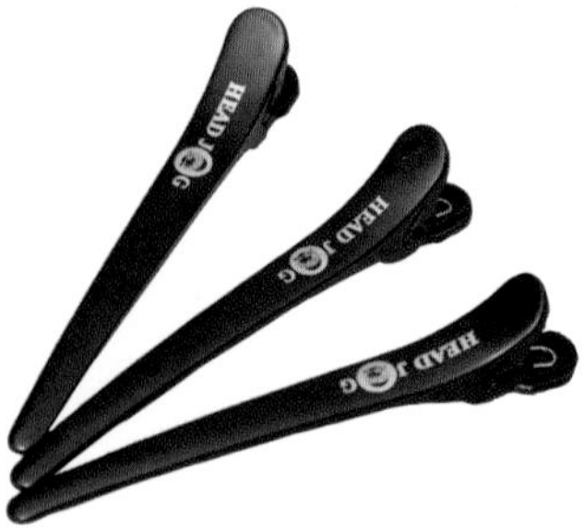	Used to keep the hair under control when you are colouring.
Bowl 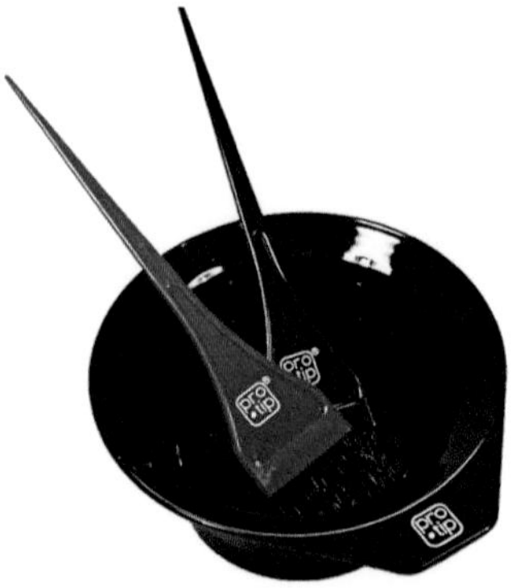	Used to hold the colour when you are applying it to the hair.
Sponge 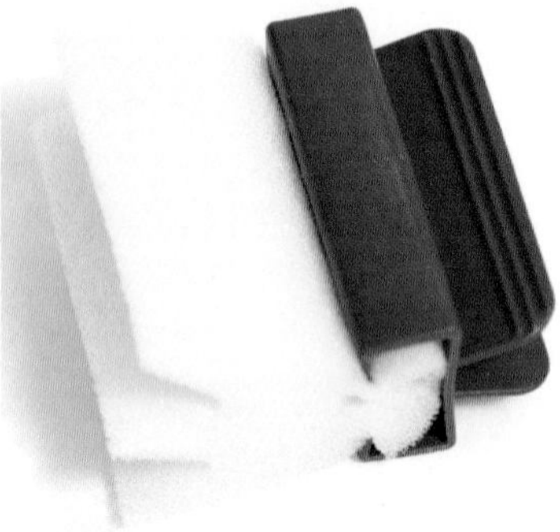	Used to apply the colour to the hair.

Tools and equipment	Use
Applicator bottle 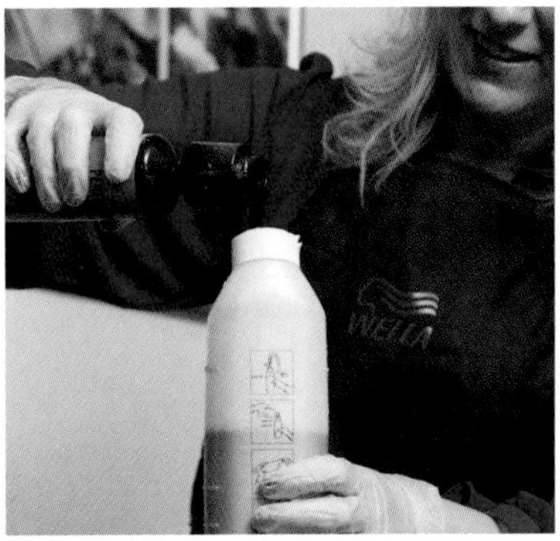	Some temporary colours come in an applicator bottle ready to apply the colour.
Colour gown 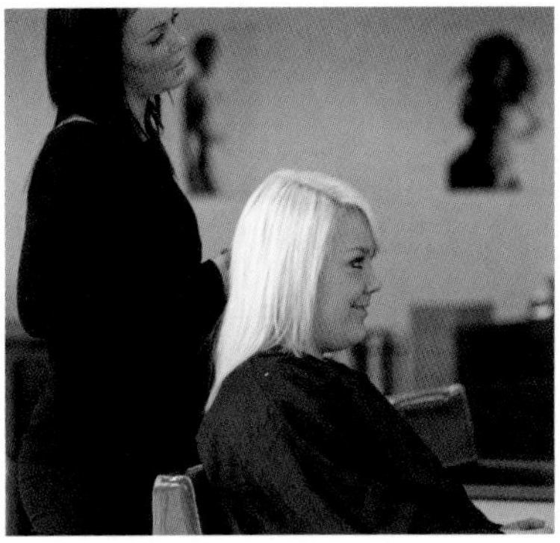	A plastic cape or apron that is waterproof. Used on top of the shampooing gown to make sure no colour gets on to the client's clothing.
Colouring towels 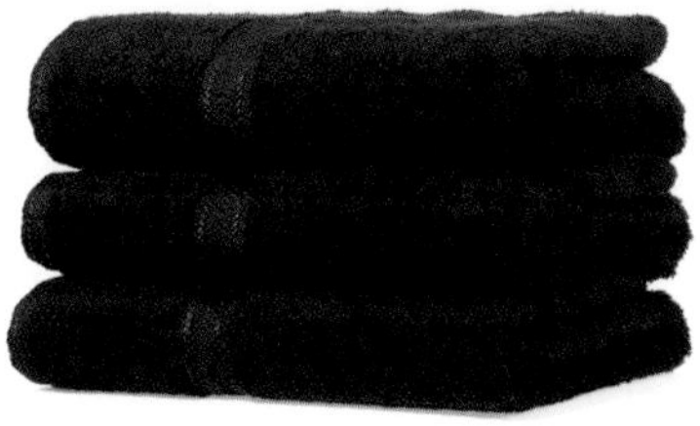	These are usually black towels so they do not show stains, which look unsightly.
Disposable gloves 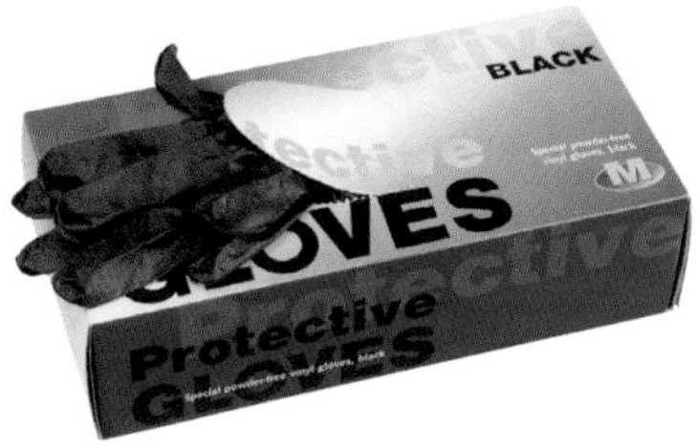	Used to protect the hands from staining and contact dermatitis.
Apron 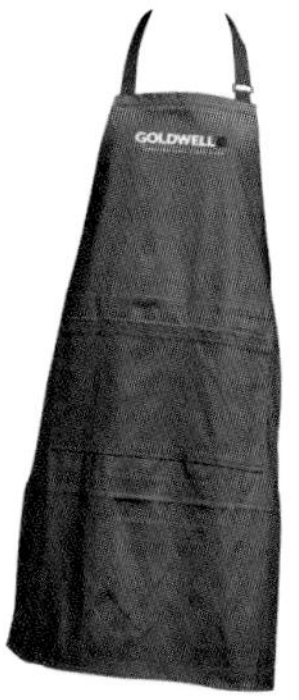	Used to protect the stylist's uniform or clothing.

PRODUCTS USED IN TEMPORARY HAIR COLOURING

Product	Use
Mousse 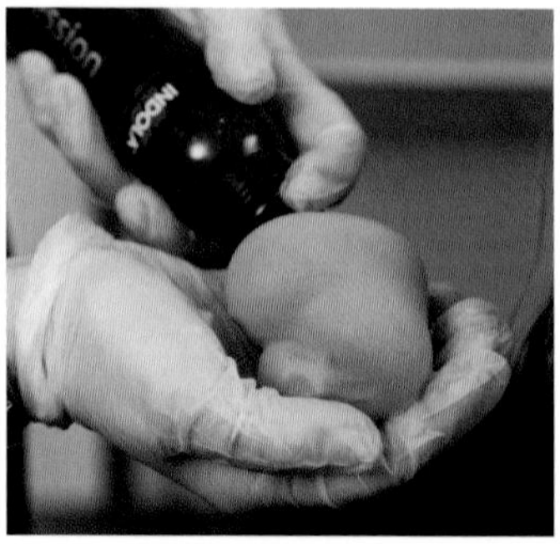	▪ Similar to mousse used in styling. ▪ Contains a colour pigment. ▪ Applied to wet hair. ▪ Also provides volume and texture.
Gel 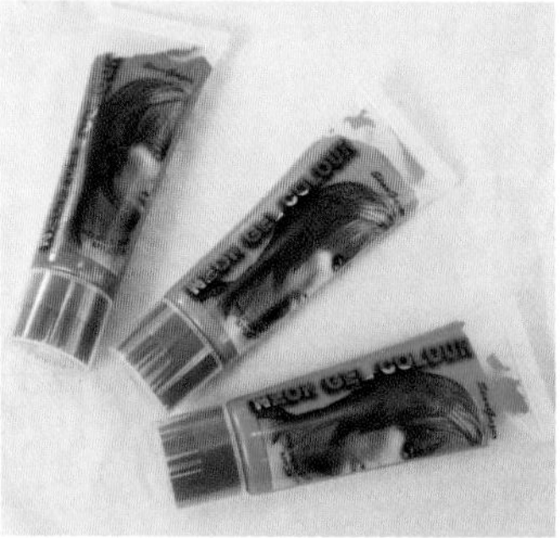	▪ Similar to setting gels but with a coloured base. ▪ Oil-based products. ▪ Applied to dry hair. ▪ Can be used for a range of effects requiring vibrant colours.
Wands 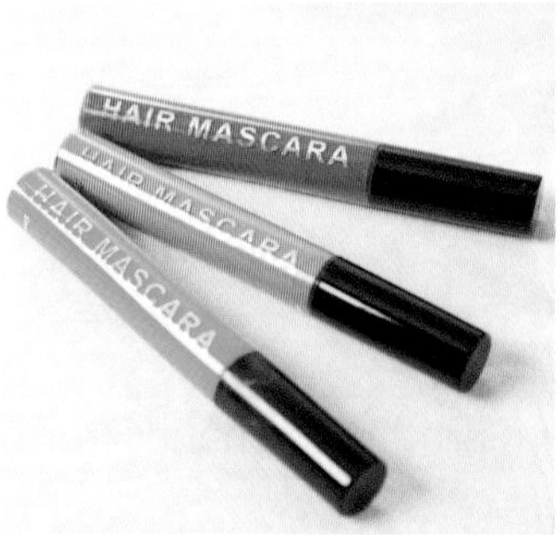	▪ 'Mascaral'-type applicator that is used to add colour to specific areas of the hair. ▪ Applied to dry hair after styling.

Product	Use
Sprays 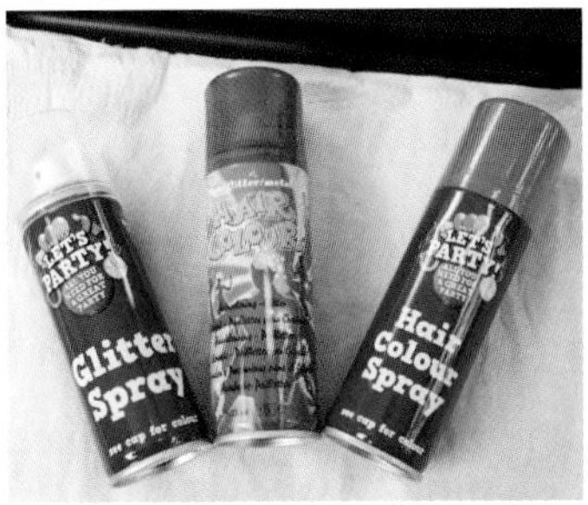	▪ Used on dry hair. ▪ The spray contains a colour pigment. ▪ The hair is sprayed when styling is finished. ▪ Used to colour parts of the hair for effect. ▪ Available in vibrant colours and as glitter spray.
Setting lotions 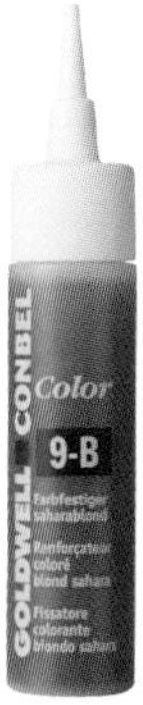	▪ These have a colour pigment added to them. ▪ Applied to wet hair before styling. ▪ Also provide hold to the hair.
Water rinses 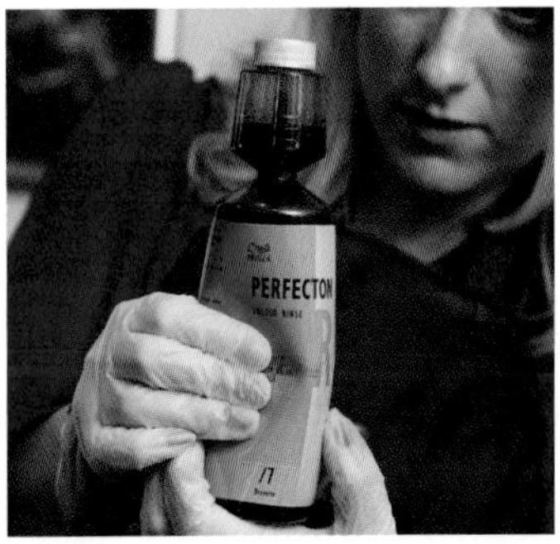	▪ Water-based colour pigment. ▪ Applied to wet hair before drying.

ACTIVITY

Working in pairs, or a small group, collect some hair cuttings that are long enough to apply colour to. Try to find a variety of colours: dark, light, and, if possible, some white or grey hair. Apply different types of temporary colour to the hair samples to see what results you get. Keep notes of what you used for each sample. Compare your results with those of other groups.

APPLY TEMPORARY HAIR COLOUR

This part of the chapter shows you how to correctly follow procedures to apply temporary colours to the hair.

PROCEDURES FOR TEMPORARY COLOUR APPLICATION

Temporary colour can be applied in many different ways. With some types of product the colour is applied to wet hair before the hair is styled. With others the colour is applied to dry hair after it has been styled.

At what point you apply the colour will depend on what finished look you want to achieve for your client:

- If you want all the hair to be coloured, apply before styling. *This is called a full-head application.*
- If you want to colour parts of the hair, applying after styling would be best. *This is called a partial-head application.*

Whichever method you choose, you must make sure you read the manufacturer's instructions carefully. They will tell you the recommended procedure for using the product.

HANDY HINTS

It is very important to read the manufacturer's instructions for all the products you use. This will ensure you use them properly and get the best results for your client.

PREPARING THE HAIR FOR COLOUR APPLICATION

For full-head applications where the colour is applied to wet hair before styling, the following procedure would be carried out:

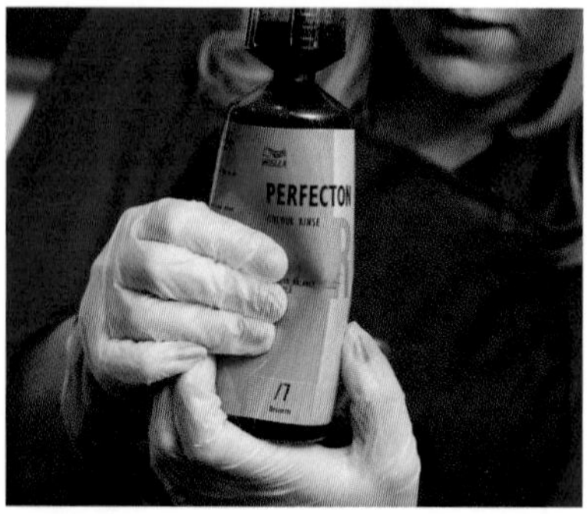

STEP 1 – Make sure you read the instructions for the colour you are using.

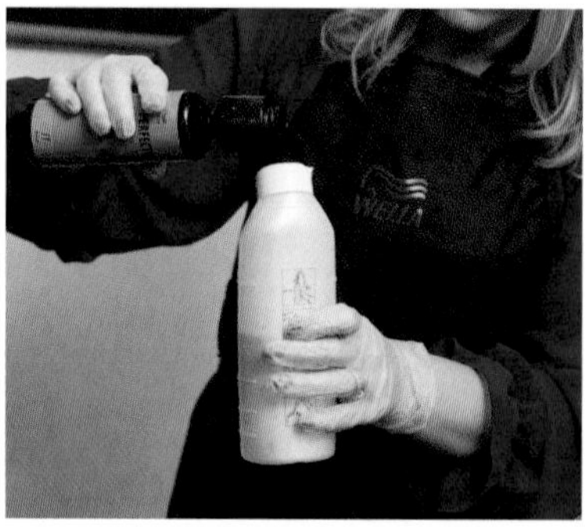

STEP 2 – Follow the instructions when you get the colour ready to apply to the hair.

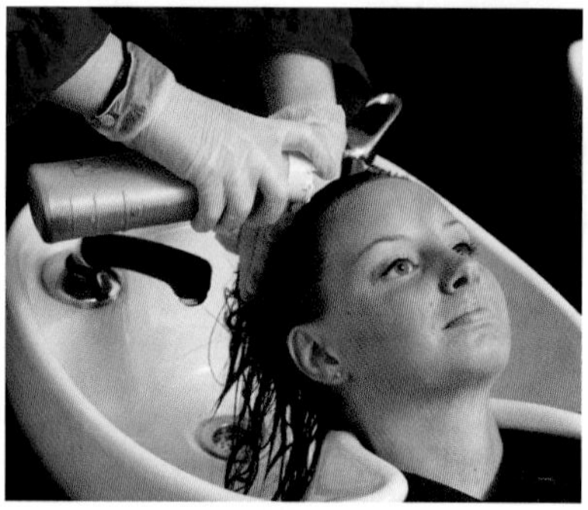

STEP 3 – Apply the colour evenly to the hair. Use your fingers to work the colour through the length of the hair.

For partial-head applications, where the colour is applied after the hair has been styled, sections are not normally used. You would apply the colour carefully to the area you have planned for your finished result.

PREPARING THE COLOUR PRODUCT

Temporary colours are ready-prepared for use. Some will need to be poured into a bowl to be applied to the hair. Some will be in an aerosol can. Others will be in an applicator bottle. Always follow the manufacturer's instructions and prepare the colour properly.

APPLYING THE COLOUR TO THE HAIR

Full-head applications

Using mousse on short to medium length hair:

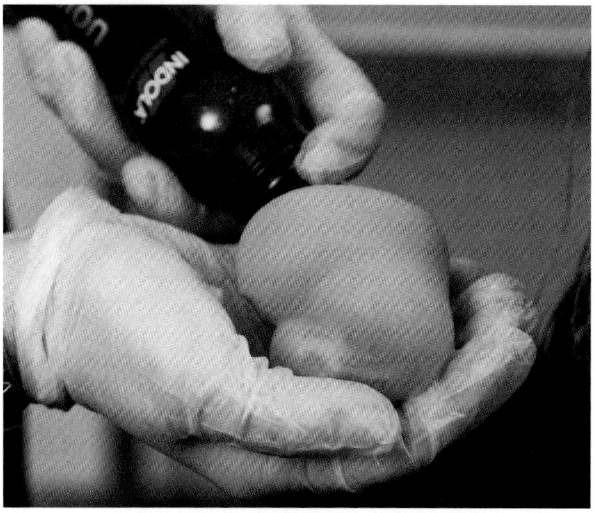

STEP 1 – Squirt the mousse into the palm of your hand. Do not use too much.

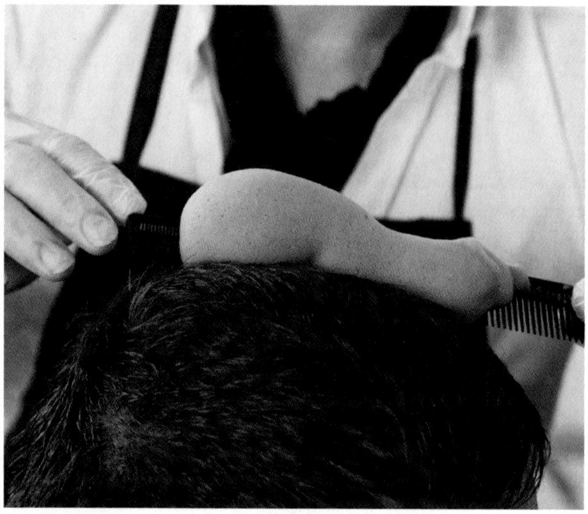

STEP 2 – Make a parting and apply the mousse with the fingers to the roots.

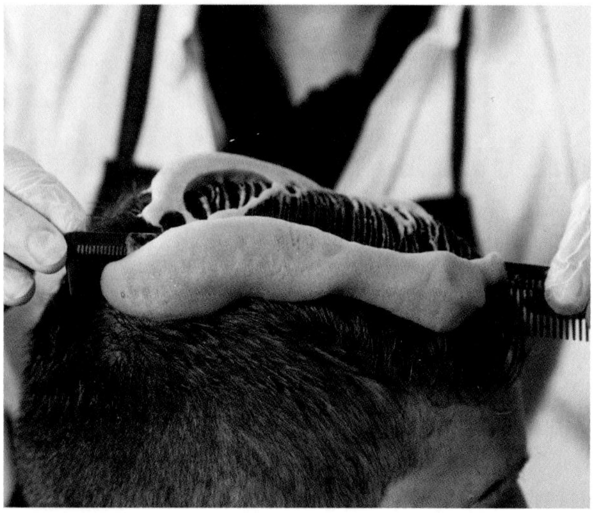

STEP 3 – Repeat until all the hair is covered. Be careful not to get any mousse on the client's face.

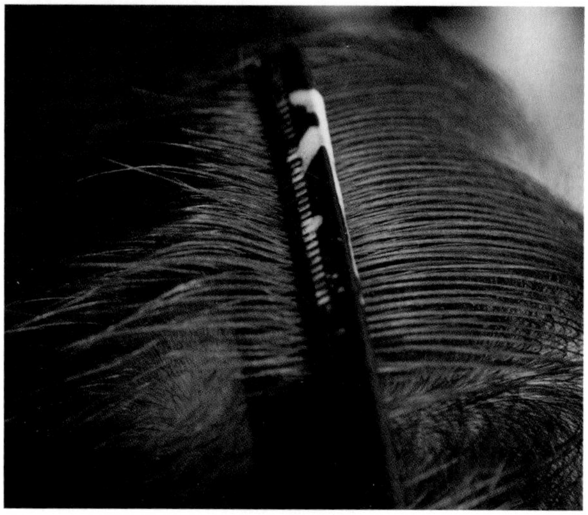

STEP 4 – Comb through the hair to make sure all the hair is covered with colour.

On long hair start the application on the nape sections:

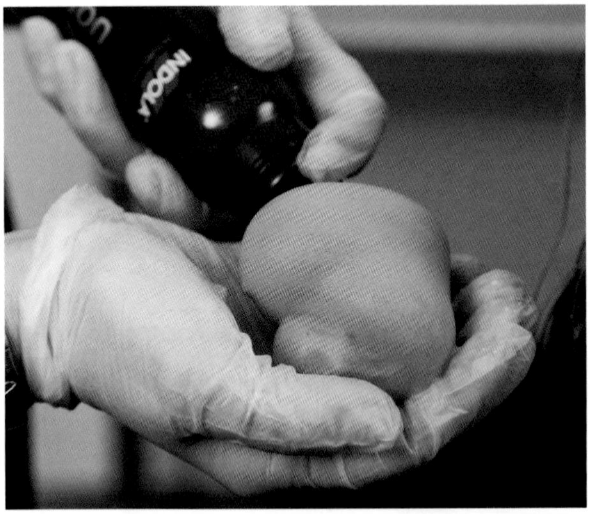

STEP 1 – For long hair you will need to use more of the product.

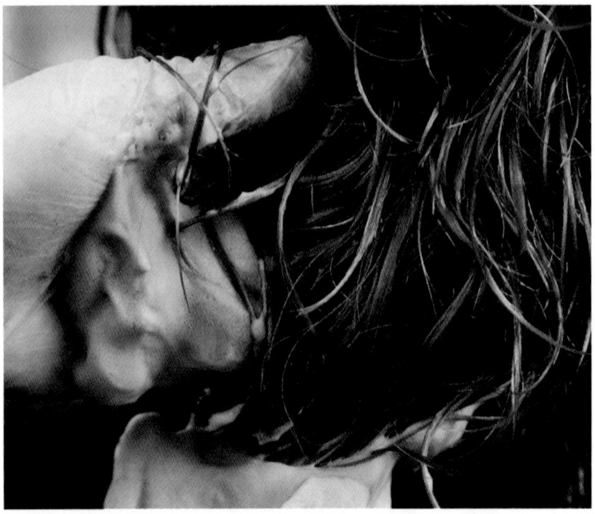

STEP 2 – Use the fingers to apply the colour to the points of the hair.

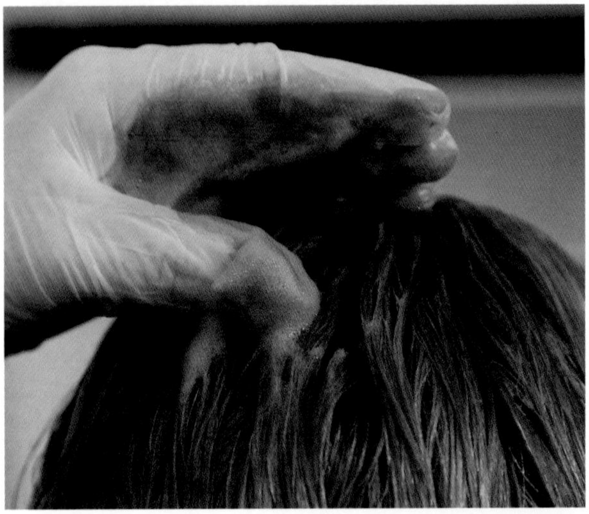

STEP 3 – Apply to the roots and comb through to make sure all the hair is covered.

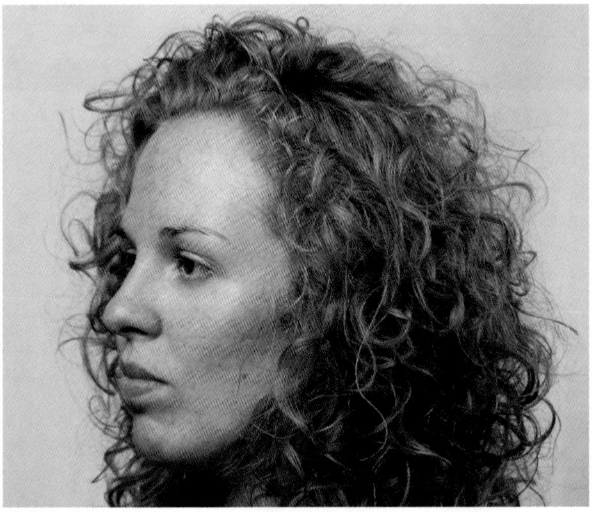

STEP 4 – The finished result.

HANDY HINTS

If you put on too much temporary colour product this is wasteful. It can also overload the hair and drip onto the client's shoulders.

If you are using setting lotion colour or water rinses they are applied in a similar way to mousse. These colours are usually in liquid form so will spread through the hair easily. They are applied by pouring a small quantity directly onto the hair at the front. You then comb through from front to crown as you did with the mousse. Repeat this process until all the hair is covered.

If the hair is long you can pour the colour into a bowl. Apply the colour to the nape sections using a sponge a little at a time. Comb through to the points and repeat as you did for using mousse on long hair.

Partial-head application

Most partial-head applications will be made after the hair has been styled. This process uses products such as gel colour, wands, sprays or colour paints.

Read the manufacturer's instructions for the recommended application procedure. The area that is to be coloured will have been planned as part of the desired look.

When the hair has been dried you can use an artist's paintbrush with colour paints or a 'mascara'-type wand to place the colour carefully where you want it.

With sprays, you can get a partial-head effect or a whole-head effect. Sprays are available in glitter or colour types. They are generally used for party styles or fashion effects.

Take care to spray only those areas you want to colour.
It is easy to colour areas you don't want coloured.

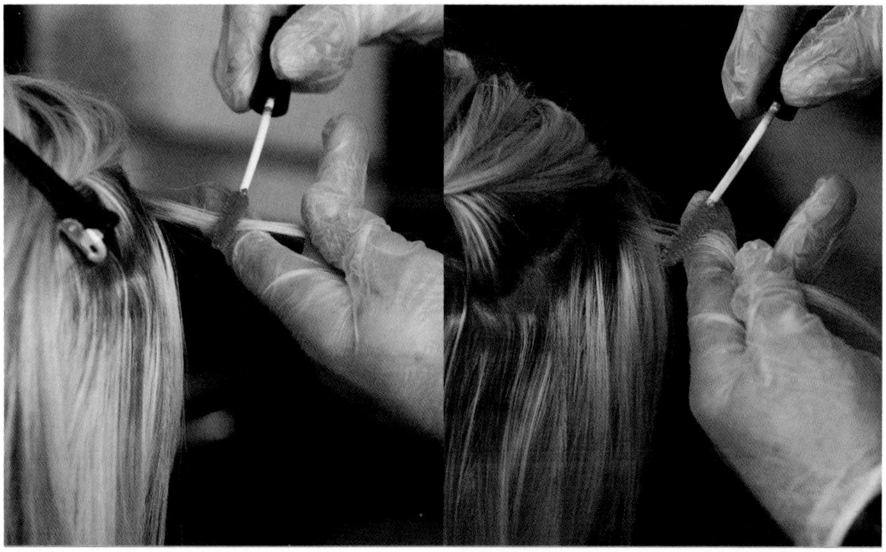

Apply colour using wand

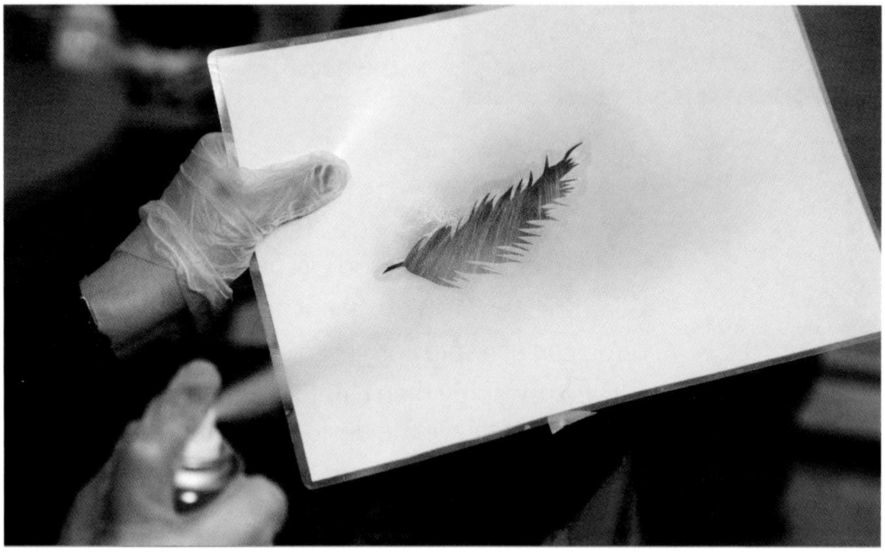

Using spray and stencil

OTHER METHODS AND TECHNIQUES

There are many other methods and techniques that you can use to apply temporary colour. Here are some examples.

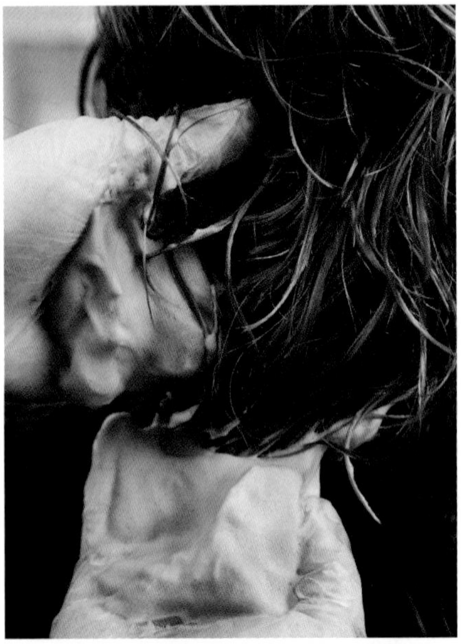

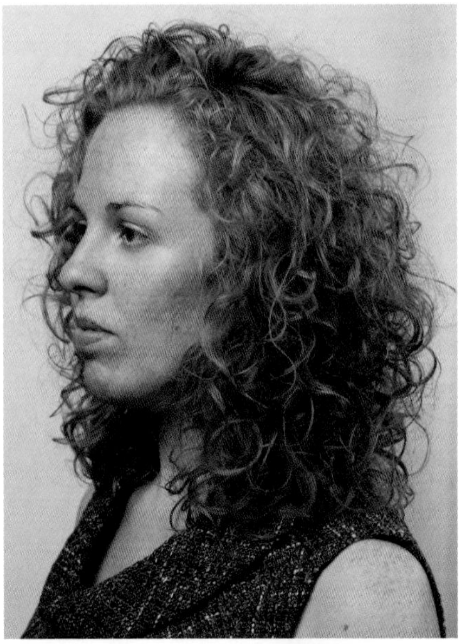

Scrunching

This could be used when you are creating a natural look to your style, usually on curly/wavy hair.

- Spread some colour on to the palm of the hand and then 'scrunch' the hair with the hand. This will spread colour onto some parts of the hair but not all.
- It will give a 'mottled' or highlighted effect on the hair.
- It can be carried out as you dry the hair using the diffuser.
- Make sure you wear gloves when you apply the colour.

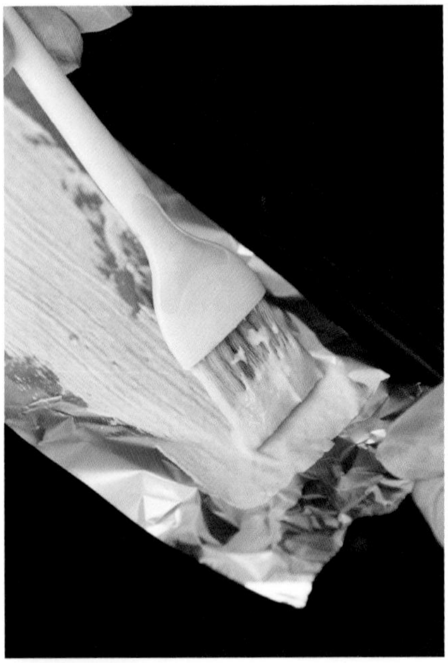

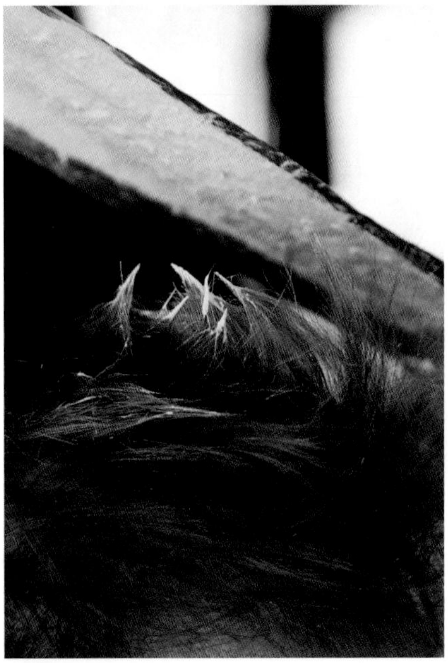

Shoe shining

This is a method of applying colour using a technique similar to shining shoes. It is best used on short hair that has a textured, spiky look.

- You will need to use gel or colour paints for this method.
- Take a strip of foil and brush some colour across the surface.
- Take the strip in both hands and lightly rub it across the surface of the hair.
- Keep the foil quite tight.
- You do not need to touch all the hair.

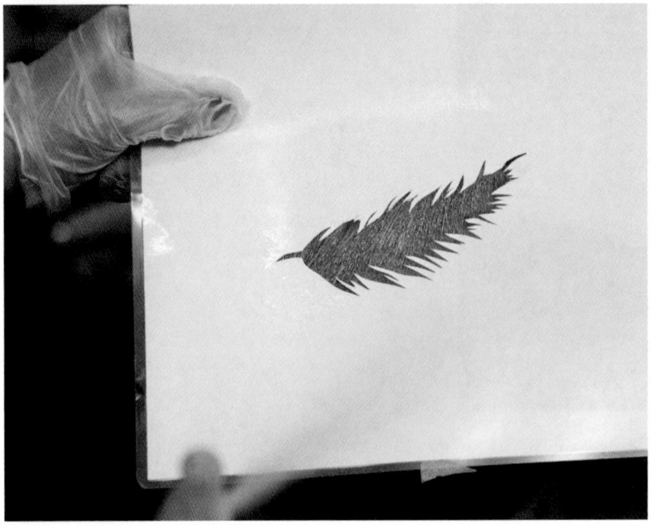

Stencilling

This is a method used to create patterns and designs on the hair. You will need a stencil with the design you want cut out. The method will be used on styled hair.

- Lay the stencil on the hair where you want it to be.
- You can use spray or gel colour.
- If you use spray then carefully spray over the stencil until you achieve the desired result.
- You could use gel colours and paint carefully, using the stencil as your guide.

REMOVING COLOURING PRODUCTS

To remove colouring products correctly you should read the manufacturer's instructions so that you follow the procedure recommended by them. Always follow instructions from the stylist when removing colour.

HANDY HINTS

Remember to check that the colour has been removed from the nape area when using a backwash basin.

HANDY HINTS

Be very careful not to let the water run down the sides of the client's face and neck when rinsing. The colour you are rinsing out of the hair may stain the clothes.

SEMI-PERMANENT COLOURS

The procedure for applying and removing a semi-permanent colour is:

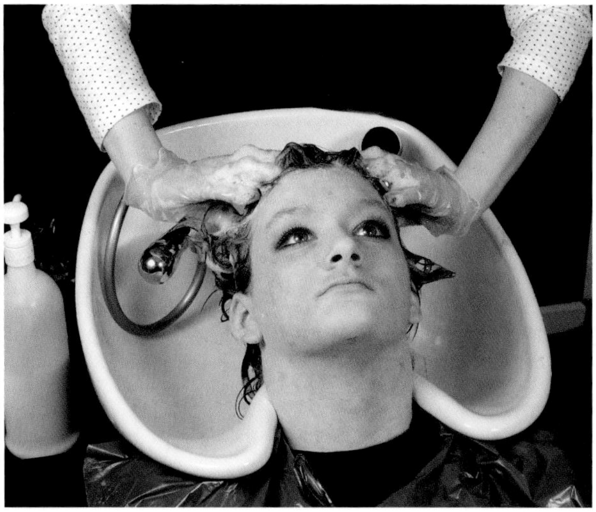

STEP 1 – Gown and protect your client and shampoo their hair.

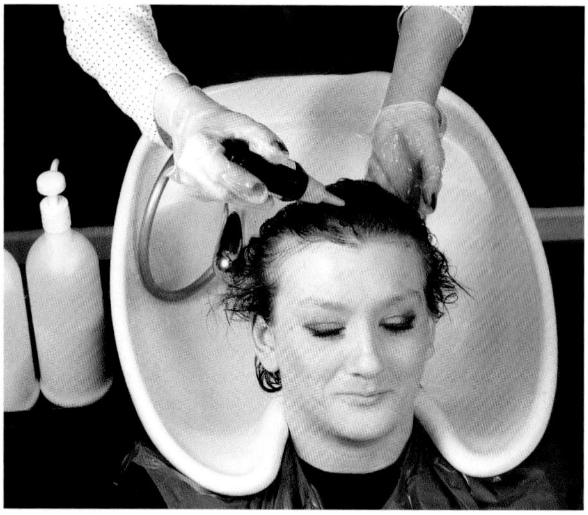

STEP 2 – Evenly apply the semi-permanent colour directly from the applicator bottle.

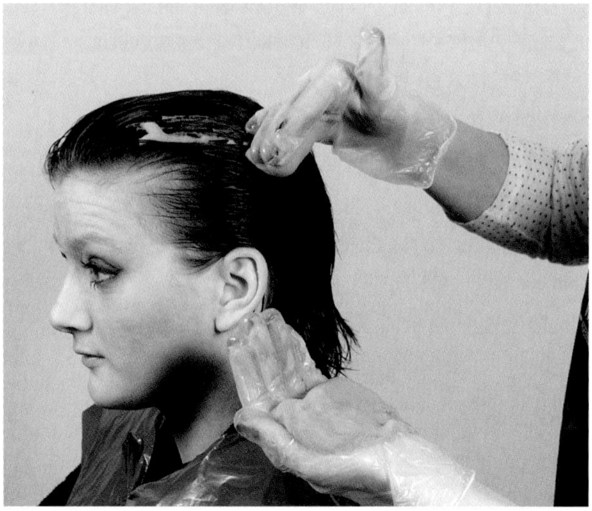

STEP 3 – Make sure the hair is covered evenly, then develop following the manufacturer's instructions.

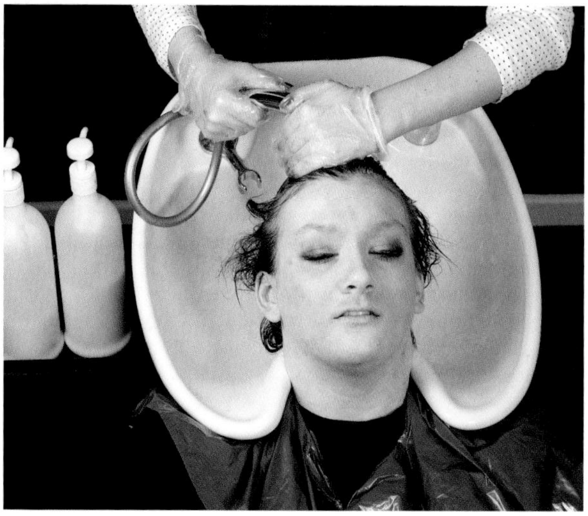

STEP 4 – Sit the client comfortably for the development time, add water to **emulsify**, then rinse thoroughly and condition the hair.

Emulsify

To combine two liquids together

PERMANENT COLOURS

Permanent colours are normally applied to dry hair. The procedure for removing the colour is:

1 Check that the gown, towel and cape are in the correct position.
2 Seat the client at the basin and make sure she is comfortable.
3 Turn on the water and check the temperature.
4 Add some water to the hair.
5 Using rotary massage, emulsify the colour and water. Make sure you cover all of the scalp to loosen the colour.
6 Check the water temperature.
7 Rinse the hair until the water runs clear. Check the nape area if you are using a backwash basin.
8 Shampoo the hair, using a shampoo for coloured hair.
9 Condition the hair using an **anti-oxidant conditioner**.

Anti-oxidant conditioner
A conditioner that stops the chemical action of colouring and lightening products

QUASI-PERMANENT COLOURS

Quasi-permanent colours are removed in the same way as permanent colours. Make sure you check that all the colour has been removed from the nape area when using a backwash basin.

LIGHTENING PRODUCTS

Bleaches and high-lift colours are removed in the same way as permanent colours.

1 Check the gown, towel and cape are in the correct position.
2 Seat the client at the basin and make sure she is comfortable.
3 Turn on the water and check the temperature.
4 Add some water to the hair.
5 If you are removing bleach products the water will loosen the bleach. Gentle massage will continue to loosen the product which can then be rinsed out of the hair.
6 If you are removing high-lift colour then use a gentle rotary massage technique to emulsify the colour.
7 Check the water temperature.
8 Rinse the hair until the water runs clear. Check the nape area if you are using a backwash basin.
9 Shampoo the hair, using a shampoo for coloured hair.
10 Condition the hair using an anti-oxidant conditioner.

HANDY HINTS

Do not use very hot water when removing the permanent colour or lightening products. The scalp may be tender after the chemical process. Cooler water will be more comfortable for the client.

APPLYING AND REMOVING COLOUR OR LIGHTENING PRODUCTS WHEN USING CAPS AND FOILS

Caps and foils are two methods of adding partial colour such as highlights and lowlights using permanent and lightening products.

Cap method

For the cap method a plastic or soft rubber cap is placed over the client's hair. The cap will have a series of holes in it. A crochet hook is used to pull small quantities of hair through each hole. The stylist will decide how much hair will be pulled through the holes and which holes are used. The hair that is pulled through is then coloured or lightened.

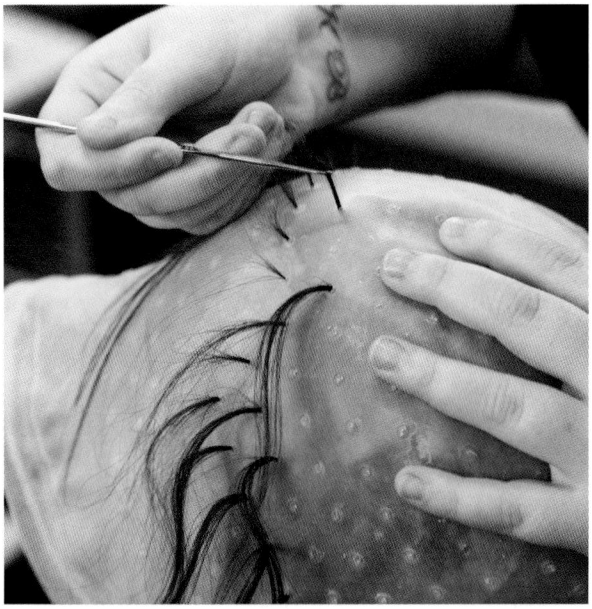

STEP 1 – Use a crochet hook to pull a small section of hair through the holes in the cap.

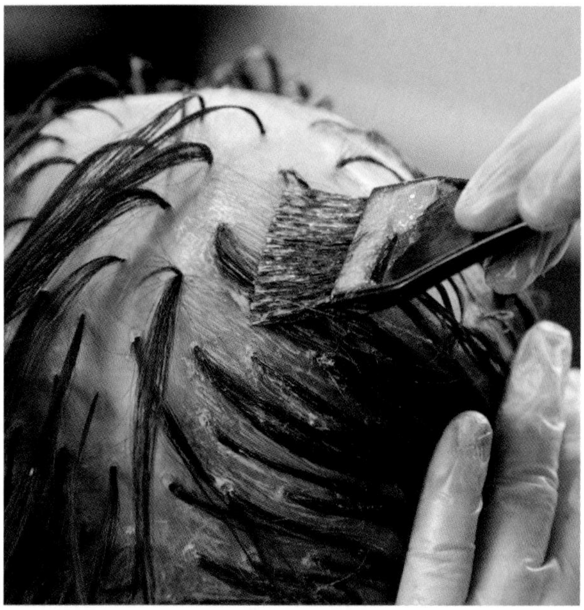

STEP 2 – Apply the colour to the sections of hair that have been pulled through the cap.

To remove the colour you should follow these steps:

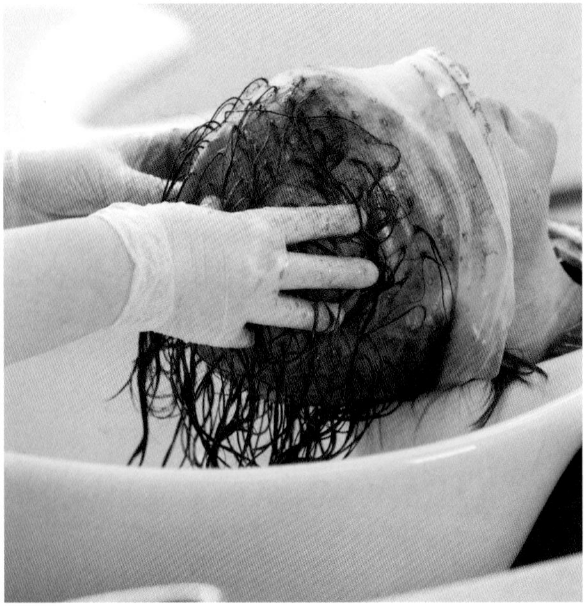

STEP 1 – Add a little water to emulsify the colour. Massage the hair to loosen the colour.

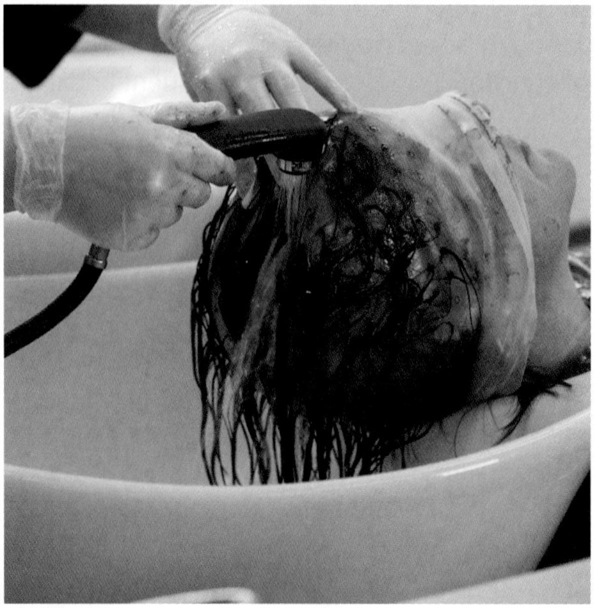

STEP 2 – Rinse the hair thoroughly to remove all the excess colour. Apply a conditioner and gently ease the cap from the hair.

HANDY HINTS

Don't forget to use a clean towel to towel dry the hair. The towel that was round the client's shoulders may be contaminated with colour.

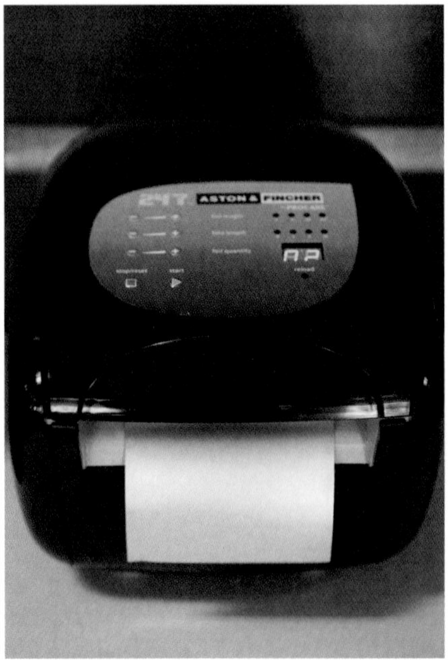

Woven method

The woven method is another method of partially colouring the hair. This can be achieved using foils, meches or wraps.

To apply colour using a meche you should follow these steps:

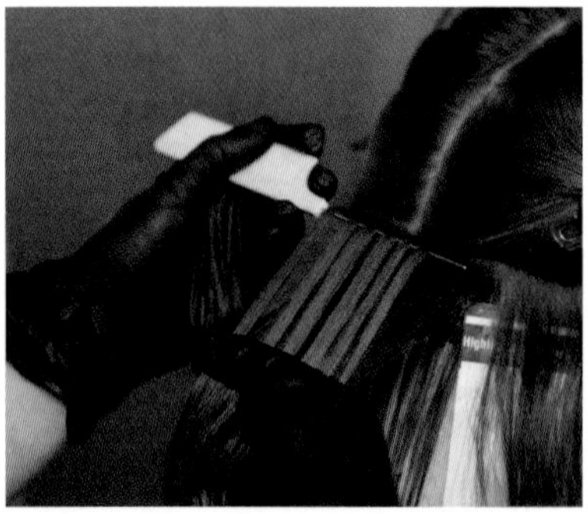

STEP 1 – Divide the hair to be coloured into manageable sections, and weave your section.

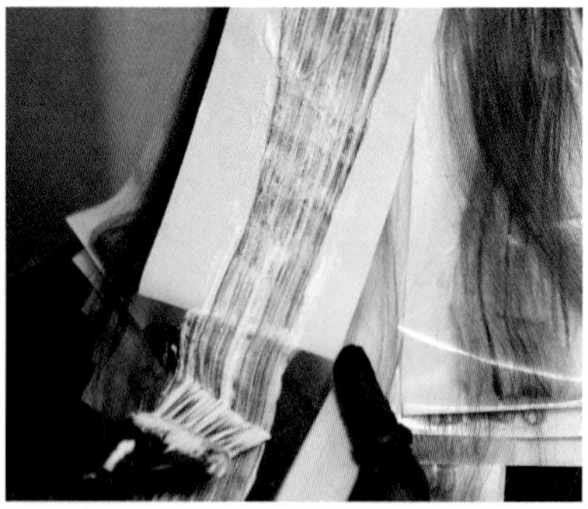

STEP 2 – Apply the product evenly without overloading the root area.

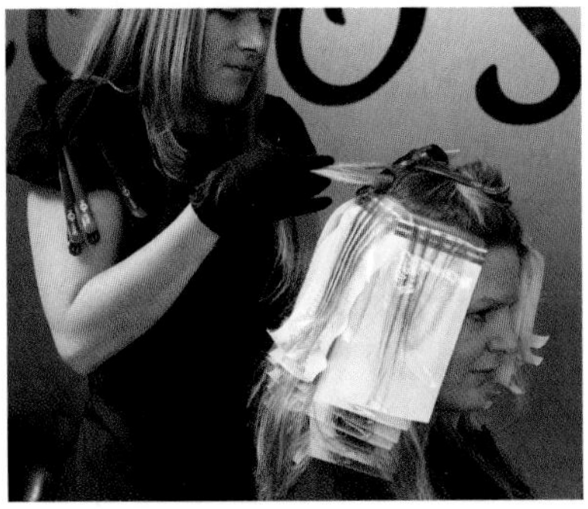

STEP 3 – Work in a methodical manner, towards the top of the head.

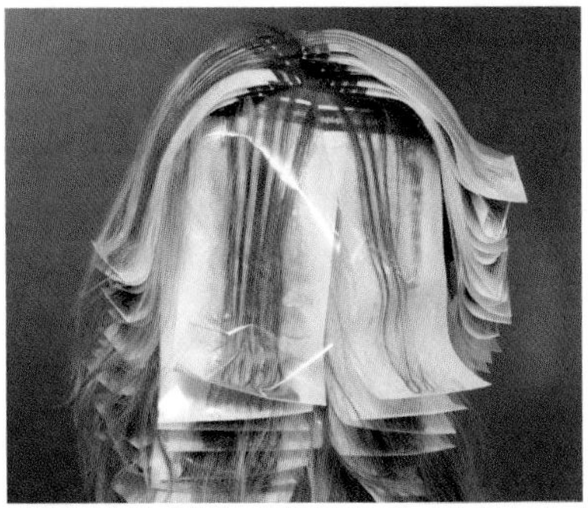

STEP 4 – When you have completed all the hair, leave it to develop.

HANDY HINTS

Always follow the instructions of the stylist when you are removing caps and foils.

ACTIVITY

In a group, make a list of the ways in which you would safely and hygienically remove foil and meche woven highlights.

IN A NUTSHELL

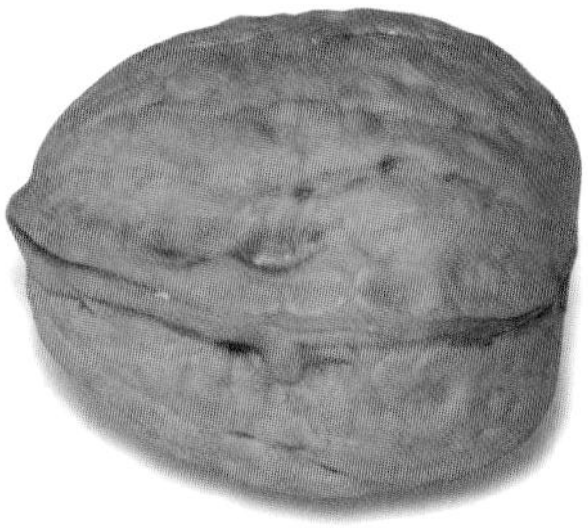

You are now at the end of the chapter. Before you test your knowledge with the revision activities, check the following list to see if you feel confident in all the areas covered. If there are still any areas you're unsure of, go back over them in the book and ask your tutor for extra support:

- the purpose and effect of colouring products
- the factors that can influence your choice of temporary colouring products and method of application
- how to prepare for temporary colouring procedures
- the different types of temporary colouring products
- the different procedures used in temporary colouring
- following safe and hygienic working practices
- the importance of good communication, behaviour and attitude
- how to apply a temporary colour
- how to remove colouring products from the hair.

REVISION ACTIVITIES

Use the questions below to test your knowledge of Chapter 111 to see just how much information you've gained. This can help you prepare for your assessments. Turn to pages 505–506 for the answers.

CROSSWORD

See if you can answer the questions and write them in the crossword.

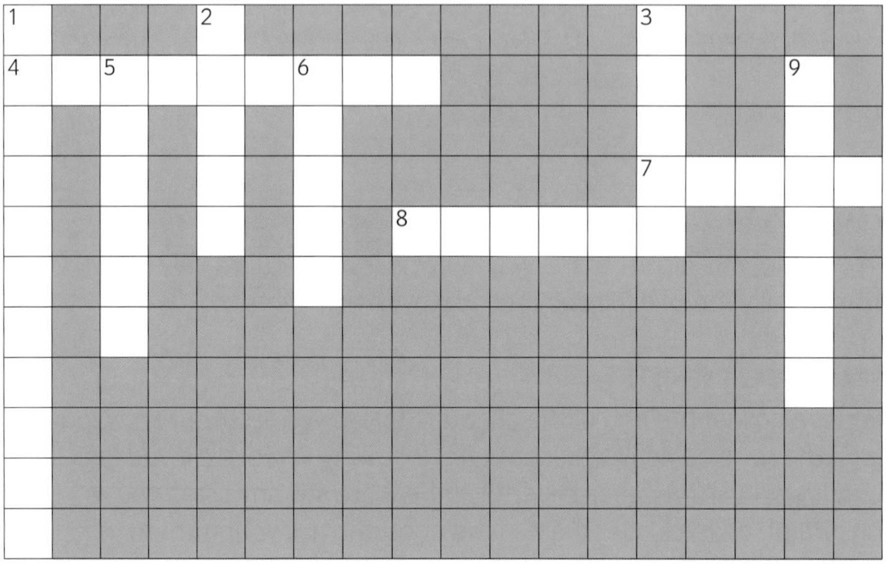

Across

4 A colour that lasts only one shampoo

7 The lightness or darkness of the client's natural colour

8 You use these to protect your hands from staining and contact dermatitis

Down

1 A method used to create patterns or designs on the hair

2 This is used to protect the client's clothes

3 'Mascara'-type applicators, used to add colour to some areas

5 This type of temporary colour is applied to wet hair

6 This is used to protect the stylist's clothing

9 The outer layer of the hair shaft

WORDS TO FIND

Copy and complete the sentences below. Use these words to help you fill in the gaps.

depth	anti-oxidant	shoe shining	porous
scrunching	wands	semi-permanent	melanin
apron	lightener	disposable gloves	colour paints

1 The pigment cells in the hair are called ______________ .

2 ______________ should be used to protect the hands when using colour.

3 An ______________ is worn to protect the stylist's clothes when colouring.

4 A ______________ colour lasts for six to eight shampoos.

5 How light or dark the hair colour is called the ______________ .

6 Hair that absorbs water easily is said to be ______________ .

7 An ______________ conditioner is used after colouring to remove oxygen.

8 ______________ is used to achieve blonde shades.

9 ______________ and ______________ are two types of temporary colour.

10 Two methods of colouring hair are ______________ and ______________ .

TEST YOUR KNOWLEDGE FURTHER

1 List the PPE that you would need to use when carrying out a temporary colour service.

2 Temporary colours can lighten a client's natural colour. True or false?

3 Why is important to behave professionally when you are working?

4 Name **three** factors that can influence your choice of temporary colouring technique.

5 Name **three** types of temporary colouring product.

6 Name **two** methods of using temporary colour for a partial-head application.

7 Name the three layers of the hair shaft.

8 How would you find out how the colour should be used?

9 Why should you wear disposable gloves when applying or removing colour products?

10 Describe briefly how you would remove a semi-permanent colour.

215 THE ART OF DRESSING HAIR

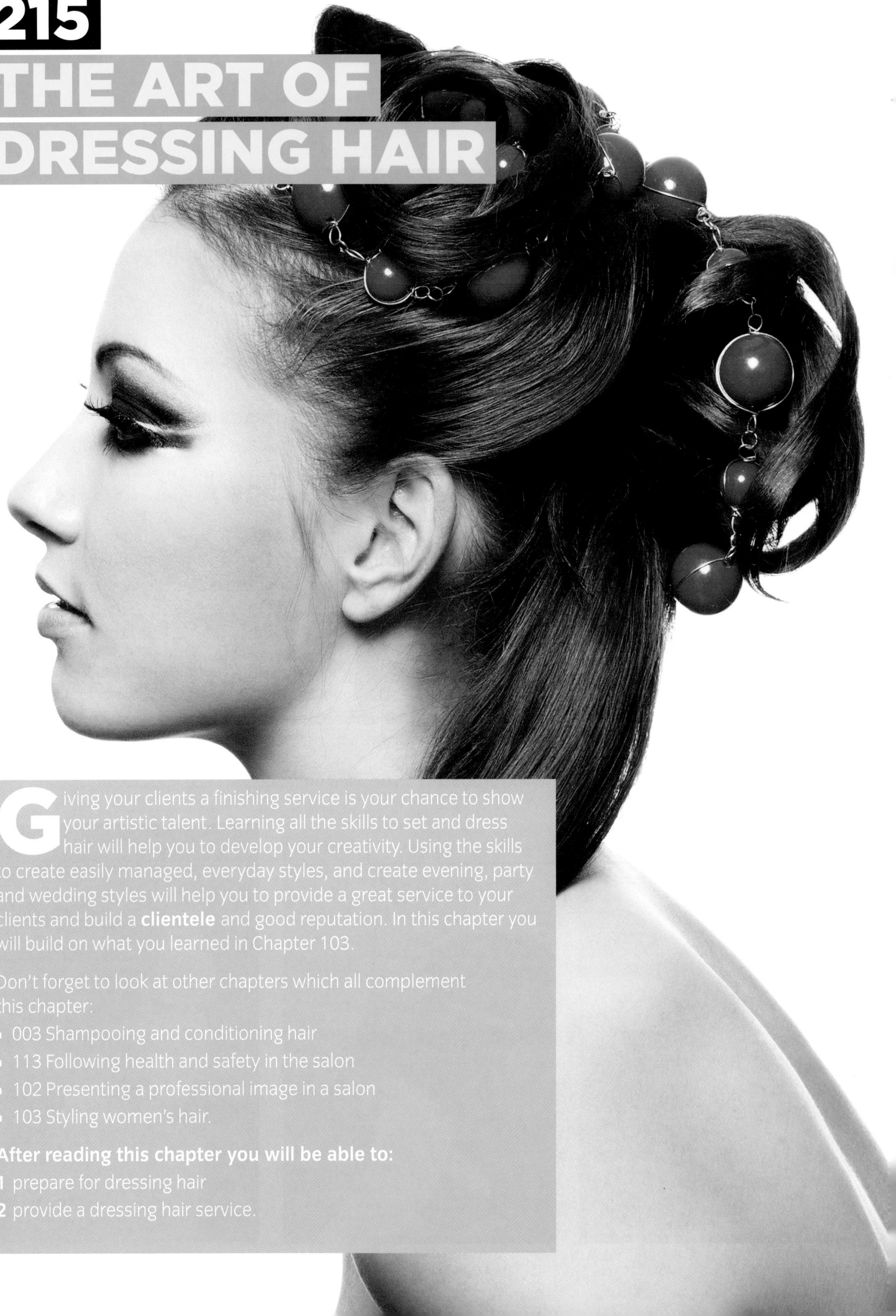

Giving your clients a finishing service is your chance to show your artistic talent. Learning all the skills to set and dress hair will help you to develop your creativity. Using the skills to create easily managed, everyday styles, and create evening, party and wedding styles will help you to provide a great service to your clients and build a **clientele** and good reputation. In this chapter you will build on what you learned in Chapter 103.

Don't forget to look at other chapters which all complement this chapter:

- 003 Shampooing and conditioning hair
- 113 Following health and safety in the salon
- 102 Presenting a professional image in a salon
- 103 Styling women's hair.

After reading this chapter you will be able to:

1 prepare for dressing hair

2 provide a dressing hair service.

HANDY HINTS

Read Chapter 103 Styling women's hair to refresh your knowledge of the basics of styling and finishing hair.

Clientele
Your customers

Chapter 103 Styling women's hair describes the basic techniques that can be used for styling women's hair. In this chapter you will learn more about styling techniques to improve your knowledge and skills in dressing hair.

PREPARE FOR DRESSING HAIR

In this part of the chapter you will build on knowledge gained from Chapter 103 and learn more about the following:

- the procedure for client preparation
- the effects of different styling techniques
- the factors that need to be considered when styling and dressing hair
- the physical effects of styling on the hair structure
- the effects of humidity on the hair structure and resulting style
- how the incorrect use of heat can affect the hair and scalp.

STYLING TECHNIQUES FOR DRESSING HAIR

BLOW DRYING

Blow drying is the most popular of all the styling techniques. Most clients will have their hair cut and blow dried. The cut puts shape and direction into the hair. Blow drying will provide the right finish to that shape. It can also enhance the shape with smoothness, lift, curl and **texture**.

Texture
What the hair feels like

The range of effects is achieved by using the different brushes available for blow drying. The 'Denman' brush is used to give a smooth finish to medium and long hair. The radial or round brush is used to give lift, curl and volume to your style.

Styling products can be used enhance the style you create.

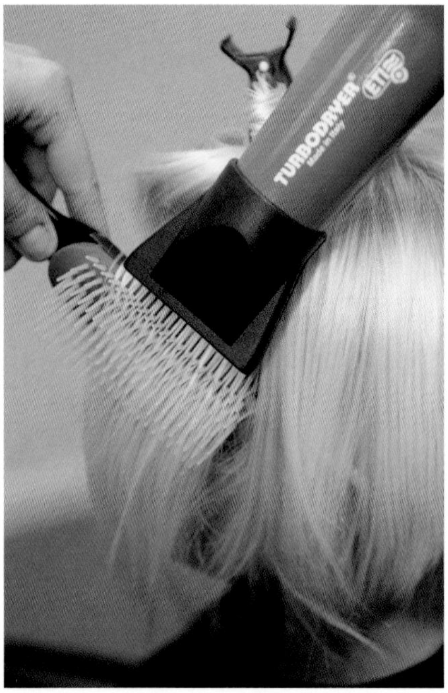

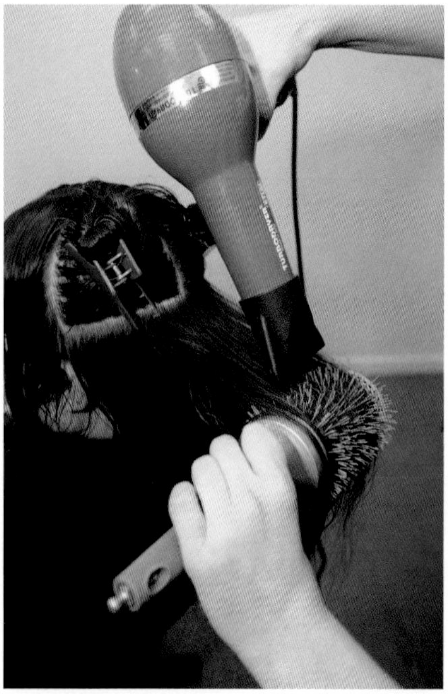

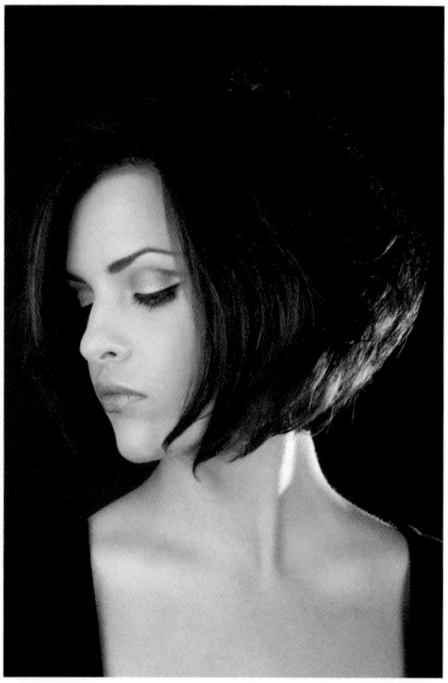

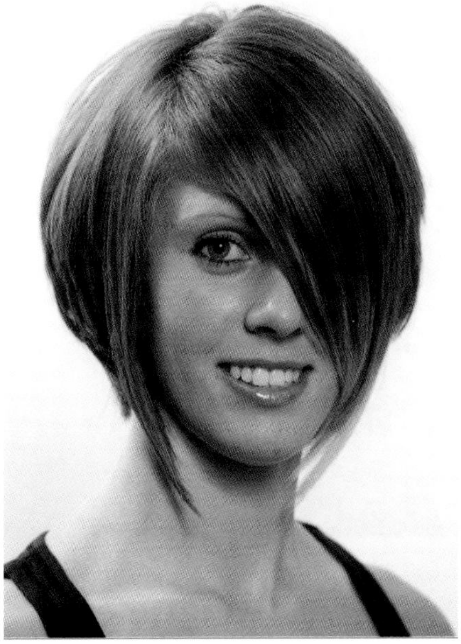

Textured short blow dry

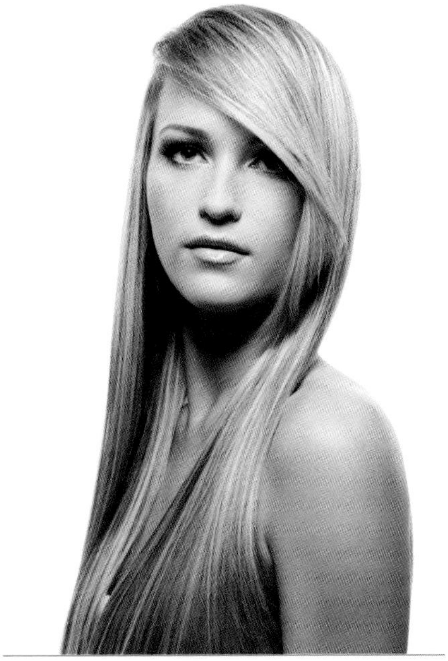

Long hair blow dry

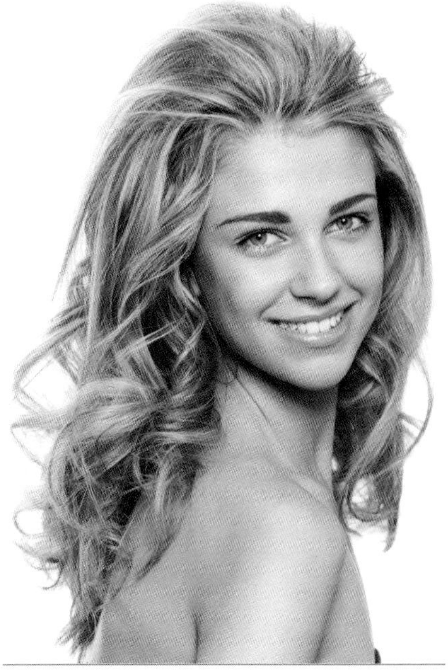

Blow dry with lift, volume and curl

FINGER DRYING

Finger drying is a technique similar to blow drying. The hair is dried using the fingers instead of a brush. It is carried out on wet hair and gives soft, natural-looking styles. This technique can be used on most lengths of hair, and works well on short hair. The fingers are used to mould the hair into shape and direction. The fingers can be used to lift the hair as it is dried to increase volume.

Lifting the hair and closing the fingers in a clawing movement will add texture and volume to the style. This is known as finger drying.

SmartScreen 215 worksheet 3

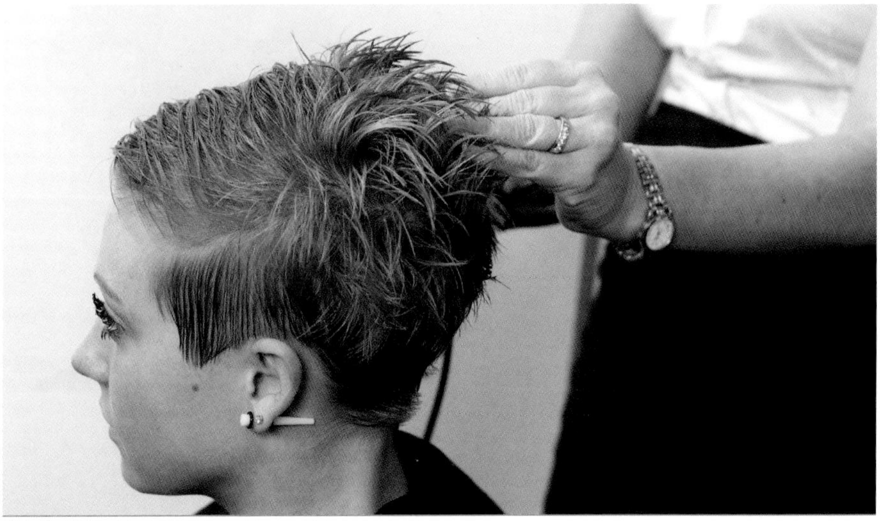

Apply the product and start to style the hair using your fingers

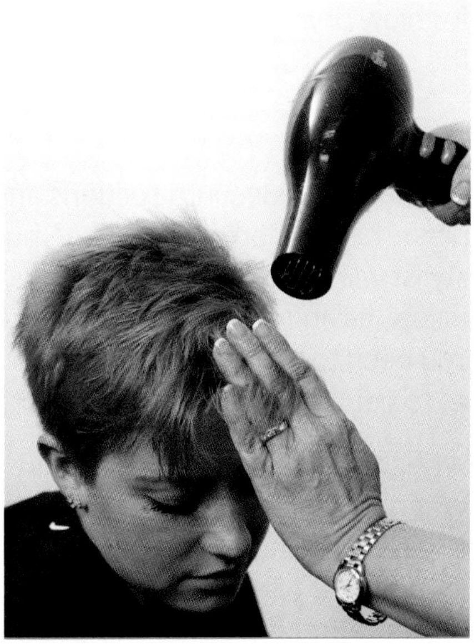

Make sure the airflow follows the direction of the hairstyle

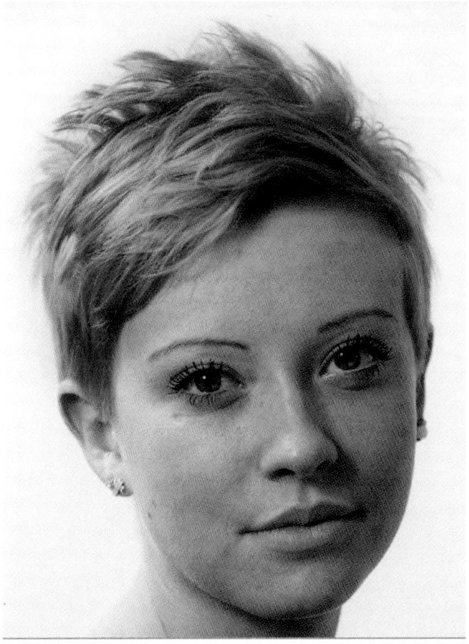

Check the client is happy with the finished look

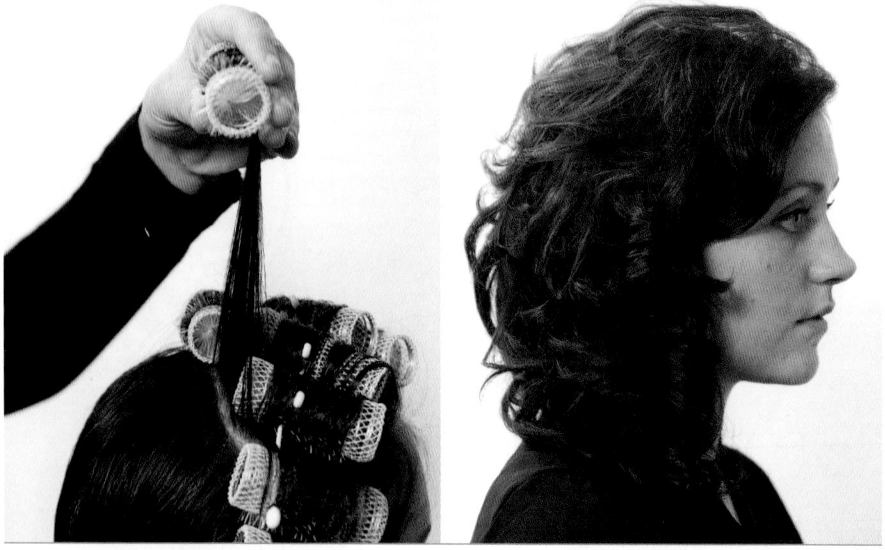

Hair set on small rollers

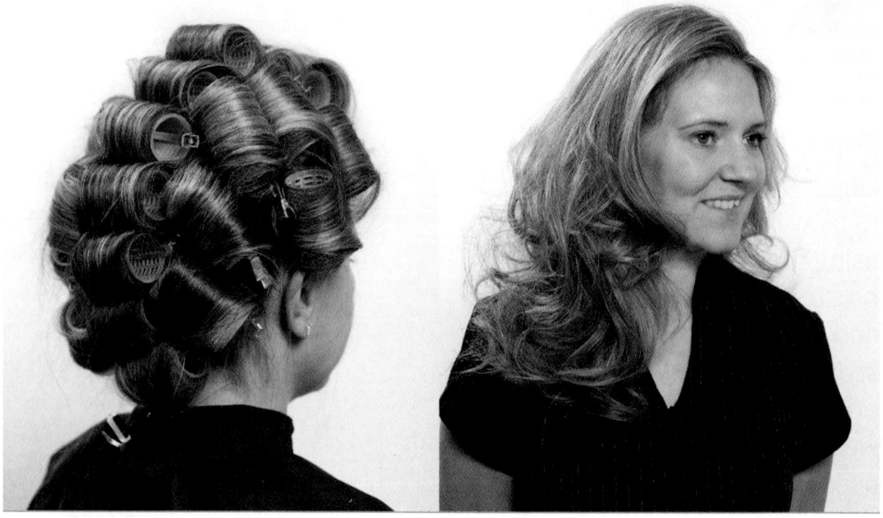

Hair set on large rollers

SETTING

Setting the hair using rollers is a widely used styling technique carried out on wet or dry hair. It is very useful on hair that is fine and not suitable for blow drying. Unlike blow drying, it does not rely on the cut to decide the shape of the finished style.

HANDY HINTS

Look back at Chapter 102 for more information on consultation techniques.

WET SETTING

The hair is divided into sections and the rollers are put in and held with pins. The position of the rollers is decided by the finished style. The stylist will decide the size of rollers and the pattern they are going to follow, having consulted with the client and agreed the finished look. You need to make sure you have put the rollers in the right place so as to get the right direction and shape when the hair is dry.

When the rollers have been put in, the hair is dried under a hood dryer. When dry and cool the rollers are removed and the hair is brushed and combed into the agreed shape. Different sized rollers are used for different effects. Small rollers are used to give tighter curls; larger rollers give softer curls. The size of curl will depend on two things: the size of the roller and the length of the hair.

Roller setting is very useful for styling longer hair and is often used for a 'hair up'. This is a style on long hair where the hair is kept in place with pins and grips. It is used to create styles for special occasions such as weddings, evenings out and parties. The rollers are used to give lift and curl to the hair. For a hair-up style the direction of the hair when it is dressed out is controlled by the grips and pins you use to keep the hair in place.

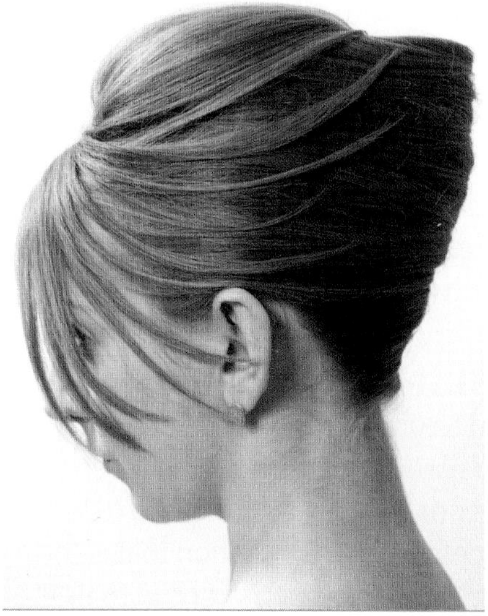

French pleat

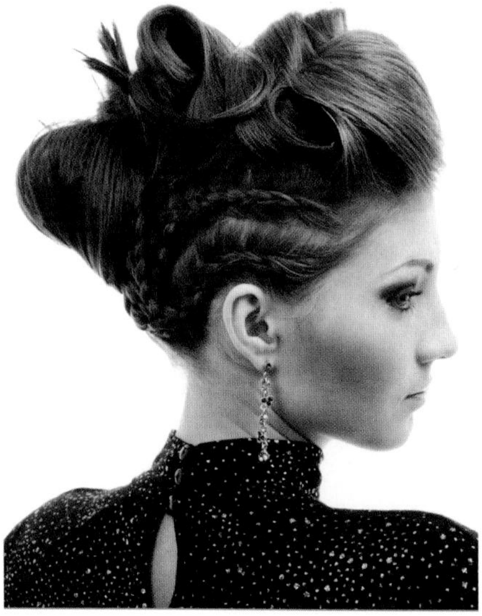

A party look

PIN CURLING

Pin curling is a method of styling where the hair is formed into a curl and then kept in place with a clip. This technique is used to achieve wave movements in the hair. It can also be used with a roller set to give some movement in the short hair in the nape area. Pin curling is carried out on wet hair. The hair is dried and then brushed and combed into shape.

There are four types of pin curl:

Barrel-spring curls

These are used to produce flat waves and curls in the hair. They are often used with roller setting to add curl to the nape area of the head if the hair is short or if you do not want any lift to that area.

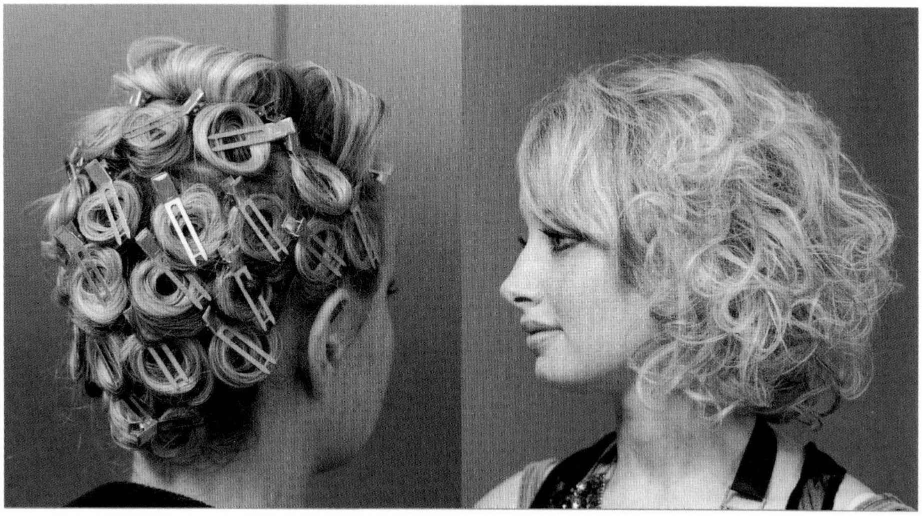

Barrel-spring curls

Barrel-spring curls can be wound in rows, one row wound to the right and the next row to the left. This will produce a wave effect with very little lift.

If the curl is secured through one side of the curl only and the other side lifted, this will produce deeper waves in the hair (this type of pin curl is known as a stand-up pin curl).

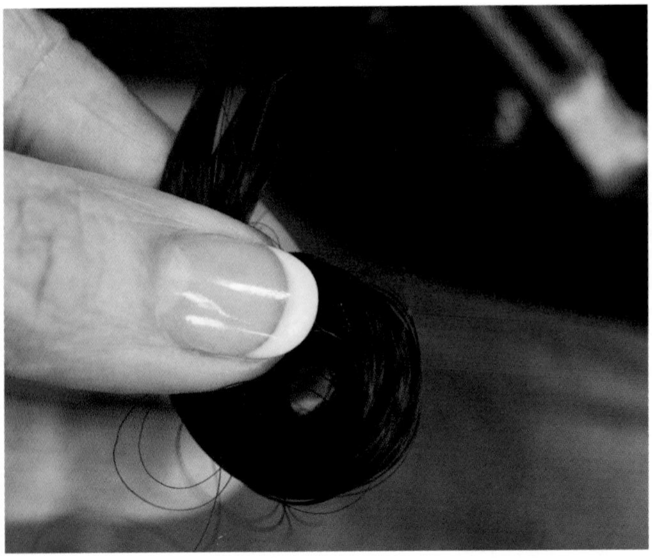

Clock-spring curls
Clock-spring curls are used to give a 'ringlet' effect. They are very useful around the hairline of a client with long hair.

Stem curls
These are made in the same way as barrel spring curls but are not wound up to the base. They are useful to give a flat curl with no lift at the roots.

BARREL CURLING

Barrel curls are used to give lift and curl in place of rollers. No two heads are the same size and when you are roller setting it is not always easy to fit the rollers exactly. You will sometimes have a section that is too small to fit the roller. You can use a barrel curl to fill the gap. They can also be used where you want changes of direction but rollers are too big. The barrel curls will need to be 'plugged' with a piece of cotton wool before drying to stop them being pushed out of shape.

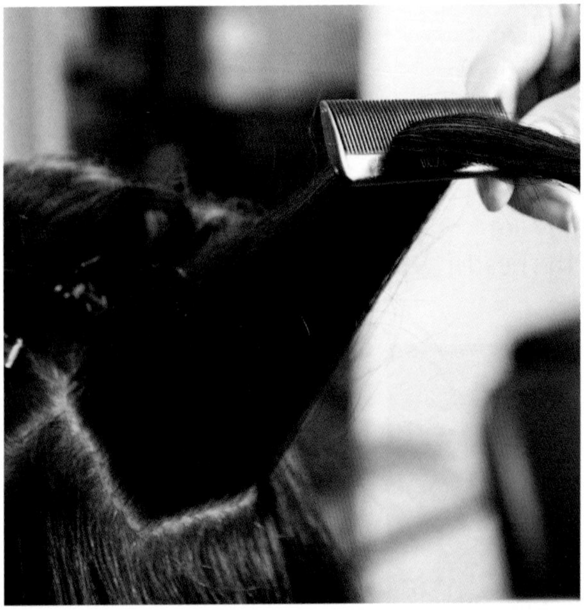

STEP 1 – Gown and prepare the client and section the hair.

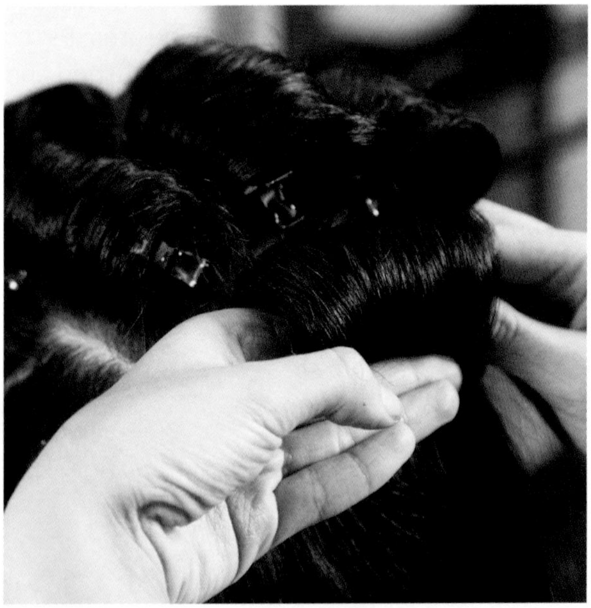

STEP 2 – Form the curl by winding the hair from the points to the roots using the fingers.

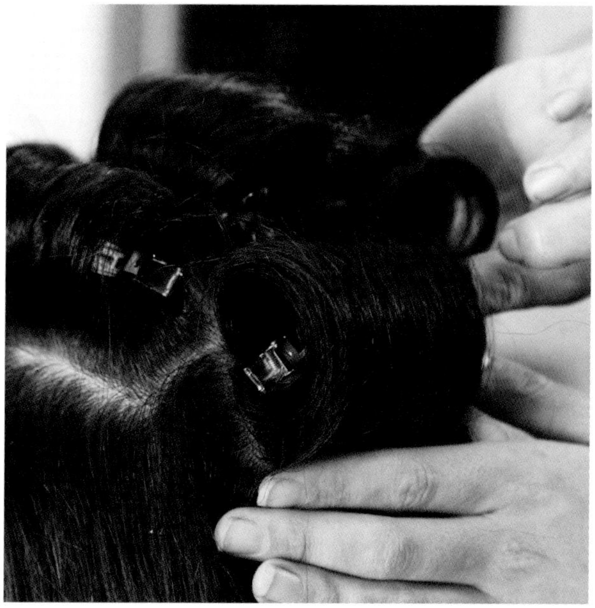

STEP 3 – Secure the curl with a pin curl clip through the base.

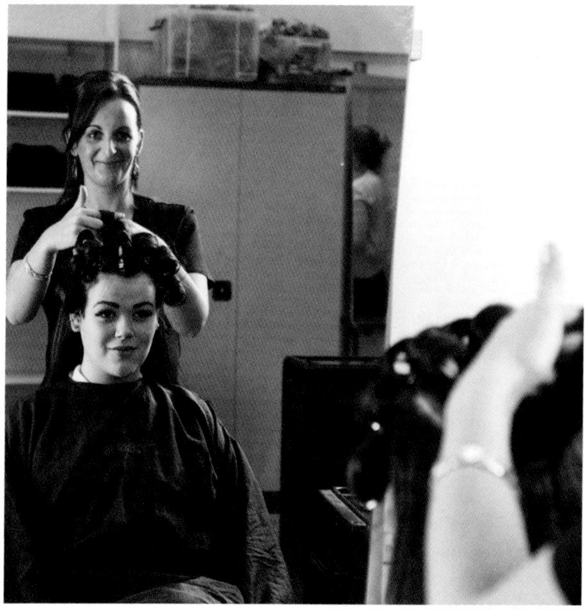

STEP 4 – Repeat the process in the direction of the style.

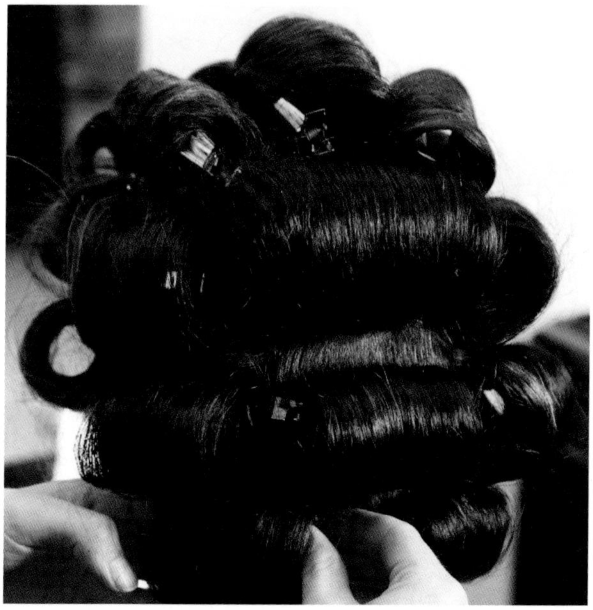

STEP 5 – Make sure the curl sits on the base and is open at the centre.

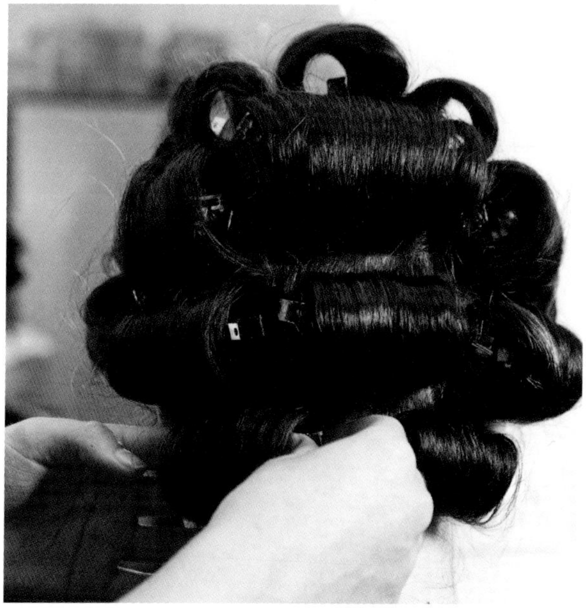

STEP 6 – Check that the curls are secure and 'plug' with cotton wool before drying if necessary.

FINGER WAVING

This is a styling technique that is used to produce a strong wave movement in the hair. The wave is made using the fingers of one hand and a cutting comb in the other.

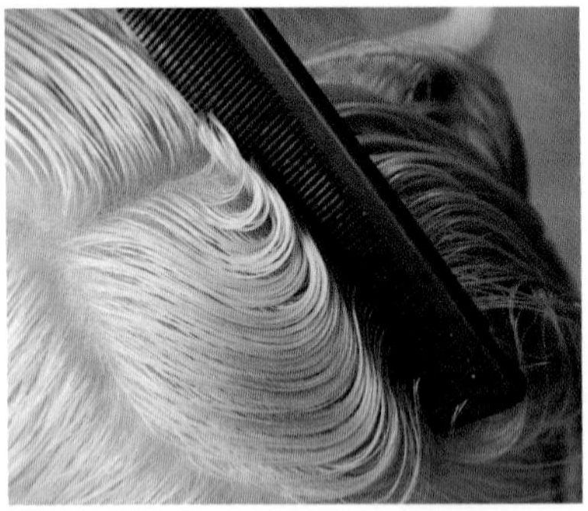

STEP 1 – Form the wave using a cutting comb and the fingers.

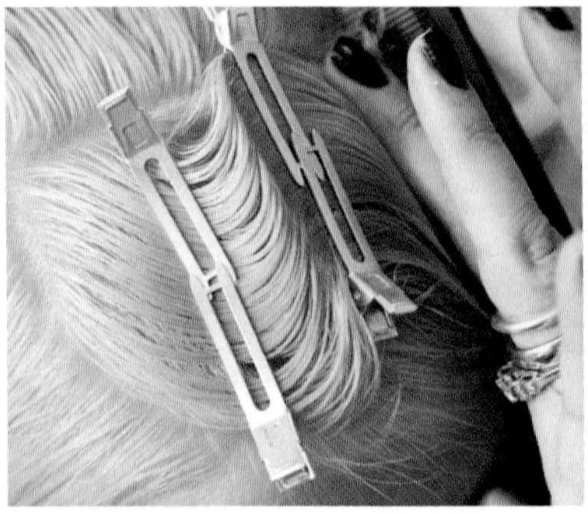

STEP 2 – Secure the wave using sectioning clips.

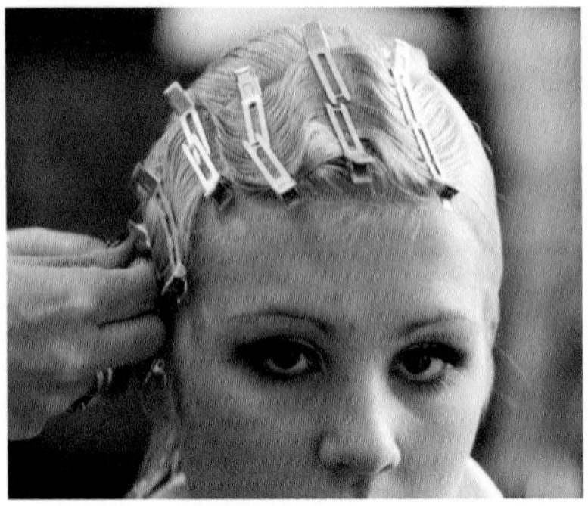

STEP 3 – Finish each section with a pin curl.

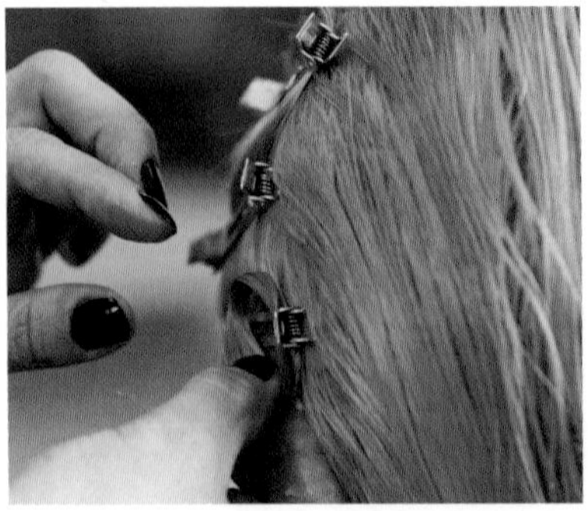

STEP 4 – Secure the pin curl with a pin curl clip.

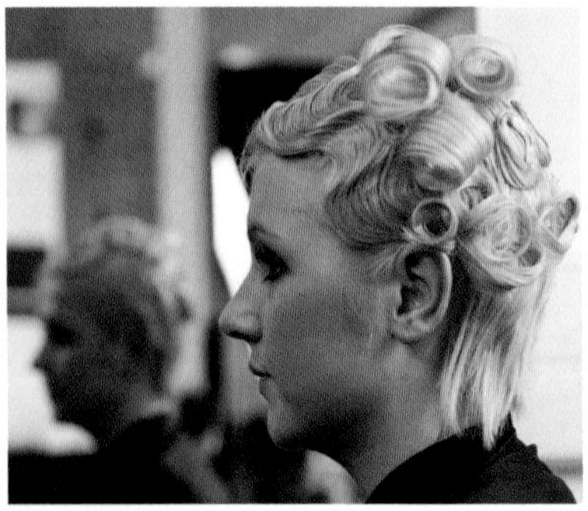

STEP 5 – Let the hair cool after drying and remove the clips.

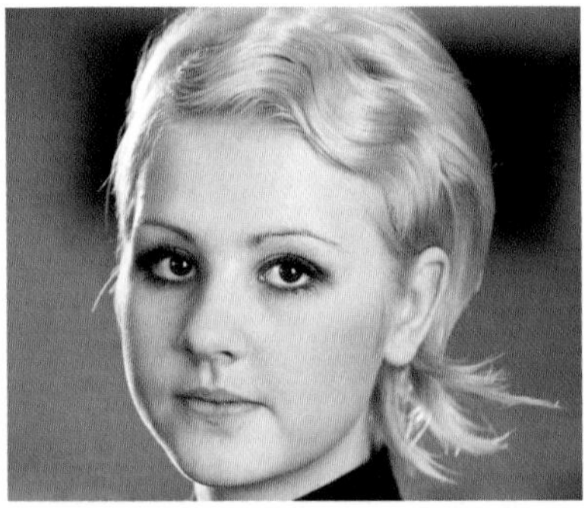

STEP 6 – The finished style.

The next group of styling methods are carried out on dry hair. They can be used on their own to style the hair or as part of other methods. The appliances used are heated and the heat produces the finish. Care must be taken to prevent damage to the hair by using too much heat.

STRAIGHTENING AND SMOOTHING

This **technique** uses straighteners to produce a straight, smooth finish. The straighteners are available in different sizes for use on different lengths of hair. It is very useful on clients with longer hair that has a natural curl. It can be used after blow drying to get a smooth finish to the style. It can also be used to prepare long hair for a 'hair-up' style.

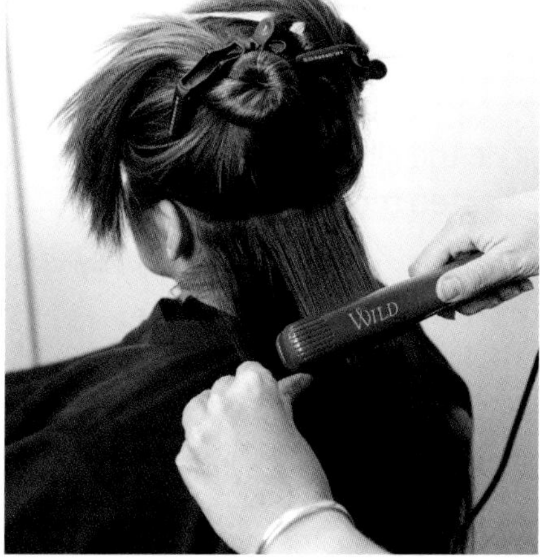

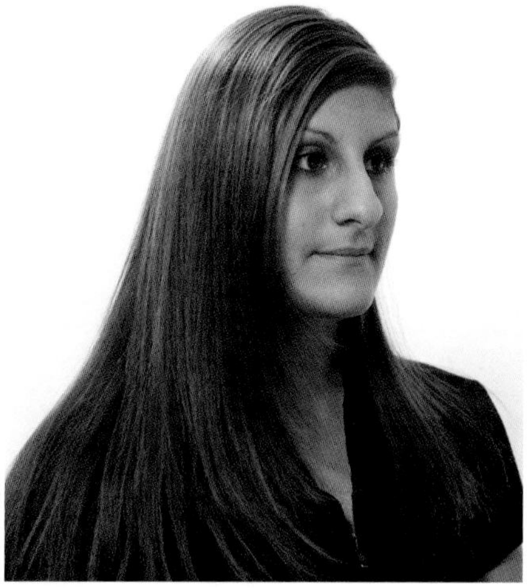

CURLING

This is a widely used technique that adds lift and curl to a blow dry. It can also be used to 'freshen up' a blow dry or set after a few days. This is a useful technique to add curl to sections of hair when you are doing a 'hair-up' on long hair. It is very useful on fine hair to give body.

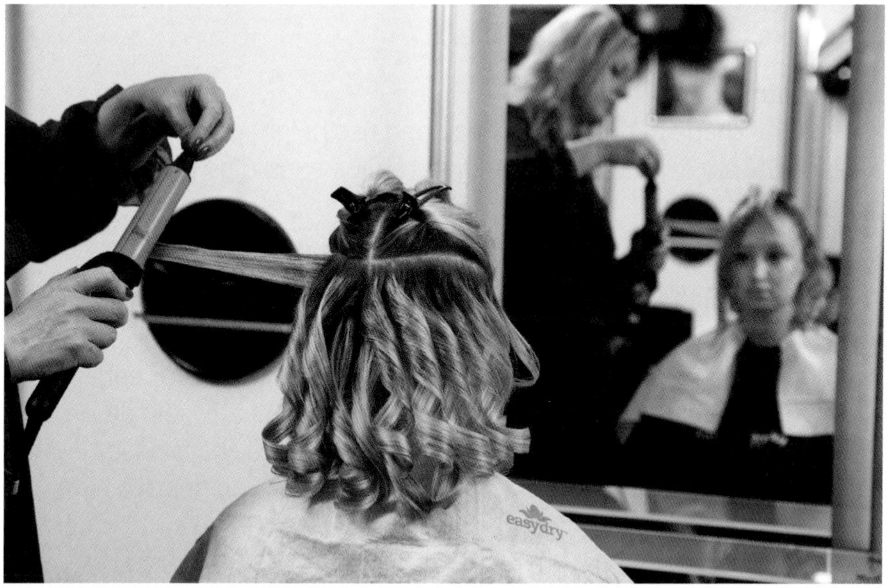

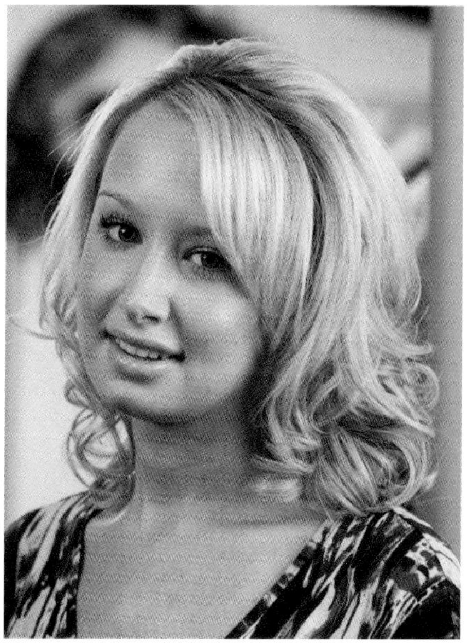

ACTIVITY

Find some pictures of styles that are achieved by these styling techniques. Make some notes of how they were done. Keep your pictures for your assignment.

Technique
Way of doing something

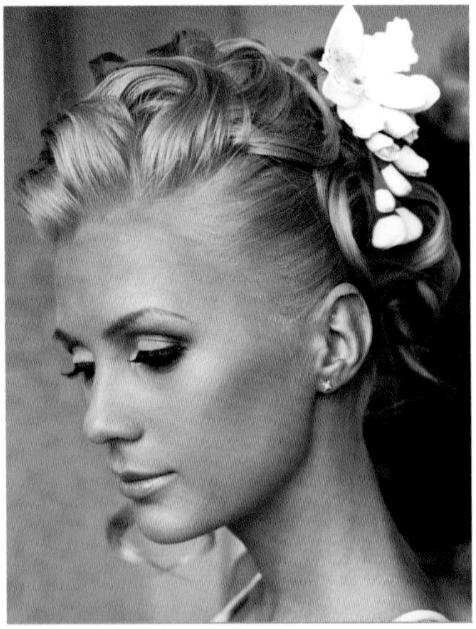
Wedding style

FACTORS THAT CAN INFLUENCE YOUR CHOICE OF STYLING TECHNIQUES

There are many factors that you will need to take into account when you are deciding which technique you are going to use to achieve the style the client wants. They will also help you decide how to use the selected technique.

THE CLIENT

The first group of factors are about the client's face shape, build and lifestyle. When you are deciding on the style you want to create for the client and the techniques and products you will need to select to achieve it, the head and face type are important. You will need to consider carefully the client's face shape, head shape, their facial features and body shape. All these things will help you design the perfect style for your client. You will want to create a style that balances features, hide some features and highlights others.

Face shape

You should always try to achieve an oval finish to the style by using height and width to adjust the actual shape of the face. For example, on round faces keep the sides of the style flatter and add some height. For square faces soften the jaw line.

Head shape

Look at the shape of the client's head and use height and width to balance the style. Face shape and head shape should be thought about together.

Facial features

The features of the face are important when you are designing a style for your client. Looking at the nose, the ears, the jaw and the eyes will help you decide if your style needs to hide certain features and/or enhance others. For example, if the client has protruding ears they should be covered. Don't use a centre parting if the client has a sharp nose. Don't choose styles that draw attention to features you need to hide.

Body shape

Look at the body shape in relation to the client's head. You are looking to balance the head and the body. If the client is very slim, using too much height, width and volume in your style can make the head look too big.

Lifestyle

The client's lifestyle is a very important factor in the styling process. Your style has to enhance their personality, their age and outlook, their clothes and make-up, and their job.

Would the style suit the job they do? Can you design a style that could be changed into something more fashionable for the client's evening and leisure time?

You will also need to think about how well the client can manage the style you are going to give them. Do they have enough time to do their hair before going to work or sorting out the family? Do they have any disabilities or conditions that may prevent them from keeping the style?

ACTIVITY

Collect a range of photos of people from magazines and on the internet. Try to work out what face shape and head shape they have, and other factors that may have had an effect on their hairstyle. Make notes about each one. Share your collection and notes with others in your group.

THE HAIR

The next group of factors are about the client's hair. You must analyse the client's hair carefully. The type of hair the client has, its texture, condition, elasticity and the density will all need to be thought about when you are deciding what you are going to do.

Texture

Hair texture is about the thickness of each individual hair:

- Fine: the individual hairs will be quite thin. You need to be careful when styling this type of hair as it may be weak. Avoid too much tension and heat.
- Medium: this texture is ideal. Is suited to long and short styles.
- Coarse: there may be too much hair for what you want to do. It can be resistant and harder to curl.

Hair condition

The condition of the hair can affect the style you suggest to the client. It can also affect the method of styling that you will use to achieve the desired result. For example, if the hair is dry or damaged, you should not use too much heat. If the hair is oily and requires frequent washing, a practical easy-to-maintain style should be considered. Using conditioners and conditioning treatments to improve the hair should be suggested.

HANDY HINTS

Read Chapter 103 for more information on hair condition.

ACTIVITY

With other members of your group, look and feel each other's hair and decide what texture the hair is. Compare your analysis with the rest of the group.

Hair density

Check the amount of hair the client has. Is there enough to achieve your planned style? Will the style last long enough for the client to be happy with it?

If the hair is sparse it will be probably be fine and weaker and will not hold the style very well. If there is lots of hair it is likely to be coarse and strong so will be hard to curl.

Hair elasticity

Hair is naturally elastic; it can stretch and go back to its original shape. If the hair is fine it may not be as elastic as coarse hair. This weakness may cause the hair to break if too much tension is put on it. Hair that has been damaged by chemical treatments such as colouring or perming will be weaker than normal hair. Using too much heat can cause the same damage.

HANDY HINTS

Read Chapter 217 to find out how to do an elasticity test.

Hair type

The client's hair will be straight, curly or wavy. If the client has straight hair you may need to add root lift and volume to your style. Straight hair tends to lie flat to the head.

With curly hair, if you want a straight, smooth style you may need to use straighteners. If your client has very wavy hair this may present some styling problems. Hair with a strong natural wave will have a strong natural shape. This will be difficult to change. You will have to go with the natural shape when you style the hair.

Hair length

Does the client have enough hair for you to achieve the style they are looking for? Does the client have too much hair? (Will the client need to have it cut?)

Very short hair will limit your choice of style. There may not be enough hair to do what the client would like. Long hair weighs more so the weight may cause the curl to drop sooner than it would with short hair.

HANDY HINTS

Don't forget, long hair will take longer to style and longer to dry. Allow extra time for this.

Hair growth patterns

You need to try to work with most hair growth patterns. Trying to work against them will be difficult. If the hair is long, then the effects of growth patterns can be avoided if the hair is kept in place with grips and pins in a hair-up style.

HANDY HINTS

See Chapter 103 for details of hair growth patterns and how to spot them.

ADVERSE SKIN, SCALP AND HAIR CONDITIONS

These are often referred to as **contra-indications**. Any disease or condition of the hair and scalp can affect your choice of styling technique and the style you decide to do. It can also decide whether or not you can carry out the service.

Check for contagious diseases such as head lice. Make sure you follow the salon's process for these situations.

Looking for diseases and conditions is a key factor of the service you provide for your client. You are able to offer the client advice in getting a condition treated. If you find bald patches on the scalp, advising the client to consult a **trichologist** may prevent the client from losing large amounts of hair permanently.

Contra-indications
Conditions that would prevent you from carrying out the service

Trichologist
Someone trained in spotting and treating hair and scalp disorders

FASHION TRENDS

Many clients want to follow fashion trends. Some clients see the latest fashion as a 'must have'. Others may just want something that is similar to the latest fashion.

The requests you get from clients will be influenced by the styles being worn by celebrities and the fashion looks they see in magazines and on TV. Your job is not just to respond to requests from clients. You need to keep up to date with fashion trends so that you can suggest styles and services to your clients.

The modern salon will use trade magazines, demonstrations and shows to help staff improve their skills. Regular staff meetings to discuss what the salon offers may also be used.

HANDY HINTS

Refresh your knowledge about adverse skin, scalp and hair conditions by reading the information in Chapter 103.

HANDY HINTS

Always get a second opinion from a senior colleague if you find anything unusual.

HANDY HINTS

You need to be tactful and careful when discussing a hair and scalp condition with a client. Make sure you do so in private, not in the main salon where others could overhear.

Meeting the client's wishes when they ask for a style worn by their favourite celebrity is not always easy. The style may be unsuitable for them when you look at all the factors you have just learned about. Try to suggest other options that would include some of the parts of the style they want.

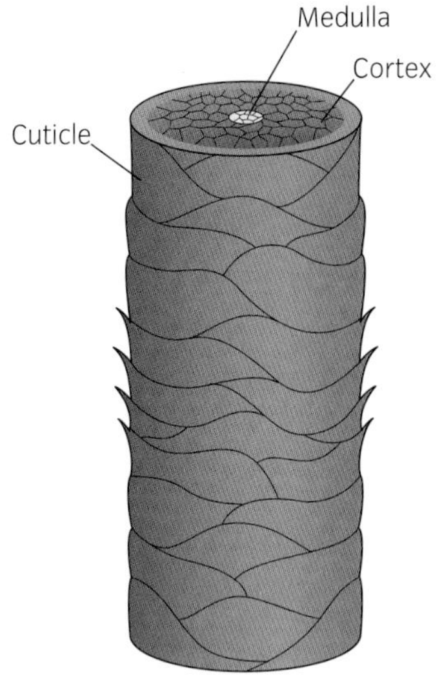

The structure of the hair

HOW STYLING AFFECTS THE STRUCTURE OF THE HAIR

In Chapter 003 Shampooing and conditioning hair you learned about the basic structure of the hair. To understand the physical effects of styling you need to learn more about the how the hair is structured.

CUTICLE

The cuticle is the outer layer of the hair which protects the cortex. When styling you need to make sure you are drying the hair in the direction that the cuticle lies.

THE CORTEX

The cortex is the largest of the three layers of the hair shaft. It contains the colour pigment of the hair. The structure of the cortex gives the hair its strength and its shape.

SmartScreen 215 handout 2

Hair is made from a hard protein called *keratin*. The keratin in the cortex is formed into long spiral chains called *polypeptide chains*. The chains run the length of the hair. To stop the hair falling apart the chains are linked together by groups of atoms called bonds or links.

There are three types of bond that join the polypeptide chains together. Each has a different job.

1 The hydrogen bond. This is made from an atom of hydrogen attracted to an atom of oxygen. It is responsible for the temporary shape of the hair. It can be broken with water. This allows the shape of the hair to be changed for a short time.
2 The disulphide bond. This bond is made from two atoms of sulphur. It gives the hair its strength and permanent shape. It is not affected by water. It can only be broken by chemical action such as that used during permanent waving. These bonds stretch when the hair is stretched.
3 The salt bonds. These bonds are made from various chemicals and do not have any effect on the strength or shape of the hair. They are usually not affected by the physical or chemical processes that we use.

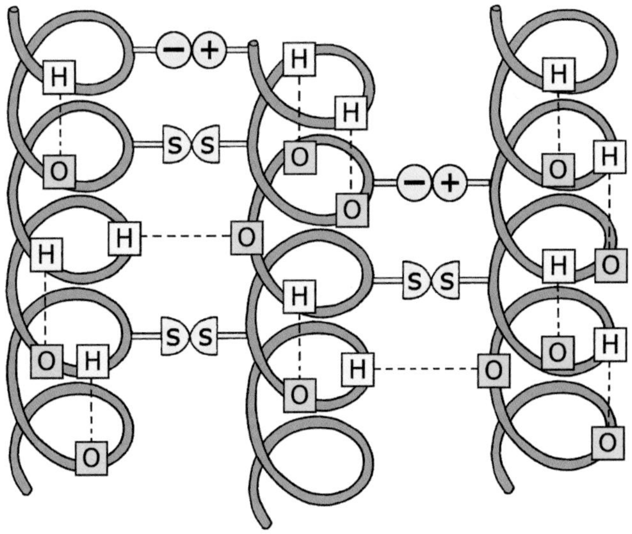
The three types of bond in the hair

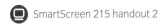

THE SHAPE OF THE HAIR

All hair has a natural shape. It will be straight, curly or wavy. The natural shape is known as the alpha keratin state. If water is added to the hair and the hair is then dried into a new shape, the new shape is known as the beta keratin state.

Changing the shape of the hair by setting or blow drying is called a *cohesive* or *temporary set*. When water is added to the hair it causes the hydrogen bonds to break and allows the hair to be stretched.

If the hair is stretched into a new shape using a brush, setting on rollers or one of the other styling techniques on wet hair, and then dried, it will remain in the new shape. As the water is dried out of the hair, the hydrogen bonds reform in new positions. This holds the hair in its new shape. When water is added to the hair again it will go back to its original shape.

We use this process to style the hair. There are two important things to remember when you are styling hair to ensure you get the best results.

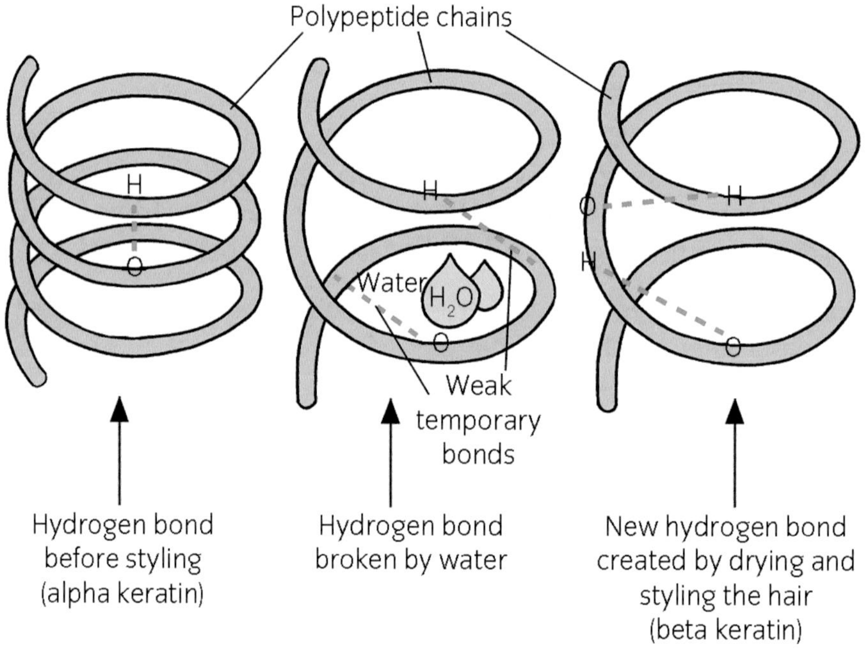

SmartScreen 215 worksheet 2

1 You must keep the hair wet as you are working. If the hair dries before you have put it in the position you want for your style you will not get a good result. The hair will have gone back to alpha keratin before you have changed it to beta keratin. This may result in your set dropping out after a short while. You may need to use tongs on your blow dry to get the lift you wanted.

2 Make sure the hair is properly dry after you have styled it. If you are setting, make sure it is dry before you take out all the rollers and clips.

HUMIDITY

Hair is hygroscopic, which means it can absorb moisture from the atmosphere. The hairstyle is therefore affected by the humidity and moisture present in the air. The hair absorbs the moisture from the air and the beta keratin state changes back to alpha keratin, because the moisture softens the temporary hydrogen bonds and the hair reverts back to its original state.

The diagram below shows the alpha to beta keratin process.

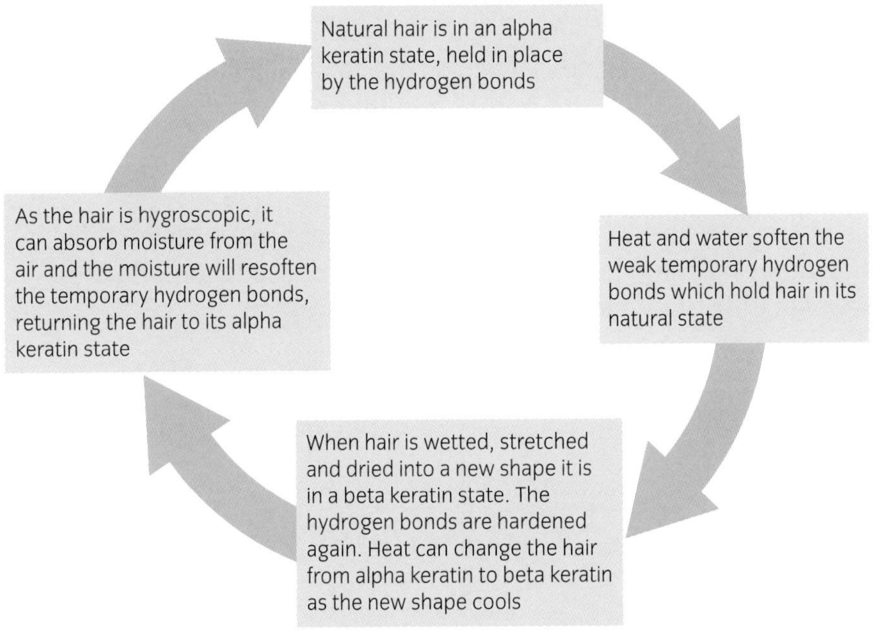

Natural hair is in an alpha keratin state, held in place by the hydrogen bonds
Heat and water soften the weak temporary hydrogen bonds which hold hair in its natural state
When hair is wetted, stretched and dried into a new shape it is in a beta keratin state. The hydrogen bonds are hardened again. Heat can change the hair from alpha keratin to beta keratin as the new shape cools
As the hair is hygroscopic, it can absorb moisture from the air and the moisture will resoften the temporary hydrogen bonds, returning the hair to its alpha keratin state

HOW THE USE OF HEAT AFFECTS THE HAIR

You have already learned how heat is used on wet hair to change the shape. Some techniques use heat directly on dry hair to style it.

Hair will always contain some moisture; it is never totally dry. Techniques including tongs, straighteners and heated rollers use the moisture in the hair to change the alpha keratin into beta keratin. They 'super dry' the hair to achieve the shape needed. Overuse of these techniques can damage the hair over time. It will look dull and straw-like, and may become so weak that it will break.

Using hand-held dryers can also lead to damage of the hair when blow drying. Using the dryer at too high a temperature for too long could lead to damage. Holding the dryer too close to the scalp or holding it still in one place for too long can cause burns to the scalp and damage to the hair.

Like tongs etc, using a hand held dryer too often can cause damage.

PREPARE THE WORK AREA

Make sure your work area is clean, tidy and organised. It will help you to work safely and hygienically. It will give the client the right impression and help you work efficiently. It will also help you to contribute to the professional standards of the salon.

GETTING THE WORK AREA READY FOR THE CLIENT

Key points to check before you bring your client to the work area.

- the work surface is clean. Wipe regularly using a suitable cleaner
- the mirror is free from smudges. Use a glass cleaner to remove smears
- your tools and equipment are in their proper place and clean. This will help you work efficiently. Make sure the tools are sterilised before use
- the floor is clean and free from hair cuttings. Sweep if necessary.

You may not be able to get all the things you need ready before the client arrives. When you have completed your consultation with the client get the rest of the products and tools you need.

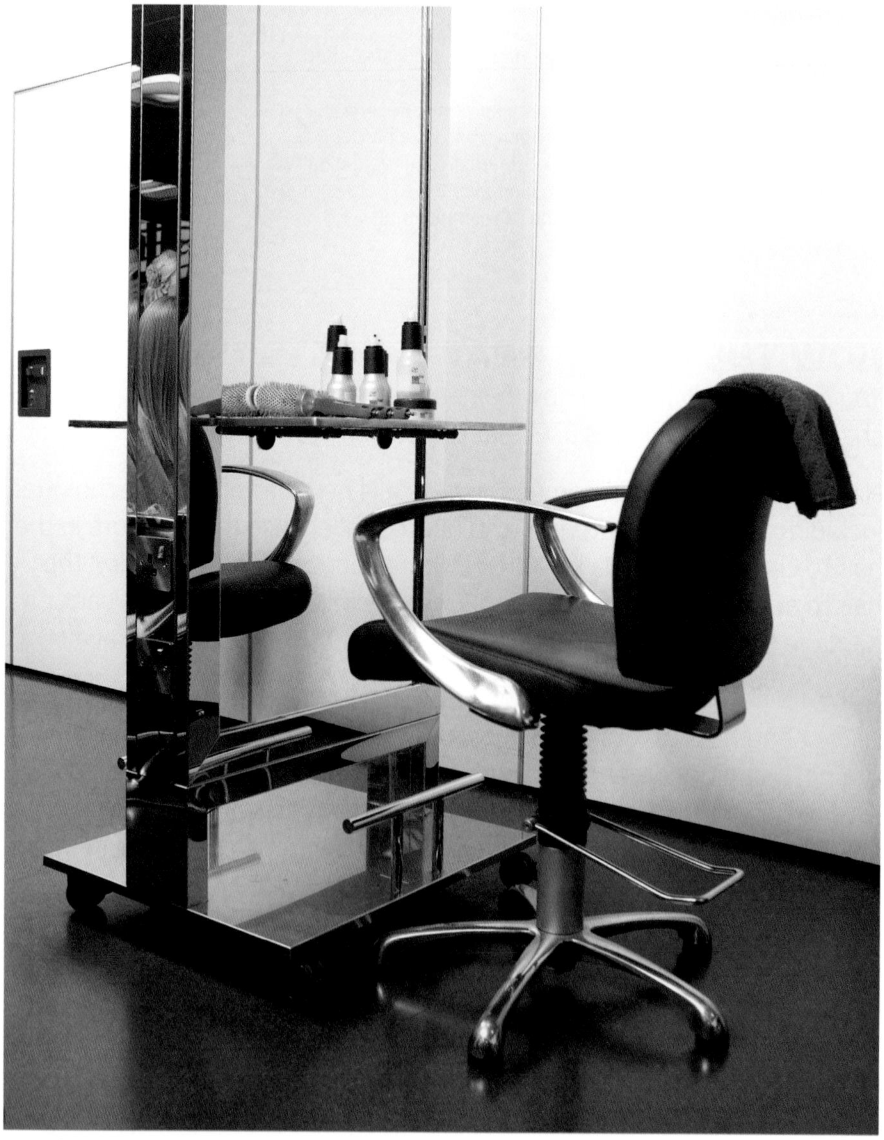

A work area set up

HANDY HINTS

Remember to make sure your appearance and your personal hygiene are up to standard. Read Chapter 102 to refresh your knowledge.

PREPARING THE CLIENT FOR A DRESSING SERVICE

Preparing the client for styling services will involve the following:

1 gowning the client to protect her clothes
2 carrying out a consultation with the client
3 shampooing and, if necessary, conditioning the client's hair.

HANDY HINTS

Read more about preparing your client in Chapter 003 Shampooing and conditioning hair.

HANDY HINTS

Check regularly that the gown is still in place and the towels are not too wet. Change the towels if you need to.

GOWNING THE CLIENT

The first part of any service will be to use the right PPE to protect the client and their belongings. For styling services, place a gown around the client to protect her clothes and a clean freshly laundered towel around her shoulders.

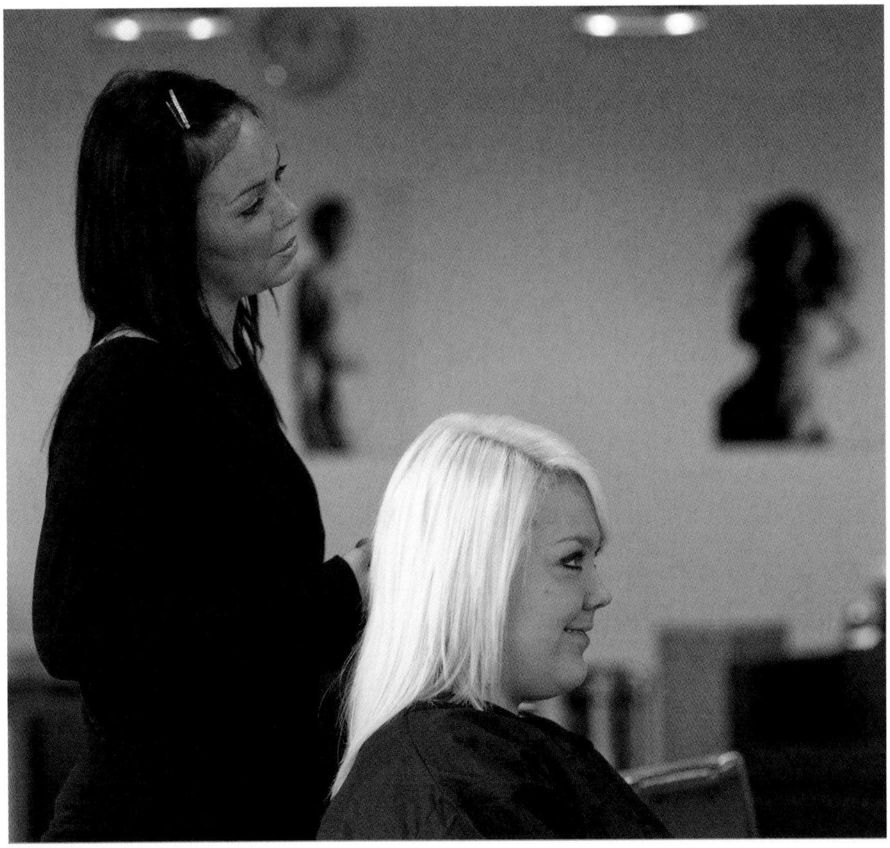

Make sure the client is wearing a gown before you start the service

SAFE AND HYGIENIC WORKING PRACTICES

Working safely and hygienically is very important. It is part of every practical skill you learn; it is part of every service you give to a client; it is part of the whole of your working day. The client will also have more confidence in you and you will look more professional.

HANDY HINTS

Read Chapter 113 Following health and safety in the salon to learn about the employer's responsibilities and your responsibilities to provide a safe and healthy working environment.

SmartScreen 215 handout 1

METHODS OF STERILISATION AND DISINFECTION

You should keep your work area tidy and use only hygienic tools and equipment. This will help to reduce the risk of harm to you and your clients and help to prevent cross-infection.

HANDY HINTS

Go to Chapter 113 and read more about methods of sterilisation.

The three principal methods of sterilising your tools and equipment are:

- Autoclave: this disinfects by using moist heat. Items should be left in for around ten minutes. Always follow the instructions. Used for metal and glass tools.
- Ultraviolet UV cabinet: this sterilises using ultraviolet radiation. Used for metal, glass and plastic items such as scissors, combs and clips. The items should be turned during sterilisation.
- Chemical immersion: this disinfects using a chemical. The chemical is often called Barbicide, which is the brand name for the solution used. It is convenient, simple and efficient, and is the most widely used method in the salon. It can be used for metal, glass and plastic, eg scissors, combs and tweezers. Always read the instructions for the solution being used.

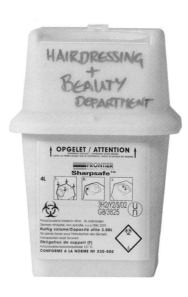

DISPOSING OF WASTE

Work in the salon will produce waste that will need to be disposed of during your work. Protecting the environment is very important. We must dispose of the waste properly. The salon will have strict procedures for getting rid of waste. You must make sure you follow them.

COSHH information for the products you use will tell you how to dispose of any waste. Sharp items such as used razor blades must be put into special sealed boxes known as 'sharps boxes'. They are usually yellow. When they are full the salon will arrange for them to be collected.

The local council may have bye-laws about waste bins and collections.

Always remember to:

- work carefully and try to reduce the amount of waste – this will help the environment and save the salon money
- dispose of the waste properly and safely by using the correct processes.

CONSULTING WITH THE CLIENT

Consulting with the client allows you to find out what the client wants. It is how you decide what you are going to do.

Chapter 003 Shampooing and conditioning hair describes how to consult with your client to find out what shampoo and conditioner you will use, and how you will carry out the service. If you are going to style the client's hair, then you need to find out more information from the client. You need to find out:

- what style the client wants and why – something easy-to-manage, fashionable or trendy?
- why the client wants it – is it for a special occasion or something else?

This will help you decide which styling techniques you will use.

The next thing to do is to look at all the factors that can influence your choice of technique, such as face shape and hair type.

COMMUNICATION

Communication and behaviour are very important when dressing hair. You may have great skills, but if you can't communicate with clients properly they won't have a good impression. In order for clients to feel happy about coming to you for dressing services, you need to feel comfortable with them, even if you haven't met them before. This starts with being confident about what you're doing, and thinking about the types of question you're asking. Refer to Chapter 102 for more details about communication and behaviour.

HANDY HINTS

Don't forget to ask the client how they look after their hair at home and what products they use.

HANDY HINTS

Make sure you check the hair and scalp for diseases and conditions. If the client has a contagious disease you may not be able to carry out the service.

SHAMPOO AND CONDITION THE CLIENT'S HAIR

When you have finished your consultation and prepared the tools and equipment you are going to need, the next step is to shampoo the hair ready for the styling service.

Remember to select the right shampoo and conditioner to prepare the hair in the way you need for the styling technique and products that you have chosen for the styling service.

SmartScreen 215 handout 3

SmartScreen 215 worksheets 1 and 4

HANDY HINTS

Read Chapter 003 Shampooing and conditioning hair to refresh your knowledge.

HANDY HINTS

When you towel dry after shampooing do not over dry the hair. For the styling process to work properly the hair should be moist but not dripping water. If the hair is too dry it will be hard to get the shape you need.

PROVIDE A DRESSING HAIR SERVICE

Before you start the styling service, check that the client is seated properly, comfortably and in the correct position for you to be able to work safely. Make sure the gown and towels are in place.

TOOLS AND EQUIPMENT USED IN BASIC STYLING TECHNIQUES

Tools and equipment	Use	Routine maintenance
Wide-toothed comb 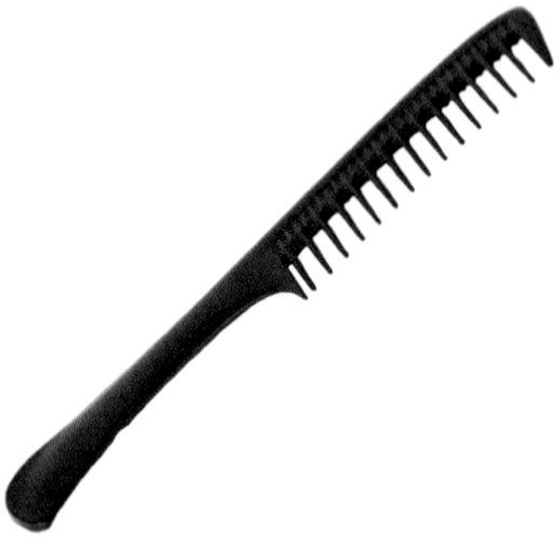	Used to detangle hair before styling.	Remove loose hair, wash in hot soapy water, dry and sterilise in chemical solution or UV cabinet. Dry before using on the client. Throw away any combs that have teeth missing.
Cutting comb 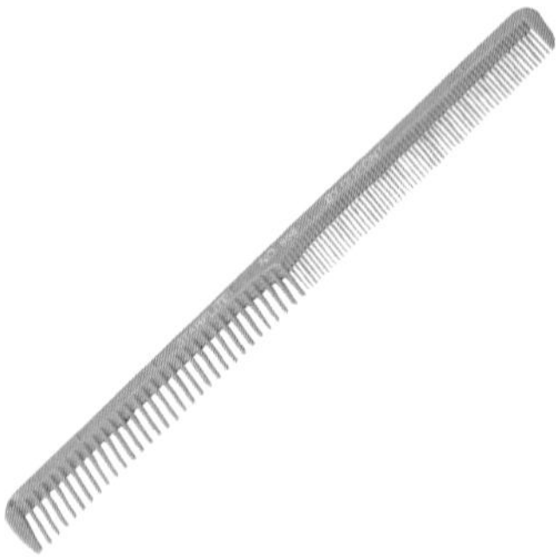	Used to split the hair into sections to keep it under control while you work.	
Tail/pintail comb 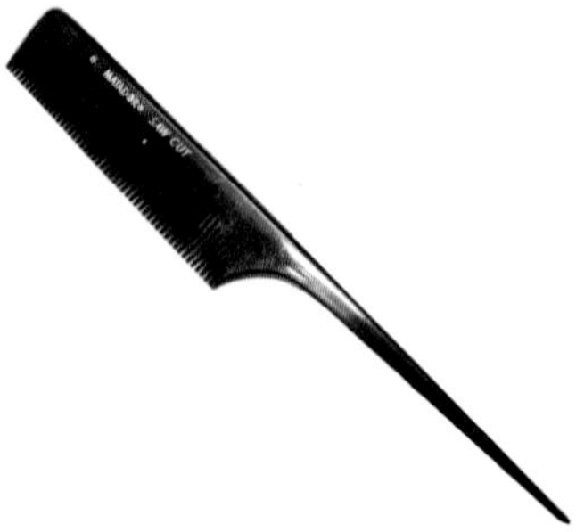	Used when setting and pin curling to make the sections to be wound on the roller or made into a pin curl.	

Tools and equipment	Use	Routine maintenance
Dressing out comb 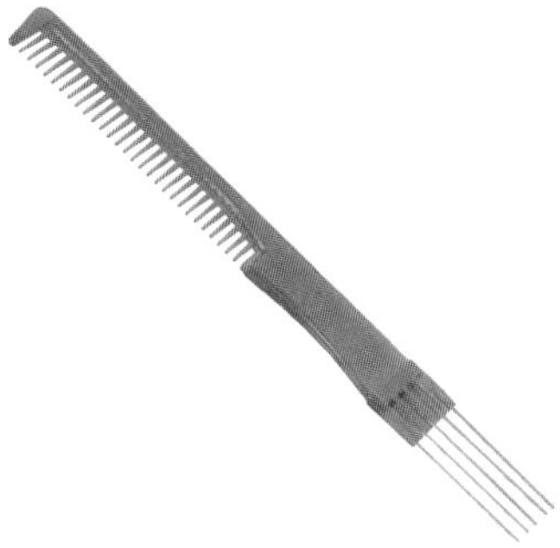	Used when the hair has been dried to backcomb and dress the hair to shape and finish the style.	Same as wide-toothed comb.
Sectioning clips 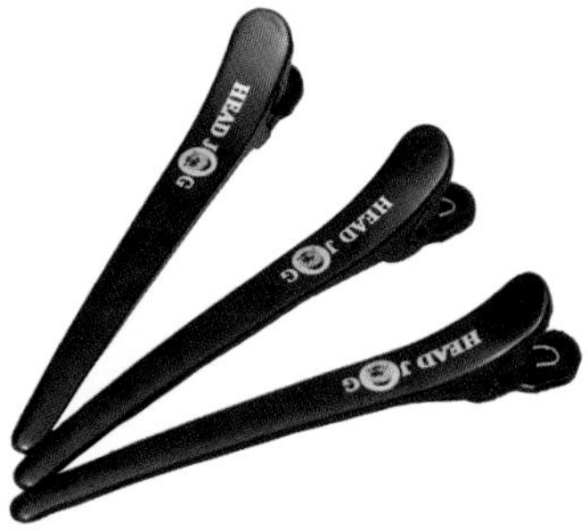	Used to keep the hair in place as you work.	Remove loose hair, wash in hot soapy water, dry and sterilise in UV cabinet.
Bristle brush 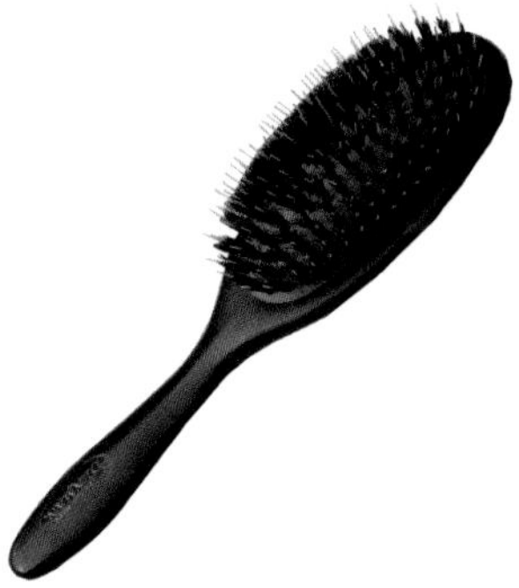	This is a soft brush used for general brushing and to remove roller marks when you are setting and dressing the hair.	Remove loose hair, wash in hot soapy water, dry and sterilise in chemical solution or UV cabinet. Dry before using on the client.
Denman brush 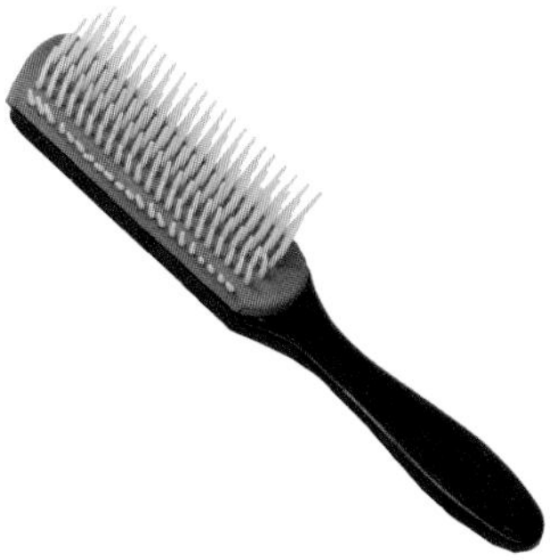	Used in blow drying to create a smooth, straight finish such as a 'bob' style.	Remove loose hair, wash in hot soapy water, dry and sterilise in chemical solution or UV cabinet. Dry before using on the client.

Tools and equipment	Use	Routine maintenance
Vent brush 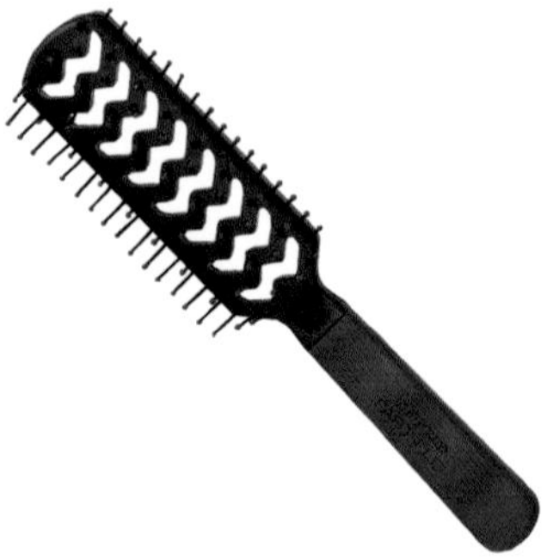	Used to create a textured straight finish when blow drying.	Same as bristle brush.
Radial brush 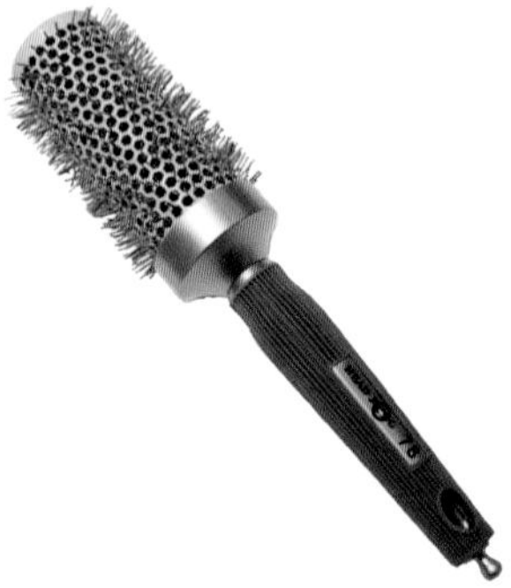	Radial brushes come in different sizes and are used to create root lift, curls and waves in hair of different lengths.	Same as bristle brush.
Rollers 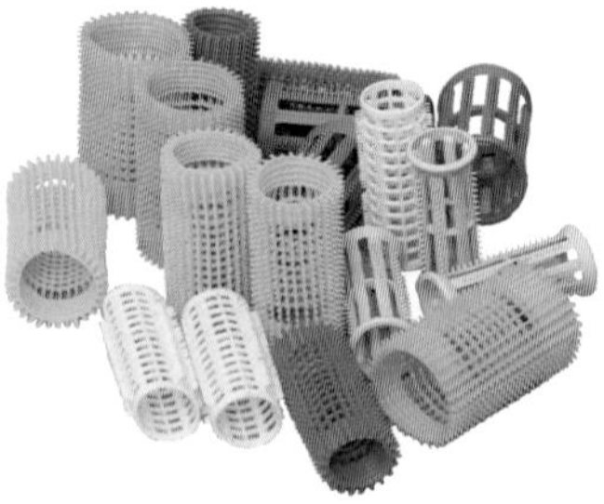	Rollers come in a range of sizes from small to large. They are used to set the hair. They produce lift, waves and curls.	Wash in hot soapy water; dry. Sterilise if required in chemical solution or UV cabinet.
Pins 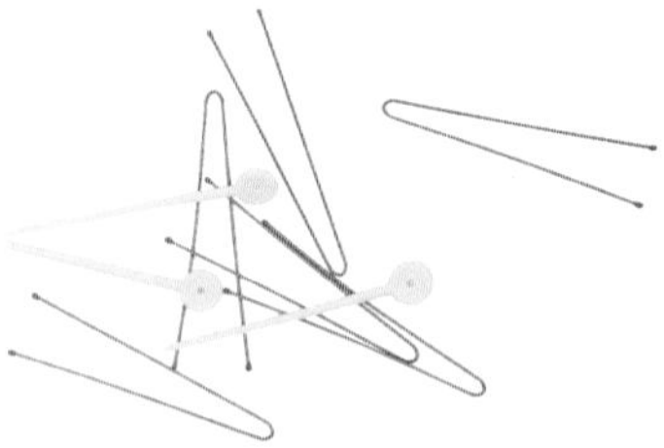	These are used to keep the rollers in place when setting the hair.	Wash in hot soapy water and dry thoroughly. Throw away any misshapen pins.

Tools and equipment	Use	Routine maintenance
Pin curl clips 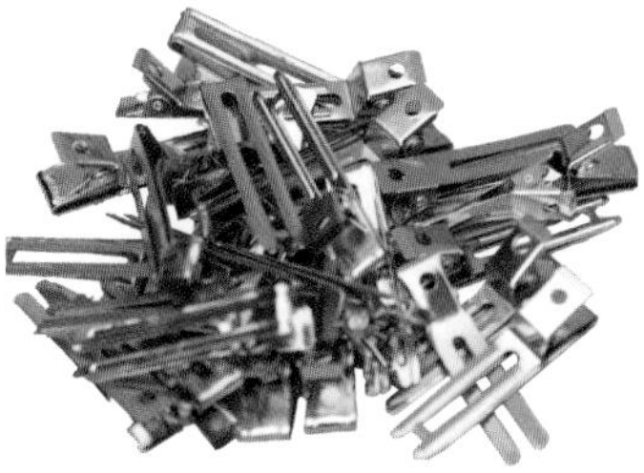	These are spring-loaded clips that are used to hold the hair in place when pin curling.	Remove loose hair, wash in hot soapy water, dry and sterilise in UV cabinet.
Grips 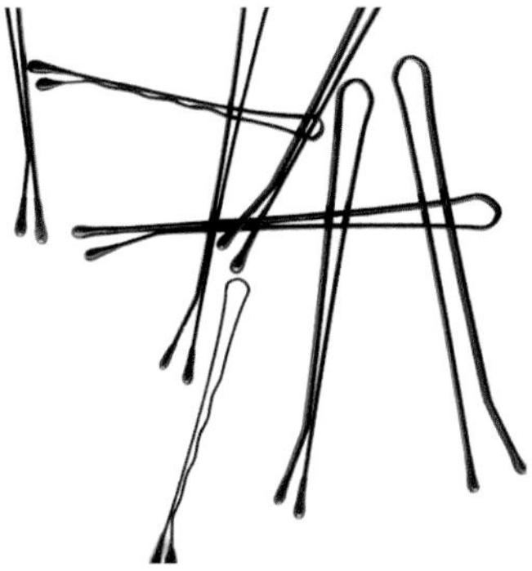	Sometimes called 'kirby' grips. They are used to hold hair in position when dressing out long hair in a hair-up style.	Wash in hot soapy water and dry thoroughly. Throw away any misshapen grips.
Hand-held dryer 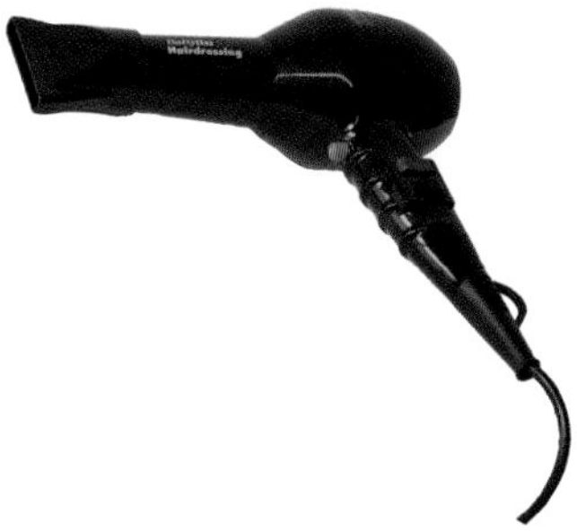	Used to dry the hair during blow drying. Has different heat settings and speeds.	Wipe the outer casing with a cleansing wipe. Do not use water. Use a disinfecting wipe if needed.
Diffuser 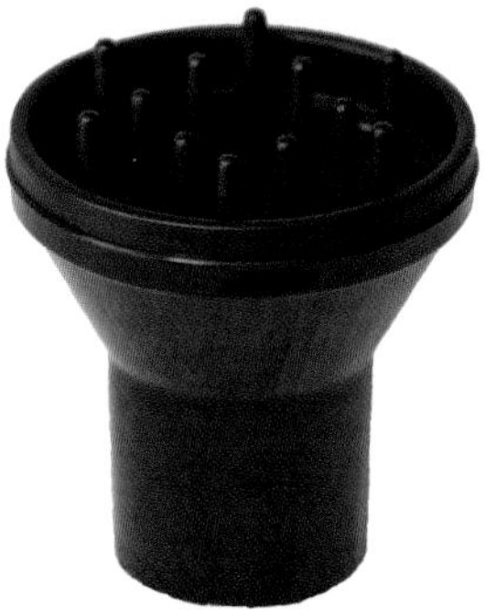	An attachment for a hand dryer used when finger drying. It spreads the airflow and decreases its force.	Wash in hot soapy water and dry before use. Use a disinfecting wipe if needed.

Tools and equipment	Use	Routine maintenance
Nozzle 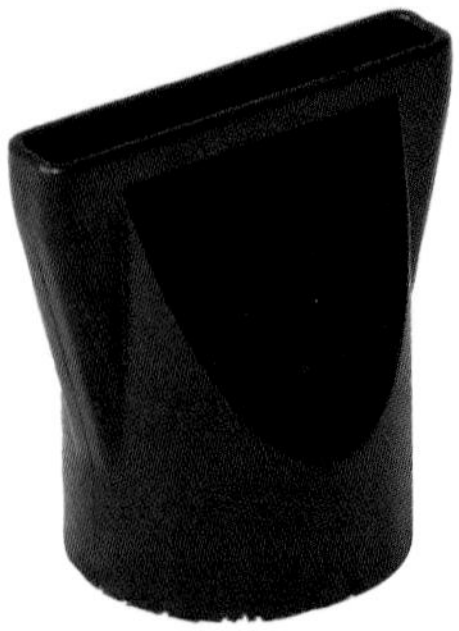	Another attachment that allows you to direct the airflow and heat more accurately when blow drying.	Wash in hot soapy water and dry before use. Use a disinfecting wipe if necessary.
Straightening irons 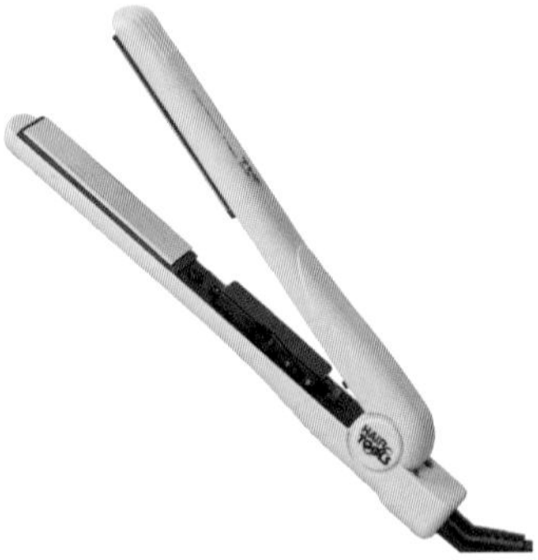	These have flat, heated surfaces that are used on dry hair to straighten and smoothe it.	Follow the manufacturer's instructions. Use the appropriate cleaner to remove product build-up. Use a disinfecting wipe if necessary.
Tongs 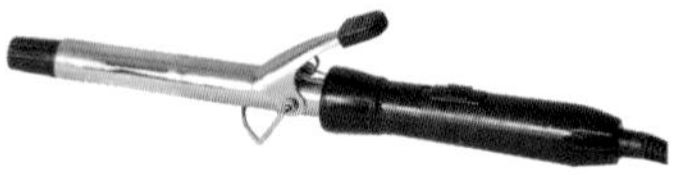	These have a round barrel shape that is heated. Used on dry hair to create curl and body.	Follow the manufacturer's instructions. Use the appropriate cleaner to remove product build-up. Use a disinfecting wipe if necessary.
Hood dryer 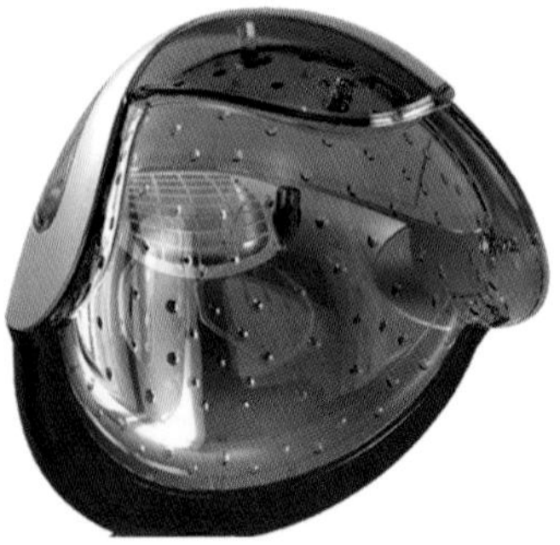	Used to dry hair that has been set.	Wipe the outer casing with a cleansing wipe. Do not use water. Use a disinfecting wipe if needed.

Tools and equipment	Use	Routine maintenance
Heated rollers 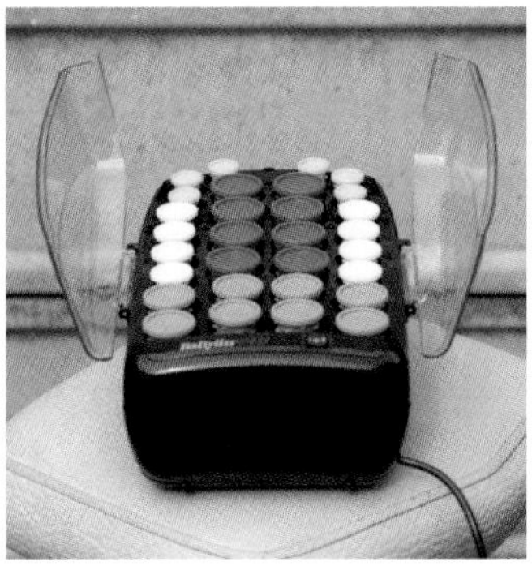	These are electrically heated rollers that are used on dry hair to refresh the style and shape.	Follow the manufacturer's instructions. Use the appropriate cleaner to remove product build-up. Use a disinfecting wipe if needed.
Gown 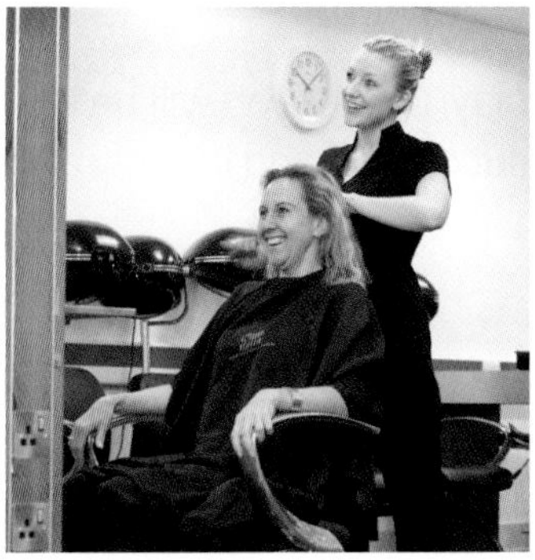	This will cover the client and help to prevent anything getting onto their clothes.	Wash the gowns after each use. Use detergent and the correct wash programme. Throw away any damaged, torn or stained gowns.
Towels 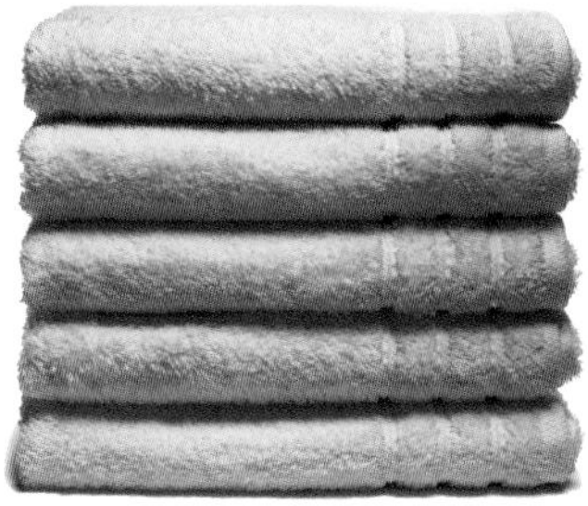	Used when shampooing and styling to prevent the client's clothing from getting wet.	Wash the towels after each use. Use detergent and the correct wash programme. Throw away any damaged, torn or stained towels.
Hand mirror 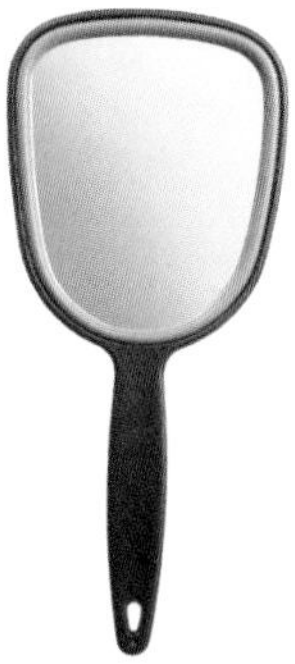	Used to show the client the back of their head so they can see the finished result.	Clean with glass cleaner and a cleansing wipe.

Tools and equipment	Use	Routine maintenance
Accessories 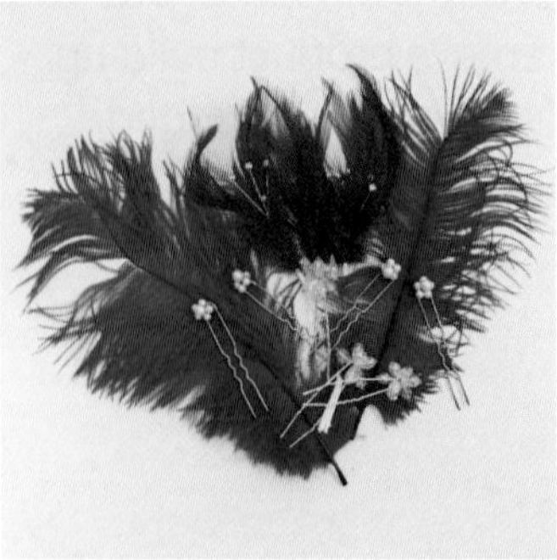	This will include feathers, ribbons, flowers, added hair and many other decorative things. They are used to enhance the style. Especially useful for weddings, parties and styles for special occasions.	Most accessories will be used on individual clients and not reused on other clients. Many items will only be used once and then thrown away.

ACTIVITY

With a partner, carry out a consultation role play. One of you will be the client, the other the barber. Discuss if it was successful and identify any areas you could improve.

STYLING PRODUCTS

Styling product	How it is used	Effect on the hair
Mousse/activator 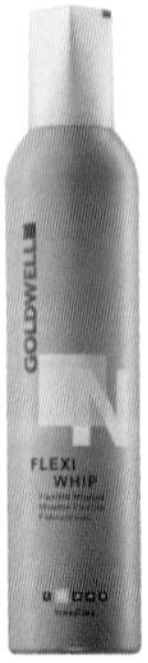	Used on wet hair before blow drying or setting. Apply to the hair and comb through evenly.	It gives support and hold to the style, making it last longer.
Gel 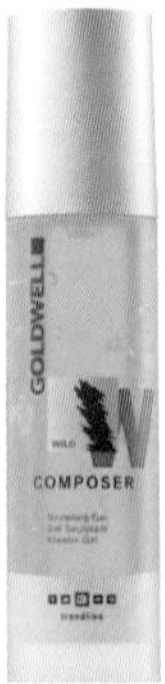	Used on wet or dry hair to provide volume and texture.	Provides an elastic effect, allowing the hair to bounce back into style. Can be used to tame or enhance curls.

STYLING PRODUCTS

Styling product	How it is used	Effect on the hair
Blow dry/setting lotion 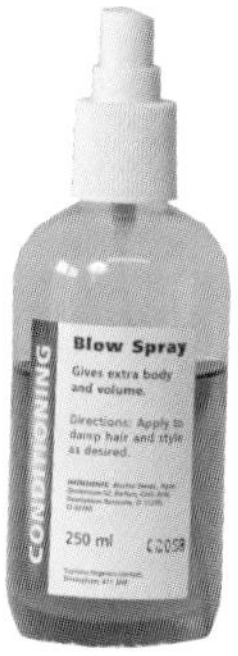	Similar to mousse but in liquid form. Used on wet hair before blow drying or setting. Carefully trickle or spray onto the hair and comb through evenly.	Gives volume, lift and support for fine hair.
Heat protectors 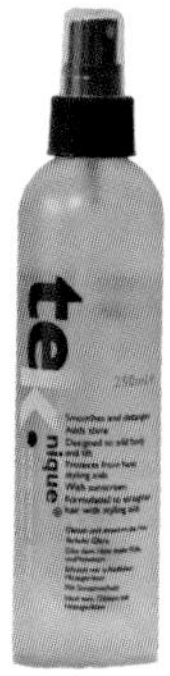	This is sprayed onto dry hair before using heated appliances such as tongs and straighteners.	Protects the hair from the effects of the heat. Prevents frizz.
Moisturisers 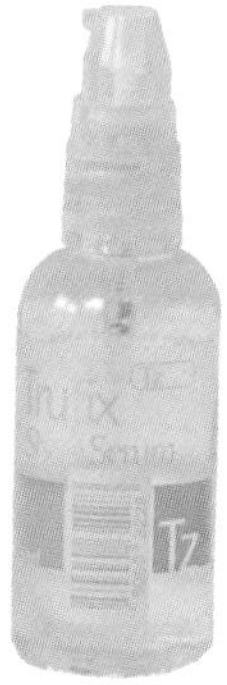	Used on wet hair when blow drying. Spray onto the hair and comb through evenly.	Will help smoothe frizzy curly hair to get a straighter look.

HANDY HINTS

Remember to position yourself correctly when you work. Move around the client as you work so you do not have to bend or twist, which can cause backache and fatigue.

FINISHING PRODUCTS

Finishing product	How it is used	Effect on the hair
Wax 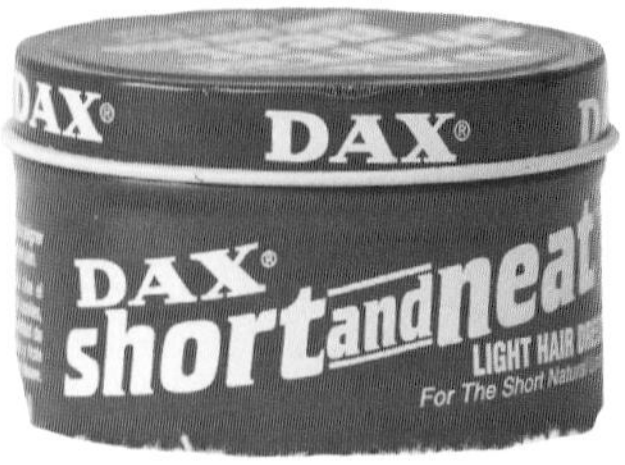	Applied to dry hair. Use the hands and fingers to work the wax through the hair. Avoid the root area.	Used to achieve a 'spiky', 'messy' look. Can also be used to smoothe flyaway hair when doing a hair up.
Hairspray 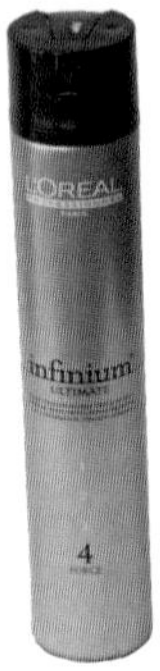	Used on dry hair. The hair is sprayed lightly when dressing or drying is finished.	It holds the hair in place and gives it shine. Helps to keep moisture out of the hair making the style last longer.
Gel 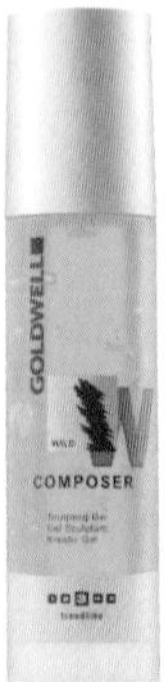	Used on dry hair. Massage a small amount into the palms of your hands and work evenly onto the hair, shaping and moulding with the fingers.	Used to give stronger hold to the hair and gain the desired finish.
Serum 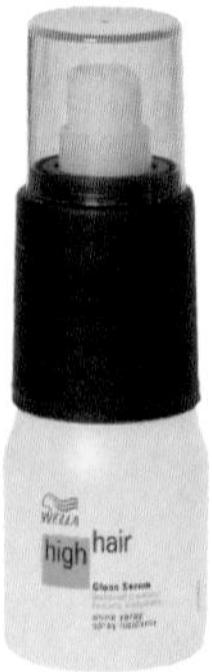	Applied to dry hair before using straighteners. Rub two to five drops on the palms of your hands and apply evenly to the hair.	Will calm frizzy and flyaway hair. Will protect from heat.

Finishing product	How it is used	Effect on the hair
Dressing cream/oil 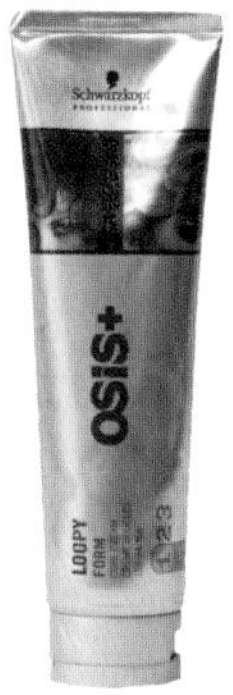	Used on dry hair. Apply a small amount to the hair using the fingers. Do not add too much as it will make the hair look greasy and flat.	Used to control the hair and achieve a smooth, slick finish. Will make the hair shine.

CARRYING OUT A STYLING TECHNIQUE

The first part of any styling technique you carry out is to apply the styling product you have selected for the technique you are going to use.

SmartScreen 215 worksheet 5

HANDY HINTS

Read the manufacturer's instructions and check any PPE you may need to use.

CONTROLLING THE HAIR

Whichever technique you are going to use, you should be able to control the hair to get the result the client wants. Work with a firm but gentle approach to the hair, using good clean sections. These will help you work around the head well. Keeping good tension when you brush or blow dry will make sure the hair goes in the direction you want it to.

If you are not in control, the hair will not do what you want it to do. Most clients will want to feel what you are doing. If you are too gentle they may think you are not doing their hair properly.

BLOW DRYING THE HAIR

The most important thing to remember when you are blow drying is to have the hair under control. If the hair is not under control you will not get the shape and finish you want. Remember to work safely. You will be using heat to dry the hair. Focus on what you are doing all the time.

HANDY HINTS

Keep the hair tight so when you put the clip in it is not loose and floppy. You will have better control and it looks more professional to the client.

Sectioning the hair

When you are blow drying medium to long hair you should divide it into sections. Use a sectioning clip to keep them in place. This will keep the rest of the hair out of the way as you dry each section. How you section will depend on the style you have chosen. The sections should follow the direction of the style.

You are now ready to blow dry the hair.

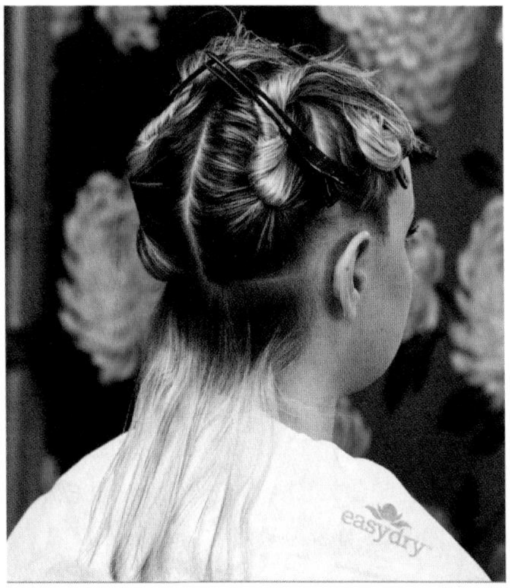

Divide the hair into sections for blow drying

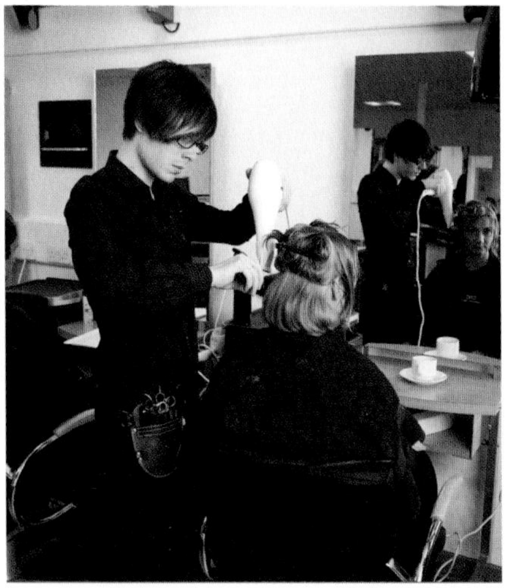

A blow drying service

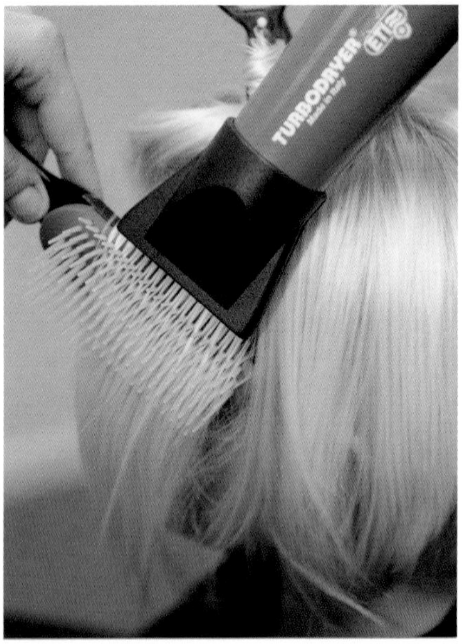

Using a Denman brush

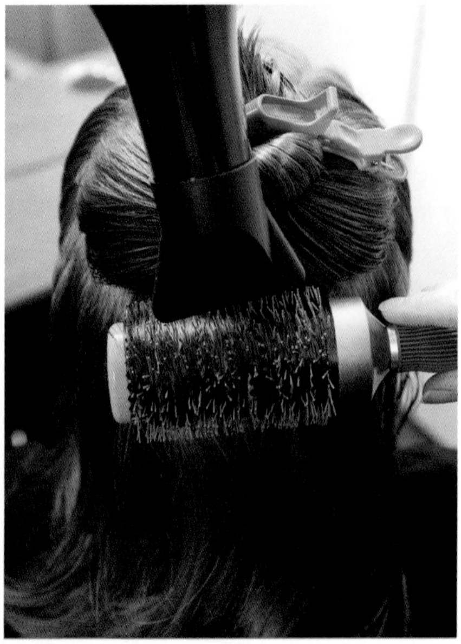
Using a radial brush

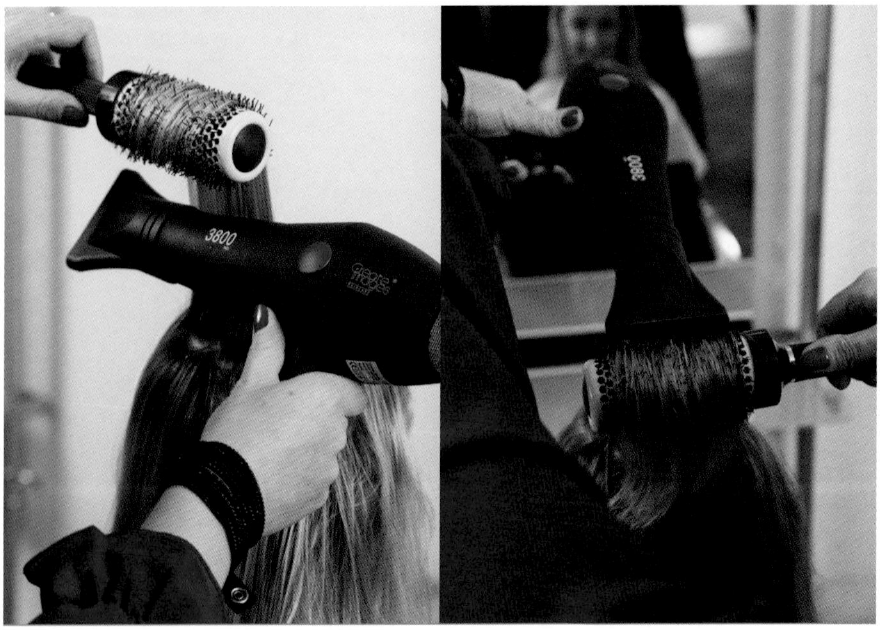

Angle the hairdryer to get the shape you want

Using the dryer

The airflow from the dryer must always be away from the client's scalp. You need to direct the airflow in the direction of the style. Hold the dryer at least 10–15 cm away from the hair as you dry it. If the dryer is too close it can damage the hair. Don't hold the dryer in one place for too long; this could burn the client's scalp.

Brushes

Your brush choice will depend on the look you want to achieve and the hair you are working with. For a straight style such as a classic bob a Denman brush would be used. A radial brush will give lift and volume.

The airflow should be directed onto the brush. Do not direct the airflow to the hair between the brush and the scalp. This will spoil the shape you are trying to get.

Tension

Keep the hair under tension as you dry it. This will give you a smoother finish. Do not use too much tension as this may cause discomfort to the client.

Angles

Changing the angle of the brush and the dryer will help you get the shape you want. You need to practise holding the dryer and brush in each hand. Holding the dryer and brush in different positions is important for a good result.

ROLLER SETTING AND DRESSING HAIR

In this technique the hair is wound on curlers of various sizes. This will give lift, curl and shape to the hair. When the hair is dry the rollers are removed and the hair is brushed and combed into shape. This is called dressing the hair.

To get different shapes and styles the rollers are placed in different patterns. When you have finished the consultation with the client you will have agreed how the finished style will look. The rollers are placed in the hair in positions that will give the direction, lift and shape that you want.

This is known as a *directional wind*. The hair is sectioned into oblongs and the rollers placed next to each other in neat rows.

A directional wind can produce gaps in the finished style where the rows join each other. To prevent this you can use a *brick wind*. Instead of neat rows the rollers are wound so that they look like bricks in a wall. You still follow the direction of the finished look. This method will reduce the problem of gaps in the finished result.

ACTIVITY

Design two styles that use roller setting. Take photos as you work, showing:

- the size of the rollers that you are using
- the roller pattern
- the styling products
- how you dressed the style after drying
- the finishing products used.

Roller setting – using a brick wind

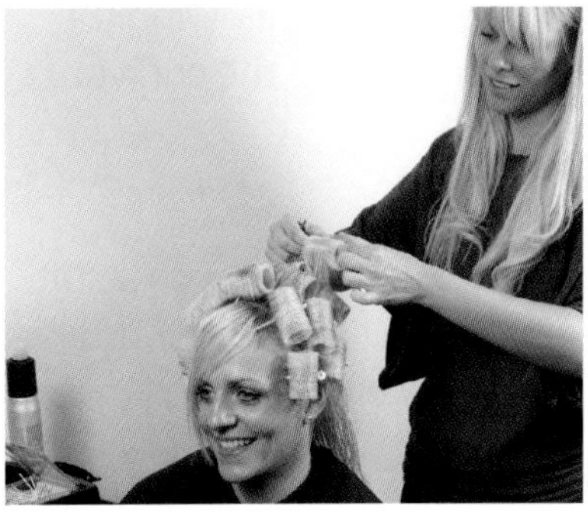

STEP 1 – Wind the rollers in a pattern that looks like bricks in a wall.

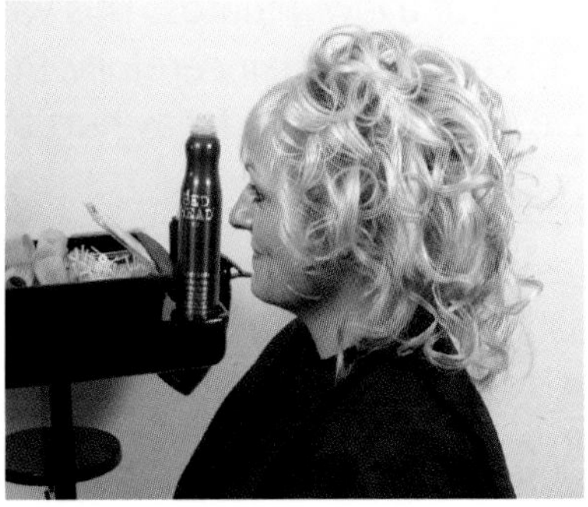

STEP 2 – Allow the hair to cool and then remove the rollers.

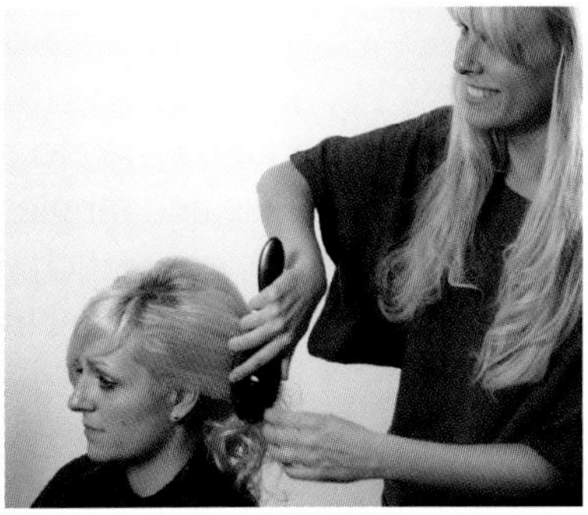

STEP 3 – Remove the roller marks with a brush and dress into the desired style.

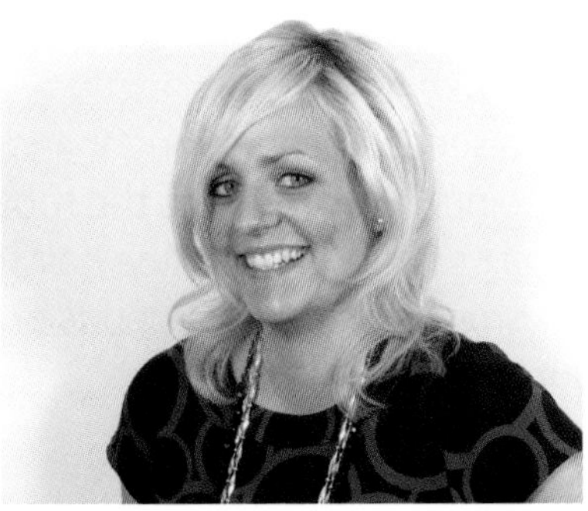

STEP 4 – Apply a finishing product if required and ensure the client is happy with the result.

HANDY HINTS

Don't forget ear pads to protect the ears.

Tension and control

Use even tension when you are putting in the rollers. This will give you the direction and finish you want. Don't fix the rollers too tightly; this can be uncomfortable for the client and can damage the hair.

Sectioning

Clean, neat and even sections are essential for achieving your style. Remember, the sections you make should not be wider or longer than the size of roller you are using.

If the section is too wide and the hair hangs off the sides of the roller the hair will go in the wrong direction when it is dry and it will be harder to get the finish you want. It will also be harder for the client to style their hair at home.

Drying the hair

Dry the hair using a hood dryer. This will take between 15 and 30 minutes depending on the length and thickness of the hair.

Make sure the hair is properly dry before you dress it out. Leave the hair to cool for a few minutes. This will make the set last longer. Wind the rollers out of the hair carefully. Pulling them can weaken the curl you have just created and may hurt the client.

Dressing out

Dressing out achieves the finish to the style. Brush the hair with a soft bristle brush. This will cause less damage to the hair than other brushes such as a 'Denman' brush. Follow the shape you want. This loosens and spreads the hair and removes any roller marks.

Use the dressing out comb to tease the hair into its final shape. This will also give you a smooth finish to your style.

Apply any finishing products to want to use, such as hairspray.

Backcombing and backbrushing

These are two techniques used to give height and volume when dressing out. They are also used to provide a firm base when dressing out long hair in a hair-up style.

Backbrushing

Hold a section of hair upright and brush the hair from about halfway to the points downwards to the root. This roughens the cuticle and tangles the hair slightly, binding the hair together for a fuller shape. How much backbrushing you do depends on how much lift and volume you want in your style.

Backcombing

Backcombing is carried out in the same way as backbrushing but using a comb instead of a brush.

It provides greater support and increased volume. It is used on long hair to provide a strong base to secure the grips and pins used in a hair-up style.

STYLING LONG HAIR

Long hair provides you with the chance to create a wide range of finishes – from simple straight flowing styles, soft curls, plaits, twists and curly styles to beautiful elegant hairstyles for special occasions.

You will use a mixture of styling techniques to achieve your desired style. The techniques can be used separately or together.

HANDY HINTS

Read Chapter 105 Plaiting and twisting hair to learn about techniques for plaiting and twisting long hair.

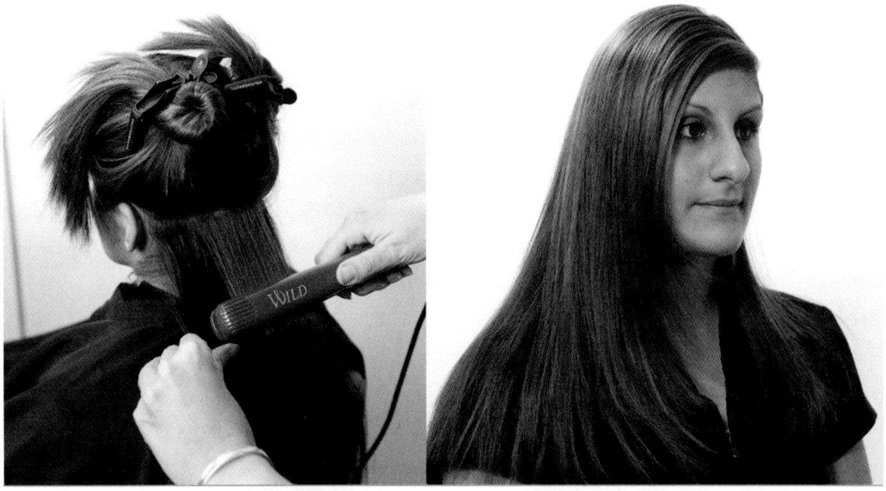

Use straighteners to achieve a straight flowing style

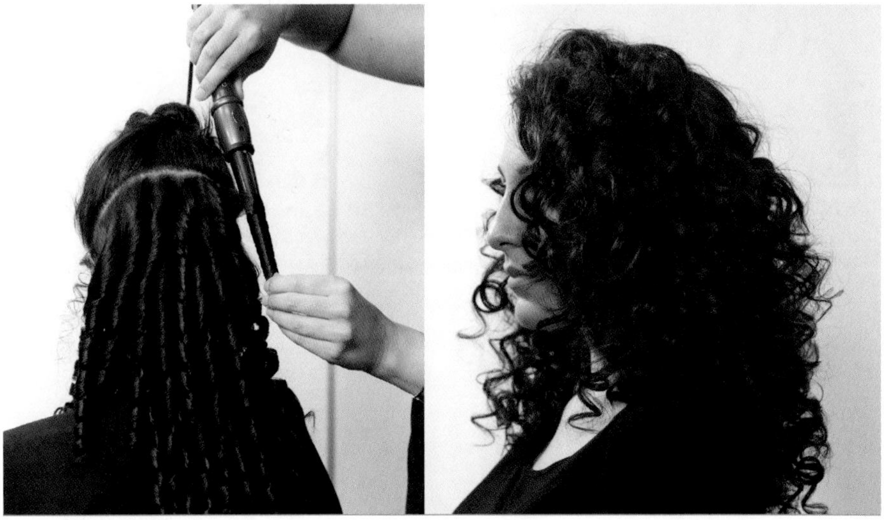

Tongs can be used to create styles with lots of curl and volume

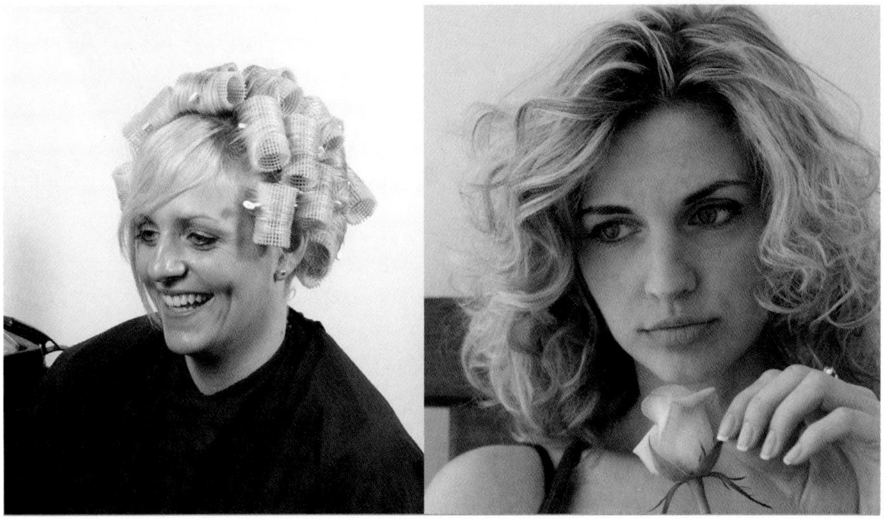

Large rollers can be used to give soft curls and movement

Avant garde
The latest fashions, new designs and techniques

DRESSING LONG HAIR UP

This is the type of style you will be asked to do for a wedding, a special occasion or a party. Styles will range from a sophisticated, elegant style to an '**avante garde**', off the wall style.

The finished look you are going to create will determine how you prepare the hair. You can:

- blow dry or use straighteners if you are looking for a flat, sleek style
- use large rollers if you need lift and curl in your style.

An example of a long hair-up style is a vertical roll or French pleat. This is a classic style that will suit many occasions. It can be enhanced by adding accessories like flowers and jewellery.

The hair should be dry and straight. The style requires using grips to provide a base on which the pleat itself is made and secured. Backcombing is used to form the base and also to add lift to any areas that need it.

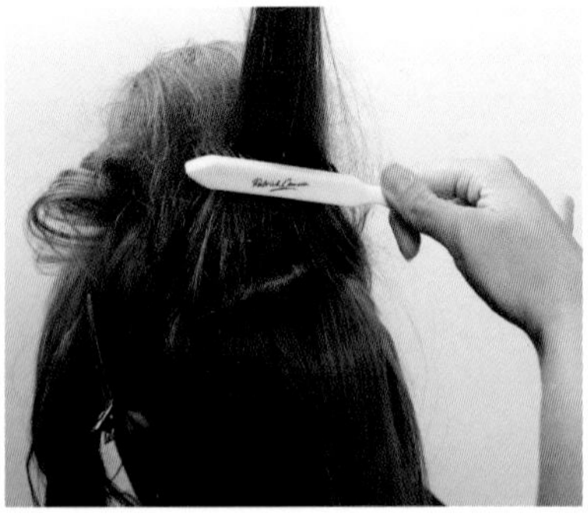

STEP 1 – Backcombing the roots after applying styling products.

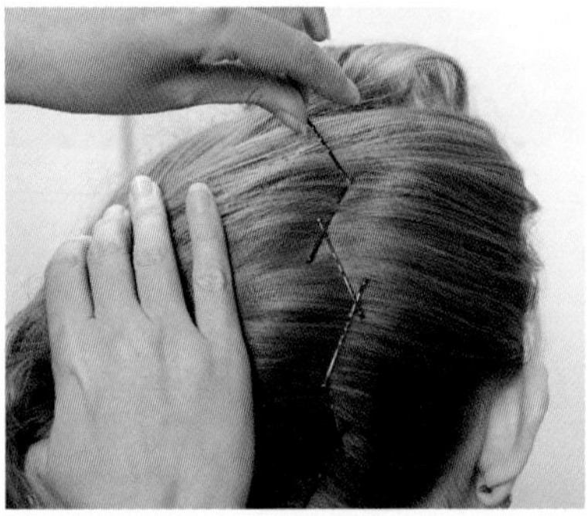

STEP 2 – Criss-crossing grips applied down the centre.

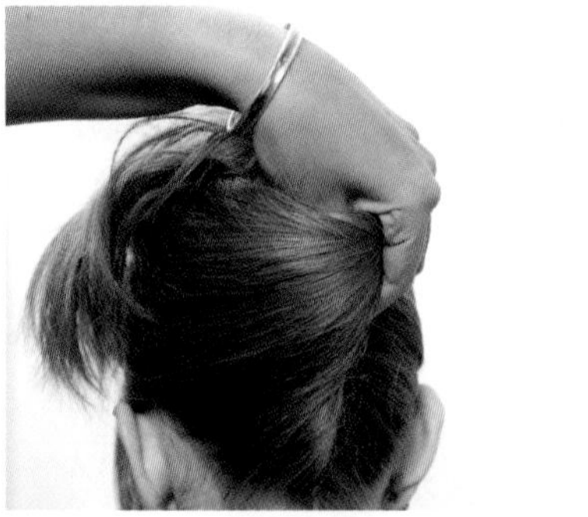

STEP 3 – The hair is folded and slightly twisted over the grips, and secured with pins.

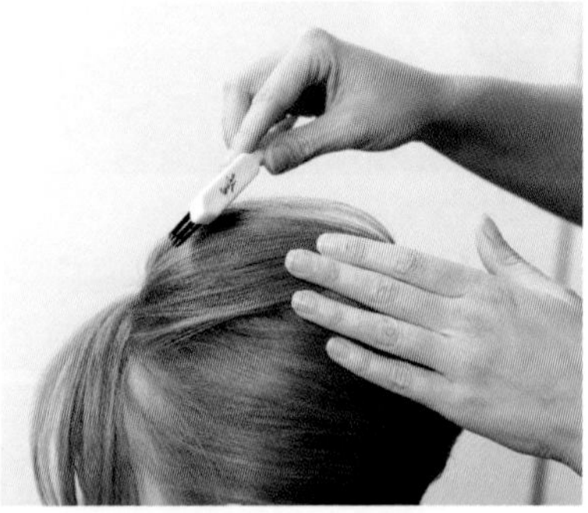

STEP 4 – The ends are tucked under the roll, the top section is smoothed over and finishing products are applied.

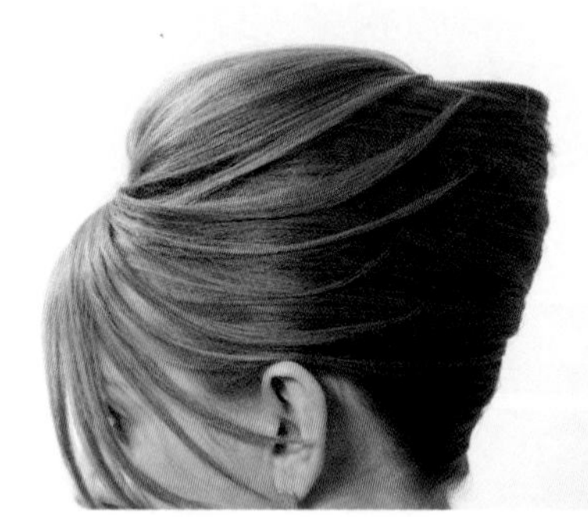

STEP 5 – The finished result.

ACTIVITY

Design two long hair styles and carry out your designs on a model or block. Make up a mood board to show how you achieved the style.

AFTERCARE ADVICE

Keeping their hair looking good is something that all your clients will want to do. Giving the clients advice about how to look after the style you have created for them at home is part of the service you give them. Your advice should include:

- what products to use
- what equipment and tools they will need
- how to use both the products and tools to maintain and recreate their style.

ACTIVITY

Practise giving aftercare advice on styling, working with a partner and taking it in turns to be the client and stylist. Discuss how successful you are.

PRODUCTS

Advise the client about the products that will be best for their hair. Talk about the products you have used in creating the style (include styling and finishing products) and how the client should use them at home. Don't forget to tell them how to remove the products correctly. Tell them about which products will keep her hair in good condition.

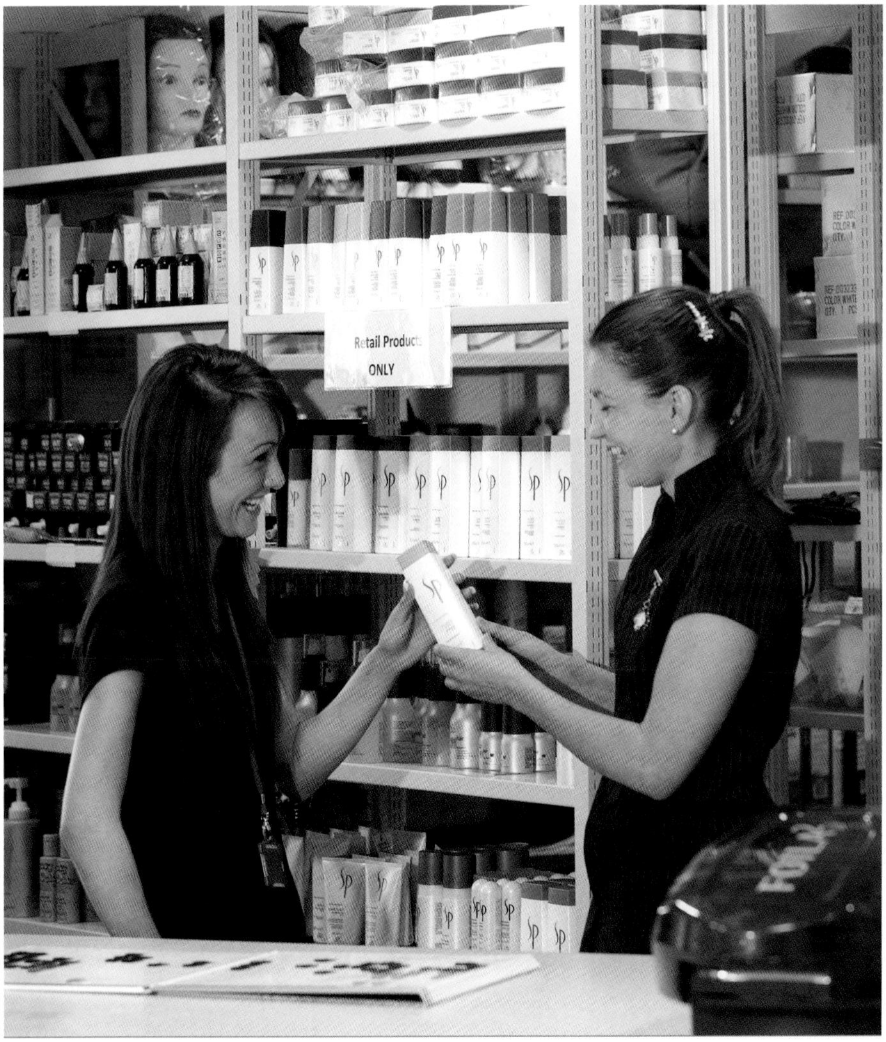

Two students getting products from the stock room

HANDY HINTS

Telling the clients about the products to use at home is a good chance to sell them your retail products.

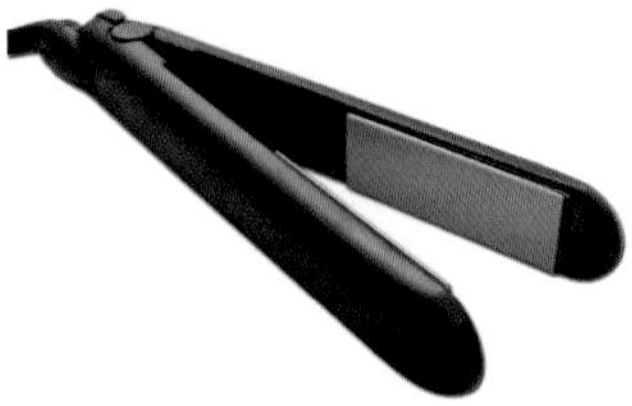
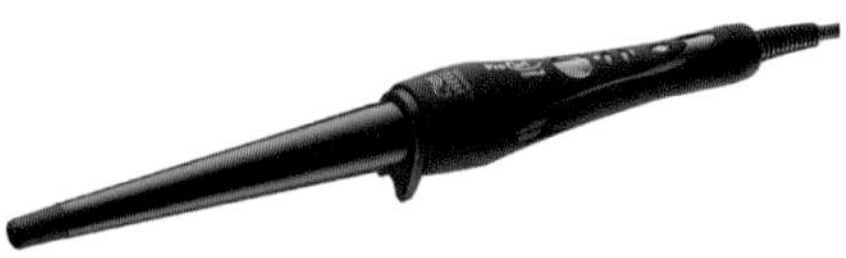
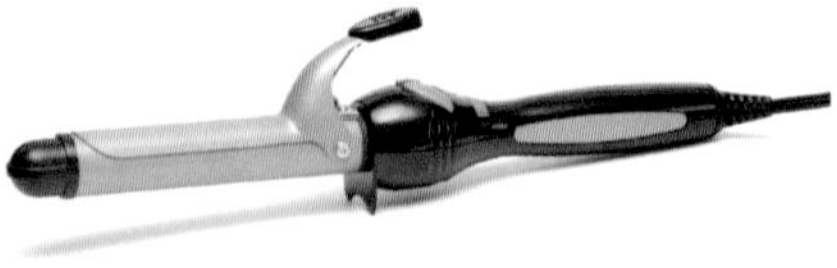

TOOLS AND EQUIPMENT

Ask the client about the combs and brushes they use at home. Advise them about which tools and equipment they should be using to keep their hair looking good and protect the condition of the hair. If you are telling the client about straighteners, tongs or other heat appliances, don't forget heat protector products to go with them. Tell the client how to use the tools properly and how to clean them.

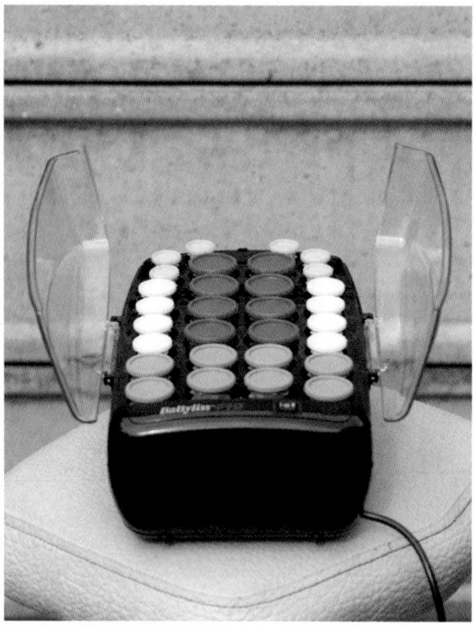

RECREATING THE LOOK

As you are working on your client, tell them how they can do it at home: how they can blow dry their hair; how to use heated rollers to refresh a style that is set; how to dress the hair; how to use tongs to quickly add some curl.

Give the client information about when they are likely to need repeat services to maintain their style, for example when it would need cutting again.

ACTIVITY

Learn about your salon's retail products so you can tell the clients about the benefits to their hair if they purchase and use the product.

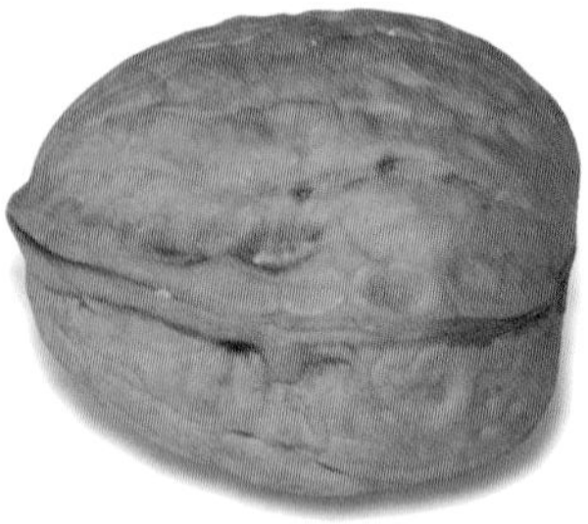

IN A NUTSHELL

You are now at the end of the chapter. Before you test your knowledge with the revision activities, check the following list to see if you feel confident in all the areas covered. If there are still any areas you're unsure of, go back over them in the book and ask your tutor for extra support:

- the techniques for styling and dressing hair
- the factors that can influence your choice of techniques
- how to prepare the client for styling and dressing their hair
- the tools, equipment and products that are used in dressing hair
- how styling affects the structure of the hair
- the effect of using heat and the effect of humidity on the hair
- following safe and hygienic working practices
- the importance of good communication, behaviour and attitude when styling women's hair
- the purpose of backcombing and backbrushing when styling
- giving aftercare advice.

REVISION ACTIVITIES

Use the questions below to test your knowledge of Chapter 215 to see just how much information you have gained. This can help you prepare for your assessments. Turn to pages 506–508 for the answers.

WORDS TO FIND

Copy and complete the sentences below. Use these words to help you fill in the gaps.

backcombing	denman	hair density	finger drying
stem	radial	head shape	hydrogen bonds
straighteners	barrel spring	face shape	cohesive
oval	on base	vent	

1 Three types of brush used in styling hair are ____________, ____________ and a ____________.

2 The perfect face shape is ____________.

3 Changing the shape of the hair by setting or blow drying is called a ____________ set.

4 ____________ and ____________ are types of pin curl.

5 ____________ is a technique that will give soft natural-looking styles.

6 When setting hair with rollers the roller should always sit ____________.

7 Using ____________ will produce smooth hair styles particularly on longer hair.

8 Factors that should be taken into account when consulting with the client include ____________, ____________ and ____________.

9 ____________ is used to give lift when dressing the hair.

10 The ____________ are responsible for the temporary shape of the hair.

TEST YOUR KNOWLEDGE FURTHER

1 Name **five** styling techniques that can be used to style and dress hair.

2 Name **five** factors that can influence your choice of technique.

3 Which bonds in the hair are changed when the hair is set or blow dried?

4 Name **three** styling products that can be used during blow drying or setting and state what they are used for.

5 Name **three** types of pin curl and state the effect they give.

6 Why is it important to listen when you are consulting with the client?

7 What PPE would you use for your client when blow drying?

8 Why should the hair be sectioned when setting and blow drying?

9 What size section should you use when putting in a roller?

10 Name **two** things that will promote a good atmosphere and image in the salon.

11 What is the purpose of backcombing the hair when dressing out?

12 Name **three** finishing products that can be used during styling and dressing out and state what they are used for.

13 Name the three things that you should include in giving aftercare advice to the client.

14 Increased humidity will make the set or blow dry last longer. True or false?

SmartScreen 215 worksheet 6

15 Closed questions require a long answer from the client. True or false?

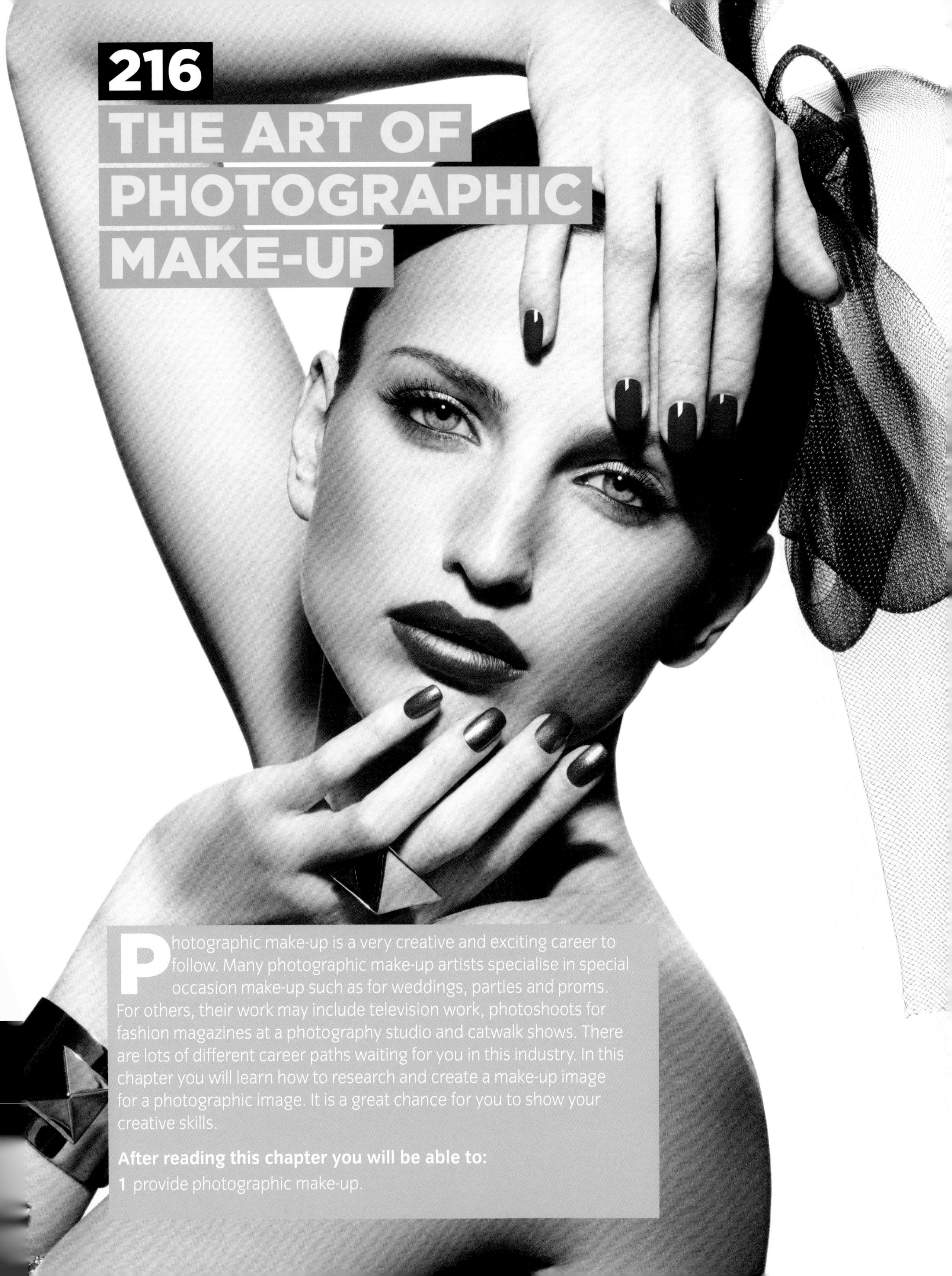

216 THE ART OF PHOTOGRAPHIC MAKE-UP

Photographic make-up is a very creative and exciting career to follow. Many photographic make-up artists specialise in special occasion make-up such as for weddings, parties and proms. For others, their work may include television work, photoshoots for fashion magazines at a photography studio and catwalk shows. There are lots of different career paths waiting for you in this industry. In this chapter you will learn how to research and create a make-up image for a photographic image. It is a great chance for you to show your creative skills.

After reading this chapter you will be able to:

1 provide photographic make-up.

PROVIDE PHOTOGRAPHIC MAKE-UP

HANDY HINTS

Look back at Chapter 113 to refresh your knowledge of health and safety.

Before you begin the photographic make-up it's important to be prepared. Health and safety requirements should be carried out for every treatment, but knowing how to set up your treatment area, getting the right products and tools together, carrying out a proper consultation and knowing about warm and cool colours are also musts for make-up services. All of these things have been discussed in Chapter 106 – please refer to that chapter for further guidance.

HANDY HINTS

If you have to travel to a different location (other than the salon) for a make-up service, it would be a good idea to carry all of your tools, equipment and products in a suitable storage bag or box. These should be strong enough to protect your kit, but also light enough for you to be able to carry everything, especially if you have to go upstairs.

SAFE AND HYGIENIC WORKING PRACTICES

As with all hair and beauty treatments, it is important for you to work in a safe and clean way. You should keep your treatment area tidy and use only hygienic tools and equipment. This will help to reduce the risk of harm to you and your clients and help to prevent cross-infection. The client will also have more confidence in you and you will look more professional.

It is your responsibility to be aware of health and safety legislation to protect yourself, your clients and your colleagues.

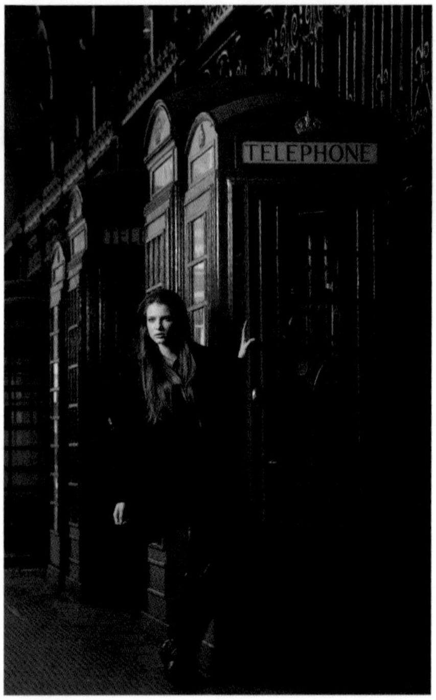

LOCATION

There are many different events where a photographic make-up service is needed. Some of them do not take place in a salon, so you will need to be prepared to move your products, tools and equipment to other **locations** to carry out the make-up service. Make sure you carry only what you can safely hold, especially if you need to carry equipment upstairs. Make sure you know the correct way of lifting and ask your tutor if you're not sure.

Location
Place

You may have to work in the following locations for photographic make-up:

- A wedding – the bride may want you to go to their house on the morning of the wedding to do their hair or make-up.
- A photoshoot – this may take place in a photography studio or at an outside location for a fashion magazine. The location will depend on the theme of the final photographic image.
- Fashion and catwalk shows – you may need to work 'behind the scenes' at the location of the fashion or catwalk show.

HANDY HINTS

You will need to read through and complete the activities in Chapter 106 Basic make-up application to help prepare you for this chapter.

HANDY HINTS

See Chapter 113 for the correct way to lift equipment.

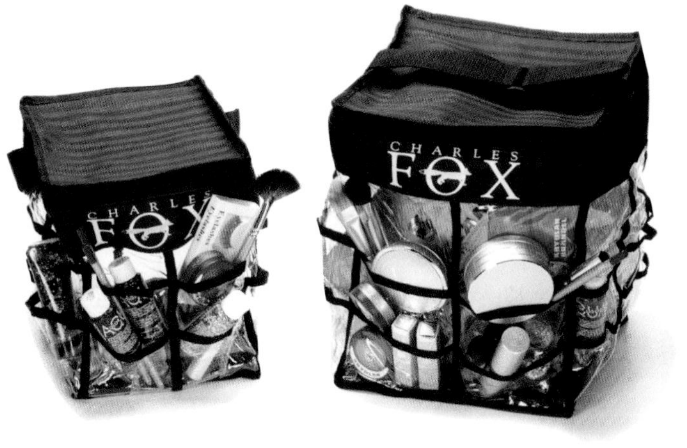

PREPARING FOR THE MAKE-UP SERVICE

Wherever the photographic make-up is taking place, it is important that you get yourself and the treatment area prepared. All of the products, tools and equipment need to be ready. This will make sure that the treatment flows well and also gives the client a positive first impression. This will also help the client to relax and have confidence in you.

SmartScreen 106 worksheet 1

HANDY HINTS

You may not be working in a salon for a photographic make-up service. Remember to check where you will be working beforehand, so that you know what you will need to take with you.

PRODUCTS USED IN A PHOTOGRAPHIC MAKE-UP SESSION

There are many products you need to learn about for a make-up treatment. Most of them have already been mentioned in Chapter 106, so please refer to that chapter for details.

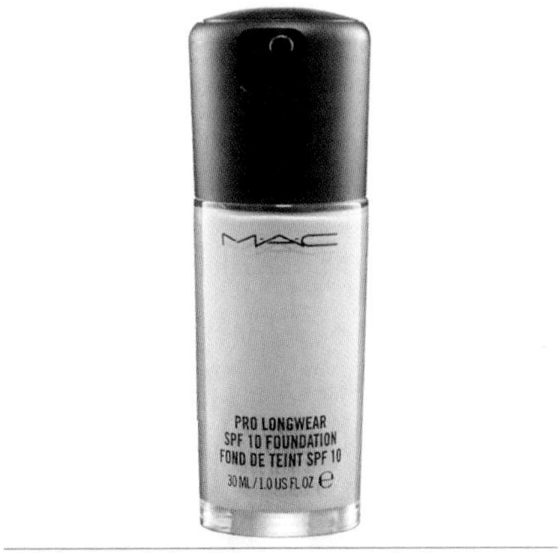

Foundation

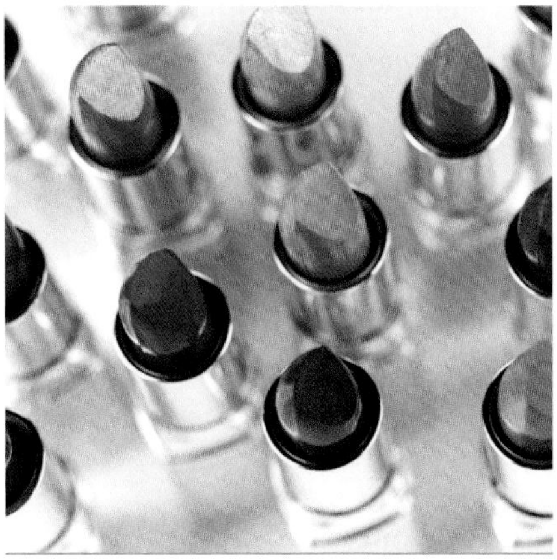

Lip products

HANDY HINTS

You can build on your basic make-up skills when learning to carry out a make-up for photography work.

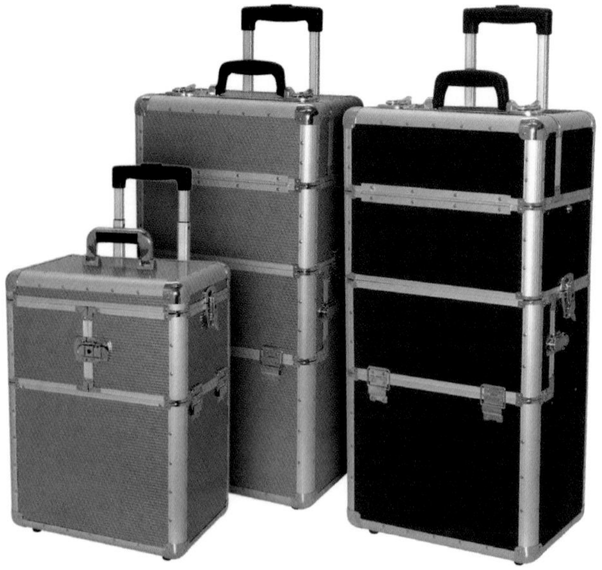

You should always carry your make-up products, tools and equipment in a carrying case if working on location

You will need to have the following products, tools and materials on your trolley:

- skin care products – cleansers, toners and moisturisers; suitable for all skin types
- make-up products – concealers, foundations, powders, blushers, lip products (lipstick, lip liners, lip gloss), eye products (eyeshadow, eye pencil, mascara)
- make-up tools and equipment – applicators, brushes, cotton wool, tissues, make-up palette
- a mirror
- a treatment plan and pen
- a treatment couch or make-up chair
- coverings for your client – headband, couch covers, couch tissue, towels and gown.

ACTIVITY

To remind you of the anatomy that you need to know for this chapter, read Chapter 106 and answer the following questions:

1 Where are the following bones found?

a mandible
b frontal
c zygomatic
d maxilla

2 Which one of the following glands (found in the skin) produces oil?

a sebaceous
b sweat

3 What are the skin's main functions? (Remember 'SHAPES'.)

4 Which **two** of the following skin conditions would prevent you from applying a photographic make-up?

a dry skin
b recent scars
c oily skin
d bruising

When you have finished, check your answers with your tutor.

HANDY HINTS

Go to Chapter 006 Skin care and read up on the different skin care products.

HANDY HINTS

For this chapter you will need to know the following anatomy:
- the bones of the face
- the structure and functions of the skin
- adverse skin conditions.

Refer to Chapter 106 Basic make-up application for this information.

CONSULTATION

Before you start the treatment you will need to carry out a consultation with the client.

HANDY HINTS

See Chapter 106 for details on how to carry out a consultation for a make-up treatment.

COMMUNICATION

Communication is very important for the consultation as you need to be able to talk to your clients. Using a range of language linked to a make-up treatment will present a professional image to the client and show that you are fully trained.

HANDY HINTS

See Chapter 106 for make-up terms which you can also use for photographic make-up.

CLIENTS FOR PHOTOGRAPHIC MAKE-UP

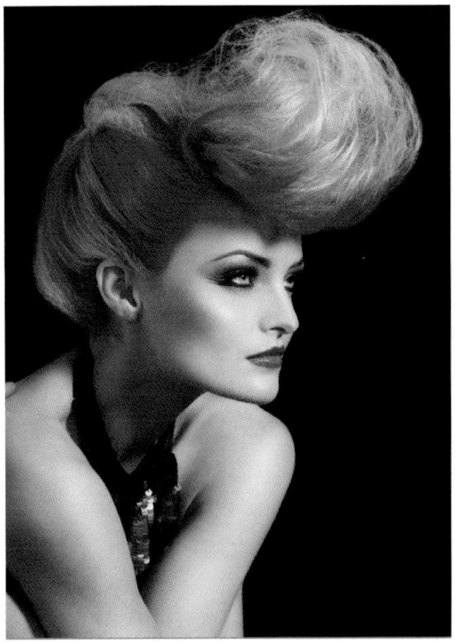

Photographic make-up

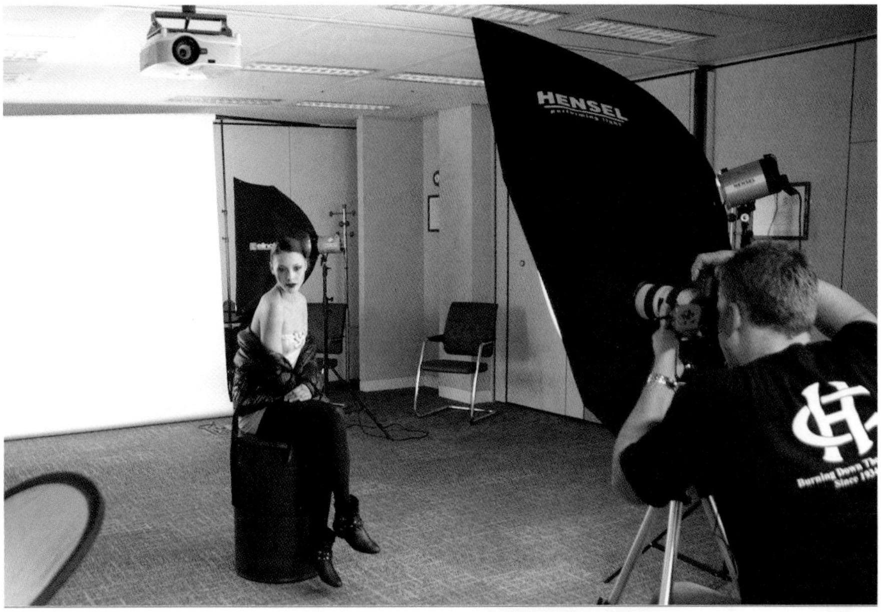

Photoshoot in a photography studio

Your 'client' or 'customer' for a photographic make-up will depend on the situation in which you are applying the make-up. For example:

- A wedding make-up will usually involve the bride, the bridesmaids and the mother of the bride as well. It may be the bride who decides on how she wants the make-up to be applied to them all and the colour of make-up used. Your 'customer' is the bride in this case.
- In a photoshoot, it is usually the photographer who decides on what make-up is to be applied to the 'model'. Your customer in this case is the photographer. They will guide you on how they want the make-up applied as they will know what effect they want to achieve in the photo.
- A fashion- or catwalk-show make-up is very like a photoshoot. Your 'customer' is usually the organiser of the show. You will need to speak to them beforehand to make sure that you know exactly what make-up look they are hoping to achieve. They will decide on what make-up they want their models to have for the overall look.

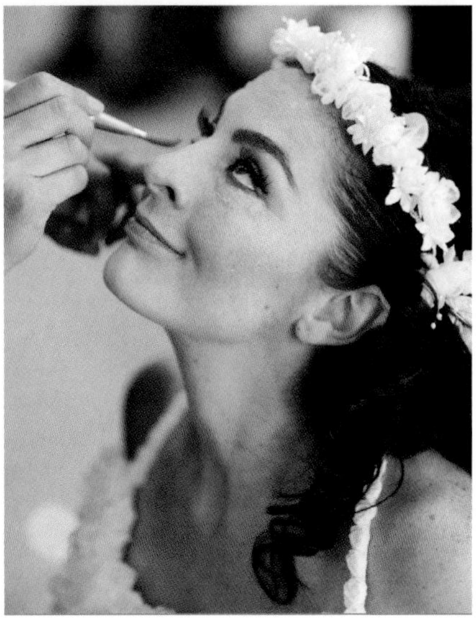

Wedding make-up

HANDY HINTS

Dealing with professional people like photographers can be difficult when you're not used to it. Make sure you ask your tutor for support.

FACTORS THAT WILL INFLUENCE PHOTOGRAPHIC MAKE-UP

There are certain factors that you will need to think about when planning your photographic make-up treatment. This will make sure that the make-up you apply is suitable for the client. Look back at the factors in Chapter 106 as these also apply to photographic make-up.

HANDY HINTS

For more information about these factors go to Chapter 106 Basic make-up application.

CONDITION OF THE SKIN

Before you begin your photographic make-up service you will need to have a look at the client's skin. This will help you to choose the most suitable make-up products for the client. You will need to think about the following factors:

- Skin type – dry or oily. Choose the best products for this type of skin, such as a cleansing cream for dry skin or cleansing lotion for oily skin.
- Condition of the skin – if it is dry, use a cream moisturiser; if it is oily, use a moisturising lotion. You may also need to apply more loose powder to oily skin to help to reduce the shine on the skin.

Expose
To show

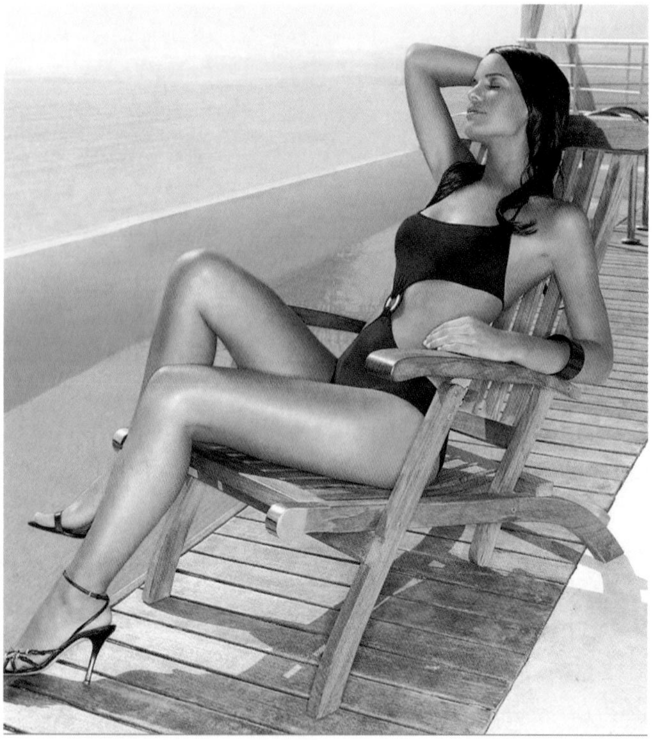

A tan may look good, but it means your skin is damaged

Effects of sunlight

When you go out in the sun you **expose** your skin to ultraviolet rays. When this happens the skin will darken in colour, which is known as a sun tan. Some people burn very easily and their skin goes red, whereas other people tan more quickly and turn brown. If you expose your skin to too much sun and over a long period of time it will age more quickly. This means that your skin will be more likely to dry out and get wrinkles. It is suggested that you use a good sun protection cream when you are out in the sun, as this will help to stop your skin from burning and looking older before its time.

Ageing

As you get older, the skin changes. For example, it becomes drier and wrinkles may form (particularly around the eyes and mouth area). There is not a lot we can do to stop this from happening, but using a moisturiser regularly will help to delay the signs of ageing, as this will keep the skin well moisturised.

ACTIVITY

Make an information leaflet that can be given to your clients, informing them of the effects of sunlight and ageing on the skin. Include some information on what the clients can do to help to protect their skin from these effects.

HANDY HINTS

Ultraviolet rays are sometimes known as 'UV' rays.

APPLYING MAKE-UP TO CLIENTS WHO WEAR GLASSES

If your client or model wears glasses, it is important to make sure that you check how the eye make-up will look when the client has the glasses on. You can do this by asking them to keep trying them on during the make-up treatment. You will need to make sure that the eye make-up colours chosen suit the colour of the frames and also the lenses (if they are tinted). If the lenses are tinted you may have to make the eye make-up colours slightly stronger so that they show up.

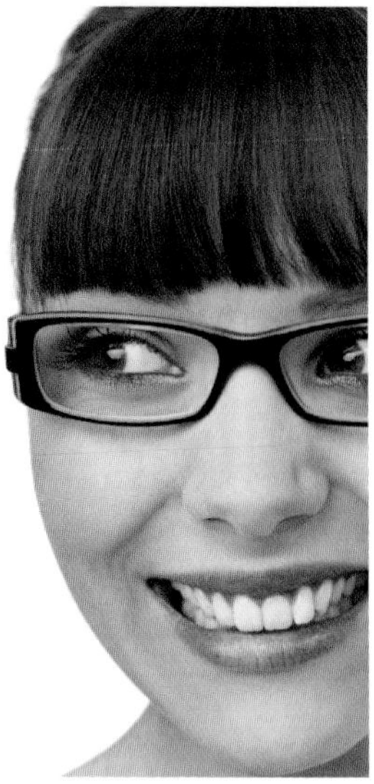

APPLYING MAKE-UP TO CLIENTS WHO WEAR CONTACT LENSES

If your client wears contact lenses, you should give them the choice of either taking them out during the treatment or leaving them in. Some people find even the slightest pressure on their eyelids very uncomfortable when they are wearing their lenses.

Whether the client is wearing them during the treatment or decides to put them in afterwards, here are some simple tips to help you:

- Be very gentle when working on and around the eye area.
- Be very careful not to get any make-up products in the client's eyes (such as eyeshadow). If you do, the contact lens will become dirty and will **irritate the eye**. If this happens, you may not be able to continue with the make-up treatment and all products will need to be removed. The client may also have to remove the lenses to clean them.
- Make sure that the client keeps their eyes closed when applying the make-up; in particular the loose powder, blusher, shader, highlighter and eyeshadows. This is because they are all powders and if they get into the eye, they may stick to the contact lens and this will irritate the eyes.

Irritate the eye
Cause the eyes to water, become red and sore

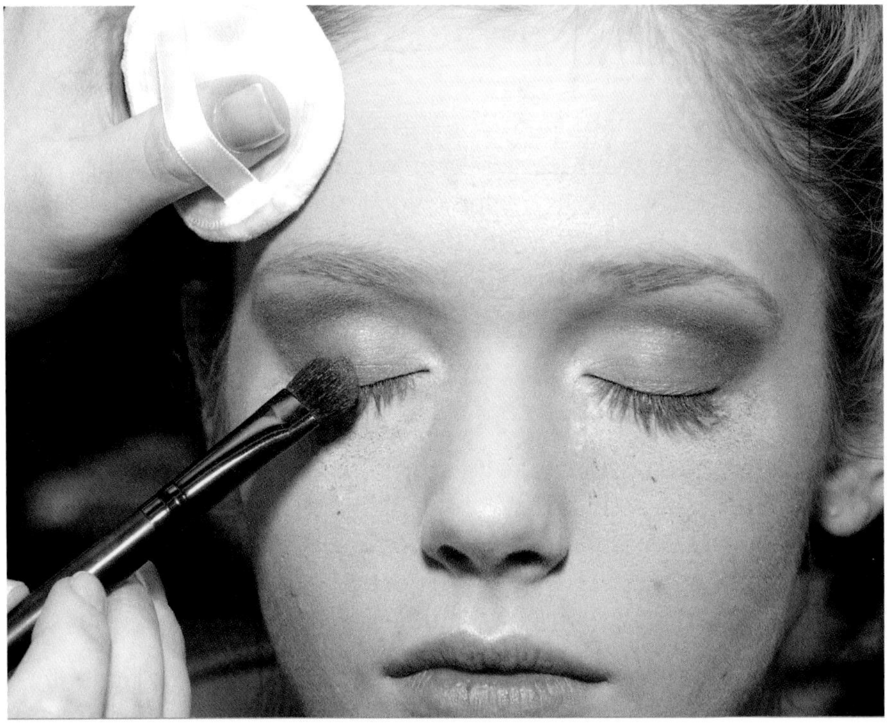

Work gently over the eye area

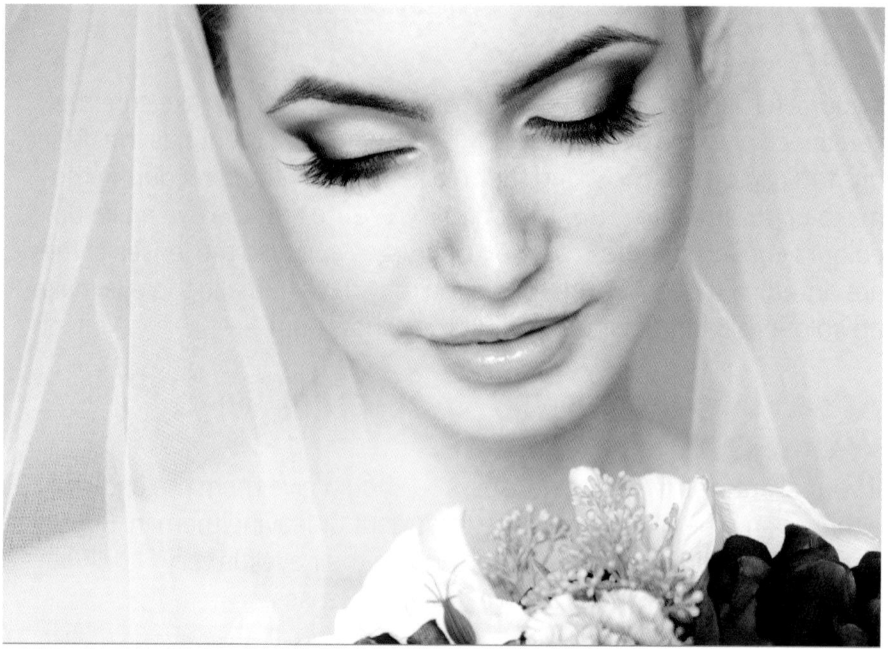
Always listen to what the bride wants for her big day

HANDY HINTS

The use of shading and highlighting products is particularly important in photographic make-up work. In black and white photographs, the make-up applied needs to make the angles of the face, such as the cheekbones and jaw line, look more **defined**. Shaders and highlighters will help to do this.

Defined

More obvious, stands out more

THE OCCASION

A wedding

Many brides will choose to have a make-up artist do their make-up for them on their big day. This is because they want to look extra special. It is important that you check the following so that it all runs as smoothly as possible:

- the date and time of the wedding
- the colour of the bridesmaids' dresses and the bride's flowers – this will help you choose the colours of the make-up, such as the lipstick and nail colours
- whether the bride is having her hair done before or after the make-up – if the hair is done afterwards, the make-up may need to be checked and corrected if needed just in case any has been washed off during the hair styling.

Sometimes a practice make-up is carried out before the wedding day. This is to make sure that the bride-to-be is happy with the make-up. You may also need to give the client some tips on how to keep the make-up looking good all day. This may include applying more lipstick.

HANDY HINTS

Refer back to Chapter 106 Basic make-up application to remind you of the correct and hygienic use of shaders and highlighters.

ACTIVITY

Design a leaflet that could be given out to clients in your salon to promote a wedding make-up service.

A photoshoot in a photography studio or for a fashion magazine

Some photography studios may have a member of staff who is trained in applying make-up. Other photographers use freelance make-up artists, who they call in when they are needed. There may even be the chance for you to work with a local studio or fashion photographer.

Photographic make-up can be very creative. There are many different effects that can be made by the photographer by using different camera angles and lighting effects.

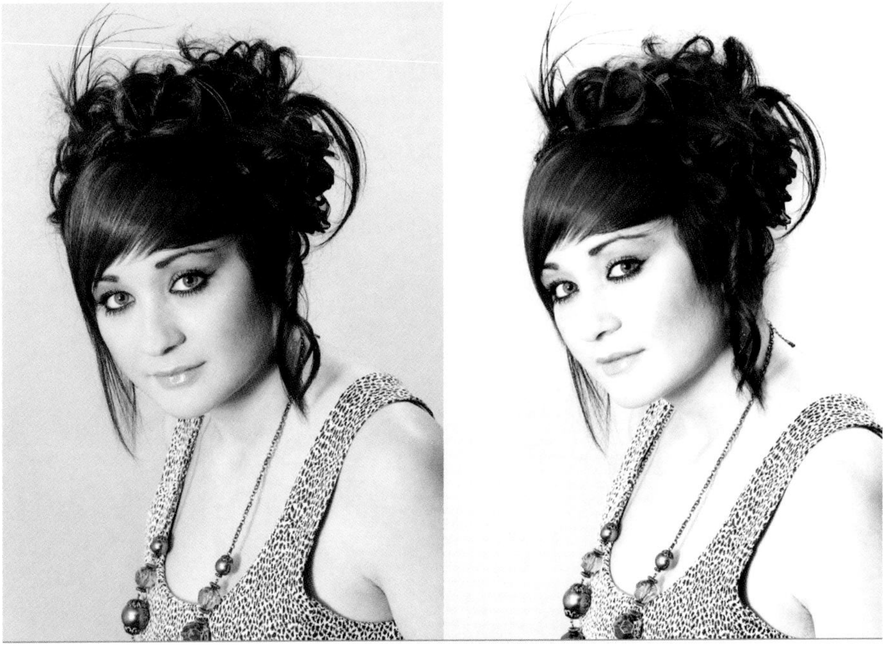

Colour and black and white photographs of the same make-up

The following points need to be thought about when applying make-up for photography work:

- Discuss with the photographer what effect they want to achieve for the photo. This may make a difference to the colours you use with your make-up. If the photo is to be a black-and-white finish, the make-up may need to be stronger.
- The lighting that is used for photography can create a lot of heat. As a result the client's skin can become warm and may **perspire**. For this reason it is important not to apply the make-up too heavily.
- You may need to re-apply the face powder during the photography session to help to reduce the shine from the skin's surface if the client gets warm.
- **Matt colours** are better for photographic work as they do not cause a shine and therefore photograph better. Any shine on the skin may cause a **reflection** on the finished photograph.
- Products should be blended really well, as failing to do so may show up on the finished photo.
- Shaders and highlighters can be used to help create and define facial features. This is particularly important if the photograph is to be in black and white.
- Avoid creamy products as these can create a shiny appearance on the photo.
- For bridal photography make-up, it is best to use powder products for shading and highlighting. This will reduce the shine on the face.

Perspire
Sweat

Matt colours
Colours that do not have a shine

Reflection
Shiny area

ACTIVITY

Compare the pictures below showing the same photos in colour and black and white.

- Can you see how strong the make-up needs to be applied for the effect needed in black and white?
- Where would you put the shader and highlighter products?

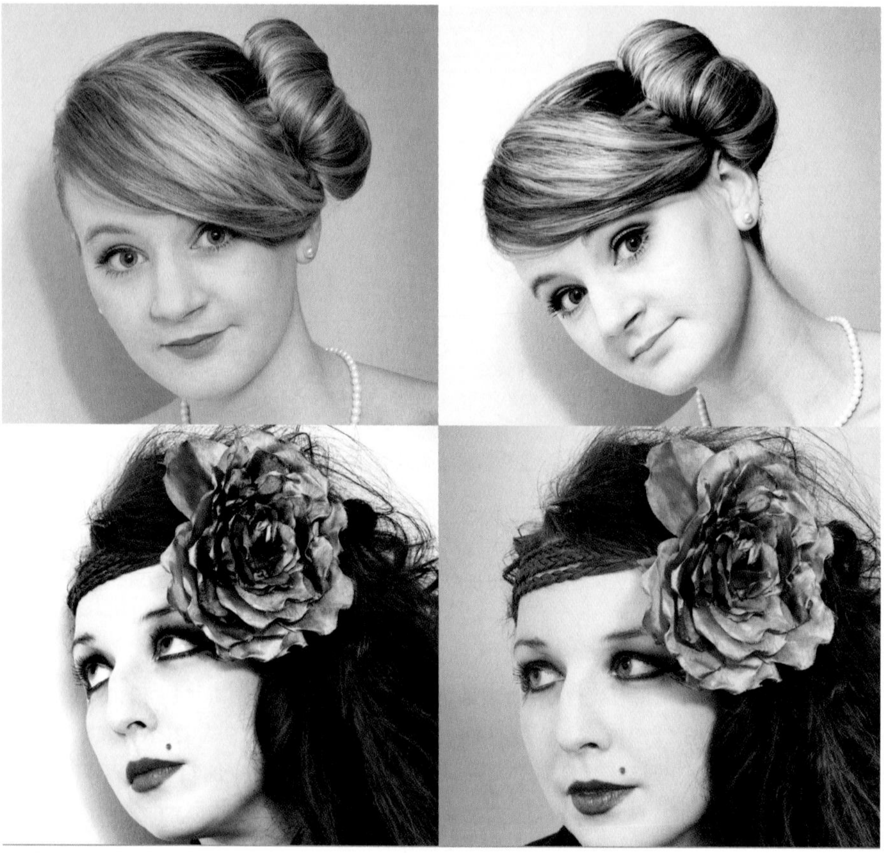

Fashion make-up

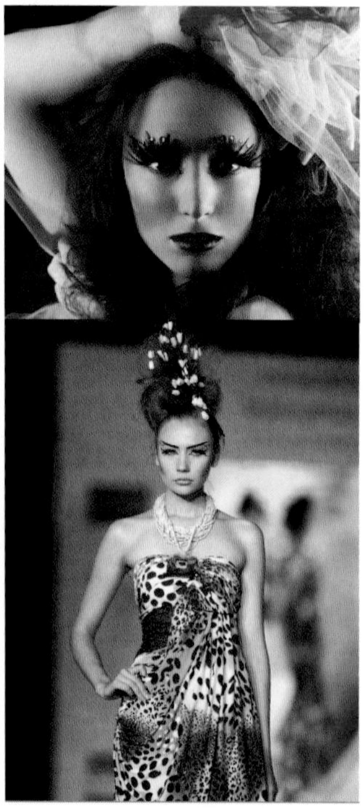

Catwalk-show make-up

ACTIVITY

Practise applying different coloured make-up looks. Take photographs of them. If you can, see what they look like in black and white and compare them with the coloured photos. Which colours stand out most when the photos are in black and white?

As with all make-up treatments, you will need to think about what the finished look will be before applying the make-up.

Fashion and catwalk shows

The lighting used for fashion and catwalk shows is often strong artificial lighting. This means that the make-up applied to the models needs to be very bold. You will need to work closely with the organiser of the show to find out what make-up they would like on the models.

HANDY HINTS

For catwalk-show make-up, you may need to apply more shader and highlighter, eyeshadow, eyebrow and lip colour to make the make-up stand out more.

HANDY HINTS

If the client becomes too hot, a refreshing fine-mist spray can be used to cool their skin.

OTHER FACTORS

The following factors also need to be taken into account when carrying out a photographic make-up service. See Chapter 106 for more information.

- Eye and lip shape – so that you know where to put the make-up to correct the shape where needed.
- Adverse skin conditions – these are conditions that would either prevent (stop) the treatment from taking place, eg a bruised eye, or restrict the treatment (so that it would need adapting). For example, if the client had watery eyes, you would need to take great care when applying the eye make-up.
- Face shape – by using blusher, shader and highlighter, you can correct different face shapes, eg applying shader to the sides of the jaw and forehead on a square-shaped face.
- Skin, eye and hair colour – you need to choose make-up colours that suit the client's natural colours.
- Fashion trends – it is important to keep up to date with the latest make-up looks, eg in magazines, on the internet, on the television. This will make sure that your photographic make-up looks are up to date.

HANDY HINTS

The make-up colours that you use may be chosen by the photographer or event organiser. It will depend on the theme for the finished look. You may not always, therefore, be able to think about the client's skin, eye and hair colour when choosing the make-up colours to apply.

HANDY HINTS

Refer back to Chapter 106 Basic make-up application and read up on these factors for more information.

PLANNING A PHOTOGRAPHIC MAKE-UP BY USING A MOOD BOARD

Mood boards can be your chance to show your ideas in a creative way. You can use written information, fabrics, pictures and many other artistic materials on your mood boards. All of these will help to get attention, which will enhance what you are trying to communicate.

Different photographic make-up looks can be easily presented on a mood board. It is a chance to link different themes (such as colours) and different make-up techniques (such as eye make-up designs).

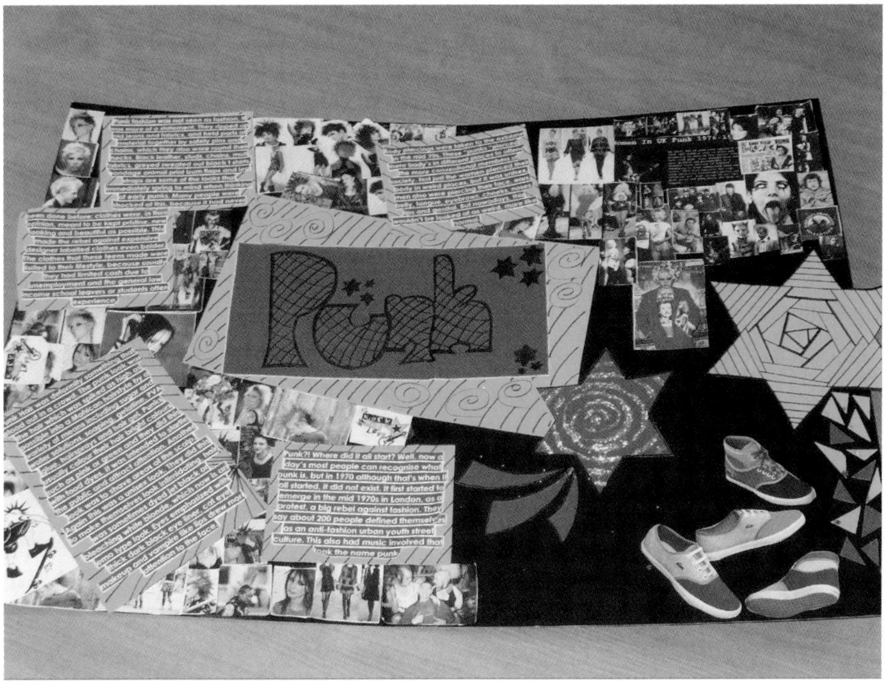

A mood board for a punk theme

HANDY HINTS

Go to Chapter 112 Creating a hair and beauty image for more information on how to create a mood board.

HANDY HINTS

After you have carried out a consultation with your client, you can present a mood board to show them how your ideas are developing, and to check that you are working as your client wants you to. Mood boards are a type of poster design that may have images, text and samples of objects. They are used to develop a design idea and to show the image to other team members or clients.

ACTIVITY

Look at how wedding make-up is different in different cultures around the world. In small groups, each choose a different culture of your own (your tutor will help you) and design a wedding look for a bride from that cultural background.

- Create a mood board to show off your designs and planning.
- Finally, carry out the make-up look. Show the looks from different groups as part of a catwalk show. The theme could be 'brides from around the world'.

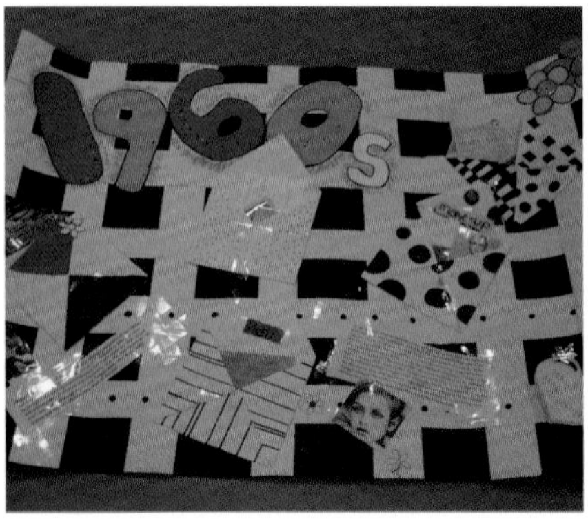

A mood board for a 1960s theme

For your mood board to work, the following factors need to be taken into account:

- Planning: prepare any information you are going to include on the mood board. You will need to be clear as to what information you are trying to get across and make sure that it is written clearly, so that it is easily understood.
- Images: choose the images carefully. Make sure that they match what you are trying to communicate.
- Colour: the colours you choose are important, particularly in make-up. Colours can also be very eye-catching and make the mood board more interesting to look at.
- Research: try to use a variety of different resources when you research your ideas (eg magazines, the internet, books, etc).
- **Verbal communication**: sometimes, you may need to talk to explain what your mood board is about. This will help with communicating your ideas.
- **Written communication**: make sure that the written information on a mood board is short and clear. It will need to be easy to read and understand. The written information should support the images and other creative materials that you have used on your mood board.
- Presentation: mood boards should be placed where people can stand and look at them. They may also be used as part of a presentation where you speak about the subject and use the mood board to support what you are saying. In a salon a mood board can be placed on the wall to promote the make-up looks you can create.

Verbal communication
Communicating through spoken language

Written communication
Communicating through the use of written words, such as on a treatment plan

ACTIVITY

Create some make-up mood boards that you could have on your salon wall. The purpose of this is to show the different looks that a client may choose for their make-up. Develop one showing warm colours and one for cool colours.

HANDY HINTS

Refer to Chapter 106 Basic make-up application for more information and examples of warm and cool colours.

APPLYING PHOTOGRAPHIC MAKE-UP

The routines for carrying out photographic make-up are the same routines as carried out in Chapter 106. Please see this chapter for details.

AFTERCARE ADVICE

After you have finished applying the make-up to your client, it is important to make sure that you give them the correct aftercare advice. Refer to Chapter 106 for details.

EVALUATING THE TREATMENT

After you have finished the treatment, make sure that you record everything you have done. This will help you to **evaluate** your work and learn from your experience before the next time you do it.

Evaluate
Assess; look back at something that you have done and think about how you could improve it

VERBAL FEEDBACK

Get verbal feedback from your client or customer, eg the bride, photographer or organiser of the fashion show. Ask them how they felt it went and whether or not you could improve on anything next time. You will then be able to think about this for any future photographic make-up treatments that you carry out.

HANDY HINTS

Keep photos of work that you have carried out in a portfolio. You can then use this to show future clients.

WRITTEN FEEDBACK

Make a note of the products and colours used on your treatment plan. This may be in the form of a letter from the show organiser, thanking you for the work that you carried out and maybe giving you some suggestions to help you improve for the future.

HANDY HINTS

Make a note of any useful hints to yourself as soon as you can after the photographic make-up service. They will then be fresh in your mind.

PHOTOGRAPHIC EVIDENCE

You may be able to take a photograph of the completed make-up that you carried out – on the bride or in the photography studio or of the models at a show. You can use these to show future clients the work that you have done. It may also help to give them ideas for their own make-up.

SELF-EVALUATION

It is a good idea to write down any helpful tips for the next time you carry out this service. An example may be to remember to check that you have a sink nearby to wash your hands in before and after applying make-up to each model at a fashion show.

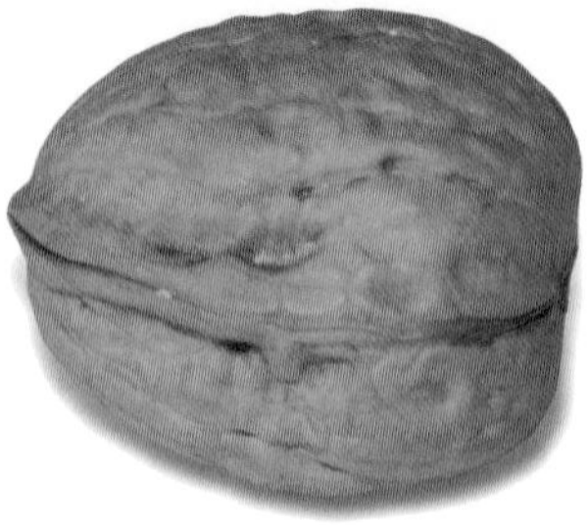

IN A NUTSHELL

You are now at the end of the chapter. Before you test your knowledge with the revision activities, check the following list to see if you feel confident in all the areas covered. If there are still any areas you're unsure of, go back over them in the book and ask your tutor for extra support:

- how to maintain safe and effective methods of working when providing a photographic make-up service
- what products, tools and equipment are required and how to use them safely and hygienically
- what factors you need to consider
- how to communicate and behave in a positive way
- the preparation needed and how to carry out a photographic make-up
- basic anatomy of the face (the structure and function of the skin, skin types and the main facial bones)
- the purpose of a mood board and how to present one
- aftercare and the different methods of evaluating the service.

REVISION ACTIVITIES

Use the questions below to test your knowledge of Chapter 216 to see just how much information you've gained. This can help you to prepare for your assessments.

Turn to pages 508–510 for the answers.

SmartScreen 106 sample questions

WORDS TO FIND

Copy and complete the sentences below. Use these words to help you fill in the gaps.

mood board	hygienic	products	highlighter
factors	tools	photographic	evaluate
make-up	equipment	shader	theme

1 You will need to be prepared to carry your products, ________ and ________ to locations outside the salon for a photographic make-up.

2 A ________ is a type of poster design that may consist of images, text and samples of objects.

3 You should keep your treatment area tidy and use only ________ tools and equipment.

4 Make sure that you record everything you have done. This will help you to ________ your performance and learn from your experience for next time.

5 A ________ is a make-up product that is used to make areas look less noticeable, such as a wide jaw line.

6 A ________ is a make-up product that is used to make areas look more noticeable, such as the cheekbones.

7 The occasion, skin type, face shape and fashion trends are examples of ________ that need to be taken into account when carrying out a photographic ________ service.

8 If you are going to a different location to carry out a ________ make-up service (other than in the salon), it would be a good idea to carry all of your tools, equipment and ________ in a suitable storage bag or box.

TEST YOUR KNOWLEDGE FURTHER

1 List **three** different occasions for which you may need to apply photographic make-up.

2 List **three** things that you need to take into account when applying make-up for photography work.

3 What is a mood board?

4 What do you need to take into account when you are designing a mood board?

217 THE ART OF COLOURING HAIR

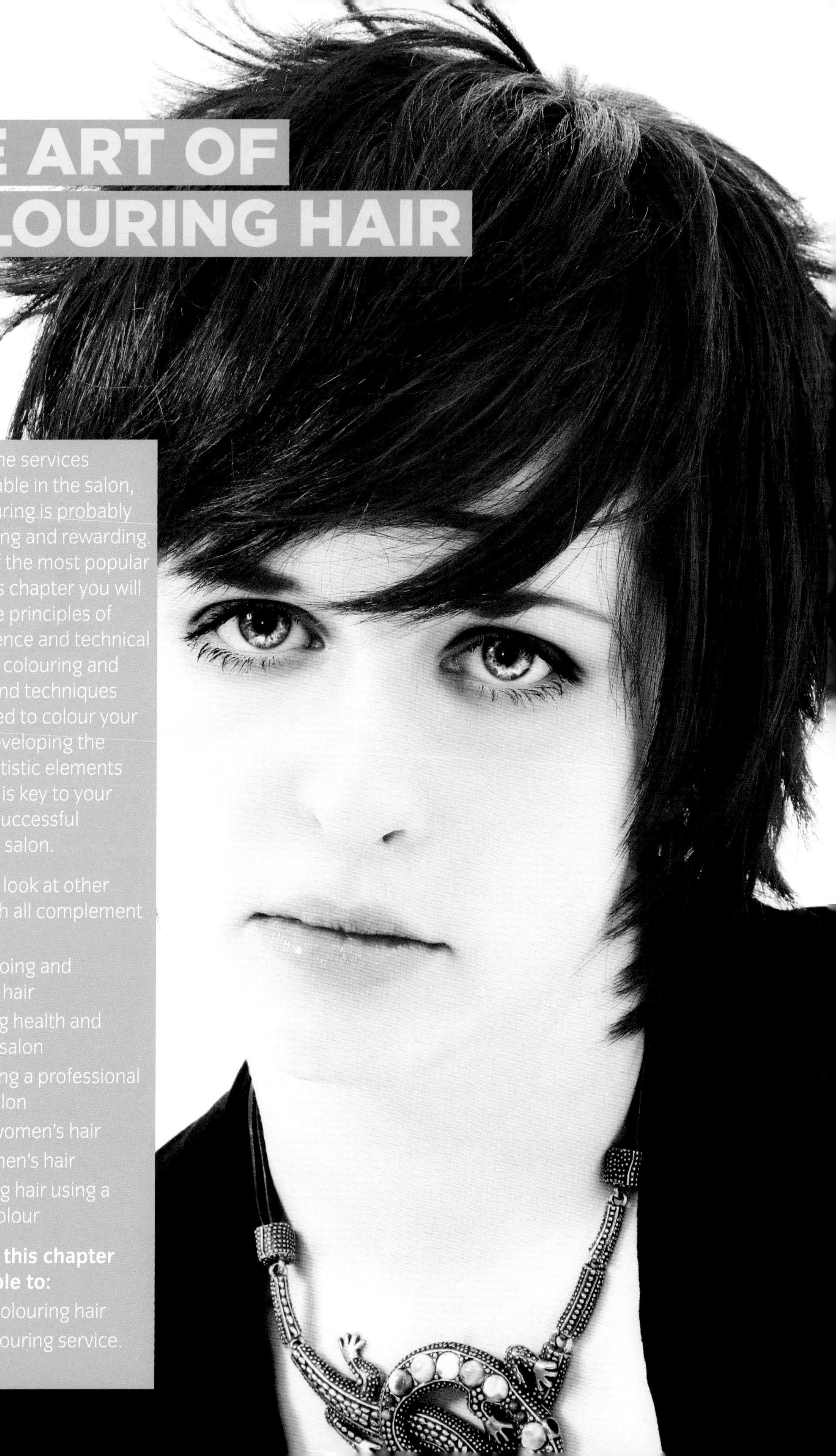

Of all the services available in the salon, colouring is probably the most exciting and rewarding. It is also one of the most popular services. In this chapter you will learn about the principles of colour, the science and technical aspects of hair colouring and the products and techniques that can be used to colour your client's hair. Developing the creative and artistic elements of the services is key to your ability to be a successful colourist in the salon.

Don't forget to look at other chapters, which all complement this chapter:

- 003 Shampooing and conditioning hair
- 113 Following health and safety in the salon
- 102 Presenting a professional image in a salon
- 103 Styling women's hair
- 104 Styling men's hair
- 111 Colouring hair using a temporary colour

After reading this chapter you will be able to:

1 prepare for colouring hair

2 provide a colouring service.

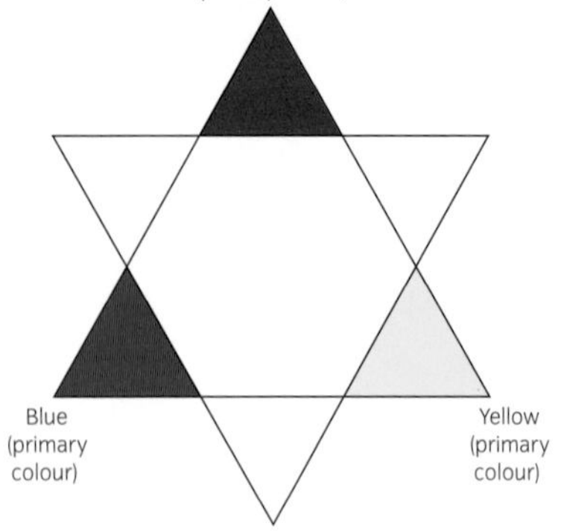

Primary colours

THE SCIENCE OF COLOUR

All the colours that we see come from red, yellow and blue. These are called the primary colours. They cannot be made from mixing other colours together.

Mixing equal quantities of two of the primary colours together will produce three more colours. Mixing red and yellow together will produce orange, mixing yellow and blue will give you green, and red together with blue will give violet. These are called the secondary colours.

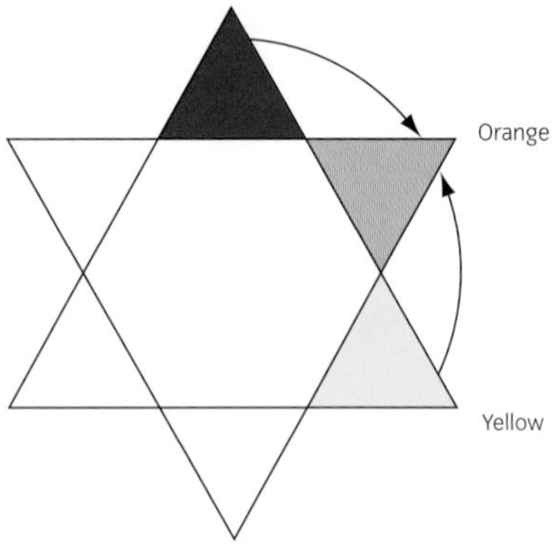

Secondary colour orange

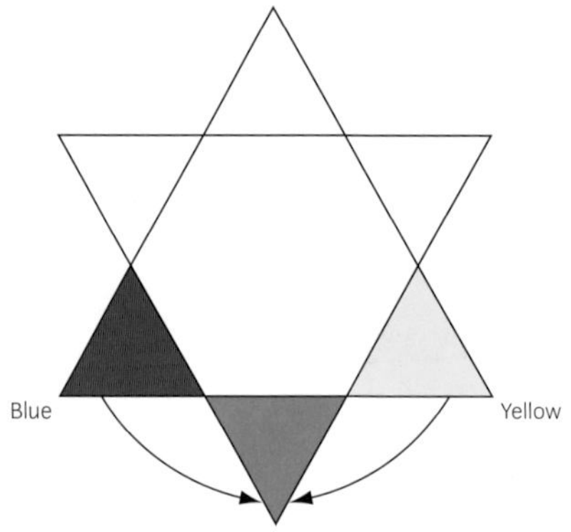

Secondary colour green

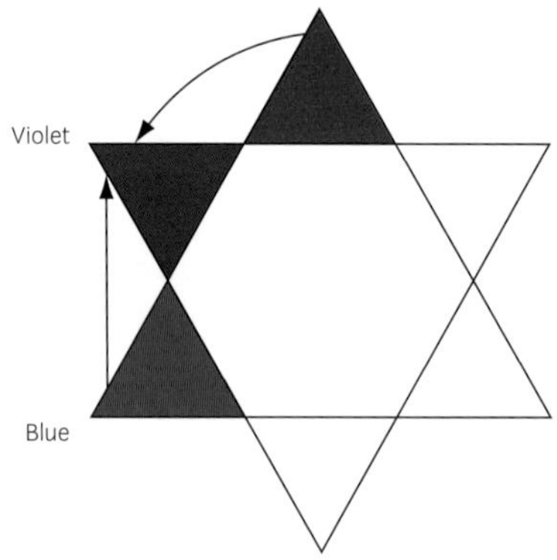

Secondary colour violet

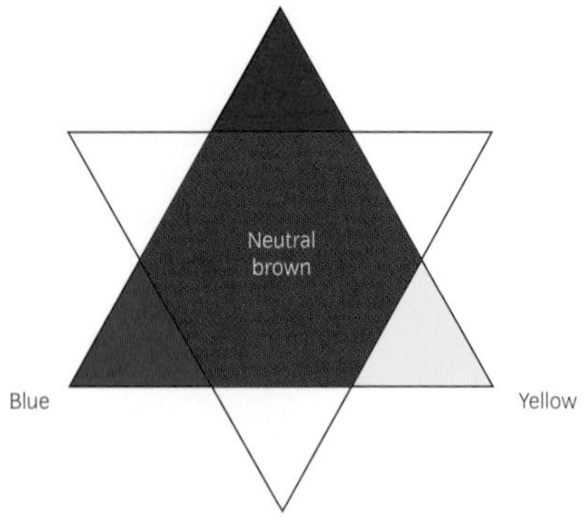

Mixing all the primary colours together gives a neutral brown shade

HANDY HINTS

To help you remember the order of the colour star, try to memorise: Richard Of York Gave Battle In Vain.

Richard	Red
Of	Orange
York	Yellow
Gave	Green
Battle	Blue
In **V**ain	Indigo/Violet

You can make lots of other colours by mixing primary colours and secondary colours together in different amounts. If you mix the three primary colours together you will get a neutral brown shade.

ACTIVITY

Try mixing water-based paints together to prove the colours you can get from the primary and secondary colours. Make a chart showing the colours you mixed, with details of which colours you mixed together and how much of each you used.

HOW LIGHT AFFECTS COLOUR

Daylight and the light we get from light bulbs will change the colour you see when you look at something. The brighter the light the brighter the colour will be. If the light is dim then the colour of things will appear to be less strong.

In certain lights a colour may appear quite different. If the light source is coloured it will change the colour of the object you are looking at.

NATURAL HAIR COLOUR

The pigments that make up the natural colour of the hair are called melanin. They are found in the cortex. There are two types of melanin in the hair:

- Eumelanin is made up of black and brown pigments. They are large colour **molecules**.
- Pheomelanin is made up of small molecules of red and yellow pigments.

Molecule
The smallest part of something

How dark or light the hair is and what shade it is will depend on how much of each of the types of melanin are in the hair.

THE INTERNATIONAL COLOUR CHART

The International Colour Chart (ICC) is the numbering system that all manufacturers follow. Everyone uses the same numbers to describe a colour's depth.

When you refer to your client's hair colour, you look at the depth and the tone of the hair. The depth is how light or dark the hair is, and the tone is the colour you see. If you describe someone as a redhead, you're describing their tone. If you describe someone as bleached blonde, you're referring to the depth of the hair.

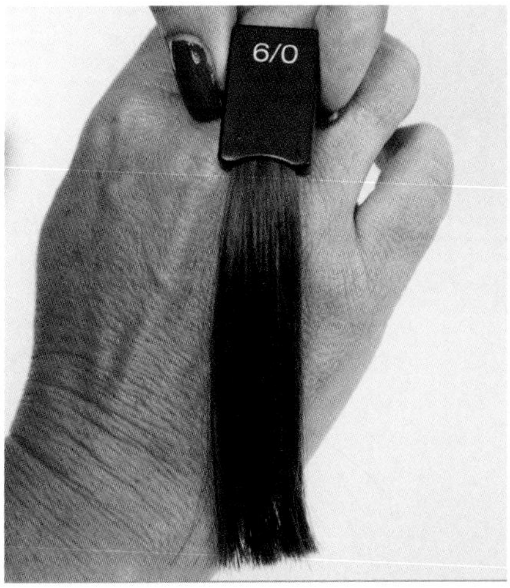

Depth of colour at 6/0

DEPTHS OF HAIR

The natural depths of hair range from 1 (black) to 10 (lightest blonde).

The range of depths, from lightest to darkest, is as follows:

10 lightest blonde
9 very light blonde
8 light blonde
7 medium blonde
6 dark blonde
5 light brown
4 medium brown
3 dark brown
2 darkest brown
1 black

TONES IN THE HAIR

The tone numbering system describes the colour you see. All manufacturers use a similar description of the tone, but the numbering system will vary. Depths and tones are usually written in numbers for the stylist's use, and given descriptive names for the client's benefit. For example: the description for depth 8 (light blonde) may be written as 8/0, 8–0, 8.0 or 8N, depending on the manufacturer. The 0 refers to the tone.

Examples of primary tones

Description of tone	Wella	L'Oréal	Goldwell
Natural	/0	/0	N – natural
Ash	/1 or /9	/1	A – ash
Blue ash	/8	/1	BV – blue violet
Green ash	/2	N/A	NA – green
Gold	/3	/3	G – gold
Red	/4	/6	R – red
Mahogany	/6	/5	RB – red brown
Brunette	/7	N/A	B – brown

In the colour chart, the first digit after the depth is the primary or stronger tonal colour. For example 8/3 is depth 8 (light blonde) with a primary tone of 3 (gold): this could be described as a light golden blonde. Primary tones are often mixed together to create secondary tones: these are indicated by the second digit.

Examples of secondary tones

Description of tone	Wella	L'Oréal (as a guide)
Natural ash	/01	/01
Natural gold	/03	/03
Copper (red and gold)	/43	/4 or /46 or /44 or /64
Copper (gold and red)	/34	/4 or /43 or /34
Violet red	/46	/56
Mahogany red	/56	/26 or /45
Golden brown	/73	/35 or/53

For example, 6/43 is depth 6 (dark blonde) with a tone of /43 (red and gold). This colour could be called dark red gold blonde or dark copper blonde.

If the mixed tone was more gold than red, it would be shown as 6/34. This would still be a dark copper blonde, but the copper tone created would not be as vibrant as 6/43.

TYPES OF COLOURING PRODUCT

There are five types of hair-colouring product that can be used to change the colour of the hair:

- temporary colour
- semi-permanent colour
- quasi-permanent colour
- permanent colour
- lighteners (hair bleach).

Each type is used for a different purpose and has a different effect on the hair.

TEMPORARY COLOURS

These products offer the client a quick colouring solution without commitment. They do not need any tests before use and can usually be removed easily. They are ideal for adding some 'life' to the colour of the hair.

	Advantages	Disadvantages
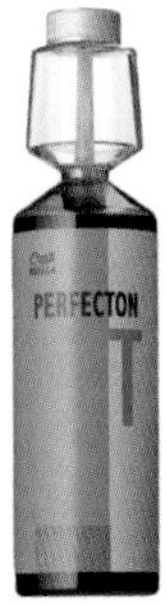	▪ No commitment ▪ Adds shine and tone ▪ Enhances natural colour ▪ Quick and easy to apply ▪ No development time ▪ Chemical free ▪ Good way to introduce the client to colour ▪ Lasts only one shampoo	▪ Only lasts for one shampoo ▪ Cannot make the hair lighter ▪ Does not colour white hair very well ▪ Colour might be uneven and difficult to remove from porous hair

SEMI-PERMANENT COLOURS

Semi-permanent colours are a useful way of introducing the client to colour. They last for up to eight shampoos so the client can change the effect more easily than with permanent colours. They do not usually require any mixing and no skin test is necessary before use. They will blend in small quantities of white hair but they will not lighten the hair. They provide a choice for clients with sensitivity or **allergy** problems. If they are used on porous hair the result can be darker or stronger than intended. The colour may also be uneven on porous or damaged hair. If the hair has serious cuticle damage the colour may be washed out of the hair more quickly.

Allergy
Where the body reacts badly to products; may cause a rash, itchiness and redness

	Advantages	Disadvantages
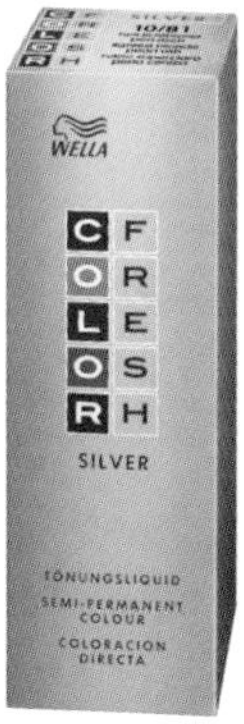	▪ No commitment ▪ Good way to introduce the client to colour ▪ Will not damage the hair ▪ Lasts between six and eight shampoos ▪ Adds shine, tone and depth ▪ Enhances current look and can refresh existing colour ▪ Blends up to 20% white hair ▪ Enhances the natural colour ▪ Can be used for fashion effects	▪ Only lasts for six to eight shampoos ▪ Colour fades with each shampoo ▪ Cannot make the hair lighter ▪ Only blends white hair ▪ Colour might be uneven and give a darker result on porous hair

QUASI-PERMANENT COLOURS

Quasi-permanent colours last longer than semi-permanents but not as long as true permanent colours – up to 24 shampoos. They can be used to produce a wide range of colour results. The colour has to be mixed with a 'developer'. This will cause a chemical process to occur and produce the result you want to achieve during the processing time. Quasi-permanent colours give better coverage of white hair than semi-permanent colours. They can be used to give up to two shades of lift to natural hair. The client must have a skin test before having a quasi-permanent colour. Quasi-permanent colours are popular as high-street retail colours for use at home. They come in cream and gel form.

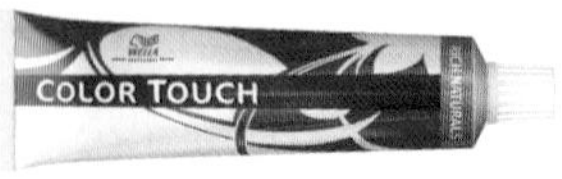

Advantages	Disadvantages
■ An introduction to permanent colour ■ Lasts up to 24 shampoos ■ Will add depth and tone ■ Can be used to lighten hair a little ■ Fashion colours ■ Will refresh faded colour ■ Will cover up to 50% white hair	■ Will leave a regrowth ■ Colours will fade more quickly on hair with a damaged cuticle ■ Will only cover 50% white hair ■ Needs a skin test before application

PERMANENT COLOURS

These are available in a wide range of shades and tones. They give a permanent result. They can be used to lighten the hair by up to four shades. They cover 100 per cent of white hair. Permanent colours can be used to produce natural, fashion and fantasy colours. They are very popular for avante garde styling. Permanent colours contain a chemical called paraphenylenediamine (usually called PPD for short). This substance can cause a skin reaction in some people. A skin test is necessary before it is used.

Hydrogen peroxide
A chemical used to bleach hair.

Permanent colours are mixed with **hydrogen peroxide** immediately before use. This will cause a chemical reaction which produces the colour during the development time. A regrowth application will be needed every four to six weeks as the hair grows.

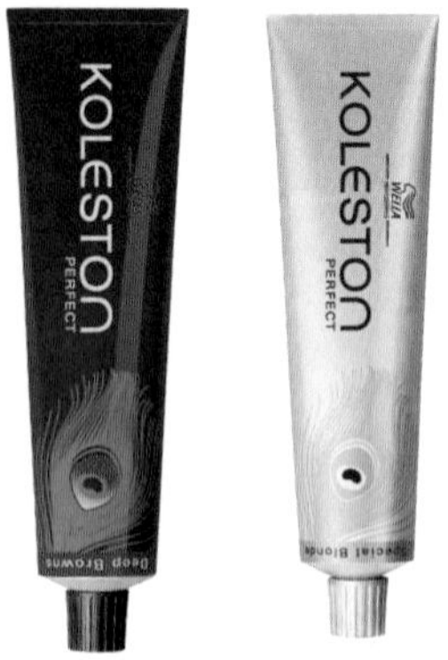

Advantages	Disadvantages
■ Will give a permanent result ■ Can be mixed to produce a huge range of colours ■ Adds tone and depth ■ Can give a complete change of image for the client ■ Covers 100% white hair ■ Can lighten hair up to four shades ■ High-lift colours can lighten the hair up to five shades ■ Can be used for fashion effects and vibrant colours, both full-head and partial-colouring methods	■ Results are permanent and not easy to change ■ Commits the client to colour when applied to the full head ■ A skin test is required before application ■ A regrowth application is required every four to six weeks ■ Can cause damage to the hair as a result of the chemical process

LIGHTENING PRODUCTS

Lightening products are used to change the client's natural colour to a lighter shade. Bleaches are products made especially to lift the natural colour of the hair. They will lighten the hair up to six shades. They are available in powder or gel/oil form.

Powder bleach

Powder bleach is mixed with hydrogen peroxide immediately before use. It is mixed to a creamy consistency that is liquid enough to spread when it is applied but not so runny that it drips everywhere and runs through the hair. This type of bleach gives the greatest degree of lift. It is generally used for partial colouring techniques with caps and foils. It can be used for full-head applications when used with lower-strength hydrogen peroxide.

Oil or gel bleach

Oil or gel bleach, sometimes called emulsion bleach, is used for full-head on scalp applications. It is mixed with low-strength hydrogen peroxide and can have 'boosters' added to give a greater degree of lift. It will give as much lift as powder bleach but does not damage the hair quite as much.

Bleach products generally produce a yellow result and anti-yellowing agents are added to reduce this effect. Sometimes the use of a toner will be needed to reduce the yellow effect. These are especially made for use on hair that has been bleached. Bleach products will damage the hair. Conditioning the hair regularly will be necessary to keep the hair in good condition.

	Advantages	Disadvantages
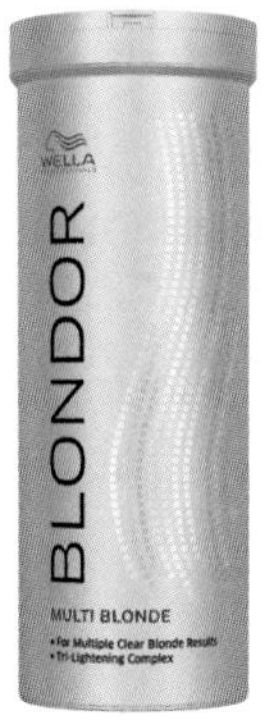	▪ Lightens the hair by up to six shades ▪ Gives a permanent result ▪ Produces fashion effects using foils and caps ▪ Gives strong contrast when used in partial application ▪ Can be used for complete change of image	▪ Results are permanent and not easy to change ▪ Commits the client to lightening product when applied to the full head ▪ A regrowth application is required every four to six weeks ▪ Some partial applications can be difficult to maintain ▪ Can cause damage to the hair as a result of the chemical process

ACTIVITY

In a group, prepare a chart showing the different types of colour, and the advantages and disadvantages of each.

HANDY HINTS

Find out if there are any shows or demonstrations being held in your area that you could go to.

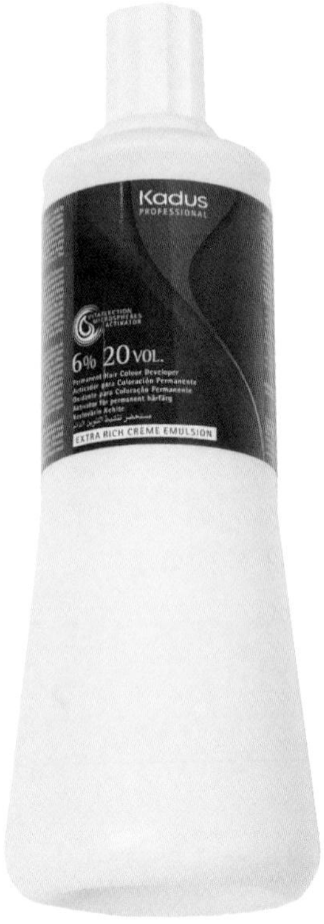

20 volume peroxide

HYDROGEN PEROXIDE

Permanent colours, high-lift permanent colours, bleaches and some quasi-permanent colours are mixed with a chemical called hydrogen peroxide immediately before they are applied to the hair.

Hydrogen peroxide has the chemical formula H_2O_2. It is a colourless liquid made from water (H_2O) which has had more oxygen (O_2) added to it.

$2H_2O + O_2 = 2H_2O_2$

When the hydrogen peroxide is mixed with permanent colour, oxygen is released. The oxygen causes a chemical reaction to occur in the colour to produce the shade required. It also affects the melanin in the cortex. When mixed with bleaching products the oxygen given off is used to lighten the hair by changing the melanin in the cortex.

Hydrogen peroxide is used in different strengths when colouring. The strength to be used is determined by the amount of lift you want to get. The greater the lift you want, the higher the strength you need to use.

The terms volume and percentage (%) are used to describe the strength. Hydrogen peroxide is usually available in the following volumes:

10 volume, 20 volume, 30 volume and 40 volume

The volume strength describes the amount of oxygen that will be given off during development.

For example, if you fill a small container with 10 volume hydrogen peroxide it will give off enough oxygen to fill the same container ten times.

20 volume hydrogen peroxide will fill the container 20 times in the same time. 40 volume will fill it 40 times.

HANDY HINTS

Hydrogen peroxide, like all chemicals used in the salon, must be handled and used safely and correctly. Refresh your knowledge of the COSHH regulations in Chapter 113 Following health and safety in the salon.

The term 'percentage' (%) describes the amount of pure hydrogen peroxide that is mixed with water to provide the amount of oxygen you need. For example:

- A 3 per cent solution would be made from 3 parts pure peroxide added to 97 parts water. This will give a strength of 10 volume.
- 6 per cent = 20 volume
- 9 per cent = 30 volume
- 12 per cent = 40 volume.

Alkali
Something with a pH over 7. An example is an alkali toothpaste

Neutralise
To make a chemical neutral

Hydrogen peroxide might not work if kept in a warm environment. It often has a weak acid added to it to make it work. This will allow it to be stored safely. Permanent colours and bleaches will have **alkalis** added to them to **neutralise** the acid in the hydrogen peroxide so the oxygen is released more easily.

USING PEROXIDE

The table below shows the different strengths of peroxide and their uses.

Percentage of peroxide	Volume of peroxide	Uses
1.5% 3% 4%	As a guide, we refer to these weak solutions as 10 volume and developers	To darken, to add tone and quasi-permanent colours
6%	20 volume	One shade of lift, to darken, to add tone, to cover 100% white hair
9%	30 volume	Two shades of lift with a normal tint, or three shades of lift with a high-lift tint
12%	40 volume	Three shades of lift with a normal tint, or four to five shades of lift with a high-lift tint

ACTIVITY

Use the salon's shade chart and identify the tone of the hair of others in your group. Make a list and then compare your results with those of the rest of the group.

USING THE COLOUR CHART

Successful colouring is based on your skills, your creativity and knowing your products. A key part of achieving that success is using the colour chart in your consultation with the client. It will help you do three things that are essential to achieving the result the client wants.

1 Deciding the depth and tone of the client's natural colour. This is your starting point. Match the client's hair to the swatches on the chart to find the one that is nearest to the natural colour.

2 Finding out the colour the client wants to go. Let the client look at the chart and discuss the colours with them to decide what colour they want to be. This is called the target colour.

3 Once you have decided **1** and **2** you need to work out the colour or colours and techniques you need to use to achieve the target colour.

HANDY HINTS

You will not be able to match the colour exactly to the chart. You need to decide on the tone that is nearest to one of the colours on the chart.

HANDY HINTS

You will learn more about colour and colour selection when you progress to Level 2 and Level 3.

HOW COLOURING PRODUCTS AFFECT THE HAIR STRUCTURE

Whatever colouring product you are going to use on a client, and whatever technique you will use, it is very important to know the effect of the colour and process on the structure of the hair.

TEMPORARY COLOURS

Temporary colours have large molecules which coat the outside of the cuticle. This puts a thin film of colour on the outside of the hair. You can still see the natural colour through the film. This will enhance the natural colour but not change it dramatically.

If the cuticle is damaged or the hair is porous then the colour molecules can enter the cortex. This is likely to produce an uneven or patchy colour and it may be harder to remove it.

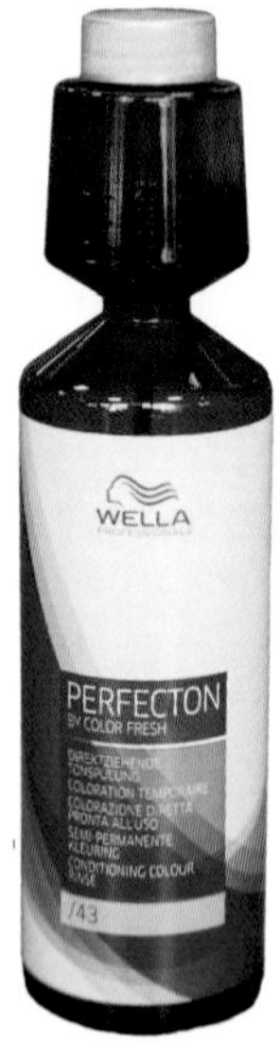

Temporary colour rinse

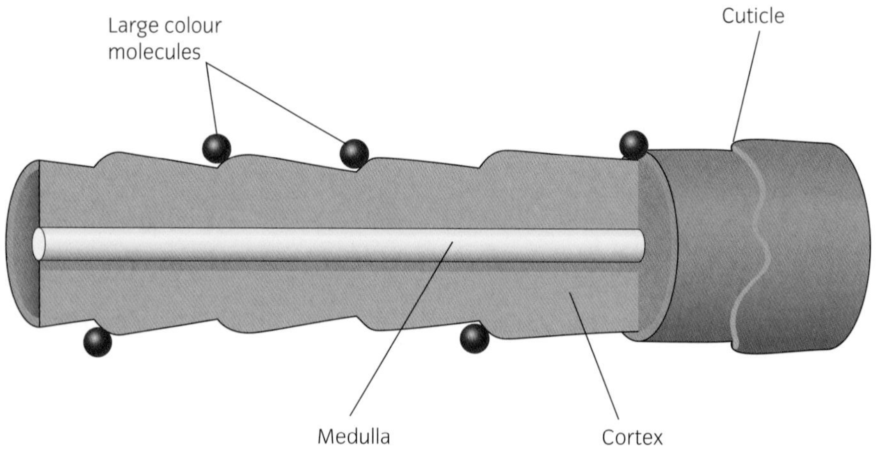

Effects of temporary colour molecules on the hair

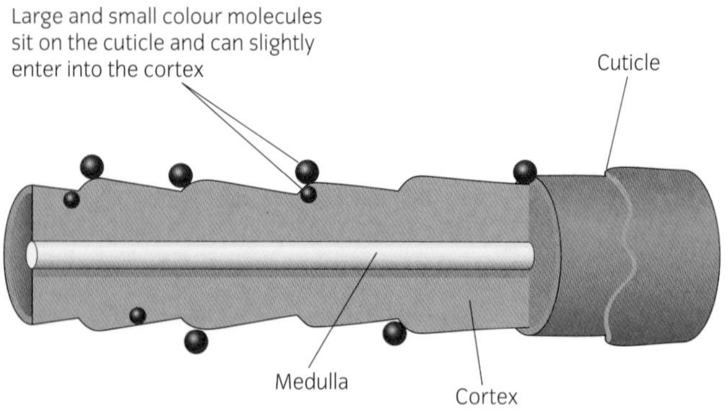

Effects of semi-permanent colour molecules on the hair

SEMI-PERMANENT COLOURS

These are made up of both large and small colour molecules. The large molecules coat the cuticle. The smaller molecules will lodge between the cuticle and the cortex. If the hair is porous then the smaller molecules can get into the cortex. This could give a patchy, uneven result which may make the hair darker than you intended.

The colour has to be left on the hair for a period of time to allow the colour to lodge between the cuticle and the cortex. This is called the development time. The manufacturer's instructions will tell you how long the development time should be.

PERMANENT COLOUR

Permanent colours contain small coloured molecules that are small enough to pass under the cuticle and into the cortex. The colour is mixed with hydrogen peroxide immediately before use. The hydrogen peroxide will give off some of its oxygen once it is mixed with the colour. The oxygen does two things: first, it will **oxidise** some of the melanin making it colourless. This also creates space for the artificial colour to go in. Second, the oxygen joins the small artificial colour molecules together and at the same time makes them coloured.

Oxidise
To add oxygen

The new large molecules are too big to come out of the hair, which is what makes the colour permanent. For a lighter result than the client's natural colour a higher volume of hydrogen peroxide is used so more of the hair's natural pigment is oxidised.

Darker permanent colour

For a colour darker or the same as the client's natural depth, the colour is usually mixed with 20 volume or 3 per cent hydrogen peroxide: 10 volume is used to oxidise the melanin and the other 10 volume reacts with the colour to make the large coloured molecules.

Lighter permanent colour

If a lighter than natural depth is required, 30 volume or 9 per cent hydrogen peroxide is used: 10 volume to produce the large colour molecules as before and 20 volume to oxidise more melanin to allow a lighter result to be achieved.

A development time is required to allow these two processes to work. The manufacturer's instructions will tell you what you have to do to get the best out of the product.

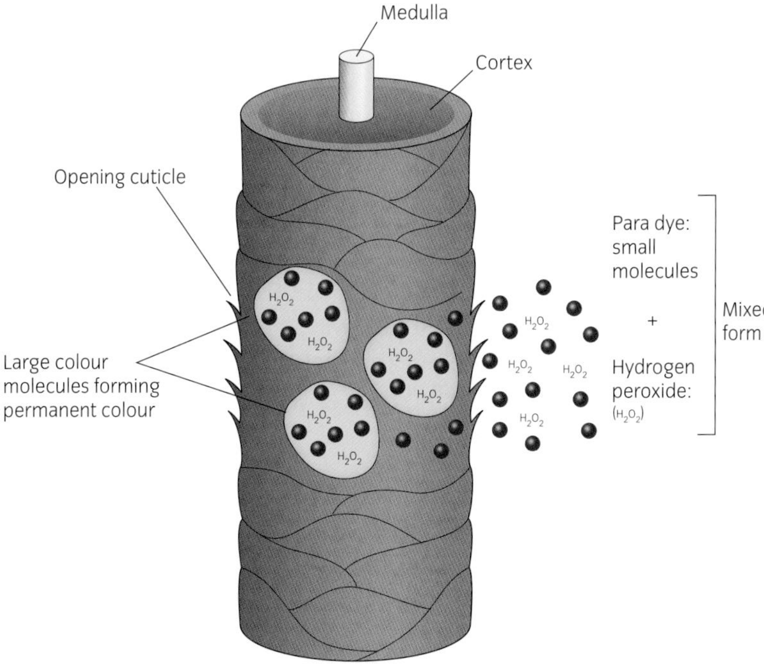

The molecules that form permanent colour

QUASI-PERMANENT COLOUR

Quasi-permanent colours are a mixture of the small colourless molecules used in permanent colour and other larger molecule pigments. They use the same process as permanent colours. Low volumes of hydrogen peroxide are mixed with the colour immediately before application. The oxygen will oxidise some of the natural melanin and change the small molecules into larger coloured ones. The other colour molecules will lodge in the edge of the cortex and will be removed a little at a time when the hair is shampooed.

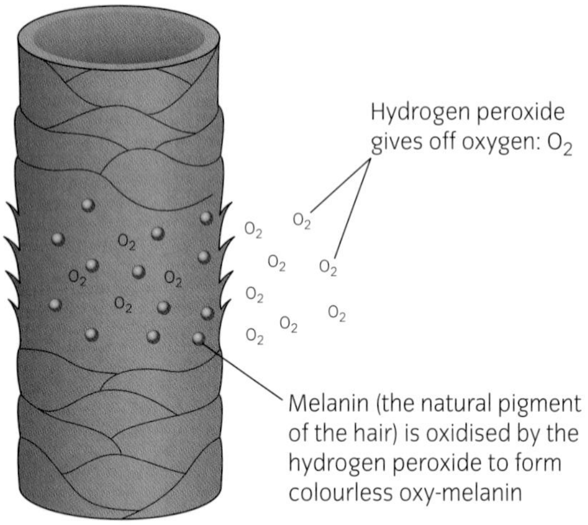
Hydrogen peroxide gives off oxygen: O2
Melanin (the natural pigment of the hair) is oxidised by the hydrogen peroxide to form colourless oxy-melanin

Effects of lightening products on the hair

LIGHTENING PRODUCTS

High-lift colours are colours that are designed to make the hair lighter. They work in same way as permanent colours but use higher volumes of hydrogen peroxide. They need to oxidise more of the natural melanin to achieve the target colour.

Bleaches are also mixed with hydrogen peroxide just before use. 20 volume (6 per cent) or 30 volume (9 per cent) are normally used.

Using 30 volume (9 per cent) hydrogen peroxide will give a lighter result. The oxygen is used to oxidise the melanin in the hair. It changes the melanin into oxy-melanin which is colourless.

The black/brown pigments (eumelanin) are easier to oxidise. The red/yellow pigments (pheomelanin) are more difficult to oxidise. This is why bleached hair often has a yellow tone to it. The yellow pigment is not always fully oxidised.

When you are colouring the hair you must remember that:

COLOUR + COLOUR = DARKER COLOUR

Colouring the hair is not like painting a wall. When you paint a wall you cover the old coat of paint with a new one. The new colour will hide the old one. You may need to use two coats but you can turn a dark-coloured wall into a light-coloured wall quite easily.

When you colour the hair the colour you put on does not hide the natural colour like paint does. What you will see is both colours mixed together. If you add colour to colour the result will always be darker than the colour you started with, no matter what shade or depth of colour you use.

To make the hair a lighter colour you need to take some of the darker natural colour away and then replace it with a lighter colour. This is how permanent colours work. Because temporary and semi-permanent colours do not oxidise the melanin in the hair they cannot lighten the hair.

You must also remember that you cannot remove permanent colour from the hair using lightening products such as high-lift colour and bleaches. They can only be removed by a colour reduction process.

FACTORS THAT NEED TO BE CONSIDERED WHEN SELECTING COLOURING PRODUCTS

There are many factors that you must consider when you are selecting colouring products and choosing techniques. Some of the factors are very important. Failing to take them into account could lead to a disaster. Ending up with the wrong colour, damaging the hair, loss of hair and even causing the client serious injury are all things that could happen.

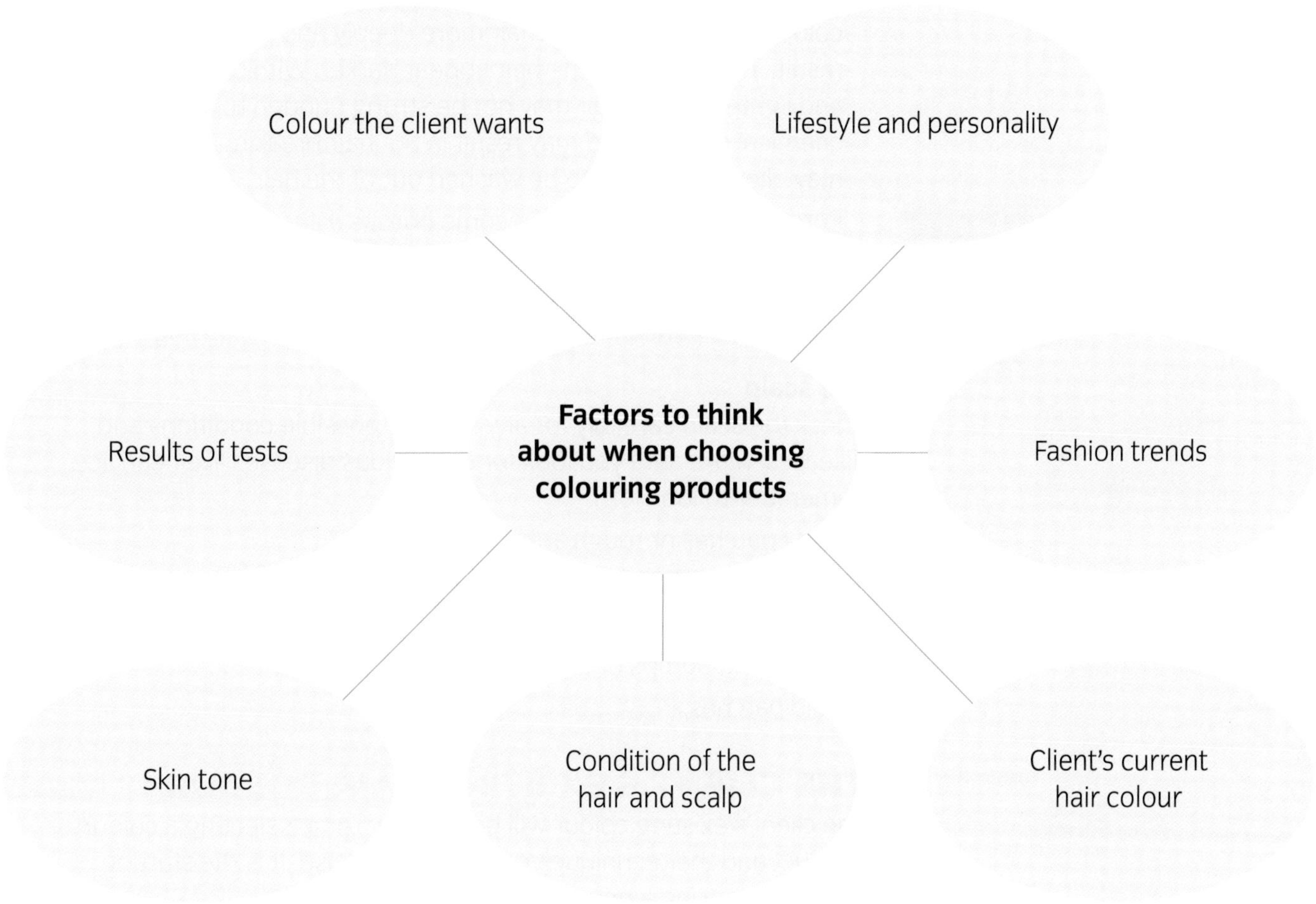

THE COLOUR THE CLIENT WANTS

Whenever you are carrying out a colour service, the first thing you need to find out is what colour the client wants to have. Finding this out will be a major factor in deciding:

- which colour product you need to use
- the technique you need to use and the actual colour you need to apply.

It may also help you decide that you cannot do what the client is asking for.

HANDY HINTS

Remember, as we get older the skin tone usually lightens and the hair will go grey. For most people the two will balance each other. Clients may often ask to have their hair coloured the shade they were when they were young. The client should be advised to have a lighter shade.

SKIN TONE

The client's skin tone is important in selecting the colour. The hair colour and skin tone must balance each other for a natural look. If you are going for a contrast it must be acceptable. For example, if the client has a pale skin then black or very dark brown will make the skin appear whiter. If the client has a 'reddish' skin tone then ash shades will make the complexion appear redder.

THE CONDITION OF THE HAIR AND SCALP

The hair

The condition of the hair is very important when you are deciding on the colouring product and technique. Things you need to look for are:

- Dry hair – the cuticle will be rough and not lie flat. This can cause temporary and semi-permanent colours to give patchy, uneven results and could lead to the colour being washed out more quickly.
- Damaged hair – with temporary and semi-permanent colours, the colour may enter into the hair more deeply and give a patchy, uneven result. This can make the hair appear darker. With permanent colour and lighteners the hair may not be strong enough to withstand the chemical process and may result in the hair breaking off. The damage may allow the colour to be washed out of the hair, causing fading.
- Porous hair – the hair will become porous if it is damaged and this will allow colour to penetrate more easily into the cortex. This can give patchy, uneven results and a darker result than you wanted. With permanent colours the colour can wash out, causing it to fade.

HANDY HINTS

Use the shade chart to find out the depth and tone of the client's hair. Do it carefully and accurately.

The scalp

Check the scalp carefully for any signs of possible conditions and diseases. Make sure you look for contagious diseases like head lice. Remember to look for:

- scaly patches or rough areas on the scalp
- red, inflamed patches
- cuts and abrasions on the skin
- lumps and bumps or raised areas
- bald patches.

THE CLIENT'S EXISTING HAIR COLOUR

The client's existing colour will be a key factor in selecting a colour product and the technique you are going to use. It is the starting point of choosing a new hair colour.

The client may not have had colour before, so the hair colour will be natural. If the client has had colouring services before, the hair may still have colour product on it. This will affect both your choice of colour product and your ability to achieve the desired result.

On a natural head you need to look at the amount of white hair the client has. Remember, some types of colour do not cover white hair very well. If the client has a lot of white hair then you will need to think about a permanent colour.

If the hair is dark, with perhaps a depth of 1 to 4, and the client wants to go very blonde, it may not be possible to achieve that amount of lift.

HANDY HINTS

Read Chapter 003 to refresh your knowledge of how to recognise head lice and what other signs to look for when you check the scalp.

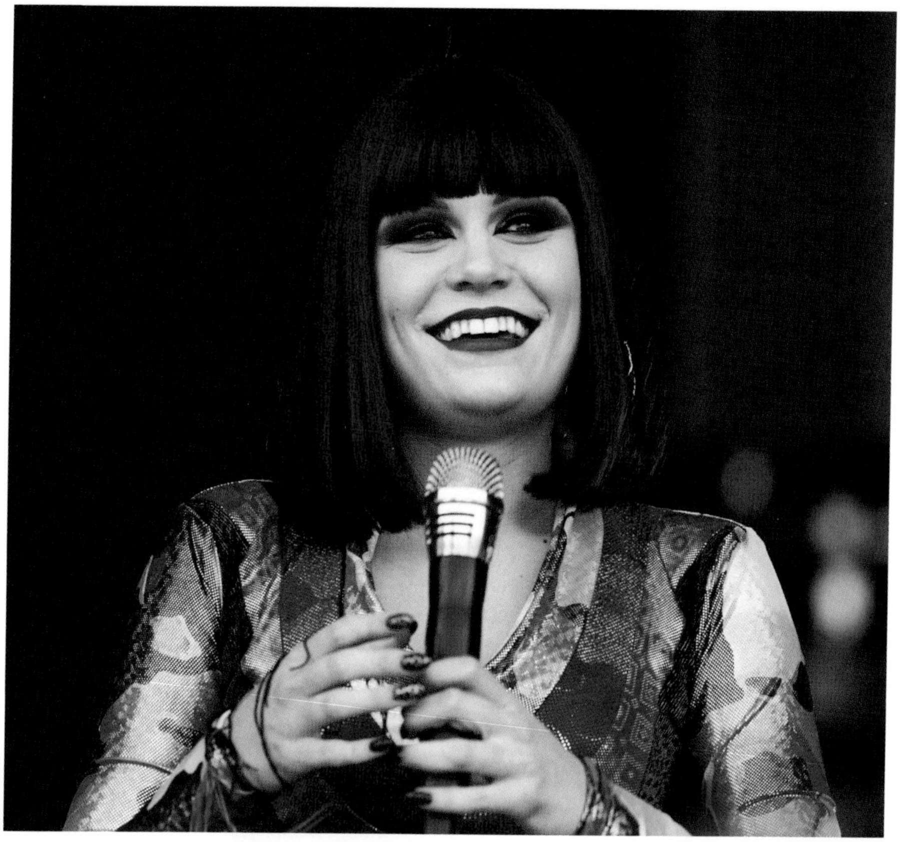

FASHION TRENDS

Colouring the hair will always follow fashion trends. Advertising plays a big part in the colour market. You will see advertisements for colour products everywhere. Magazines for both men and women will carry advertisements for them, featuring branded products, many of which you will be familiar with.

Other media forms will also have items on fashions in colour and the latest looks. TV programmes and features in newspapers will show the latest styles and techniques. TV and media coverage of celebrity events is massive and will be watched by all sorts of people. Clients will see a look that they like, be it the latest fashion 'must have' or a style and colour on an actor or actress in a TV programme, and ask you to achieve that on their hair. You will then have the task of deciding whether the look the clients want will suit them, and whether their hair will be suitable and strong enough to withstand the products required. Many of the advertisements you will see are intended for home use. You will need to explain to the client your choice of professional product and why you are recommending it.

ACTIVITY

In groups, discuss which pop stars are setting fashion trends.

LIFESTYLE AND PERSONALITY

Clients will want their hair coloured for many different reasons. When you find out from the client what they want, you need to consider how their lifestyle and personality will impact on their choice.

Take into account the style and type of clothes they wear. If they wear old-fashioned clothes, bright vibrant colours will look out of place. Their job may be one where bright, striking colours would be inappropriate.

The client's personality is also important: are they quiet and reserved, bright and bubbly, confident or nervous? A bright, bubbly client may not be happy with plain colours. How long the client has been thinking about a colour is important. Is their request a spur of the moment thing? If it is and they have asked for something bright and image changing, they may not like it when it is done. They may realise they have gone too far. People on holiday will often ask for things they would never consider when they are at home. We all tend to be more daring at times and then realise we have made a mistake.

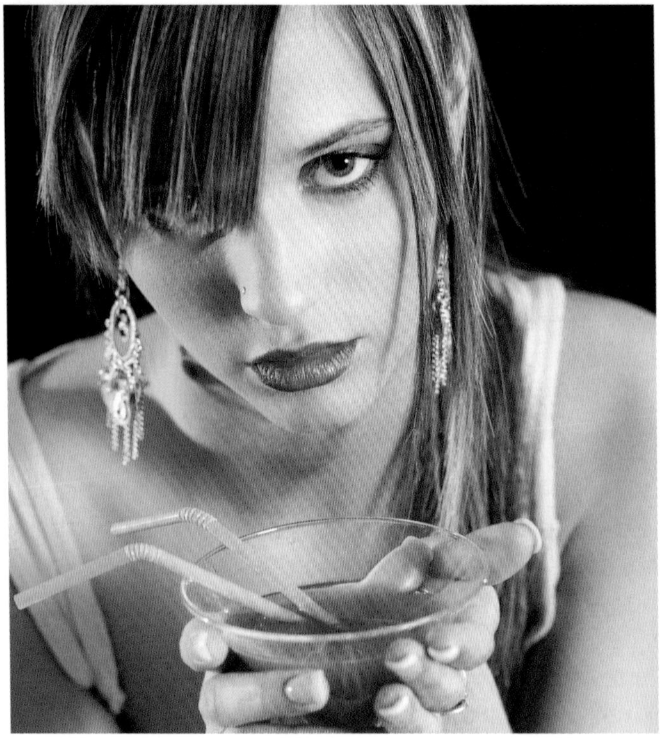

RESULTS OF TESTS

Because hairdressing services can require the use of chemical processes in order to work, making sure the result of the service meets both the client's and the salon's expectation is essential. Colouring the hair is one of those services. You need to make sure that:

- the hair is in good enough condition to have the colour done
- your selection of product is the right one to achieve the desired result
- the client is not allergic to the colour product
- the development time is enough to get a good result.

To find these out you will need to carry out some tests before and during the colouring service.

Skin test

What is the test for?

To find out if the client is allergic to the ingredients of the colour. The test must be carried out if you are using permanent or quasi-permanent colours that contain **PPD**, at least 48 hours before the colour service is to be carried out.

PPD

This stands for paraphenylenediamine. It is in most hair dyes

How is the test carried out?

A skin test is usually carried out on the soft skin just behind the ear or on the inside of the elbow.

1 Always follow the manufacturer's instructions.

2 Clean the area and make sure it is dry.

3 Mix a small quantity of the colour you have selected with hydrogen peroxide and apply a small amount to the cleaned area. Leave it to dry.

4 Explain to the client what you are doing. Tell the client that they should try to avoid touching or washing the area.

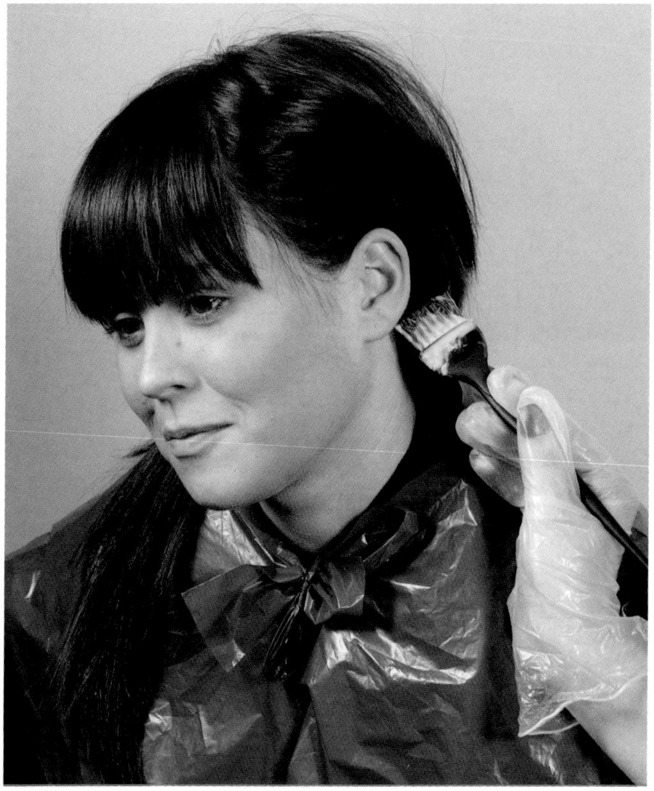

Always do a skin test before using permanent or quasi-permanent colour

The results of the test

If the skin where the test was carried out is red and inflamed, or has sore areas that are weeping and itchy, this means the client has reacted to the colour. They should NOT have the colour service carried out. This is known as a *positive* result.

If there is no change to the skin where the test was carried out it will be safe to carry out the colour. This is a *negative* result.

What could happen if the test is not done?

If the client is allergic to colour and you do not do the test, the results could be very serious. The client's scalp can be badly affected, becoming red and inflamed. Weeping sores could lead to blood poisoning. There could be severe swelling to the face and neck. The client would need medical treatment straight away.

You cannot tell if a client is allergic to colour other than by doing a skin test. Clients who have had colour for many years can suddenly develop an allergy.

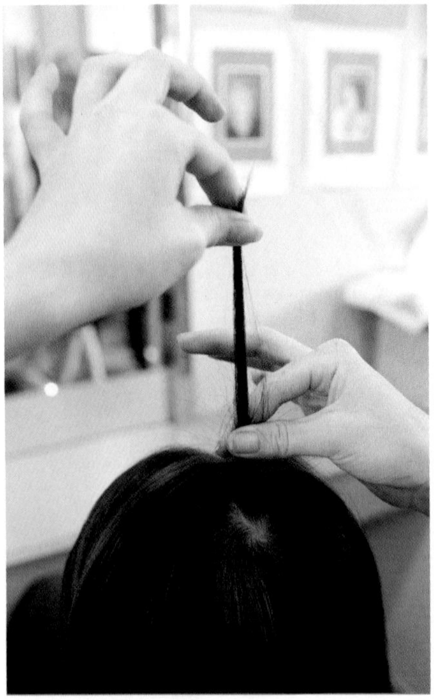

A porosity test

Porosity test

What is the test for?

To find out if the hair is porous, and likely to soak up or 'grab' the colour you are going to apply. This is particularly important for temporary or semi-permanent colours. It can also affect permanent colours.

How is the test carried out?

1 Take a few strands of dry hair and hold away from the head and under tension.
2 With the fingers of the other hand, gently slide them down the hair shaft from point to root.
3 It is important to keep the hair under tension when you do the test and not to use too much force when you slide your fingers along the hair shaft.

The results of the test

If the hair is porous it will feel rough and bumpy as you slide your fingers along the hair shaft. If the hair feels smooth it is not seriously porous. If the hair is porous you may need to change your selection of product and colour, or not carry out the service.

What could happen if the test is not done?

If you do not do the test and the hair is porous, the colour you use will penetrate more easily and in greater quantity than you intended. This could lead to a patchy or uneven colour, especially when using temporary or semi-permanent colours.

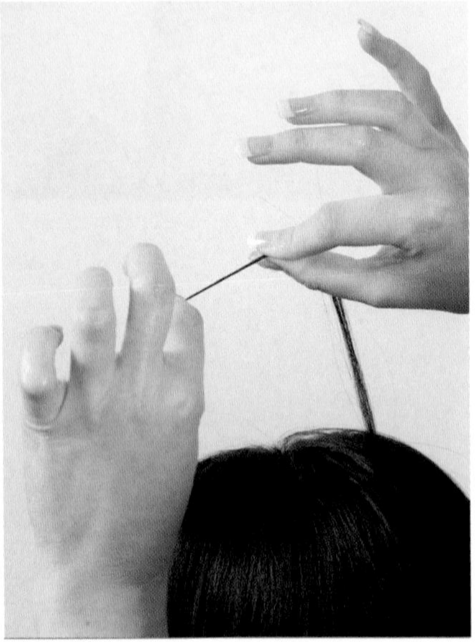

An elasticity test

Elasticity test

What is the test for?

To find out if the hair is strong enough to have the colour done. This is particularly important for permanent colours and lighteners, where a chemical process will be part of the service. It is not so important for temporary or semi-permanent colours.

How is the test carried out?

1 Take one or two hairs and dampen them with warm water.
2 Once they are wet, hold the hair between the thumb and forefinger about a third of its length from the points (less if the hair is long).
3 With the thumb and forefinger of the other hand, hold the points of the hair and gently pull the hair and then release. Do this at least twice.

The results of the test

Hair is elastic, which means it will stretch and return to its original length. Hair that is in good condition will stretch to half its length again and then return to its original length without damage. If it is in poor condition the elasticity will be low, so when you pull the hair it might break or it will go out of shape and not return to its original shape. If the hair is weak you may have to change the type of colour or not carry out the colour service.

What could happen if the test is not done?

If you do not do the test and the hair is weak then the colour process could cause it to break off, or the condition of the hair will become much worse. Hair with low elasticity is also likely to be porous.

Colour test (sometimes called a test cutting)

What is the test for?

To see if the colour you have selected will give the colour you and the client have agreed on. The test can be done using several possible choices to see which one gives the best result.

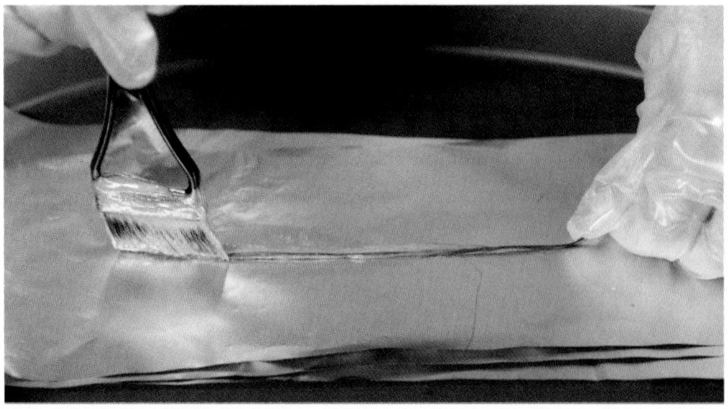

A colour test

How is the test carried out?

1. Cut a small quantity of hair from the back of the client's head.
2. Apply the selected colour to the cutting and leave it to process.
3. If more than one colour is to be tested you will need enough hair to do all the tests. You need to keep them separated from each other.

The results of the test

When you have finished applying the colour, carefully wash off the colour as you would if you were removing the colour from the head. Carefully dry the sample and look at the result. If you have carried out more than one test, compare the results of all the tests side by side to see which one gives the best result.

HANDY HINTS

No matter how experienced at colouring you are, testing is very important and should always be used to make sure you get the right result.

What could happen if the test is not done?

You might not get the result you want to achieve. The client may be unhappy with the colour they end up with.

Colour development test (sometimes called a strand test)

What is the test for?

This test is carried out during the development of the colour. It will tell you how the colour is processing and how it may be affecting the hair condition.

How is the test carried out?

1. Carry out the test at regular intervals during processing.
2. Pick up a small strand of hair and carefully wipe off the colour.
3. Look at the hair to see the colour that has been achieved so far.
4. With lightening products, because they can damage the hair, do a gentle elasticity test (pull the hair) to check on its condition.
5. If further development time is needed then carefully replace the colour or lightener and continue processing, repeating the test until the result is satisfactory.

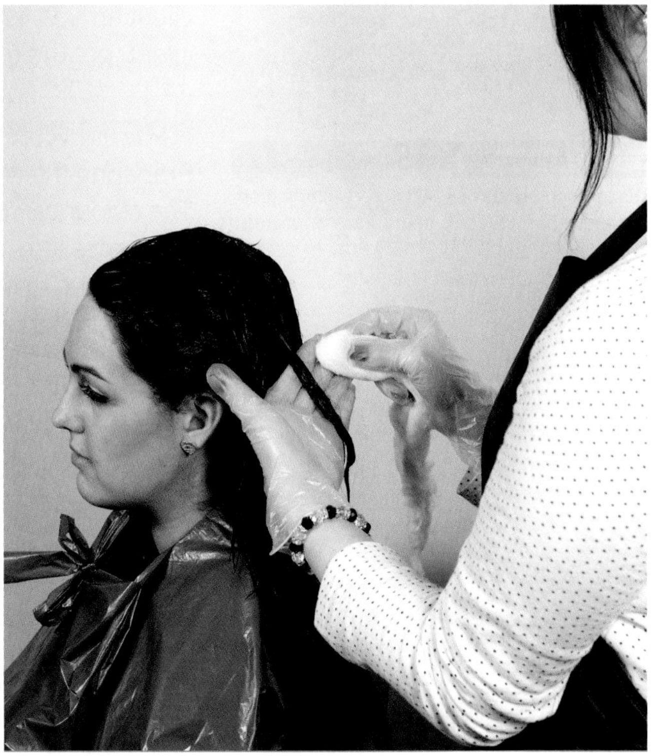

A colour development (strand) test

The results of the test
When development is finished you should have achieved the desired result with no serious damage to the hair.

What could happen if the test is not done?
The colour may not be satisfactory because it could be under- or over-processed. When using lightening products, damage can occur with over-processing which could cause the hair to break.

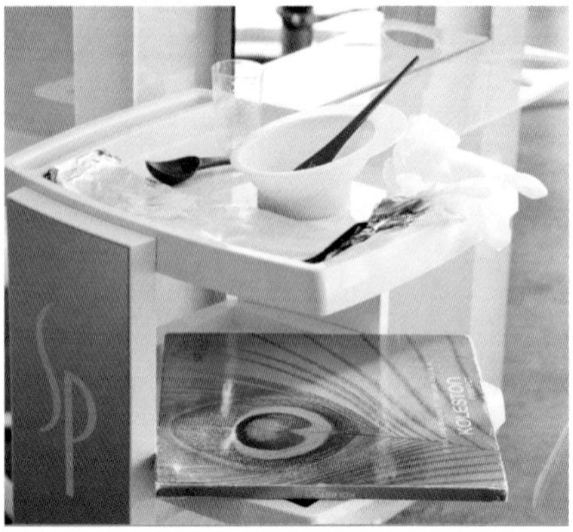
Set-up for a colouring service

ACTIVITY

Working in pairs, practise carrying out the tests on each other. Discuss your results with the rest of the group.

PREPARE FOR A COLOURING SERVICE

When colouring services are to be carried out you need to prepare the work area, the client and yourself.

THE WORK AREA

Work surfaces should be clean with tools and equipment in their proper place. Make sure they are clean and sterilised where necessary, ready for use. Remember, this will help prevent the transfer of infection. Mirrors should be clean with no smudges. The floor must be swept, with no loose hair or rubbish, and the chair must be clean.

You may not be able to get all the things you need ready before the client arrives. When you have completed your consultation with the client, get the rest of the products and tools that you need.

HANDY HINTS

Remember to make sure your appearance and your personal hygiene are up to standard. Read Chapter 102 to refresh your knowledge.

HANDY HINTS

Read Chapter 103 or 104 for more information on the importance of preparing the work area.

PREPARING THE CLIENT

Preparing the client properly for colouring services is important. The colour can cause damage to the client's clothing and belongings if it comes into contact with them. This could cost the salon money if they have to be replaced. Always make sure you follow the salon's procedure for client preparation.

If the colour is to be applied to dry hair:

- Use a standard gown first.
- Place a colour towel around the shoulders.
- Next, use a plastic or nylon colour gown.
- Place another colour towel around the shoulders.

Make sure the gowns are properly fastened and cover all the client's clothes.

If the client's hair needs to be shampooed before the colour is applied, prepare the hair for shampooing and then follow the procedure for colour.

HANDY HINTS

Refresh your knowledge by reading Chapter 003 Shampoo and conditioning hair.

PREPARING YOURSELF

Make sure you always prepare yourself correctly when using colour.

- Always wear non-latex gloves when applying, removing or testing. Permanent colours contain PPD which can cause serious skin conditions.
- Make sure you wear an apron to protect your clothes. Clients do not want to see stained clothes as it gives the wrong impression.

SAFE AND HYGIENIC WORKING PRACTICES

As you have learned in other chapters, working safely and hygienically is very important. It is part of every practical skill you learn, part of every service you give to a client, and part of the whole of your working day.

You should only keep your work area tidy and use only hygienic tools and equipment. This will help to reduce the risk of harm to you and your clients and help to prevent cross-infection. The client will also have more confidence in you and you will look more professional.

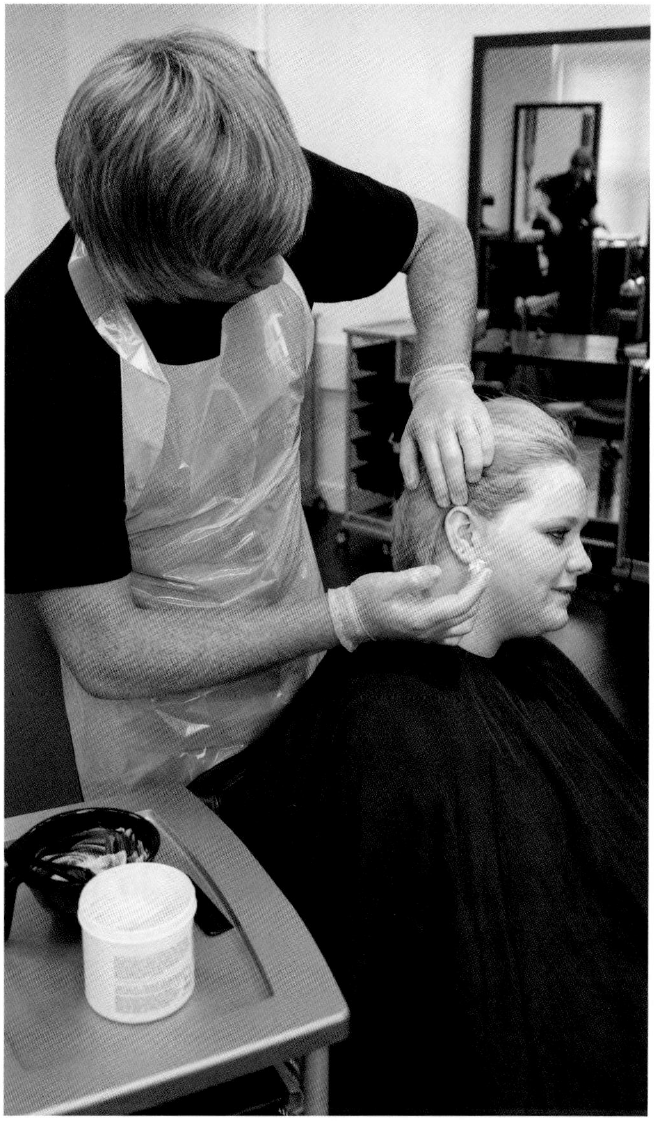

ACTIVITY

Read Chapter 113 Following health and safety in the salon to learn about the employer's responsibilities and your responsibilities to provide a safe and healthy working environment.

HANDY HINTS

Make sure the client is seated correctly and is comfortable. Don't forget your own posture and stand upright. Move around the client as you work.

- **PPE** – personal protective equipment: you will need a freshly laundered gown and clean towels for the shampoo; colouring towels and a plastic gown or cape for the client when you carry out the colour. You will also need non-latex gloves and an apron for yourself. Make sure you follow the manufacturer's instructions.
- **COSHH** – Control Of Substances Hazardous to Health: these regulations cover how to safely use any products that may be partof the service. They will also include using a disinfectant safely when using it to clean tools and equipment.
- **HASAWA** – Health and Safety at Work Act: check the work area for any hazards before you start work on the client. Check that all the equipment, tools and products are clean and safe to use on the client.
- **Electricity at Work Regulations:** check all the electrical equipment you will use in the styling process before you start.

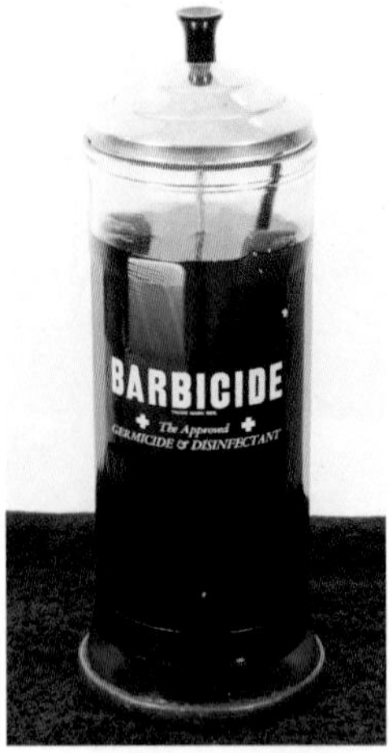

Barbicide

HANDY HINTS

Go to Chapter 113 and read more about methods of sterilisation.

HANDY HINTS

Refresh your knowledge about consulting with the client for shampooing and styling services. Read Chapter 003 Shampoo and conditioning hair, and Chapter 103 Styling women's hair or Chapter 104 Styling men's hair.

Don't forget to check that all the tools are sterilised, ready to start work. Methods of sterilisation in a colouring service include using a disinfectant such as Barbicide for combs.

ACTIVITY

Go to Chapter 113 Following health and safety in the salon and list all of the health and safety laws that you should follow when carrying out a colouring service.

HYGIENE WHEN USING COLOUR

The following table is a guide for keeping your tools and equipment ready for use:

Tools/equipment	Hygiene advice
Towels and gowns	Machine wash on a high temperature.
Plastic cape and apron	Wash in hot soapy water, rinse and dry.
Combs and brushes	Wash in warm, soapy water. Place in sterilising jar.
Bowls and brushes	Wash thoroughly after use to remove all traces of colour.
Clips	Wash, dry, then place in the sterilising jar or the UV cabinet.
Disposable gloves	Throw away after use. Use a new pair for each client.

PROVIDE A COLOURING SERVICE

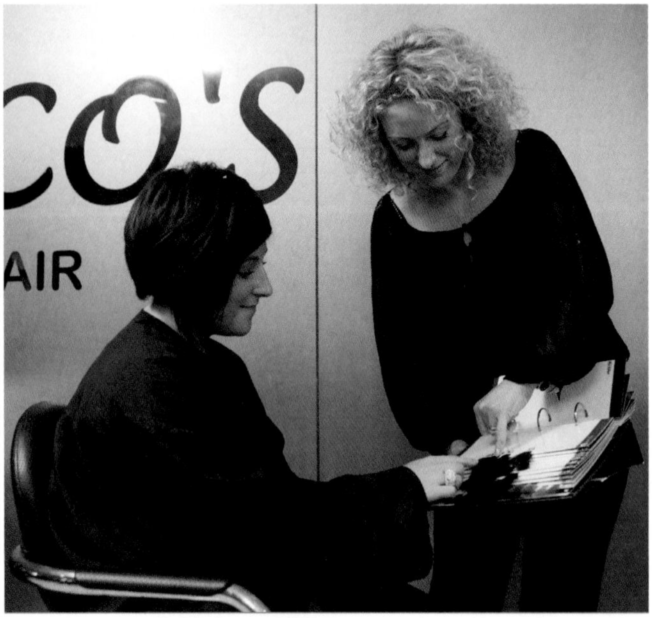

A consultation for a colouring service

In this part of the chapter you will learn how to select and use the correct application method, products, tools and equipment to provide a temporary and semi-permanent hair colour service.

CONSULTATION

Consulting with the client allows you to find out what the client wants. It helps you decide what you are going to do. Consultation is always carried out before the hair is shampooed.

When you consult with the client about the colour service you will also consult with them about the styling service and the shampoo.

If you are going to carry out a colour, then you need to find out certain information from the client:

- The first thing you must find out is what effect the client is looking to achieve. You also need to find out why the client wants their hair coloured.
- Have they really thought about it?
- Can they cope with the commitment?
- Can they live with the result?
- Are they being daring?
- They may not be able to cope with the reality of what you have done. Make sure you explain everything to the client so they fully understand what the outcomes of the colouring that you are going to do are.
- Now look at all the factors that can influence your choice of colour and technique. When you have looked at these factors you need to decide whether you can achieve what the client has asked for. If you can't then you will need to suggest other options.
- Next, select the products to use – colour, shampoo, conditioner and finishing products.
- Last of all, decide how you will carry out the technique and the tools and equipment you will need to use.

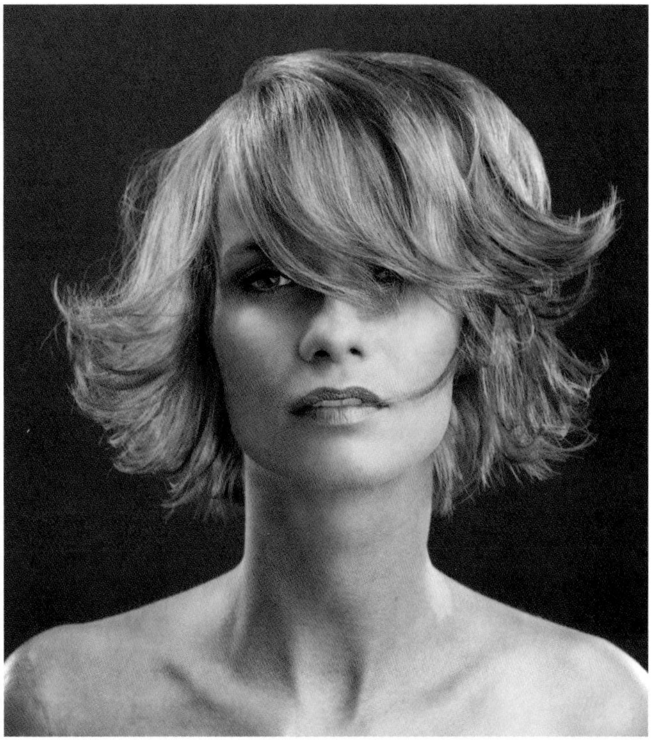

ACTIVITY

Prepare questions that you could use to find out why your clients want colour. Try out the questions on one of your colleagues and see if they work. Discuss with the rest of the group which questions worked and which didn't.

HANDY HINTS

The instructions for some products may say 'Apply the colour to wet hair without shampooing' in which case just wet the hair with warm water.

HANDY HINTS

Refer to Chapter 102 for more details about communication and behaviour.

COMMUNICATION

Communication and behaviour are very important when colouring. You need to be good at talking to people, including those you may not have met before. This starts with being confident about what you're doing, and thinking about the types of question you are going to ask.

CARRYING OUT A TEMPORARY COLOUR

The procedure for carrying out a temporary colour is described in Chapter 111 Colouring hair using temporary colour. Refer to this chapter for details.

HANDY HINTS

Check that the gown and towels are properly in place.

HANDY HINTS

Read Chapter 003 Shampoo and conditioning hair to refresh your knowledge of the procedure.

HANDY HINTS

Read the manufacturer's instructions for all the ranges of colour used in the salon. This will improve your knowledge of the products that you will use and enable you to consult with your clients more confidently.

CARRYING OUT A SEMI-PERMANENT COLOUR

It is essential to read the manufacturer's instructions for the brand of colour you are going to use. The instructions are intended to help you get the best result from the product. They will tell you:

- whether the hair should be shampooed before the colour is applied
- how to apply the colour
- the development time required to get the best result
- how to remove the colour from the hair
- what, if any, aftercare products may be useful
- how to use the product safely (COSHH requirements).

ACTIVITY

Find out the precautions that you should take when using a semi-permanent colour.

SHAMPOO THE CLIENT'S HAIR

When you have finished your consultation, the next step is to shampoo the hair ready for the colouring and finishing service. Chapter 003 Shampoo and conditioning hair describes the method of shampooing the hair ready for other services.

TOOLS AND EQUIPMENT FOR COLOURING SERVICES

Tools and equipment	Use
Wide-toothed comb 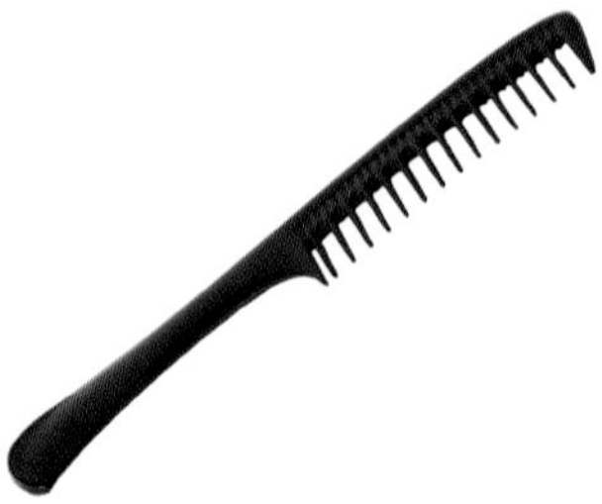	Used to remove tangles from the hair before shampooing and to prepare the hair for the colour after it has been shampooed.
Tail/pintail comb 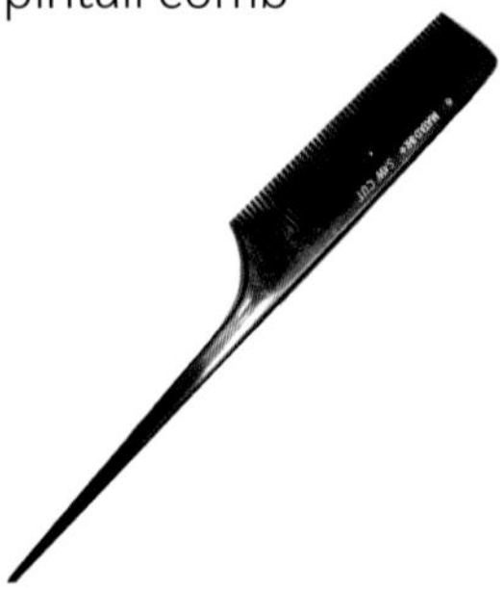	Used to make sections in preparation for colouring.

Tools and equipment	Use
Sectioning clips 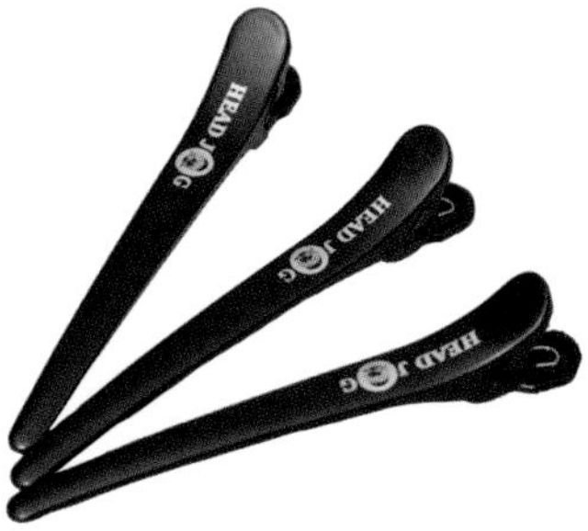	Used to keep the hair under control when you are colouring.
Bowl 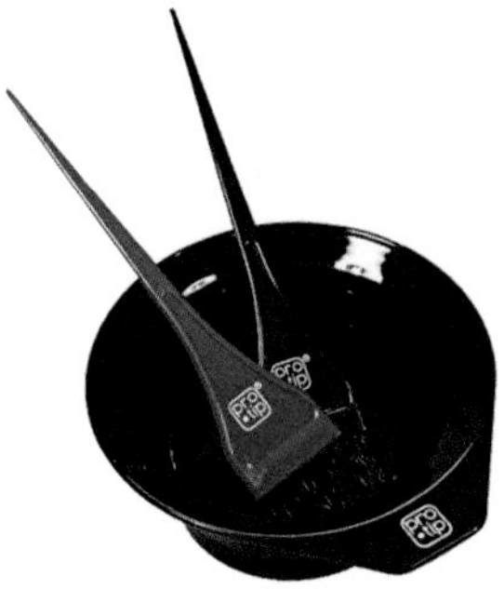	Used to hold colour when you are applying it to the hair.
Tinting brush 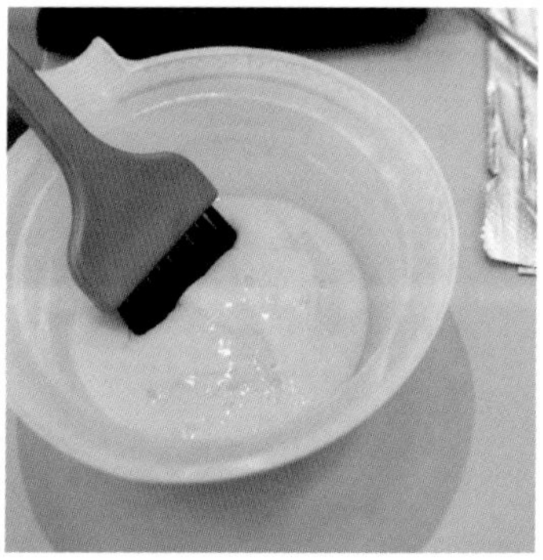	A small flat brush with a pointed handle. The brush is used to apply colour to the hair. The pointed handle is used to make sections.
Sponge 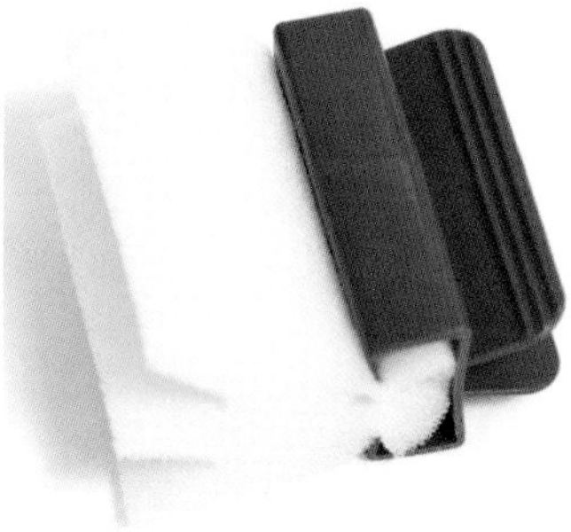	Used to apply colour to the hair.

Tools and equipment	Use
Applicator bottle	Some temporary and semi-permanent colours come in an applicator bottle ready to apply the colour.
Colour gown 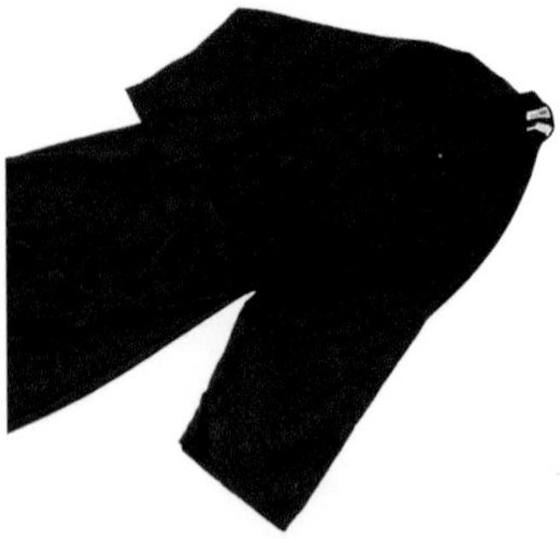	A plastic cape or apron that is waterproof. Used on top of the shampooing gown to make sure no colour gets onto the client's clothing.
Colouring towels 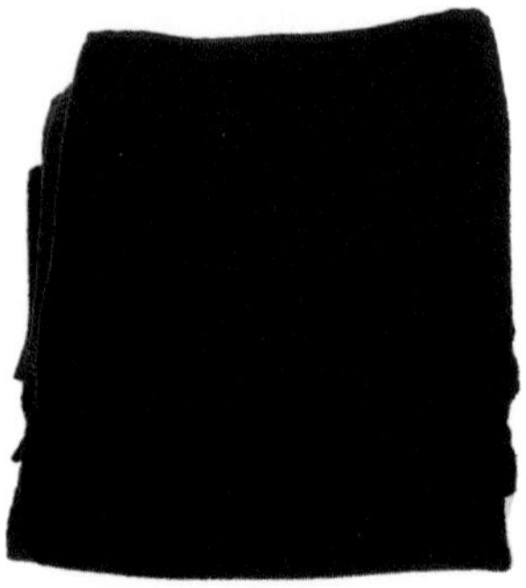	These are usually black towels so they do not show stains, which look unsightly.
Trolley 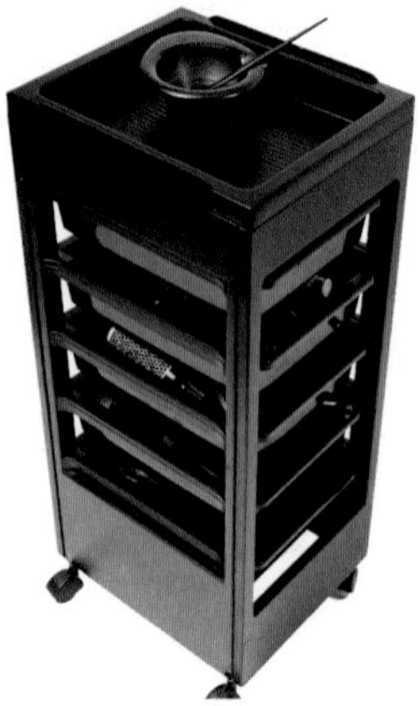	This is used to put the colour bowl and other tools on so that you can work around the client and have the things you need close to you.

Tools and equipment	Use
Disposable gloves 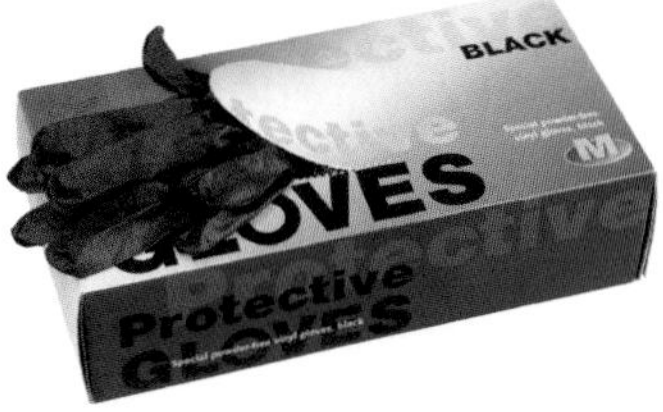 	Used to protect the hands from staining and dermatitis.
Apron 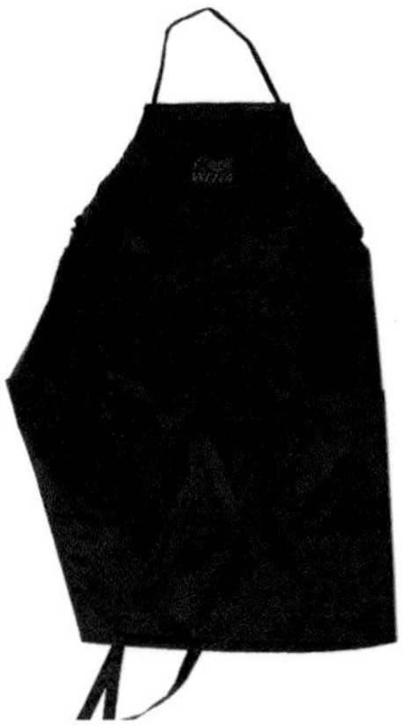	Used to protect the stylist's uniform or clothing.
Climazons and rollerballs 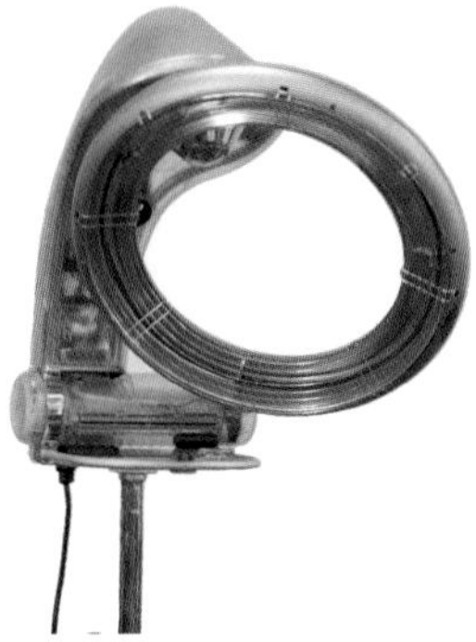	These machines produce heat, which is used to help colour development. The heat is passed to the hair by radiation and not hot air as a dryer would use, so it doesn't disturb the hair.

COLOUR TECHNIQUES

There are a wide variety of techniques that you can use to achieve the result the client wants. New methods are being devised all the time. Keep up to date with new fashions and methods by reading trade magazines, manufacturers' information and attending demonstrations and shows.

The more widely used colour techniques include the following:

FULL-HEAD APPLICATIONS

This technique is used for temporary and semi-permanent colour application or when the client is having permanent colour or lightening products for the first time. The colour will be applied to all the hair. The hair should be sectioned into four quarters. Small sections between 1 cm and 2 cm wide are then taken and the colour applied. The manufacturer's instructions will tell you how the colour should be applied.

PARTIAL-HEAD APPLICATIONS

Partial-head applications are made when you want to colour only parts of the hair. Clients who have quasi-permanent, permanent colour and lighteners will need to have the roots of the hair coloured at regular intervals as the hair grows. This is called a 'regrowth' or 'retouch' application. Apply the colour to the root area that has grown since the colour was last done. Section the head into four using small sections as you did for the full-head application. The colour is applied just to the root area. Be careful not to let the colour overlap the hair that is already coloured. This could darken that area causing a 'banded' look.

As well as regrowth applications, many other effects can be achieved using partial-head applications. These include:

Highlights

This is a popular effect where sections of hair are coloured lighter than the natural colour to give a contrasting effect. The sections can be small or large, and all over the head or in parts. The stylist would plan where and what size the highlights would be.

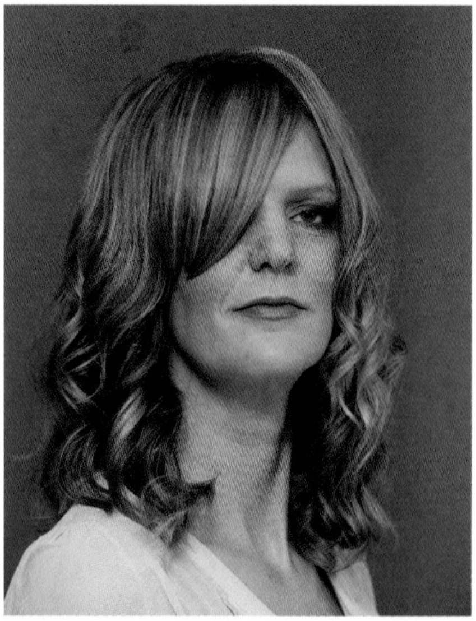

Lowlights
Lowlights are another popular effect, which is the opposite of highlights. The sections of hair are coloured darker than the natural colour.

The range of effects you can get with highlights and lowlights is only limited by your creativity and your client's requirements. You can put in both highlights and lowlights. You can use bright, vibrant colours for maximum contrast. You can use large sections just in the front of the head. Many clients will want very light blonde highlights. Some will want more subtle colours, perhaps the same depth as their natural colour but with more tone.

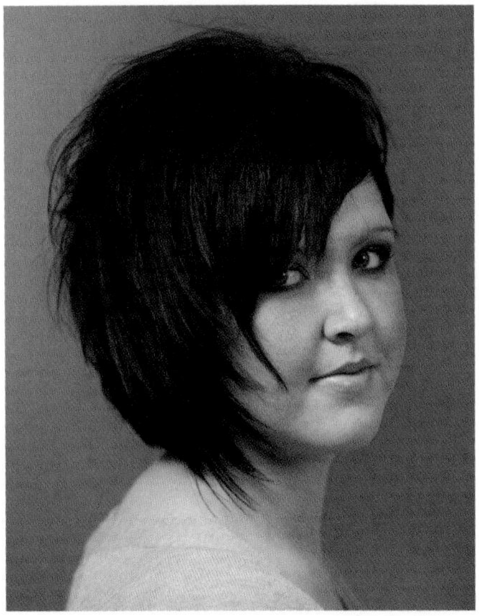

The techniques you can use to achieve these effects include:

Foils
This technique uses aluminium foil.

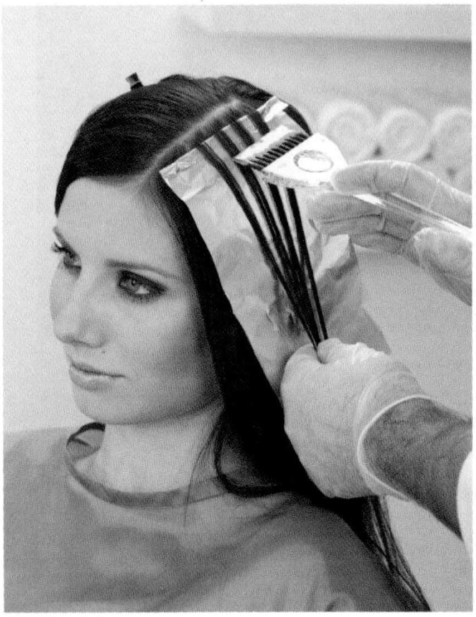

Colour cups

Colour cups can be used to create multi-coloured highlighting effects. It works best on short to medium-length hair.

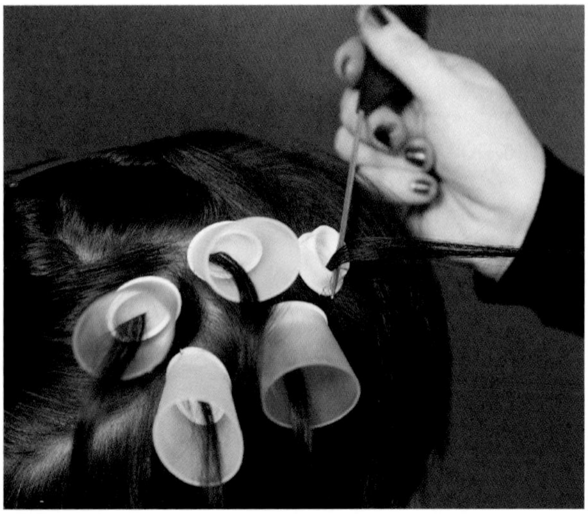

STEP 1 – The cap is placed over the client's scalp.

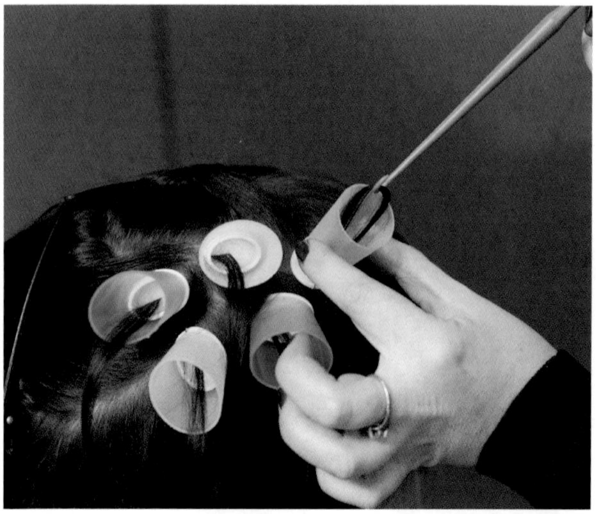

STEP 2 – A crochet hook is then used to pull a small quantity of hair through the pre-formed holes where the stylist wants them to be.

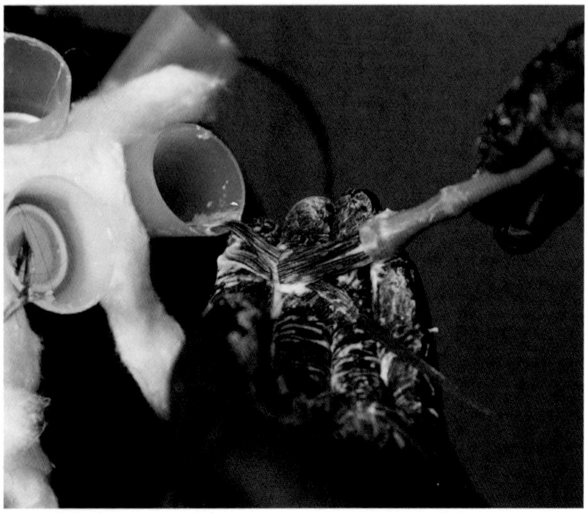

STEP 3 – When all the hair required has been pulled through the colour or lightener is applied to it. Development will then take place.

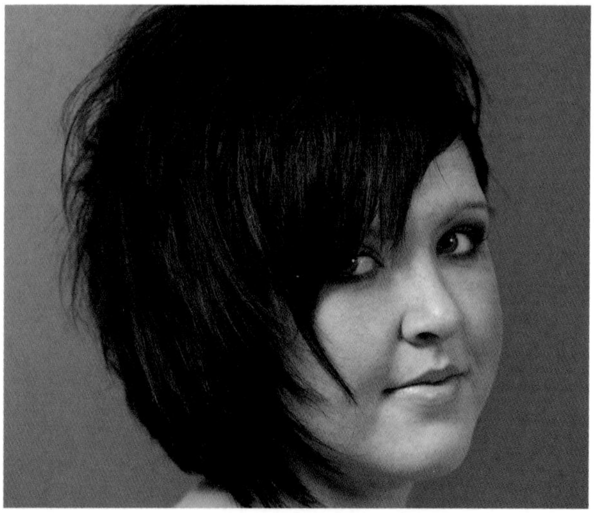

STEP 4 – The finished result.

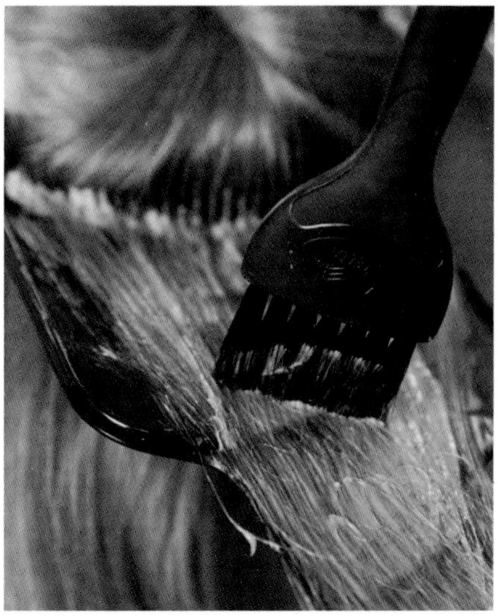

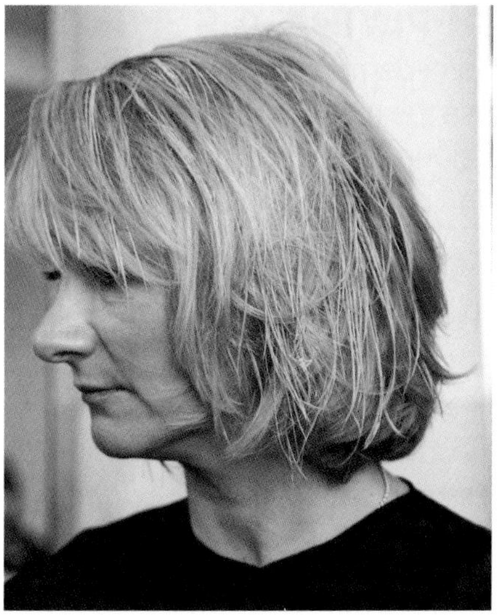

Spatula

This is a quick technique for highlights or lowlights. A spatula is used to apply colour to the hair. The spatula is designed to colour only parts of a section. It is best used for adding tone at the same depth as the natural colour. It should not be used with bleach products as the colour may run, which would result in a bigger highlight than you want.

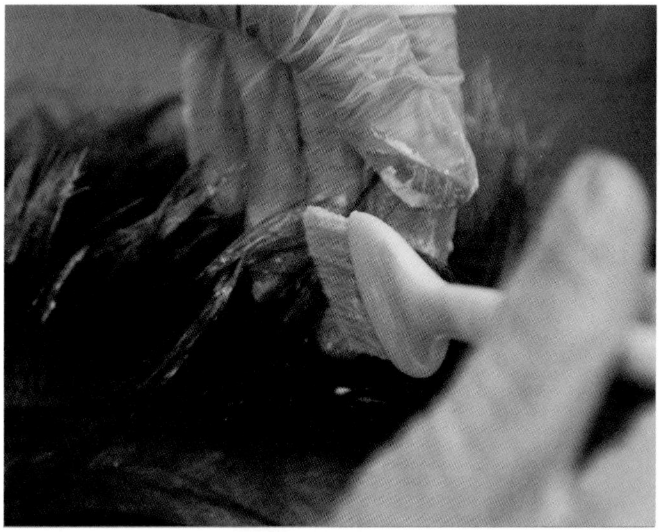

The freehand technique

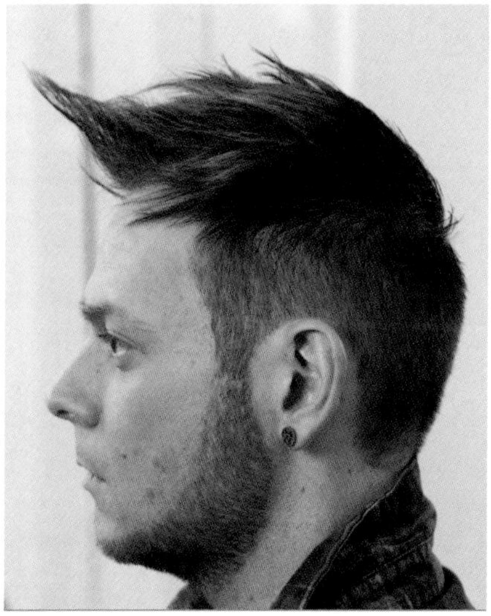

After using the freehand technique

Freehand

Freehand is a technique where you apply the colour randomly to the hair. You can use a brush or your fingers to apply the colour. This method can be used to give a particular effect to a style.

ACTIVITY

In your group, prepare a chart describing the results that can be achieved when using the different colouring techniques.

APPLYING A SEMI-PERMANENT HAIR COLOUR

Semi-permanent colour can be applied in many different ways. Always use the method recommended by the manufacturer. Semi-permanent colours are normally applied to all of the hair (a *full-head application)*, and before styling and finishing.

You can also use a *partial-head application* where you apply the colour to specific parts of the hair.

PREPARING THE HAIR FOR COLOUR APPLICATION

The hair should be towel dried after the shampoo so it is damp but not dripping with water. Do not overdry the hair.

The manufacturer's instructions may give a suggested method of application. The salon may have its own procedure. If it does then you should follow it.

If you are going to use a brush or a sponge to apply the colour, then sectioning of the hair will be used to make sure you get even coverage of all the hair. It will create the right impression with the client.

Sectioning for a semi-permanent colour

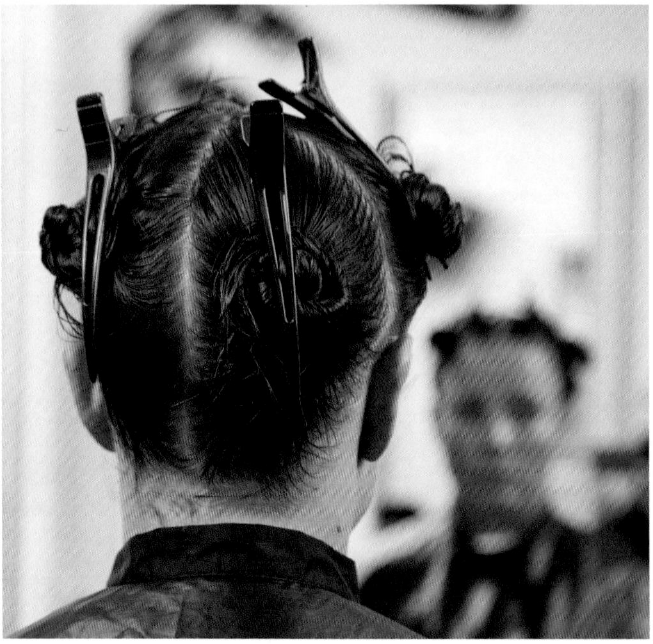

1 Using a tail comb, make two partings, one from the centre of the forehead to the centre of the nape and one from ear to ear over the crown. Secure each of the four sections with a sectioning clip.
2 Make a horizontal section between 1 and 2 cm wide in one of the two back sections. If the hair is thick or long use 1 cm sections. If the hair is medium to short or fine then use 2 cm sections.

ACTIVITY

With a partner as your client, practise sectioning the hair for a semi-permanent colour. (You can practise applying the colour using conditioner instead if you wish.)

HOW TO CARRY OUT A SEMI-PERMANENT COLOURING SERVICE

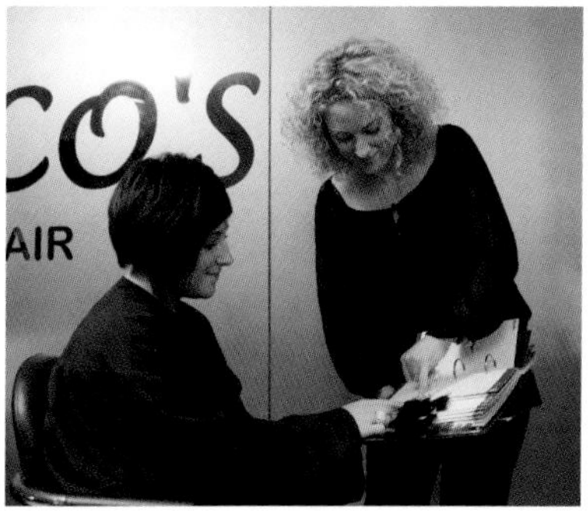

STEP 1 – Confirm with the client the choice of colour; gown and protect the client.

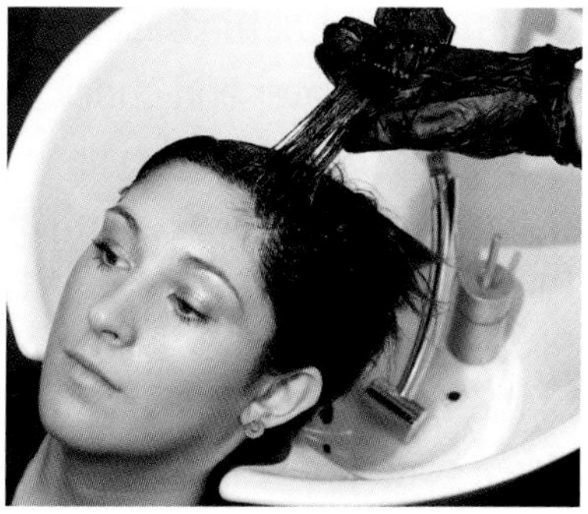

STEP 2 – Shampoo the hair and towel dry then apply the semi-permanent product.

HANDY HINTS

Semi-permanent colour must be applied to pre-shampooed hair.

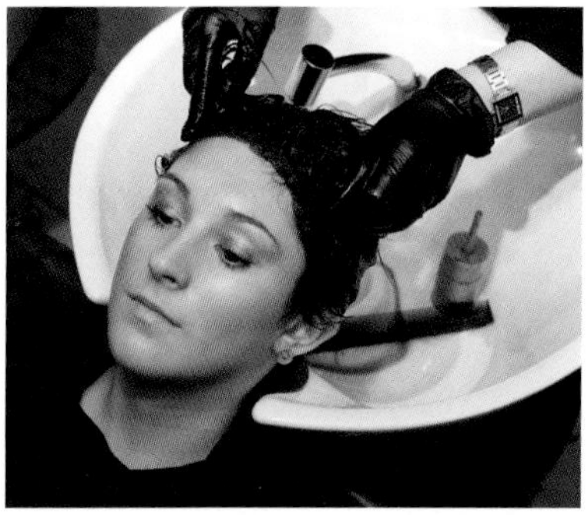

STEP 3 – Apply evenly through the hair.

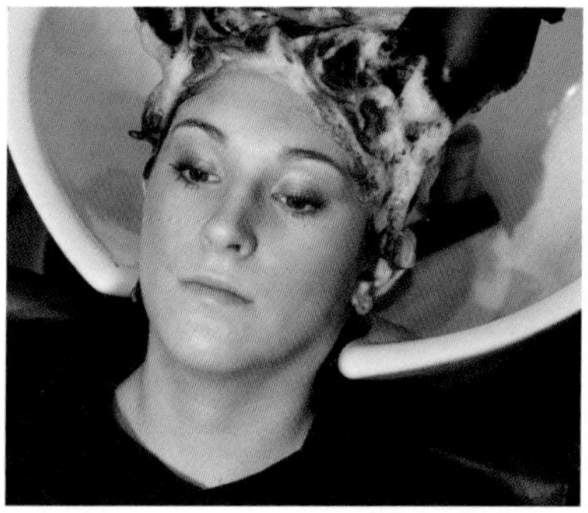

STEP 4 – After the development time, add some water, emulsify and rinse thoroughly. Then shampoo and condition the hair.

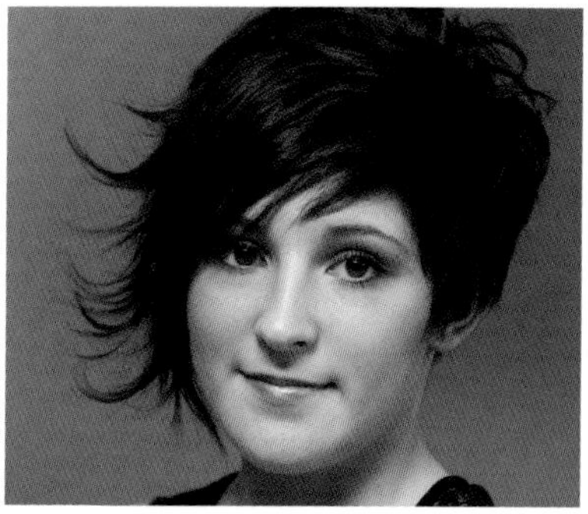

STEP 5 – The finished result.

Semi-permanent colours must be rinsed off the hair thoroughly at the end of the development time, followed by applying a conditioner.

REMOVING A SEMI-PERMANENT COLOUR

The procedure for removing a semi-permanent colour is as follows:

1 Check that the gown, towel and cape are in the correct position.

2 Seat the client at the basin and make sure they are comfortable.

3 Turn on the water and check the temperature.

4 Add some water to the hair.

5 Using rotary massage **emulsify** the colour and water. Make sure they are cover all of the scalp to loosen the colour.

6 Rinse the hair thoroughly until the water runs clear. Make sure all of the colour is removed.

7 Use a conditioner if necessary to smoothe the cuticle.

8 Towel dry the hair using a clean towel. The towel around the shoulders may be contaminated with colour.

9 Carefully comb through the hair to prepare it for the finishing service.

The client is now ready for the styling and finishing service.

Emulsify
To combine two liquids together

HANDY HINTS

Remember to check that the colour has been removed from the nape area when using a backwash basin.

HANDY HINTS

Be very careful not to let the water run down the sides of the client's face and neck when rinsing. The colour you are rinsing out of the hair may stain the clothes.

COMPLETE THE RECORD CARD

Keeping a record of what you do to the client's hair is essential to providing a professional service to the client. It is especially important for services that use chemicals on the hair. The information you keep will have many uses:

- You will know the products the client has had which will be useful for their next visit.
- You will have a record of how a service was done so if there is a problem you can use the record to help resolve the problem.
- You can see when the client last had some services and you can recommend when they are due to have them again.
- You can record the result of the service and the client's comments at the time.

A record card for a client having semi-permanent colour should include:

- the client's details
- your analysis of their hair and scalp
- details of all the factors that can affect the colour choice and method
- details of any tests you did and their results
- the colour product you selected and the technique you decided to use
- shampoo used
- how the colour was applied
- the development method and time
- any products that were used during removal
- what the result was
- any comments from the client.

ACTIVITY

Working with a colleague, make a list of things that you need to record using the list above. In a group discussion compare your list with the rest of your group. Agree as a group a list of information required for a semi-permanent colour service.

PROVIDING AFTERCARE ADVICE

Giving the client advice about how to look after the colour at home is part of the overall service. Semi-permanent colours last between six and eight shampoos. If the client washes their hair every day the colour will not last very long. Explain how shampooing less will help make the colour last longer. Conditioning the hair will keep the cuticle closed.

Informing the client when the colour would need to be repeated will make them aware of both costs and the need to make another appointment for colour services.

Aftercare advice does not need to be given after the colour and finishing service has been completed. You can give it as you work, using your work to demonstrate things to the client. Don't forget to recap when you have finished.

ACTIVITY

In a small group, or with a partner, make a list of all the things that you should tell the client when giving aftercare advice.

ACTIVITY

In a small group, make a list of the ways in which you worked safely and hygienically when colouring the hair with a semi-permanent colour.

IN A NUTSHELL

You are now at the end of the chapter. Before you test your knowledge with the revision activities, check the following list to see if you feel confident in all the areas covered. If there are still any areas you're unsure of, go back over them in the book and ask your tutor for extra support:

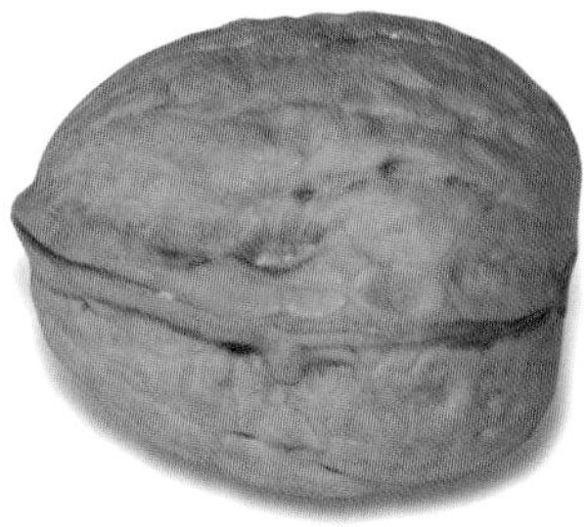

- the types of colouring product and colouring technique
- the factors that need to be considered when selecting colouring products
- the tests that need to be carried out before and during colouring service
- the science of colour
- the International Colour Chart (ICC)
- how colouring products affect the hair structure
- the use of hydrogen peroxide in the colouring process
- how to consult with the client for colouring services
- how to prepare the client for temporary and semi-permanent colours
- how to select the application method and the tools and equipment required for temporary and semi-permanent colours
- how to apply a temporary colour
- how to remove colouring products from the hair
- how to prepare the hair for semi-permanent colour application
- the development process
- how to remove the colour
- the importance of keeping a record card
- the aftercare advice that should be given to a client.

REVISION ACTIVITIES

Use the questions below to test your knowledge of Chapter 217 to see just how much information you have gained. This can help you prepare for your assessments. Turn to pages 510–512 for the answers.

WORDS TO FIND

Copy and complete the sentences below. Use these words to help you fill in the gaps.

strand test	hydrogen peroxide	skin test	hair texture
lifestyle	highlights	primary	contact dermatitis
skin tone	target colour	foils	secondary
colour chart	eumelanin		

1 Red, yellow and blue are called ______ colours; green, orange and purple are called ______ colours.

2 A ______ should be given before each application of permanent colour.

3 The black/brown pigments in the hair are called ______ .

4 A ______ is used to find out the client's natural colour.

5 ______ and ______ are methods of partial colouring.

6 Permanent hair colour is mixed with ______ before it is applied to the hair.

7 If a client is allergic to 'para' dyes a condition called ______ can develop.

8 A ______ is carried out during development of the colour to find out if processing is complete.

9 The colour that the client wishes to go is called the ______ .

10 ______ , ______ and ______ are factors that should be taken into account when consulting with the client.

TEST YOUR KNOWLEDGE FURTHER

1 What colour do you get if you mix the three primary colours together?

2 Pheomelanin is made up of black and brown pigments. True or false?

3 Name **four** factors to be considered when you are selecting a colour product.

4 Name **three** advantages of a permanent colour.

5 How many shades of lift can be achieved using bleach on the hair?

6 What percentage solution of hydrogen peroxide is equal to 20 volume?

7 Name **two** partial-head hair colour techniques.

8 Name the nine shades of depth on the International Colour Chart.

9 Finish this statement: colour + colour = ?

10 Name **three** tests that should be carried out before and during the colour service.

11 A positive result from a skin test means it is safe to colour the client's hair using a permanent colour containing PPD. True or false?

12 What size section of hair should you take when applying a semi-permanent colour?

13 Where would you find information about how to use a colouring product?

14 Name **four** things that should be filled in on a record card when a client has a colour service.

15 Name **two** things you would tell the client when giving aftercare advice.

REVISION ACTIVITIES ANSWERS

101 INTRODUCTION TO THE HAIRDRESSING AND BEAUTY SECTOR

Wordsearch

									Q	W									
									D	E									
								K	X	J	A								
								N	L	P	Z								
							Q	W	I	E	X	X							
							K	K	R	R	U	B							
W	B	A	R	B	E	R	L	B	T	M	J	W	A	X	I	N	G	D	R
I	E	E	T	W	O	S	T	Y	L	I	S	T	B	C	O	L	O	U	R
	N	Z	T	B	A	A	T	S	N	N	U	I	Y	W	T	U	L	E	
		M	V	A	H	E	H	V	B	G	Y	D	W	J	F	T	J		
			S	R	E	C	E	P	T	I	O	N	I	S	T	K			
				D	P	Q	R	Y	C	X	W	I	O	U	H				
			W	J	J	Q	A	M	A	N	I	C	U	R	E	F			
			E	P	A	P	P	N	K	H	S	A	L	O	N	A			
		W	R	Q	H	W	I	A	Q	F	V	N	A	I	L	C	P		
		B	U	T	Q	Y	S	Q			E	A	J	R	R	I	M		
	I	X	F	S	K	F	T					R	H	Q	O	A	V	Z	
	U	Y	M	C	U									I	G	L	B	B	
B	S	U	G													C	Q	G	Y
U	U																	P	T

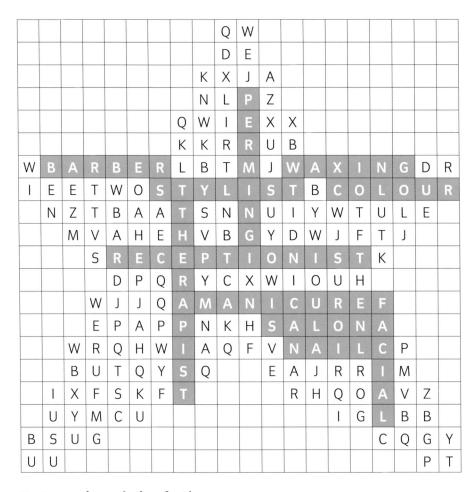

Test your knowledge further

1. List **eight** job opportunities in the hairdressing and beauty sector.
   Any eight from the following: salon junior; hair stylist; barber; beauty therapist; make-up artist; nail technician; salon manager; receptionist; salon owner; colour technician; session stylist; product technician; manufacturer's sales rep; spa therapist; beauty consultant; trainer; assessor; tutor.

2. What is the name of the regulations that cover working hours and breaks?
   Working Time Regulations

3. List **three** things that you should do to keep fit and healthy.
   Any three from the following: eat properly; get enough rest; exercise regularly; wear the right shoes; pay attention to your personal hygiene.

4 Give **two** reasons why being flexible is necessary for a hairdresser, barber, beauty therapist or nail technician.
Any two from the following: You cannot finish work until you have finished the client. You may need to do extra work if one of your fellow workers is ill. You may need to delay your lunch break in order to fit in another client.

5 Name **eight** places you could work when you have finished your training.
Any eight from the following:
- hairdressing salon
- barber's
- beauty salon
- nail bar
- specialist salon/spa
- clinic
- health hydro/farm
- health and fitness club
- leisure centre and hotel
- cruise liner
- theatre, film or television studio
- fashion and photography studio
- hospital
- mobile salon
- freelance.

6 Name **two** organisations that could give you information about qualifications.
Habia, City & Guilds

7 List **six** services provided by a hairdressing salon.
Any six from the following: shampoo and blow drying; shampoo and setting; dressing hair for a special occasion; cutting; gents cutting; full head colouring; temporary colouring; highlighting or lowlighting; perming; hair extensions.

8 List **four** services provided by a beauty salon.
Any four from the following: manicure and pedicure; waxing; eye treatments; make-up for all occasions; facial; body massage; aromatherapy; electrical epilation; body therapy treatments.

102 PRESENTING A PROFESSIONAL IMAGE IN A SALON

Words to find

1 Presenting a **professional image** to your client is very important.

2 Using **body language** will help you communicate effectively with your client.

3 Wearing **flat shoes** will prevent backache and fatigue.

4 To be effective in your work you must know the **salon procedures** used in your place of work.

5 A well balanced diet, regular exercise and enough sleep are essential parts of your **personal wellbeing**.

6 **Speaking** and **listening** will help you communicate effectively with the client.

7 Using **deodorant** will help prevent body odour when you are working.

8 **Open** and **closed** are types of question you can use when consulting with the client.

9 A good stylist/therapist will always **follow instructions** from their salon manager.

10 Good **behaviour** and **attitude** will help to give your clients the right impression of you.

Test your knowledge further

1 Name the four things that are important to your professional image.
Personal appearance; personal health and hygiene; behaviour and attitude; communicating with others.

2 Why is it important for your hair or your make-up to look good in the salon?
It is an advert for the salon.

3 Why should you keep your nails short and well-manicured when working in the salon?
So they look good and do not cause injury to the client.

4 Why is it important to keep your hands dry and moisturised?
To reduce the risk of dermatitis.

5 What is using facial expression and gestures called?
Body language.

6 Why is it important to listen when you are communicating?
So you can understand what the client is saying and what they want.

7 Why is it important to keep good eye contact with your client when you are talking to them?
To show that you are paying attention to them.

8 What are questions that require a short answer called?
Closed questions.

9 What type of question would you use if you needed to find out about products and equipment the client has used at home?
Open questions.

10 Name **two** things that will promote a good atmosphere and give a good impression in the salon.
Any two from the following: following instructions; working co-operatively with others; following salon procedures.

112 CREATING A HAIR AND BEAUTY IMAGE

Words to find

1 You can get ideas for your hair and beauty image from places such as books, films, in **magazines**, fashion shows, the television and from the **internet** (using search engines such as 'Google').

2 In order to create a **hair** and beauty **image**, it is important to think about what the theme will be.

3 When you have decided on the theme, you will need to be clear about the purpose for the hair and **beauty** image.

4 Examples of when a hair and beauty image may be used are for a **competition** (that may be judged), a **photoshoot** for a magazine picture, for a catwalk show or for a mood board.

5 In order to **create** your overall image, you will also need to take into account the clothing and accessories needed, the make-up colours and the hairstyle.

6 A **mood board** is a type of poster that may contain images, text and samples of objects. It is used to **plan** and develop a design idea.

Test your knowledge further

1 List **three** reasons why a stylist or beauty therapist may need to create an image?
Any three from the following: to promote a new service or treatment to clients; to give a client a new image; for photographic pictures in magazines; for fashion or catwalk shows; for television work; as part of a competition.

2 When you are deciding on your theme, where can you get information from to help you?
The internet; fashion magazines; photographs; sketches; textbooks; television/DVDs/films; image libraries; fashion shows.

3 What are some of the different ways that you could present the images of your theme?
A competition; a photoshoot; an advertisement of treatments and services to clients; in a magazine; at a catwalk show; on a mood board.

4 What is a mood board?
A type of design that may consist of images, text and samples. It is used to develop a design idea and to communicate the image to other team members or clients. It might be a poster or scrapbook.

113 FOLLOWING HEALTH AND SAFETY IN THE SALON

Words to find

1 Clothing that is used to protect the stylist when they are working is often called **PPE**.

2 Good **ventilation** will provide a healthy working environment.

3 The **COSSH** Regulations give information about how to use products safely and how to dispose of them.

4 If the fire alarm goes off you should evacuate the premises and go to the **assembly point**.

5 Combs can be sterilised in a jar filled with **Barbicide**.

6 **Non-latex gloves** should be used to protect your hands when using chemicals.

7 It is important to **sterilise** all your tools before they are used on a client.

8 If someone is hurt at work the **accident book** must be filled in.

9 Something that could cause injury or hurt someone is called a **hazard**.

10 To reduce the possibility of someone being injured in the salon a **risk assessment** is carried out.

Test your knowledge further

1 Whose responsibility is it to provide personal protective equipment?
The employer's.

2 Describe your duty under the Health and Safety at Work Act.
Not to do anything that may cause harm to yourself or others while at work.

3 What is a hazard?
Something that could cause harm to someone.

4 What is a risk?
The likelihood of the harm occurring.

5 Name **two** methods of sterilisation.
Any two from the following: autoclave; ultraviolet cabinet; chemical immersion.

6 Name **two** things that can be used to protect a client.
Any two from the following: gown; towels; cape; cutting collar.

7 What is the name of the test required by the Electricity at Work Regulations?
PAT or portable appliance test.

8 Name **two** things that would cause the salon to be evacuated.
Any two from the following: fire; flood; bomb alert.

9 Why should you not move someone who has slipped over in the salon?
Because you may cause them more harm.

10 What is the first thing you should do if you discover a fire in the salon?
Tell the person in charge (the boss or the manager).

114 SALON RECEPTION DUTIES

Words to find

1 A junior should always **follow instructions** given to them by the stylist.

2 The reception area should always be clean and tidy to create the right **first impression** when a client enters the salon.

3 **Cheques** and **credit cards** are methods the client may use to pay their bill.

4 The receptionist should always present a **positive image** to the client.

5 **Magazines** can be offered to a client if they have to wait for their appointment.

6 A good **retail display** can help sell products to the client.

7 It is important that the **appointment book** is filled in correctly so that the stylists know when their clients are expected.

8 Always **meet and greet** the client as soon as they enter the salon.

9 Accurately recording **messages** will make sure the right information is given to the stylist.

10 The receptionist should always speak clearly and use the right tone when answering the **telephone**.

Test your knowledge further

1 Name the four things that will provide a positive image when you are working on reception.
Personal appearance; behaviour; communication; efficient service.

2 Why is it important to have your hair and make-up looking good when you are working?
They are adverts for the salon. They show the quality of the salon's work.

3 Name **four** things that you should do to keep the reception area clean and tidy.
Any four from the following: tidy and clean the desk; top up the stationery; check and clean the waiting area; tidy the magazines; check and tidy the cloakroom; check crockery and drinks; check and tidy the retail display.

4 When should you greet a client who has just arrived at the salon?
b As soon as possible.

5 List **three** things you should do when a client arrives for their appointment.
Any three from the following: greeting the client; checking their appointment; seating them in the waiting area; taking their coat; offering a magazine; telling the stylist they have arrived; providing a drink.

6 Why is important to write clearly when taking a message?
So that other people can read it and understand it.

7 What should you do if you cannot deal with a client's request?
Get someone else to come and deal with the client as soon as possible.

8 List **three** methods of payment that a client could use to pay their bill?
Any three from the following: cash; credit or debit card; cheque; voucher.

9 When making an appointment for a client, what information do you need from them?
The service they want; when they would like it done; who they would like to do their hair or treatment; whether there are any other days and times they could make.

10 Why do you need to know how long a service takes when making an appointment?
So that you can book the correct amount of time out for the stylist/therapist to do the service.

115 WORKING WITH OTHERS IN THE HAIR AND BEAUTY SECTOR

Words to find

1 Talking is a form of **verbal** communication.

2 When we communicate, 50 per cent is through our **body language**, 40 per cent is through our tone of voice and 10 per cent is through the words that we say.

3 Ways that you can show good **communication** skills include smiling, being polite, making good eye contact and having a relaxed posture.

4 An example of good **teamwork** is everyone working together.

5 If you speak with the same **tone** to your voice, it will sound very boring.

6 Smiling, nodding your head and having good eye contact are all examples of **non-verbal** communication.

7 It is important for a hairdresser or beauty therapist to have good **listening** skills so that they hear what the client is saying to them.

8 If staff are happy in their work then they will feel **motivated** to do their job well.

Test your knowledge further

1 When staff get along and help each other get work done, everybody benefits.
True

2 An example of good teamwork is when everyone completes their own jobs.
False

3 Sharing ideas is not good teamwork.
False

4 Smiling is an example of verbal communication.
False

5 Rudeness is an example of negative behaviour.
True

6 Listening is an example of positive communication.
True

003 SHAMPOOING AND CONDITIONING HAIR

Crossword answers

	1 R			2 M										
3 C	O	R	T	E	X									
	T			D		4 T	R	5 E	A	T	M	E	N	T
	A			I				F						
	R			C				F						
	Y			A				L						
		6 C	U	T	I	C	L	E						
				E				U						
				D			7 D	R	Y					
								A						
								G						
		8 S	U	R	F	A	C	E						

Words to find

1 Effleurage, rotary and friction are the massage movements used in shampooing and conditioning.

2 It is important to test the water temperature before using it on the hair.

3 A wide-toothed comb is used to remove tangles from the hair before shampooing.

4 The three parts of the hair shaft are called the cuticle, cortex and medulla.

5 The cuticle of the hair can be smoothed using a surface conditioner.

6 Drying the hands and using hand cream will help prevent dermatitis.

7 Liquid and cream are types of shampoo used to clean the hair.

8 To protect the client's clothing a gown and towels are used.

9 The type of shampoo that will be used on the client will be decided during the consultation.

10 The hair should be rinsed thoroughly to remove all traces of the shampoo.

Test your knowledge further

1 Name **two** reasons for shampooing and conditioning the hair.
Any two from the following: to clean the hair; to improve the condition; to prepare the hair for the next service; to relax the client.

2 Why is it important to stand properly when shampooing?
To prevent backache and tiredness.

3 Why should floors be swept regularly?
To remove anything that might cause someone to slip and hurt themselves; to keep the salon looking neat and tidy.

4 Name the three parts of the hair shaft.
Cuticle; cortex; medulla.

5 Name **three** things you need to find out when consulting with your client before shampooing.
Any three from the following: what services the client wants and how they want their hair to look like afterwards; what the client has had done to their hair recently; what hair type the client has; what the texture of the hair is; what products the client has used on their hair; any hair and scalp conditions that that might affect the services you have to give.

6 Why is it important to rinse your hands thoroughly during the shampooing service?
To help prevent contact dermatitis.

7 List **three** things that will help you present a professional image.
Any three of the following:

- Treat the client with politeness and respect.
- Give the client your undivided attention when working on them.
- Make sure the client has everything they need during their visit.
- Communicate with the client positively and clearly.
- Make sure your body language is positive and conveys the right messages.
- Make sure your appearance and behaviour are up to standard.
- Respect client confidentiality (don't tell others what the client tells you).
- Talk to the client while you are working on them.

8 Name the three massage movements used in shampooing.
Effleurage; rotary; friction.

9 What effect do surface conditioners have on the hair?
Smoothe the cuticle; make the hair shine.

10 Name the massage movement used in conditioning.
Petrissage.

004/105 PLAITING AND TWISTING HAIR

Words to find

1 Twists and plaits should be secured using **professional bands**.

2 The client's **face shape** will determine whether plaits or twists will suit them.

3 The **elasticity** of the hair describes how the hair will stretch.

4 If there are bald areas just inside the hairline it could be a sign of **traction alopecia**.

5 The section taken for 'on scalp' plaits is called a **channel**.

6 **Cross-infection** is the term used to describe the transfer of a disease from one client to another.

7 **Serum** is a product that can be used when plaiting.

8 **Cornrows** and **twists** are examples of 'on scalp' plaiting.

9 A **tail comb** is used to make partings and split sections.

10 A **three-stem** plait and a **French** plait are 'off scalp' plaits.

Test your knowledge further

1 French plaiting is an 'on scalp' method of plaiting. True or false?
False

2 Name **four** factors that can influence your choice of plaiting or twisting technique.
Any four from the following: head shape; face shape; body shape; lifestyle; hair growth patterns; hair growth cycle; hair length; hair condition; hair texture; elasticity; adverse hair and scalp conditions.

3 Why is it important to prepare your work area before you start work on the client?
To give the client the right impression/to present a professional image; to be able to work efficiently and safely.

4 Name **three** styling products that can be used during plaiting or twisting and state what they are used for.
Any three from the following: gel – used on wet or dry hair to provide volume and texture; serums – these are oil-based products, they help smoothe the hair and prevent it tangling when you are sectioning; blow dry/setting lotion – used on wet hair before blow drying, gives volume lift and support for fine hair; hairspray – used on dry hair to add shine, be careful not to use too much; spray moisturisers – used on dry hair to add shine, be careful not to use too much.

5 Name **four** tools or pieces of equipment that can be used for plaiting or twisting.
Any four from the following: wide-toothed comb; tail comb; sectioning clips; bristle brush; Denman brush; grips; pins; hand-held dryer; straighteners; tongs; bands; accessories; decorations.

6 What can happen if too much tension is used in plaiting or twisting?
It can cause traction alopecia; it can be uncomfortable for the client.

7 What face shape is ideal for plaiting and twisting styles?
Oval

8 What should be used to secure a cornrow plait?
A professional band

9 Name **two** things that can be used to enhance plaiting and twisting styles.
Any two from the following: jewellery; fabrics; flowers; beads; threads.

10 Name **two** things that you should tell the client when giving aftercare advice.
Any two from the following: to avoid rubbing or massaging the hair; to avoid using too much aftercare product; how to remove the bands or grips. (Use a tail comb to gently unpick the plait, starting at the points, or unwind the twist from the point. Brush the hair with a bristle brush to remove tangles after unpicking. Use a good cleansing shampoo to remove product build-up. Use a conditioner to restore the condition of the hair.)

005 CREATING AN IMAGE USING COLOUR FOR THE HAIR AND BEAUTY SECTOR

Words to find

1 Red, blue and yellow are known as **primary** colours.

2 Orange, purple and green are known as **secondary** colours.

3 The colour green is made by mixing blue and **yellow** colours together.

4 When you mix red and blue together, the colour produced is **violet**.

5 **Complementary** colours are colours that are opposite the primary colours on the colour star.

6 The colour **spectrum** is made up of the following colours: red, **orange**, yellow, **green**, **blue**, indigo, violet

7 Having a good understanding of **colour** is important in the hair and beauty industries. It is taken into account when choosing hair, make-up and nail enamel products.

Test your knowledge further

1. Name the three primary colours
   Red; yellow; blue.

2. Is it possible to mix colours together to get primary colours?
   No.

3. What are secondary colours?
   These are the colours that you get when you mix primary colours together.

4. Name the three secondary colours.
   Violet; orange; green.

5.

yellow	+	blue	=	green
blue	+	red	=	violet/purple
red	+	yellow	=	orange

6. What are complementary colours?
   These are colours that are opposite each other on the colour star.

7. Copy and complete the table below to find the complementary colours for the three primary colours.

Primary colour	**Which two primary colours are mixed together to get the complementary colour?**	**What complementary colour is produced from mixing them together?**
Red	Blue and yellow	Green
Yellow	Red and blue	Purple
Blue	Red and yellow	Orange

8. Which of the primary and secondary colours are classed as 'warm colours'?
   Red; yellow; orange.

9. Which of the primary and secondary colours are classed as 'cool colours'?
   Blue; purple; green.

10. How is the colour spectrum used in the hairdressing and beauty therapy industries?
    In hair colouring and hair colour correcting; in make-up treatments, face painting and manicure treatments (nail varnish and nail art).

006 SKIN CARE

Words to find

1 If you use tools and equipment that are clean, this is an example of good **hygiene**.

2 A product that is used to remove facial make-up is called a **cleanser**.

3 A **spatula** is used to hygienically remove products from jars or pots.

4 After you have applied the toner, a **tissue** is used to blot the skin dry.

5 Before your client arrives, **preparation** of all of your tools, equipment and products is important. This will make sure that you have everything ready for the treatment.

Test your knowledge further

1

Skin care product	Type of skin care product	Which skin types it is suitable for
Cleansers	Face wash	Oily and combination skin types
	Lotion	Oily, combination and normal skin types
	Milk	Oily, combination and normal skin types
	Cream	Normal and dry skin types
Toners	Freshener	Dry and normal skin types
	Toner	Normal skin type
	Astringent	Oily and combination skin types
Moisturisers	Lotion	Oily and combination skin types
	Mousse	Normal skin type
	Cream	Normal and dry skin types

2 For what reason would you use a blanket in a treatment?
To keep the client warm; to help them to relax.

3 a What does a cleanser do?
Removes make-up and surface dirt from the skin.

b What does a toner do?
Refreshes the skin; removes the last traces of the cleanser; tightens the pores.

c What does a moisturiser do?
Helps to stop the skin from drying out; makes the skin feel soft and supple.

Skin type description	Which skin type is this describing?
▪ Usually dry cheeks and oily skin on the 'T' zone (forehead, nose and chin)	Combination
▪ Even skin texture ▪ Feels soft ▪ Skin colour is even ▪ Does not feel tight ▪ Feels firm to touch	Normal
▪ Shiny ▪ Spots ▪ Blackheads ▪ Large pores	Oily
▪ Flaky patches ▪ Dull ▪ Feels tight ▪ Small pores ▪ Whiteheads	Dry

5 Name **two** positive ways in which you can communicate with your client.
Any two from the following: smile; sit or stand upright; listen to them.

6 Why is it important to smile at your client?
It makes the client feel welcome.

7 Why should you not ask the client questions during the lip cleanse?
The cleanser may go into their mouth.

8 During a skin care treatment, which do you apply first – the toner or the cleanser?
Cleanser

9 Give **two** reasons why a client may have a skin care treatment.
Any two from the following: to relax them; to improve their skin condition; to learn about which products suit their skin type.

007, 109, 110 HAND CARE AND PROVIDING BASIC MANICURE AND PEDICURE TREATMENTS

Crossword

			[1]P							[2]C					
[4]F	I	L	E							O					
			D							N				[3]B	
[6]M	A	N	I	C	U	R	E			[5]S	Q	U	A	R	E
			C							U				I	
		[7]C	U	T	I	C	L	E		L				T	
			R							T				T	
			[8]E	[9]R	Y	T	H	E	M	A				L	
				I						T				E	
				D						I					
				G						O					
[10]B	A	C	T	E	R	I	A			N					
				S											

Words to find

1 A **manicure** is a treatment that cares for the hands.

2 During the consultation, it is important to check whether your client has any **allergies** to the products that you are using. This will help to stop any adverse reactions from happening.

3 Nail **enamel** is applied to the **nail** plate to give it colour.

4 If you apply a **base** coat before the nail enamel, it will help to stop the nail enamel from staining the nail plate.

5 A **pedicure** is a treatment that cares for the feet.

6 A **top coat** is applied after the nail enamel and will help to protect the enamel and prevent it from chipping.

7 The skin around the base of the nail is called the **cuticle**.

8 A nail **file** is used to shorten and shape the nails.

9 Oval, rounded, pointed, squoval and **square** are all types of nail shape.

Test your knowledge further

1 The spatula and orange stick can be placed in Barbicide during the treatment.
True

2 Towels should be machine washed at a high temperature.
True

3 Nail-varnish remover is applied onto the nails with a tissue.
False

4 A treatment plan should include details of the treatment, such as the colour of enamel used.
True

5 Cuticle cream helps to remove nail varnish.
False

6 Massage will make the skin feel dry.
False

7 Good communication will help to relax the client.
True

8 A top coat is applied before the nail varnish.
False

9 An oval shape is good for short fingernails.
False

10 Erythema is an example of a contra-action.
True

11 After soaking, the cuticles can be gently eased back using a spatula.
False

12 A good therapist will ensure that the treatment area is prepared before the client arrives.
True

13 Dry cuticles would benefit from a manicure/pedicure treatment.
True

103 STYLING WOMEN'S HAIR

Words to find

1 A **double crown** and a **cowlick** are both types of growth pattern.

2 Tools used in styling hair can be sterilised using **Barbicide** or an **autoclave**.

3 **Anagen**, **catagen** and **telogen** are the three stages of the growth cycle of hair.

4 If the hair grows to a point in the middle of the forehead this is called a **widow's peak**.

5 When you are blow drying the hair should be **sectioned** to keep it under control as you work.

6 The client's clothes should be protected by using a **gown** and **towels**.

7 **Coarse**, **medium** and **fine** are all types of hair texture.

8 Something that would prevent you from carrying out the service is called a **contra-indication**.

9 Questions that start with 'why', 'what', 'where' and 'how' are **open** questions.

10 Using even **tension** when you are putting in the rollers will give you the direction and finish you want.

Test your knowledge further

1 Name **four** basic styling techniques that can be used to style women's hair.
Any four from the following: blow drying; straightening and smoothing; roller setting; finger drying; curling; hair up; pin curling.

2 Name **four** factors that can influence your choice of technique.
Any four from the following: head shape; face shape; body shape; lifestyle; hair growth patterns; hair growth cycle; hair length; hair condition; hair texture; elasticity; adverse hair and scalp conditions.

3 Why is important to prepare your work area before you start work on the client?
To give the client the right impression/to present a professional image; to be able to work efficiently and safely.

4 Name **three** styling products that can be used during styling and state what they are used for?
Any three from the following: mousse; gel; setting lotion; hairspray; moisturiser; wax; heat protectors.

5 Name **four** tools or pieces of equipment that can be used for blow drying.
Any four from the following: wide-toothed comb; sectioning clips; 'Denman' brush; vent brush; radial brush; hand-held dryer; diffuser; nozzle.

6 Why is it important to listen when you are consulting with the client?
So that you can understand what they are saying; this helps you to find out what they want.

7 What PPE would you use for your client when blow drying?
A clean gown and freshly laundered towels.

8 Why should the hair be sectioned when blow drying?
To keep the hair under control while you work.

9 What size section should you use when putting in a roller?
The section should not be wider or longer than the roller being used.

10 Name **two** things that will promote a good atmosphere and image in the salon.
Any two from the following: following instructions; working co-operatively with others; following salon procedures.

104 STYLING MEN'S HAIR

Crossword

1 S													
T				2 W									
3 R	A	D	I	A	L								
A				X									
I					4 M								
G				5 C	O	W	L	I	C	K			6 D
H					U						7 D		E
T		8 C	O	N	S	U	L	T	A	T	I	O	N
E					S						F		S
9 N	O	Z	Z	L	E						F		I
E											U		T
R											S		Y
S			10 B	A	R	B	I	C	I	D	E		
											R		

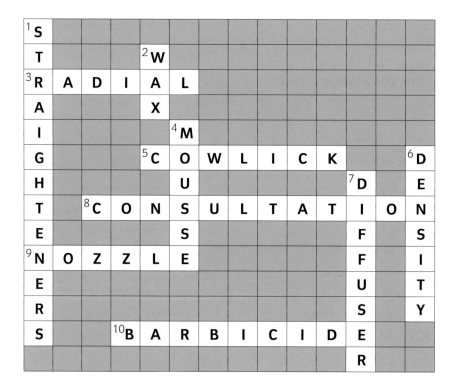

Test your knowledge further

1 Name **three** basic styling techniques that can be used to style men's hair
Any three from the following: blow drying; straightening and smoothing; finger drying; curling; pin curling.

2 Name **four** factors that can influence your choice of technique.
Any four from the following: head shape; face shape; body shape; lifestyle; hair growth patterns; hair growth cycle; hair length; hair condition; hair texture; elasticity; adverse hair and scalp conditions.

3 Why is important to prepare your work area before you start work on the client?
To give the client the right impression/to present a professional image; to be able to work efficiently and safely.

4 Name **three** styling products that can be used during styling and state what they are used for.
Any three from the following: mousse; gel; setting lotion; hairspray; moisturiser; wax; heat protectors.

5 Name **four** tools or pieces of equipment that can be used for blow drying.
Any four from the following: wide-toothed comb; sectioning clips; 'Denman' brush; vent brush; radial brush; hand-held dryer; diffuser; nozzle.

6 Why is it important to listen when you are consulting with the client?
So that you can understand what he is saying. This helps you find out what he wants.

7 What PPE would you use for your client when styling?
A clean gown and freshly laundered towels.

8 Why should the hair be sectioned when finger drying?
To keep the hair under control while you work.

9 What would wax be used for when styling men's hair?
Applied to dry hair to achieve a textured finish to the style. Often used to get a 'spiky', 'messy' look.

10 Name **two** things that will promote a good atmosphere and image in the salon.
Any two from the following: following instructions; working co-operatively with others; following salon procedures.

106 BASIC MAKE-UP APPLICATION

Crossword

	[1] B					[2] S	E	B	U	M	
	[3] L	I	L	A	C						
	U										
	S			[4] F							
	H			[5] O	V	A	L				
	E			U							
[6] G	R	E	E	N							
				D							
		[7] B		A		[8] H					
[9] P	A	L	E	T	T	E					
		U		I		A					
		E		O		D					
				N		B					
						A					
						N					
						D					

Words to find

1 A green **concealer** is used to cover up redness on the skin.

2 An example of good **hygiene** is washing your hands at the beginning and at the end of a treatment.

3 **Blusher** adds warmth and colour to the cheeks.

4 An example of good **communication** is speaking slowly and clearly to the client.

5 **Foundation** is applied after the concealer and before the face powder.

6 A day **make-up** usually uses lighter colours than an evening one.

7 A make-up **palette** can be used to mix colours on and also to apply make-up in a hygienic way.

8 An example of an adverse skin condition is a **stye**. If a client has one of these, you will not be able to apply the make-up.

9 A **headband** is used to keep the client's hair off their face during the treatment.

10 The make-up **brushes** should be thoroughly cleaned between each client to avoid cross-infection.

11 An ultraviolet cabinet is used to store brushes in a hygienic way.
True

12 Towels, gowns and headbands should be machine washed at a low temperature.
False

13 Foundation is applied onto the face with a tissue.
False

14 A treatment plan has details of the client's name and address only.
False

15 Green concealer is used for covering redness in the skin.
True

16 A toner is used to cleanse the face of make-up and surface dirt.
False

17 A shader is used to draw attention to areas or make them look more obvious.
False

18 Mascara adds thickness, colour and length to the lashes.
True

19 An oval-shaped face does not need any correcting with a shader.
True

20 A good therapist will ensure that the treatment area is prepared after the client has gone.
False

21 Conjunctivitis is a contra-indication to a make-up treatment.
True

22 It is better to use cream make-up products for a photographic make-up.
False

23 Examples of warm colours are orange, yellow and cream.
True

Test your knowledge further

1. How do you clean your eye pencils between clients?
   Sharpen them with a pencil sharpener.

2. When do you use face powder? What does it do?
   It is applied after the foundation. It sets the foundation.

3. What does mascara do?
   It adds thickness, colour and length to the eyelashes. It may also help to curl the eyelashes.

4. How can you correct a square face shape?
   Apply shader to the sides of the jaw and forehead.

5. What is the main difference between a day and an evening make-up?
   A day make-up is usually lighter than an evening one.

6. Give an example of how a therapist can behave in a positive way.
   Any example from the following: be friendly; be polite; smile.

7. When would you apply face powder?
   After foundation.

8. How do you apply lipstick in a clean and hygienic way?
   By using a disposable lip brush.

9. What is the natural oil of the skin called?
   Sebum.

10. Name the bone found in the forehead area.
    Frontal bone.

107 THEMED FACE PAINTING

Words to find

1. A **headband** is used to keep the client's hair off their face during a treatment.

2. A **sponge** is used to apply face painting over large areas of the face.

3. **Brushes** are used to apply the face painting when more detail is needed in the design (such as a line or dots).

4. To stop you getting backache, you should have a good **posture**.

5. An example of good **communication** is smiling and listening to the client.

6. Face paints can be mixed on a **palette** before being applied to the face.

7 Gems can be stuck onto the face to make the face-painting design look more effective.

8 You need to ask the client for what occasion they are having their face painted. You can then choose the most suitable design.

9 Face paint is a water-based product.

10 Washing your hands before and after the treatment is an example of good hygiene.

Test your knowledge further

1 Face paints are water-based products.
True

2 Gems are used to give sparkle to a face-painting design.
True

3 Face painting can be carried out on a mask, mannequin or a client.
True

4 An example of a face-painting design on a 3D surface is a picture on a piece of paper.
False

5 Examples of face-painting themes are animals and nature.
True

6 Face painting is an opportunity for you to be creative.
True

7 A consultation is carried out to find out what face-painting design the client wants.
True

8 Face paints come only in three colours – red, yellow and blue.
False

9 Face painting is popular for fancy-dress parties.
True

108 NAIL ART APPLICATION

Words to find

1 Nail art often needs a colour base of nail enamel before applying the nail art design.

2 Your products, tools and equipment should be clean and hygienic for each client.

3 Transfers come in two different types: peel off and soak off.

4 Apply a thin layer of adhesive before you rub the **foil** onto the nails.

5 An example of good **communication** is smiling and listening to the client.

6 Water-based acrylic paints can be mixed on a **palette** before being applied to the nail using a **striping** brush.

7 You need to ask the client what **occasion** they are having the nail art service for. You can then choose the most suitable design.

8 **Nail art** is often applied to the nails after a manicure or pedicure treatment.

Test your knowledge further

1 The salon should be well ventilated.
True

2 Nail art is only applied to artificial nails.
False

3 Polish secures produce a 3D effect on the nails.
True

4 It is important to choose the correct size brush for the nail art design you want to achieve.
True

5 Orange sticks can be used for striping designs.
False

6 Another name for a foil is a metallic wrap.
True

7 Tweezers can be used to help apply peel-off transfers to the nail.
True

8 Colour blending is where two or more colours are used.
True

9 Poor communication will help to promote a professional image for the salon.
False

111 COLOURING HAIR USING TEMPORARY COLOUR

Crossword

1 S				2 G									3 W				
4 T	E	5 M	P	O	R	6 A	R	Y					A			9 C	
E		O		W		P							N			U	
N		U		N		R							7 D	E	P	T	H
C		S				O		8 G	L	O	V	E	S			I	
I		S				N										C	
L		E														L	
L																E	
I																	
N																	
G																	

Words to find

1 The pigment cells in the hair are called melanin.

2 Disposable gloves should be used to protect the hands when using colour.

3 An apron is worn to protect the stylist's clothes when colouring.

4 A semi-permanent colour lasts for six to eight shampoos.

5 How light or dark the hair colour is called the depth.

6 Hair that absorbs water easily is said to be porous.

7 An anti-oxidant conditioner is used after colouring to remove oxygen.

8 Lightener is used to achieve blonde shades.

9 Colour paints and wands are two types of temporary colour.

10 Two methods of colouring hair are shoe shining and scrunching.

Test your knowledge further

1 List the PPE that you would need to use when carrying out a temporary colour service.
Disposable gloves; apron.

2 Temporary colours can lighten a client's natural colour.
True or false?
False

3 Why is important to behave professionally when you are working?
To give the client the right impression/to present a professional image; to be able to work efficiently and safely.

4 Name **three** factors that can influence your choice of temporary colouring technique.
Any three from the following: hair condition; porosity; dry, flaky scalp; natural hair colour; fashion trends; desired finished look.

5 Name **three** types of temporary colouring product.
Any three from the following: mousses; gels; wands; spray colour; spray glitter; setting lotions; water rinses; colour paints.

6 Name **two** methods of using temporary colour for a partial-head application.
Any two from the following: scrunching; shoe shining; stencilling.

7 Name the three layers of the hair shaft.
Cuticle; cortex; medulla.

8 How would you find out how the colour should be used?
Read the manufacturer's instructions.

9 Why should you wear disposable gloves when applying or removing colour products?
To help prevent dermatitis; to stop your hands from being stained.

10 Describe briefly how you would remove a semi-permanent colour.
Seat client comfortably. Add water to the hair. Emulsify the colour using rotary massage. Rinse thoroughly until water runs clear.

215 THE ART OF DRESSING HAIR

Words to find

1 Three types of brush used in styling hair are **Denman**, **vent** and a **radial**.

2 The perfect face shape is **oval**.

3 Changing the shape of the hair by setting or blow drying is called a **cohesive** set.

4 **Barrel spring** and **stem** are types of pin curl.

5 **Finger drying** is a technique that will give soft natural-looking styles.

6 When setting hair with rollers the roller should always sit **on base**.

7 Using **straighteners** will produce smooth hair styles particularly on longer hair.

8 Factors that should be taken into account when consulting with the client include **face shape**, **head shape** and **hair density**.

9 **Backcombing** is used to give lift when dressing the hair.

10 The **hydrogen bonds** are responsible for the temporary shape of the hair.

Test your knowledge further

1 Name **five** styling techniques that can be used to style and dress hair.
Any five from the following: blow drying; straightening and smoothing; roller setting; finger drying; curling; hair up; pin curling.

2 Name **five** factors that can influence your choice of technique.
Any five from the following: head shape; face shape; body shape; lifestyle; hair growth patterns; hair growth cycle; hair length; hair condition; hair texture; elasticity; adverse hair and scalp conditions.

3 Which bonds in the hair are changed when the hair is set or blow dried?
Hydrogen bonds.

4 Name **three** styling products that can be used during styling and state what they are used for.
Any three from the following: mousse – it gives support and hold to the style making it last longer; gel – provides volume and texture; setting lotion – gives volume, lift and support for fine hair; hairspray; moisturiser – will help smoothe frizzy curly hair to get a straight appearance; wax; heat protectors – protects hair from the effects of the heat and prevents frizz.

5 Name **three** types of pin curl and state the effect they give.
Any three from the following: barrel-spring curl – gives a flat, waved effect; clock-spring curl – gives a ringlet effect; stem curl – a flat wave with curl at the points; barrel curl – curl with lift.

6 Why is it important to listen when you are consulting with the client?
So that you can understand what they are saying. This helps you to find out what they want.

7 What PPE would you use for your client when blow drying?
A clean gown and freshly laundered towels.

8 Why should the hair be sectioned when setting or blow drying?
To keep the hair under control while you work.

9 What size section should you use when putting in a roller?
The section should not be wider or longer than the roller being used.

10 Name **two** things that will promote a good atmosphere and image in the salon.
Any two from the following: following instructions; working co-operatively with others; following salon procedures.

11 What is the purpose of backcombing the hair when dressing out?
To give lift and support to the style and to provide a secure base for grips and pins when doing a hair up.

12 Name **three** finishing products that can be used during styling and dressing out and state what they are used for.
Any three from the following: hairspray – it holds the hair in place and gives it shine, helps keep moisture out of the hair, making the style last longer; wax – used to achieve a 'spiky', 'messy' look, can also be used to smoothe flyaway hair when doing a hair up; gel – used to give stronger hold to the hair, and achieve the desired finish; serum – will calm frizzy and flyaway hair and protect from heat; dressing creams/oils – used to control the hair, achieve a smooth slick finish and make the hair shine.

13 Name the three things that you should include in giving aftercare advice to the client.
Products; tools and equipment; recreating the look.

14 Increased humidity will make the set or blow dry last longer. True or false?
False

15 Closed questions require a long answer from the client. True or false?
False

216 THE ART OF PHOTOGRAPHIC MAKE-UP

Words to find

1. You will need to be prepared to carry your products, **tools** and **equipment** to locations outside the salon for a photographic make-up.
2. A **mood board** is a type of poster design that may consist of images, text and samples of objects.
3. You should keep your treatment area tidy and use only **hygienic** tools and equipment.
4. Make sure that you record everything you have done. This will help you to **evaluate** your performance and learn from your experience for next time.
5. A **shader** is a make-up product that is used to make areas look less noticeable, such as a wide jaw line.
6. A **highlighter** is a make-up product that is used to make areas look more noticeable, such as the cheekbones.

7 The occasion, skin type, face shape and fashion trends are examples of factors that need to be taken into account when carrying out a photographic make-up service.

8 If you are going to a different location to carry out a photographic make-up service (other than in the salon), it would be a good idea to carry all of your tools, equipment and products in a suitable storage bag or box.

Test your knowledge further

1 List **three** different occasions for which you may need to apply photographic make-up.
Any three from the following: a wedding; a photoshoot in a photography studio or for a fashion magazine; fashion and catwalk shows; a special occasion such as a party or prom.

2 List **three** things that you need to take into account when applying make-up for photography work.
Any three from the following:

- Do not apply the make-up too heavily as the lighting may make the client warm.
- Re-apply the face powder during the photography session to help to reduce the shine from the skin's surface if the client gets warm.
- Matt colours are best for photographic work as they do not cause a shine and therefore photograph better. Shine on the skin may cause a reflection.
- Blend products really well, as failing to do so may show up on the finished photo.
- Shaders and highlighters can help create and define facial features, particularly for black and white photos.
- Creamy products can create a shiny appearance on the photos, so avoid these.
- It is best to use powder products for shading and highlighting when shooting bridal photos. This will reduce the shine on the face.

3 What is a mood board?
A mood board is a type of poster design that may consist of images, text and samples of objects. It is used to develop a design idea and to communicate the image to other team members or clients.

4 What do you need to take into account when you are designing a mood board?

- Planning – prepare any information you are going to include on the mood board. Be clear about what information you are trying to get across and make sure that it is written clearly so that it is easily understood.
- Images – choose the images carefully. They must match what you are trying to communicate.
- Colour – the colours you choose are important, especially make-up colours. Colours can make the mood board more interesting to look at.
- Research – use a variety of different resources when you research your ideas, such as magazines, the internet, books, etc.
- Verbal communication – sometimes you may need to explain what your mood board is about using verbal communication. This will help with communicating your ideas.
- Written communication – make sure that the written information is short and clear on a mood board. It must also be easy to read and understand. The written information should support the images and other creative materials that you have used on your mood board.
- Presentation – mood boards should be placed where people can stand and look at them. They may also be used as part of a presentation where you discuss the subject and use the mood board to support what you are saying. In a salon a mood board can be placed on the wall to promote the make-up looks you can create.

217 THE ART OF COLOURING HAIR

Words to find

1 Red, yellow and blue are called **primary** colours; green, orange and purple are called **secondary** colours.

2 A **skin test** should be given before each application of permanent colour.

3 The black/brown pigments in the hair are called **eumelanin**.

4 A **colour chart** is used to find out the client's natural colour.

5 **Highlights** and **foils** are methods of partial colouring.

6 Permanent hair colour is mixed with **hydrogen peroxide** before it is applied to the hair.

7 If a client is allergic to 'para' dyes a condition called **contact dermatitis** can develop.

8 A strand test is carried out during development of the colour to find out if processing is complete.

9 The colour that the client wishes to go is called the target colour.

10 Hair texture, lifestyle and skin tone are factors that should be taken into account when consulting with the client.

Test your knowledge further

1 What colour do you get if you mix the three primary colours together?
Brown

2 Pheomelanin is made up of black and brown pigments. True or false?
False

3 Name **four** factors to be considered when you are selecting a colour product.
Any four from the following: the colour the client wants to go; skin tone; the condition of the hair and scalp; the client's existing hair colour; fashion trends; lifestyle and personality; results of tests.

4 Name **three** advantages of a permanent colour.
Any three from the following: will give a permanent result; can be mixed to produce a huge range of colours; adds tone and depth; can give a complete change of image for the client; covers 100 per cent white hair; can lighten hair up to four shades; high-lift colours can lighten the hair up to five shades; can be used for fashion effects and vibrant colours; both full-head and partial colouring methods.

5 How many shades of lift can be achieved using bleach on the hair?
Up to six shades.

6 What percentage solution of hydrogen peroxide is equal to 20 volume?
6 per cent

7 Name **two** partial-head hair colour techniques.
Any two from the following: foils; cap; spatula; freehand.

8 Name the nine shades of depth on the International Colour Chart.
Black, dark brown, medium brown, light brown, dark blonde, medium blonde, light blonde, very light blonde, lightest blonde.

9 Finish this statement: colour + colour = ?
Darker colour

10 Name **three** tests that should be carried out before and during the colour service.
Any three from the following: skin test; porosity test; elasticity test; test cutting; colour development test or strand test.

11 A positive result from a skin test means it is safe to colour the client's hair using a permanent colour containing PPD. True or false?
False

12 What size section should you take when applying a semi-permanent colour?
Between 1 and 2 cm.

13 Where would you find information about how to use a colouring product?
The manufacturer's instructions.

14 Name **four** things that should be filled in on a record card when a client has a colour service.
Any four from the following: the client's details; your analysis of their hair and scalp; details of all the factors that can affect the colour choice and method; details of any tests you did and their results; the colour product you selected and the technique you decided to use; shampoo used; how the colour was applied; the development method and time; any products that were used during removal; what the result was; any comments from the client.

15 Name **two** things you would tell the client when giving aftercare advice.
Any two from the following: what shampoos and other products to use; how to use them; when the colour may need to be done again.

INDEX

D

E

F